Quality of Life Assessments
in Clinical Trials

Other Books by Bert Spilker

Guide to Clinical Studies and Developing Protocols
(Raven Press, 1984)

Guide to Clinical Interpretation of Data (Raven Press, 1986)

Guide to Planning and Managing Clinical Studies
(Raven Press, 1987)

*Multinational Drug Companies: Issues in Drug Discovery
and Development* (Raven Press, 1989)

Inside the Drug Industry (with Pedro Cuatrecasas,
Prous Science Publishers, 1989)

Presentation of Clinical Data (with John Schoenfelder,
Raven Press, 1990)

Quality of Life Assessments in Clinical Trials

Editor

Bert Spilker, PhD, MD

Executive Director, Orphan Medical, Minnetonka, Minnesota;
Adjunct Professor of Pharmacology and Adjunct Professor of Medicine,
University of North Carolina;
Clinical Professor of Pharmacy,
University of North Carolina School of Pharmacy, Chapel Hill, North Carolina;
and, Adjunct Professor,
Duke University, Fuqua School of Business, Durham, North Carolina.

Raven Press 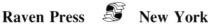 New York

Raven Press, Ltd., 1185 Avenue of the Americas, New York, New York 10036

Made in the United States of America

Library of Congress Cataloging-in-Publication Data

Quality of life assessments in clinical trials / editor, Bert Spilker.
     p.   cm.
  Includes bibliographical references.
  ISBN 0-88167-590-3
  1. Clinical trials—Social aspects. 2. Quality of Life—
Evaluation. I. Spilker, Bert.
  [DNLM: 1. Clinical Trials. 2. Quality of Life. WA 30 Q105]
R853.C55Q35 1990
615.5—dc20
DNLM/DLC
for Library of Congress   89-70022
                                          CIP

9 8 7 6 5 4 3 2

**To all clinical researchers who are working
to improve the quality of life of patients.**

Preface

The impetus for this book arose because no comprehensive books exist for clinical investigators who conduct quality of life assessments. A few books focus on either a single therapeutic area (e.g., cardiology, oncology) or on selected therapeutic areas. A more comprehensive book which emphasizes the various perspectives both globally and in more detail was needed. This book was designed to meet those needs. It discusses the tests that are available to assess quality of life and the pros and cons of each test, and it also comments on the appropriateness of these tests. Authors were chosen who are acknowledged experts in their field to make this book as authoritative as possible.

The intended audience for this book is primarily the academic, government, or pharmaceutical investigator who is planning to conduct a quality of life trial or to include quality of life assessments as part of a larger trial. The contents of this book will also be of interest to others who plan, conduct, analyze, interpret, review, or otherwise use results of quality of life trials. This includes psychologists, sociologists, statisticians, research assistants, nurses, and numerous other health professionals. Readers are encouraged to review chapters outside their usual areas of interest, because many chapters make important points that are likely to stimulate creative ideas and approaches to those working in other areas.

This book addresses the following basic questions:

1. What are the available tests and methods to use in measuring quality of life?
2. Which tests and methods are validated for use and how may other scales be validated?
3. How does an investigator choose which specific tests to use in specific situations for specific purposes?
4. What is the state-of-the-art in various therapeutic areas' quality of life?

The first section provides an overall perspective on quality of life issues. Specific chapters describe definitions, concepts, appropriate approaches, and basic issues in this area. Section II presents standard scales, tests, and approaches by focusing on the individual component categories (i.e., domains) of quality of life: economics, social interactions, psychological well-being, and physical function. Section III focuses on a number of special perspectives that are pertinent for viewing this field: cultural aspects, marketing, drug industry, and regulatory considerations. The fourth section concerns special patient populations and approaches. These include pediatric, geriatric, drug abuse, rehabilitation, chronic pain, and surgery patients. The fifth and final section discusses specific problems and diseases in a wide variety of therapeutic areas.

There is a certain degree of overlap between chapters in the five sections. This is intentional, because it allows the reader to approach any specific question or situation in multiple ways (e.g., from the perspective of the disease, type of parameters measured, purpose of the study, nature of the patient). Thus, the separate sections are intended to create a whole that is greater than the sum of the individual components.

Bert Spilker

Acknowledgments

The editor wishes to acknowledge useful discussions with and help from Dr. Luigi Cubeddu in the early stages of this work. Most of the authors have also provided advice during the numerous stages of this book. Mrs. Joyce Carpunky provided technical assistance throughout this project and Mrs. Brenda Price assisted with typing. Their help is gratefully acknowledged.

Contents

Contributors

John P. Anderson, PhD *Associate Medical Specialist, Division of Health Care Sciences, Department of Community and Family Medicine, M-022, School of Medicine, University of California, San Diego, La Jolla, California 92093*

Roger T. Anderson *Health Program Specialist, Federal Building, Room 216, Behavioral Medicine Branch, National Heart, Lung, and Blood Institute, National Institutes of Health, Bethesda, Maryland 20892*

Ivan Barofsky, PhD *Institute of Social Oncology, 14912 McIntosh Court, Silver Spring, Maryland 20904*

Gregory Burke, MD, PhD *Acting Director, Division of Oncology and Pulmonary Drug Products, Center for Drug Evaluation and Research, Food and Drug Administration, Rockville, Maryland 20857*

Barbara J. Burns, PhD *Professor of Medical Psychology, Department of Psychiatry, Duke University Medical Center, Box 3930, Durham, North Carolina 27710*

David Cadman, MD, MSc, FRCP(C) *Associate Professor, Departments of Clinical Epidemiology and Biostatistics, and Pediatrics, McMaster University, 1200 Main Street West, Hamilton, Ontario L8N 3Z5, Canada*

Stuart S. Campos *Graduate Student, Department of Anthropology, Southern Methodist University, Dallas, Texas 75275-0336*

Jennifer Clinch, MA *Senior Research Analyst, WHO Collaborating Centre for Quality of Life Studies in Cancer, St. Boniface General Hospital, 409 Tache Avenue, Winnipeg, Manitoba R2H 2A6, Canada*

Susan Czajkowski, PhD *Social Science Analyst, Federal Building, Room 216, Behavioral Medicine Branch, National Heart, Lung, and Blood Institute, National Institutes of Health, Bethesda, Maryland 20892*

Atara Kaplan De-Nour, MD *Professor and Chairman, Department of Psychiatry, Hadassah University Hospital, Post Office Box 12000, Jerusalem 91120, Israel*

Andrew Dorr, MD *Senior Investigator, Medicine Section, Cancer Therapy Evaluation Program, Division of Cancer Treatment, National Cancer Institute, National Institutes of Health, Bethesda, Maryland 20892*

Douglas A. Drossman, MD *Associate Professor of Medicine, Division of Digestive Diseases and Nutrition, Department of Medicine, University of North Carolina at Chapel Hill, CB 7080 326 Burnett-Womack Building, Chapel Hill, North Carolina 27599-7080*

David Feeny, PhD   *Professor of Economics and Clinical Epidemiology and Biostatistics, Centre for Health Economics and Policy Analysis, Department of Clinical Epidemiology and Biostatistics, McMaster University, 1200 Main Street West, Hamilton, Ontario L8N 3Z5, Canada*

Marsha D. Fretwell, MD   *Head, Program in Geriatric Medicine, and Assistant Professor, Program in Medicine, Brown University, Roger Williams Hospital, 825 Chalkstone Avenue, Providence, Rhode Island 02910*

Michael A. Friedman, MD   *Associate Director, Cancer Therapy Evaluation Program, Division of Cancer Treatment, National Cancer Institute, National Institutes of Health, Bethesda, Maryland 20892*

James F. Fries, MD   *Associate Professor of Medicine, Department of Medicine, HRP Building, Room 109, Stanford University School of Medicine, Stanford, California 94305*

Curt D. Furberg, MD, PhD   *Director, Center for Prevention Research and Biometry, The Bowman Gray School of Medicine, Winston-Salem, North Carolina 27103*

John W. Garrett, MD   *Clinical Instructor, Division of Digestive Diseases and Nutrition, Department of Medicine, University of North Carolina at Chapel Hill, CB 7080 326 Burnett-Womack Building, Chapel Hill, North Carolina 27599-7080*

Katherine S. Ginsburg, MD, MPH   *Research Associate, Departments of Rheumatology/Immunology and Medicine, Robert B. Brigham Multipurpose Arthritis Center, Brigham and Women's Hospital, Harvard Medical School, Boston, Massachusetts 02115*

Christopher G. Goetz, MD   *Professor of Neurology, Department of Neurological Sciences, Rush University, Rush-Presbyterian St. Lukes Medical Center, 710 S. Paulina Street, 8 North, Chicago, Illinois 60612*

Henry G. Grabowski, PhD   *Professor of Economics, Department of Economics, Duke University, Durham, North Carolina 27706*

Edward Guadagnoli, PhD   *Assistant Professor of Health Care Policy, Department of Health Care Policy, Harvard Medical School, 25 Shattuck Street, Parcel B-1st Floor, Boston, Massachusetts 02115*

Gordon H. Guyatt, MD, FRCP(C)   *Associate Professor, Departments of Clinical Epidemiology and Biostatistics, and Internal Medicine, Room 2C12, McMaster University Health Sciences Centre, 1200 Main Street West, Hamilton, Ontario L8N 3Z5, Canada*

Ronald W. Hansen, PhD   *Associate Dean for Academic Affairs, Simon Graduate School of Business Administration, University of Rochester, Rochester, New York 14627*

Doug Henderson-James, MHA   *Senior New Product Forecasting Analyst, Glaxo, Inc., Five Moore Drive, Research Triangle Park, North Carolina 27709*

Roman Jaeschke, MD, FRCP(C)   *Clinical Scholar, Department of Internal Medicine, McMaster University Health Sciences Centre, St. Joseph's Hospital. Fontbonne Building, 50 Charlton Avenue E., Hamilton, Ontario L8N 4A6, Canada*

Thomas M. Johnson, PhD   *Assistant Professor of Anthropology, Department of Anthropology, Southern Methodist University, Dallas, Texas 75275-0336*

Robert M. Kaplan, PhD   *Professor and Acting Chief, Divison of Health Care Sciences, Department of Community and Family Medicine, M-022, School of Medicine, University of California, San Diego, La Jolla, California 92093*

Jeffrey N. Katz, MD   *Research Associate, Departments of Rheumatology/ Immunology and Medicine, Robert B. Brigham Multipurpose Arthritis Center, Brigham and Women's Hospital, Harvard Medical School, Boston, Massachusetts 02115*

Haresh Kirpalani, BM, MRCP   *Assistant Professor of Neonatology, University of Toronto; and Staff Neonatologist, Department of Pediatrics, Hospital for Sick Children, 555 University Avenue, Toronto, Ontario M5G 1X8, Canada*

Roberta Labelle, MA   *Assistant Professor of Clinical Epidemiology and Biostatistics, Centre for Health Economics and Policy Analysis, Department of Clinical Epidemiology and Biostatistics, McMaster University, 1200 Main Street West, Hamilton, Ontario L8N 3Z5, Canada*

Karen T. Labuhn, RN, PhD   *Senior Research Associate, Kaiser-Permanente Center for Health Research, 4610 SE Belmont Street, Portland, Oregon 97215-1795*

Victor C. Lee, MD   *Assistant Professor of Anesthesiology, Department of Anesthesiology, Pain Management Center, University of Virginia Health Sciences Center, Charlottesville, Virginia 22908*

Anthony F. Lehman, MD, MSPH   *Associate Professor of Psychiatry, Department of Psychiatry, University of Maryland Medical Center, 645 West Redwood Street, Baltimore, Maryland 21201*

Robert J. Levine, MD   *Professor of Medicine and Lecturer in Pharmacology, Yale University School of Medicine, Room IE-48 SHM, 333 Cedar Street; and Attending Physician, Yale-New Haven Hospital, New Haven, Connecticut 06510*

Matthew H. Liang, MD, MPH   *Associate Professor of Medicine, Harvard Medical School, and Director, Robert B. Brigham Multipurpose Arthritis Center, Brigham and Women's Hospital, Boston, Massachusetts 02115*

Robin S. McLeod, MD, FRCS(C)   *University of Toronto, Toronto General Hospital, 200 Elizabeth Street, 9-242 North, Toronto, Ontario M5G 2C4, Canada*

A. John McSweeny, PhD   *Associate Professor of Psychology, and Director, Psychology Center and Neuropsychology Laboratory, Medical College of Ohio, Toledo, Ohio 43699*

David S. Metzger, PhD   *Center for Studies on Addiction and Department of Psychiatry, University of Pennsylvania School of Medicine, 3910 Chestnut Street, Philadelphia, Pennsylvania 19104*

Vincent Mor, PhD   *Associate Professor of Medical Science and Director, Center for Gerontology and Health Care Research, Brown University, Providence, Rhode Island 02912*

Louis A. Morris, PhD   *Acting Director, Division of Drug Advertising and Labeling, Food and Drug Administration, 5600 Fishers Lane, Rockville, Maryland 20857; and Scholar-in-Residence, Center for Marketing Policy Research, The American University, Washington, D.C. 20016*

Albert Oberman, MD, MPH   *Professor and Director, Division of General and Preventive Medicine, Department of Medicine, 608 Medical Education Building, University of Alabama at Birmingham, Birmingham, Alabama 35294*

Charles P. O'Brien, MD, PhD   *Director, Center for Studies on Addiction, University of Pennsylvania School of Medicine, Chief of Psychiatry, Philadelphia Veterans Administration Medical Center; and Vice Chairman, Department of Psychiatry, University of Pennsylvania School of Medicine, 3910 Chestnut Street, Philadelphia, Pennsylvania 19104*

Donald L. Patrick, PhD   *Professor, Department of Health Services, School of Public Health, University of Washington, Seattle, Washington 98195*

Valerie Powell, SRN, SCM, RN   *Data Manager, Quality of Life, Section of Oncology, Manitoba Cancer Treatment and Research Foundation, Winnipeg, Manitoba R3E 0V9, Canada*

James M. Raczynski, PhD   *Associate Professor and Co-Director, Behavioral Medicine Unit, Division of General and Preventive Medicine, Department of Medicine, 101 Medical Towers Building, University of Alabama at Birmingham, Birmingham, Alabama 35294*

Peter Rosenbaum, MD, FRCP(C)   *Professor of Pediatrics, Department of Pediatrics; 2nd Affiliate Member, Department of Clinical Epidemiology and Biostatistics; and Faculty of Health Sciences; McMaster University, 1200 Main Street West, Hamilton, Ontario L8N 3Z5, Canada*

John Rowlingson, MD   *Professor of Anesthesiology and Director, Pain Management Center, University of Virginia Health Sciences Center, Charlottesville, Virginia 22908*

Harvey Schipper, MD, FRCP(C)   *Head, Hematology/Oncology Service; Director, WHO Collaborating Centre for Quality of Life Studies in Cancer, St. Boniface General Hospital; and Associate Professor of Medicine, University of Manitoba, St. Boniface General Hospital, 409 Tache Avenue, Winnipeg, Manitoba R2H 2A6, Canada*

Dale Shoemaker, PhD   *Chief, Regulatory Affairs Branch, Cancer Therapy Evaluation Program, Division of Cancer Treatment, National Cancer Institute, National Institutes of Health, Bethesda, Maryland 20892*

Sally A. Shumaker, PhD   *Health Scientist Administrator, Federal Building, Room 216, Behavioral Medicine Branch, National Heart, Lung, and Blood Institute, National Institutes of Health, Bethesda, Maryland 20892*

William D. Spector, PhD   *Service Fellow, Long Term Care Studies Program, National Center for Health Services Research, Rockville, Maryland 20857*

Bert Spilker, PhD, MD   *Executive Director, Orphan Medical, 13911 Ridgedale Drive, Minnetonka, Minnesota, 55391*

Patricia W. Spitz, RN, MHRS   *Research Associate, Department of Medicine, HRP Building, Room 109, Stanford University School of Medicine, Stanford, California 94305*

Paul H. Sugarbaker, MD   *Medical Director, Cancer Institute, Washington Hospital Center, 110 Irving Street NW, Washington, D.C. 20010*

Robert Temple, MD   *Director, Office of Drug Review I, Center for Drug Evaluation and Research, Food and Drug Administration, Rockville, Maryland 20857*

George W. Torrance, PhD   *Professor of Management Science and Clinical Epidemiology and Biostatistics, Centre for Health Economics and Policy Analysis, Faculty of Business, Department of Clinical Epidemiology and Biostatistics, McMaster University, 1200 Main Street West, Hamilton, Ontario L8N 3Z5, Canada*

Ralph R. Turner, PhD   *Senior Research Investigator, Pfizer Central Research, Eastern Point Road, Groton, Connecticut 06340*

Nanette K. Wenger, MD   *Professor of Medicine (Cardiology), Emory University School of Medicine, Grady Memorial Hospital, Atlanta, Georgia 30303*

T. Franklin Williams, MD   *Director, National Institute on Aging, National Institutes of Health, Building 31, Room 2C-02, 9000 Rockville Pike, Bethesda, Maryland 20892*

Robert S. Wilson, PhD   *Associate Professor of Psychology, Rush Alzheimer's Disease Center, Rush-Presbyterian St. Luke's Medical Center, 710 S. Paulina Street, 8 North, Chicago, Illinois 60612-3864*

Quality of Life Assessments in Clinical Trials

I

Introduction to the Field of Quality of Life Trials

Quality of Life Assessments in Clinical Trials, edited by B. Spilker. Raven Press, Ltd. New York © 1990.

1

Introduction

Bert Spilker

Project Coordination, Burroughs Wellcome Co.,
Research Triangle Park, North Carolina 27709

Quality of life has become a relevant measure of efficacy in clinical studies. Its use is spreading and its importance is growing as a valid indicator of whether or not a medical treatment is beneficial. Quality of life may be viewed in terms of the individual, group, or large population of patients. Each of these groups is discussed in this book.

One of the major reasons for confusion when people approach this field is that different groups of authors who write about quality of life issues (and use the same terms) are often speaking about totally different topics that emerge from different perspectives. The purpose of this brief introduction is to provide an overall frame of reference that may be used to approach both the chapters in this book and articles in the literature.

USES OF QUALITY OF LIFE DATA

One of the most important and basic questions about quality of life is why it should be studied or used. This question may be addressed at the patient, physician, pharmacy, company, or country level. At the individual patient level the answer is most obvious, i.e., to improve the quality of that patient's treatment. At the level of an entire drug or therapy, quality of life trials may differentiate between two therapies with marginal differences in survival or different types of morbidity. Quality of life studies may also compare outcomes between two different treatment modalities, such as using a drug or surgery to treat a disease.

After quality of life studies are published, the data might be used for practical or commercial purposes. Certain pharmacies might stock a wider selection of drugs. This greater availability of certain drugs will benefit those patients who desire specific drugs to improve, it is hoped, their quality of life. Physicians might alter their prescribing habits, and companies developing drugs might focus more efforts on finding drugs that improve patients' quality of life. Other commercial advantages for a company, such as getting a drug onto a formulary (e.g., hospital, health maintenance organization), are described in Chapter 15, "An Industry Perspective." For a country, the most important use of quality of life data is to improve the allocation of health care resources.

LEVELS OF QUALITY OF LIFE

Quality of life must be viewed on a number of levels. Although the exact number and definition of levels may vary among authors, the model shown in Fig. 1 provides a basic approach to the topic.

The overall level of assessment is defined by Shumaker et al. in Chapter 9 as "an individual's overall satisfaction with life, and one's general sense of personal well-being." This overall assessment may be measured by summing the scores of an index test that evaluates each individual domain, or by simply asking patients, "On a scale of 1 to 10 (or 1 to 100, or by descriptive categories), how would you assess your overall well-being?" In the clinical trial literature, this is referred to as Clinical Global Impression. Several variations of this question exist. Given the highly personal way that patients judge their quality of life, it may readily be seen that this Clinical Global Impression question is best answered by the patient and not by the physician. A Clinical Global Impression question that assesses disease severity, however, is best answered by the physician. This question lies in the realm of clinical domains and not quality of life domains.

The middle level of broad domains in Fig. 1 is discussed by most authors in this book. The exact number and identity of quality of life domains vary from approximately three to six, depending on which authors are read. Nonetheless, both the number and general identity of these domains are similar. This topic is discussed more fully later in this and other chapters in the book.

The lower level of Fig. 1 includes all aspects of each domain that are specifically assessed by quality of life tests and scales. Choosing how to evaluate these aspects depends on whether a single index or a battery of tests is used to evaluate the

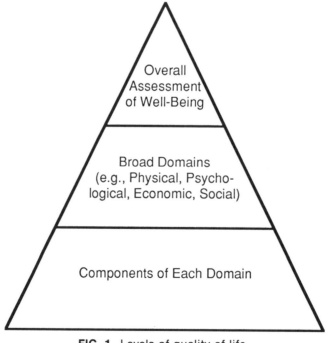

FIG. 1. Levels of quality of life.

components of one (or multiple) domain(s). Even when a single index is created to evaluate a single disease, the developers of validated tests have used widely differing compositions of factors and differing balances of the contributions of each factor. This is well illustrated in Table 3 of Chapter 31 by Barofsky and Sugarbaker.

One or more specific parameters or questions may be used in a clinical trial to evaluate a single component of a domain. Those parameters or questions may be highly important measures of the particular component, but do not represent a validated test of quality of life. Nonetheless, their importance for assessing quality of life is often clear and it is appropriate to include pertinent questions in clinical trials.

DOMAINS OF QUALITY OF LIFE

The major domains of quality of life generally referred to include the following categories:

1. Physical status and functional abilities
2. Psychological status and well-being
3. Social interactions
4. Economic status and factors

Some authors describe their own research or clinical studies as dealing with quality of life issues when in fact they study only one of these broad domains. Others study two or more domains. Although it is not necessary for an investigator to study all domains in any one trial or research program, trials that evaluate only one domain should be distinguished from those that evaluate several domains.

Modifications of these categories are sometimes used by the authors in this book, but there is general agreement in most chapters about the appropriateness of these broad domains. The definitions of these categories are subject to some debate, however, and Chapter 2 discusses this issue further.

COMBINING QUALITY OF LIFE DATA FROM MULTIPLE DOMAINS OR TESTS

A matrix may be described for the four domains and the specific instruments or tests that are used to evaluate them. Quality of life tests measure specific or general aspects of one to four domains. If a single test that measures each of the domains (and is validated for each of those domains) is used, then an aggregate overall assessment of quality of life may generally be obtained to compare different drugs or treatments. One problem with obtaining a single overall score for quality of life is that different domains may yield different results (e.g., treatment A was better than treatment B in two domains, but the opposite result was obtained in the other two domains). Even within a single domain it is common for different components to yield different results. If a battery of validated tests is used to evaluate a single domain (or all domains), it is impossible to combine all test score results. Individual test results may be aggregated, however, by presenting them in a comparative manner. Investigators must establish the relative importance of each individual test used to measure one or more aspects of quality of life prior to conducting the trial. This practice insures that data obtained from tests defined as minor are not later used to claim that a certain treatment is more (or less) effective than another.

Different types of tests and scales may be required to measure specific aspects of each category, depending on the type of patients being evaluated and the interests of the investigators. Moreover, different weights may be assigned to each of the four broad categories based on the patients' beliefs as influenced by their disease severity and nature, background, religion, plus many other factors. In addition, there is no *a priori* reason to state that each of these (or other) categories must be measured and combined to understand changes in a patient's quality of life. One domain or component of a domain may reflect a clinical situation better than the combination of several or many separate measures.

Assessment of quality of life requires input from patients to insure that the patients' perceptions are included and are accurate. A recent study compared physician and patient perceptions of quality of life using several different scales and found that correlation between the two was poor (1). This supports the view that physicians cannot accurately assess a patient's quality of life in all, or perhaps most, situations. This may result from the fact that physicians usually judge patients' clinical responses rather than how clinical responses are filtered through a patient's values and beliefs. This topic is discussed later in this introduction.

DEFINITION OF QUALITY OF LIFE

In editing this book it was necessary to decide whether to insist on a common definition of quality of life. The alternative was for each author to define quality of life on his or her own terms. The problem with the first approach is that no single, universally accepted definition exists. Moreover, because the field is diverse and changing, it would be unfair to limit the authors to a specific, narrow definition. Besides, a single definition would likely yield a stilted book that could not reflect the richness of diversity present in the field.

The problem with allowing each author carte blanche to use his or her own definition is that the book could lose the unity and cohesiveness desired. It would become merely a collection of loosely connected chapters. A compromise was reached where a general definition, based on that of Schipper et al. (see Chapter 2), was proposed to each author as a basis for his or her chapter. The fact that some authors adopted this definition while others used alternatives is viewed as a strength of the book.

RELATIONSHIP OF CLINICAL SAFETY AND EFFICACY DATA TO QUALITY OF LIFE

How does a medical treatment's benefits or adverse reactions affect quality of life?

On first consideration it appears that adverse reactions diminish a patient's quality of life and beneficial effects enhance it. But, either positive or negative clinical changes are generally judged in comparison with other benefits or problems of the treatment and with other treatments the patient has received. The patient's values and beliefs determine how a few or many different factors of a treatment's benefits and problems sum together and also whether the net change represents a positive or negative effect on his or her quality of life. The net result of a treatment on a patient's quality of life often cannot be predicted by the physician. The assessment of whether the change in quality of life is positive or negative is often a complex

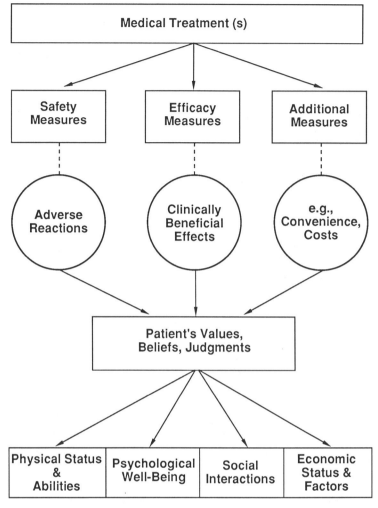

FIG. 2. Model of how clinical aspects of efficacy (i.e., benefits), safety (e.g., adverse reactions), or other factors filter through the patient's values and beliefs to influence his or her quality of life domains.

judgment that may differ for each of the broad domains or for each component of a single domain. Moreover, within each domain some components may be more positive as a result of a specific treatment, whereas other components become more negative.

Severe adverse reactions usually decrease a patient's quality of life and marked efficacy benefits usually increase it. But there are exceptions to both situations because of the patient's values that influence this assessment. For example, severe adverse reactions that are accompanied by clinical improvement may result in a net improvement in quality of life as judged by one patient, and the opposite conclusion may be reached by another patient experiencing similar effects. These points are illustrated in the model shown in Fig. 2. A corollary of this model is that one cannot simply measure adverse reactions or assess clinical benefits of a medical treatment and reach any firm conclusions about how a patient's quality of life is affected. It is necessary to measure one or more quality of life domains for a specific patient, or group of patients, to assess and document how the benefits and/or adverse reactions have been filtered through the patient's values, beliefs, and judgments. Some parameters of clinical efficacy are very closely related to quality of life (e.g., chronic pain), whereas others have an extremely weak association (e.g., reduction of non-symptomatic risk factors).

Although only one direction of arrows has been used in Fig. 2, there is a bidirectional flow under certain circumstances. For example, changes in one or more quality of life domain(s), independent of medical treatment a patient is receiving, may affect the patient's compliance with treatment and thereby influence its effectiveness. A person who loses a job or is hurt in an accident also may not have enough money to purchase medical treatment.

A figure similar to Fig. 2 could be constructed for a broad patient population or health care sector. This level is of paramount importance to health care planners who allocate resources to those medical treatments that provide the greatest benefit in clinical terms and, it is hoped, in terms of quality of life. In a population-oriented model, consideration of resource availability, allocation, and consumption would have to be included, as well as the impact of a patient's quality of life on the community.

FUTURE ISSUES TO ADDRESS

The quality of life field is a rapidly changing and developing medical area. The standards developed over the next several years will probably have a major influence on this area for a long period. It is presently premature to define many golden rules of this field, though one of the most important is that only validated scales should be used in clinical studies. A few major issues for future discussion are mentioned briefly in this section.

Using disease-specific versus general non–disease-specific scales to evaluate quality of life has proponents on both sides. This issue is currently being debated, and many experts challenge the view that each disease should be ideally evaluated with validated instruments specific to that disease. They state that well-validated general instruments may be used to evaluate patients with many types of diseases. Several chapters present views on this subject.

Specific scales used to evaluate quality of life are not always disease-specific. Some are function-specific (e.g., sexual or emotional function) or population-specific (e.g., geriatric). Many disease-specific scales are fairly general in the type of information they elicit and therefore bridge the gap between general and disease-specific scales (e.g., Health Assessment Questionnaire for arthritis, Quality of Life Index for cancer). This topic is discussed in greater detail by Patrick and Deyo (2). The choice of using a single index test to evaluate two or more domains versus using a battery of tests may never be settled by consensus. A number of authors in this book discuss this issue and many of the trade-offs involved (e.g., see Chapter 9 by Shumaker et al.).

The number of scales available for incorporation into clinical trials to evaluate quality of life issues is huge. Many of these tests have been validated in one or more patient populations. A consensus may be reached in the future on a few widely accepted scales for each domain. Other scales may be viewed as less credible, and many may eventually be rejected for quality of life assessments. Several authors in this book have already honed down the large number of possible scales and tests to a small number that are reviewed in their chapters.

A related subject is obtaining better identification of specific conditions under which individual scales should be used. At a more detailed level, specific questions relate to whether tests should (a) quantitate events or assess how patients value those events; (b) measure what patients *actually do* (i.e., activities) versus what they *can do* (i.e., capabilities); (c) use concomitant control groups, historical controls, or use the patient as his own control; and (d) assess the last 24 hours for evaluation versus considering the previous week (or other period).

If several people administer a test in one clinical trial, interrater reliability must be assessed. Some experts have also questioned whether it is necessary to train and certify individuals who administer various quality of life tests. If this is perceived to be a problem, then more attention will likely be paid to this issue. The qualifications and training of those who interpret test results is a related issue that should be discussed, especially for those scales involving subjective responses (e.g., given through interview methods).

A final issue concerns choosing which aspects of quality of life should be measured and which parameters should be used to assess these aspects. This is an important issue, because it is often possible to choose for measurement just those aspects and parameters that are most likely (or even known) to show the changes desired. This is stacking the deck before the game is played. This quasi-ethical approach to evaluating quality of life will be prevented when some or all of the earlier issues mentioned in this section are resolved. An example involves the choice of parameter(s) to demonstrate cost-effectiveness. Many different parameters exist and may be used to show that almost any treatment is better than a comparison under certain conditions. Once standards are established that describe appropriate means of evaluating cost-effectiveness, people will not be able to stack the deck in their favor as readily.

It is hoped that this book will help advance quality of life assessments by (a) helping to standardize definitions and approaches, (b) indicating which tests are validated, (c) identifying the state-of-the-art for measuring quality of life in many patient populations, and (d) stimulating wider use of these measures in clinical trials.

REFERENCES

1. Slevin MR, Plant H, Lynch D, Drinkwater J, Gregory WM. Who should measure quality of life, the doctor or the patient? *Br J Cancer* 1988;57:109–112.
2. Patrick DL, Deyo RA. Generic and disease-specific measures in assessing health status and quality of life. *Med Care* 1989;27:S217–S232.

Quality of Life Assessments in Clinical Trials, edited by B. Spilker. Raven Press, Ltd. New York © 1990.

2

Definitions and Conceptual Issues

* Harvey Schipper, † Jennifer Clinch, and
‡ Valerie Powell

* Department of Oncology, *† WHO Collaborating Centre for Quality of Life Studies in Cancer, St. Boniface General Hospital, University of Manitoba, Winnipeg, Manitoba, R2H 2A6 Canada; ‡ Manitoba Cancer Foundation, Winnipeg, Manitoba, R3E 0V9 Canada

"Quality of life" as a scientific outcome measure represents a new paradigm. For some time we have been seeking a way to describe the overall results of our diagnostic and treatment efforts in a way that makes sense to both patients and health professionals. The conceptual formulation which has emerged, and which is gaining acceptance, defines quality of life functionally by patients' perception of performance in four areas: physical and occupational function, psychologic state, social interaction, and somatic sensation. In this model the patient serves as his own control, the comparisons being made against expectation of function. Quality of life will fluctuate over time, the result of changes in any or all of its component parts. This is an intensely patient-centered approach. In some respects it is a departure from our more accustomed outcome measures.

The purpose of this discussion is to set the context for the ensuing chapters by introducing the reader to the concept. We begin with a brief historical overview. This is followed by a discussion of a number of approaches that consider quality of life from different perspectives, leading to the emergence of the paradigm as it is now understood.

Experience gained through the development of several modern measurement tools makes clear that the paradigm has operational properties which are unique, and which materially affect the design and interpretation of trials. These will be discussed, and tactical suggestions for the conduct of quality of life studies will be offered.

To conduct valid quality of life studies, a clear definition of quality of life, broadly accepted and understood by those doing quality of life research, is essential. At the present time most so-called quality of life studies utilize this terminology without definition. The result is that the rubric has become a catchall for inconsistently designed trials, many of which have unclear goals. For example, investigators may focus on the rate of wound healing, or sexuality, or financial concerns, and correlate that directly with quality of life (1–3). Although many of these individual issues may be significant contributors to quality of life, in the absence of a consistent definition it is not possible to draw other than the most limited conclusions about a patient's overall function when examining a single variable.

Subset components of overall quality of life vary according to time and circumstance. The ability to ride a bicycle may be very important to a younger person, but with increasing age or a change in habitus or social circumstance, the ability to perform that skill may take on a very different meaning. As we shall see later, examination of individual components of patient function may play a valuable role in elucidating the impact of a disease and its treatment on overall quality of life.

In the past physicians have generally viewed with suspicion the subjective assessment of treatment outcome by the patient. The reasons for this attitude are multiple and include the belief that the process of medical research is and should be identical to that of the so-called "hard" sciences such as physics, meaning the rigorous application of the Scientific Method to the processes in question. Other reasons include the belief that psychosocial parameters are of secondary importance compared to the physiologic mechanisms of illness, concern about the lack of a pragmatic definition, and unfamiliarity with psychosocial methodologies.

TOWARD A DEFINITION OF QUALITY OF LIFE

The conceptual formulation of quality of life is the result of a global consensual process, a brief review of which offers insight into the strengths and weaknesses as well as the future direction of the quality of life research effort. Karnofsky first proposed a nonphysiologic outcome parameter for cancer in 1947 (4). What it lacked in conceptual underpinnings, it made up for in the perforce logic and simplicity of its application. Only recently validated (5), and clearly representative of physical function only, the Karnofsky Scale remains a hallmark of cancer therapy trials to this day. (The New York Heart Association functional cardiac classification [6] has a similar history.) After Priestman and Baum (7) published a more broadly based breast cancer quality of life index, again purely empirically based, researchers began to ask whether it might be possible to develop a conceptual definition of quality of life accepted broadly enough to form the basis of a rigorous standard for the emergence of useful measures of quality of life. At first the concept was considered too vague and too individual to be generalized. However, five concepts emerged which contribute to the evolution of our current understanding: the psychological approach; the time trade-off or utility concept; Ware's (8) community-centered concept; the reintegration concept; and Calman's (9) Gap Principle.

The Psychological View

Psychologically and anthropologically speaking, quality of life reflects the patient-perceived, illness side of the distinction between illness and disease (10). Physicians concentrate upon the disease process (the pathophysiology) and attempt to resolve it, often paying less attention to patients' perceptions of the disease, which are the experience of illness. Many variables contribute to this experience: the perception of symptoms, the way in which the patient labels them and communicates the distress they cause, the experience of being unable to function normally, and the methods of coping used by patients and families to gain some control over the disorder. In the chronically ill, dealing strictly with the disease process may be inadequate because the disease problems are often amplified by the psychosocial response to symptoms.

Psychological variables have been shown to be a factor in some disease states; for example, stress plays a role in the development of hypertension and the relative risk of developing heart disease in different personality types (11). This has led to a greater acceptance of the relevance of psychological variables in the etiology and treatment of disease, especially since a possible mechanism for this process has been discovered in the demonstration of the effect of certain psychological states on the function of the immune system (12).

Operationally, this means that physiologic and psychologic states are not independent. One may directly influence the other. Equally important, the apportioning of disability from the point of view of quality of life rests as much on a patient's perception as on some "objective" measure of psychologic state. Early in their careers, clinicians experience the humbling lack of correlation between how such a patient should behave, based on a "medical" assessment, and his actual demonstrated ability to carry on in the community.

The importance of this psychologic approach is its dual emphasis; first on patient perception, and second on the psyche as an overt contributor to physiologic outcome.

"Utility"—the Trade-Offs We Make

Related to the relevance of certain quality of life domains to subsets of individuals, is the concept of trade-offs in quality and quantity of life. Some individuals may prefer survival at any cost, whereas others would not consider life to be worth living under certain circumstances. McNeil (13) presented groups of normal individuals with two treatment alternatives for laryngeal cancer. The first was laryngectomy, which offers longer survival. The second was radiation therapy with the attendant risk of shorter survival, but with voice preservation. On average, individuals indicated that they would trade off 14% of their full life expectancy to avoid loss of speech. The two groups were executives and firefighters, and although there was no significant difference noted in the number of years they would be willing to trade off to retain normal speech, executives on average would have been willing to trade off 17% of their full life expectancy versus only 6% for firefighters. Obviously executives placed a higher value on retaining normal speech. The group differences might have been expected on common sense grounds, but such preferences may not always be obvious, especially to researchers working in different cultural settings where different values apply.

There are numerous examples of the utility concept. Most of the studies that have been done pose hypothetical trade-offs in an attempt to put some value on an organ or functional capability. At its most primitive, the utility concept is rather like an accident insurance policy; so much for one arm, a little more for an eye and a leg, and so on. Used with the insight of Torrance (14) or McNeil (13), one begins to understand how people accommodate impairment or loss of a part of themselves.

Working daily with quality of life data, one senses these utility trade-offs being made all the time as patients seek to maximize quality of life. On one occasion, a patient in our palliative care unit observed that she could no longer work and that at intervals the pain was terrible. However, she was also able to be with friends, to talk, to reminisce, and, in her phrase, "to consolidate." She knew nothing of our arcane quality of life construct. Involuntarily she had traded off occupational function for social interaction. When she went on to say that what she had lost in the ability to work she had more than made up for by the opportunity to consolidate and to share, she epitomized for us the ceaseless trade-offs we make.

Toward a Broader View: A Community-Centered Concept

Ware proposed another way of organizing the variables that constitute health status and quality of life concepts which provides a sense of the impact illness has on the broader community (8). In his conceptualization, the variables can be grouped in concentric circles starting with the physiologic parameters of disease in the center and spreading out in turn to personal functioning, psychological distress/well-being, general health perceptions, and finally social/role functioning.

As discussed previously, the variables which measure disease are physiological and highly specific to the disease in question. Personal functioning is defined as the performance or capacity to perform everyday tasks including self-care, mobility, and physical activities. Such measures of functional status are commonly used with the chronically ill, but are often insensitive to disease status and are only weakly related to emotional functioning. Therefore they cannot be used alone to provide a comprehensive picture of the degree of health and well-being.

The third level of health status is psychologic, which is important not only as a disease category in its own right, but also because it interacts with physical disease and response to treatment. It is clear that it affects and is affected by both. Psychological well-being is included with psychological distress, because most existing measures concentrate on the distress end of the continuum and are not sensitive to changes that occur at the well-being end. It may be that reduction in psychological well-being rather than overt distress is more likely to reflect the response to physical disease or its treatment.

General health perception is the fourth circle because it is felt to encompass the individual's evaluation of the three preceding concepts. However, the correspondence is far from perfect: there is clearly more involved in a general self-rating of health status, perhaps the personal values put upon each concept. The final circle is social/role functioning, which refers to an individual's capacity to perform activities associated with his or her usual role, including employment, school work, or homemaking.

Ware's concept emphasizes a hierarchy by placing physical illness at the center of the circle. Thus it opens the issue of weighting, apportioning relative values to the component parts of the quality of life construct. Also implicit in Ware's model is the effect of illness upon a community. More than a single patient's quality of life is affected by an illness. Thus, in measuring quality of life, how far must we extend our reach?

Reintegration to Normal Living

The concept "reintegration to normal living" has been proposed as a proxy for quality of life (15). The definition offered was the reorganization of physical, psychological, and social characteristics of an individual into a harmonious whole, so that well-adjusted living can be resumed after an incapacitating illness or trauma. The domains discovered during the process of developing an index to measure this concept were: mobility, self-care abilities, daily activities, recreational activities, social activities, family roles, personal relationships, presentation of self, and general coping skills. Although certain areas usually covered by quality of life measures were not included, such as symptoms and emotional functioning, they were thought to be subsumed under the more global items. Two subscales were developed and found to correlate to some extent with appropriate groupings of items from Spitzer's Quality of Life Index (16). Hence this concept, although related to the quality of life concept, is by no means identical to it.

In spite of the differences in domain definition between reintegration to normal living and quality of life, the occasions on which it would be appropriate to measure either concept coincide. Reintegration means the ability to do what one has to do or wants to do, but it does not mean being free of disease or symptoms. Thus it is an appropriate measure for treatment outcome in chronic diseases where no cure is expected and the patient has to learn to live with the disease. The extent to which this is achieved can be thought of either in terms of reintegration, or quality of life, or both.

Calman's Gap: Quality of Life Compared to What?

To this point, our conceptual discussion has focused on three issues: quality of life is multidimensional; each dimension changes over time; and it is a patient-perceived entity. The next question concerns scalar values. Against what standard do we measure quality of life?

Calman (9) defined quality of life as the gap between the patient's expectations and achievements. Thus the smaller the gap, the higher the quality of life. Conversely, the less the patient is able to realize his expectations, the poorer his quality of life. In his analysis, Calman showed that the gap between expectations and achievement may vary over time as the patient's health improves or regresses in relation to the effectiveness of treatment or progress of disease. He emphasized that the goals set by the patient must be realistic in order to thwart undue frustration. He noted that here the professional may temper the patient's expectations and prepare him for the changes and limitations that will ensue as the disease progresses. The "impact of illness," Calman's term, may vary depending on the patient's perception of his quality of life when he is given a diagnosis. Thus a person who had been losing weight and becoming fatigued during the months prior to diagnosis may have prepared himself psychologically, and already reduced his expectations.

Another gap which reflects a further component of quality of life is that between the patient's actual achievements and his or her potential achievements (a third person estimation) (17). Andrews and Stewart (18) studied day hospital patients seen following inpatient care in a stroke unit and found that there was an important difference between the patient's potential achievements, as shown in the objective day hospital Activities of Daily Living (ADL) assessments, and the patient's actual achievements as measured by the same observers when assessing these patients at home. Channer et al. (19) showed, in patients presenting with chest pain but found not to have any evidence of ischemic heart disease, that the explanation of this fact to the patient failed to prevent further chest pain in 70% of the subjects. Both these studies are examples of a gap between the patient's actual achievements (poor ADL function and persistent restricting chest pain, respectively) and the patient's potential achievements. Both led to a diminution of quality of life: in the first study, diminution according to the external observer; in the second study, diminution according to the subject's own experiences. By potential achievements we do not mean those that are theoretically possible, but those shown actually to occur, albeit under certain conditions. Wood (20) drew attention to the importance of increasing the patient's appraisal and coping skills to enhance quality of life rather than just aiming at increasing patient satisfaction and happiness.

QUALITY OF LIFE: A DEFINITION

The quality of life rubric which has emerged from these conceptual discussions represents an attempt to define, in scientifically analyzable terms, the patient's functional outcome of a disease and its treatment. What emerges is a functional definition of quality of life, measurable and evaluatable over time. The patient serves as his own internal control. The questions to be included in the assessment may be drawn from the experience of patients, relatives, and health care providers, but they are to be answered from the perspective of the patient. This is not to deny the impact of disease on a patient's relatives or the community at large. This approach is accepted as a necessary pragmatic compromise so that meaningful studies can reasonably be undertaken. We are generalizing from the specific physiologic or biochemical parameters of a disease to an attempt to encompass the overall impact of the disease and its treatment on a particular patient. We want to know what happens to a patient in a functional way.

Intrinsic to this definition is a definition of health. One possibility is to base our model on the World Health Organization definition: "A state of complete physical, mental and social well-being and not merely the absence of disease or infirmity." This is a commendable definition, but it includes elements that are beyond the purview of traditional, apolitical medicine. Opportunity, education, and social security are important overall issues in the development of community health, but they are beyond the immediate goal of our assessment, which is treating the sick. We have chosen instead a second pragmatic definition of quality of life, that emphasizes the day-to-day comings and goings of a free, living individual. "Quality of Life" represents the functional effect of an illness and its consequent therapy upon a patient, as perceived by the patient. Four broad domains contribute to the overall effect: physical and occupational function; psychologic state; social interaction and somatic sensation. This definition is based on the premise that the goal of medicine is to make the morbidity and mortality of a particular disease disappear. We seek to take away the disease and its consequences, and leave the patient as if untouched by the illness.

THE DOMAINS OF QUALITY OF LIFE

Over the past several years a broad consensus has emerged as to the components of this overall gestalt (21,22). Though terminology may differ, there are four: physical function, psychologic state, social interaction, and somatic sensation. Some investigators, particularly in the United States, add a separate financial component (23). We think this is an inappropriate and possibly distorting addition. Although the financial consequences of an illness are clearly important, their effect upon a patient, and the community as a whole, is dependent on the structure of community social support programs rather than the biology of the disease. The financial costs that are incurred in the course of an illness fall into two categories; namely the direct costs of medical supplies and services, and the employment-related opportunity costs. The former is a social policy issue, likely not comparable from one community to another, let alone across national boundaries. This latter component is reflected in the physical function part of the quality of life measure.

It is appropriate to explore further the four domains which contribute to quality of life. If overall quality of life is somehow the combined effect of these four components, it may be that interventions specifically focused on one or more of the contributory factors will significantly change a patient's quality of life. We usually think in terms of radiotherapy or chemotherapy as therapeutic interventions for cancer. If we are looking for objective tumor response as measured traditionally, then these are the appropriate measures to consider. On the other hand, if we broaden our horizons to include overall quality of life, it may be that at a given point in the natural history of a particular disease or in a particular patient, a "nonmedical" intervention may make a more significant contribution to a patient's quality of life than conventional medical therapy. Likewise, a treatment may offer benefit when measured according to one set of parameters, for example survival or disease-free survival, but may be a disadvantage when viewed from the prospect of quality of life or its component parts.

Physical and Occupational Function

Physical and occupational function is the quality of life factor most nearly approximating the outcome measures physicians traditionally use. Questions about strength, energy, and the ability to carry on expected normal activities are typical questions asked. They correlate reasonably with physician estimates of patient well-being and function (24). To a certain extent, they follow objective measures of tumor response or physiology, but the correlation is not strong. Questions should elicit responses uninfluenced by age, sex, or by geographical habitus. A question asking about difficulty climbing stairs is of little relevance in those parts of the world where there are no stairs. Likewise, questions in this domain must be answerable by both those who have traditional occupations such as steelworkers and accountants, and housewives who might interpret such questions as having something to do with employment.

One of the subtleties implicit in the design of such instruments is that they are constructed so as to provide a scalar representation of the severity of impairment. A difficulty often encountered, particularly when borrowing from other detailed evaluations of physical or occupational function, is the truncation artifact (24). Many of these measures are designed and validated in institutionalized populations. The top level on such scales often represents the minimum functional state required for self-care. If such measures are transposed to quality of life studies, particularly when examining ambulatory populations, everyone answers at the top of the scale, and discriminant function is seriously compromised. Analogous problems have also been encountered at the lower limits of such scales when they are applied in the terminal care setting (25).

Psychologic Function

Psychologic function is relatively comfortable territory for psychologists and psychometricians, but is frequently problematic for physicians. Numerous studies show that doctors involved in traditional medical care are poor estimators of a patient's psychological state (26,27). Not surprisingly, nurses, social workers, and psychologists do better. Operationally this provides an important rationale for establishing a clinic environment where both the attending physician and the nurse have individual opportunities to speak with each patient.

Of the many psychological parameters that have an impact on quality of life, the most studied are anxiety, depression, and fear. From a number of studies there seems to be an underlying natural pattern of emotions encompassing depression and anxiety at the time of diagnosis, anxiety with each approaching reassessment, and fear at moments of diagnostic or therapeutic uncertainty (28–30). The psychometric measures employed in quality of life studies may be simple questions inquiring directly as to mood, anxiety, or depression, or they may be more sophisticated borrowings from the large psychometric testing literature.

Of substantial concern, however, is the fact that the study population we are targeting, namely chronically ill patients, comes from neither of the populations for whom these tests were initially devised. Many tests draw norms from a healthy population. Other measures have been developed to assess persons with diagnosed mental or psychiatric disabilities. Their scalar properties are often adjusted to evaluate the severity of pre-existing psychiatric conditions. Thus the validity of the psychological component in a quality of life measure tends to be held hostage to the developmental root of its questions, and is not readily transposed to another use, such as quality of life assessment. Our experience, and that of our European Organization for Research and Treatment of Cancer (EORTC) colleagues, suggests that straightforward questioning with a small number of items provides quite reasonable correlation with more detailed psychologic and psychometric examinations (24,31). However, these analyses should not be extended to making specific psychologic diagnoses, but rather serve as a broad indicator of overall psychologic function.

Social Interaction

The third quality of life composite factor is social interaction. This refers to a patient's ability to carry on the person-to-person interactions that form the core of communal living. These interactions are traditionally thought of as forming a hierarchy: family, close friends, work and vocational associates, and the general community. The importance of this parameter has long been underestimated.

Somatic Sensation

Somatic sensation is the fourth quality of life domain. The rubric encompasses unpleasant physical feelings which may detract from someone's quality of life. They include pain, nausea, and shortness of breath, among others. Of particular interest to a number of observers is the role that the attribution of discomfort has on overall quality of life. Though the data are not conclusive, many believe that unpleasant somatic sensations associated with therapy have a less deleterious effect on quality of life than similar sensations of like duration and intensity which must be attributed to the disease (32). Particularly for pain, duration and intensity appear to interact. Ventafridda suggests that multiplying the intensity of pain by its duration offers an accurate estimate of a patient's reserve (33). He goes further to suggest that the relief of pain may directly prolong life (Ventafridda, *personal communication*).

PROPERTIES OF THE QUALITY OF LIFE PARADIGM

The quality of life paradigm has a number of operational characteristics different from the clinical outcome measures to which we are accustomed (22). It is important to understand these differences in order to avoid pitfalls in clinical trials design. There are numerous examples of well-intentioned trials whose outcome and interpretation are suspect because the investigators were unfamiliar with the benefits as well as the limitations of the methodology. Four important properties merit discussion: the quality of life parameter is multifactorial; it is patient self-administered; its value is variable over time; and it is subjective.

Multifactoriality

It is apparent at a glance that the quality of life parameter measures more than a single aspect of a patient's overall function. Having defined quality of life operationally as the synthesis of four domains (physical and occupational function, psychologic state, social interaction, and somatic sensation), one needs to be satisfied that enough of a patient's overall daily living is encompassed by these measures that the score is truly representative of the whole process. This is analogous to determining how representative either the blood glucose, or the hemoglobin A1C, is of the overall diabetic process. The reader may be reassured by reference to the literature on the evolution of early quality of life indices, that a number of techniques including factor analysis, multiple observer interview studies, etc., suggest that these domains taken together offer a good approximation of a patient's functional quality of life.

The next question to ask is whether the brief inquiries into each quality of life domain adequately reflect their target. It is clear that one cannot make a detailed psychosocial or occupational evaluation out of four or five questions. However, correlation studies comparing quality of life, on a factor by factor basis, with much more detailed measures representing each factor provide much reassurance about their validity. The correlations tend to be high, and when factor analysis is used as a statistical technique, the factor groupings are orthogonal, suggesting, for the well-designed indices, that the questions point to specific factors rather than being vague probes of well-being (21,34).

Numerous investigators have now tried to develop cancer-specific global quality of life indices (24,34–40). In attempting to provide a compact index of broad applicability, repeatable at frequent intervals, some compromise has been made. In particular, the analysis of specific somatic disability has been abbreviated. It simply is not feasible to ask every patient, at every intervention, about a vast range of symptoms and side effects which may have little relevance to the particular clinical situation. In an attempt to resolve this difficulty, Neil Aaronson at the World Health

Organization (WHO) Quality of Life Collaborative Centre in Amsterdam has proposed a "Core Plus Module" approach (31). The essence of the idea is that one
administers both a global quality of life index and a smaller additional module that
is disease-specific. In principle this allows one to make consistent overall quality of
life assessments, while at the same time dissecting the dysfunctions identified with
measures specific to each disease. The WHO Quality of Life Index, under development, represents something of an integration of indices like the Functional Living
Index—Cancer (FLIC) (24) and the EORTC Core Plus Module approach (31).

The related weighting problem is more vexing and largely unresolved. How does
one weight the individual domain scores so as to arrive at a reasonable overall quality
of life score? At the present time no studies resolve the issue. It may be that the
relative weightings of quality of life domain scores are themselves variable over
time, and hence not amenable to fixed weighting. This means that before comparing
quality of life outcomes of different trials, one is required to take into account differences in domain weightings among the quality of life measures used. It may serve
as an enlightening historical aside to note that when the FLIC was first devised, we
tended to provide an overall quality of life score because we lacked confidence that
the factor scores were representative (24). Many researchers are now more confident
in the use of quality of life subscores as probes (not as diagnostics), and suggest that
an assessment of quality of life may include both an overall score, as defined precisely
for the instruments being used, and component subscores.

From an analytic point of view, this makes it possible to begin to dissect out
component factors of quality of life and the variable impact treatment may have on
each. Implicit in this strategy is the large volume of data that flows from a quality
of life study. Several variables are measured at each encounter and patients are
followed for a considerable time. In addition to the usual clinical information, several
items of quality of life data will be collected. This has clear workload implications.

Self-Administration

Most, but not all, quality of life indices are patient self-administered. Some, such
as Spitzer's Quality of Life Index, are designed to be administered by third parties
(16). The evidence suggests that physicians tend to focus on physiologic data and
measure it well. Nurses, social workers, family, and patients tend to place more
emphasis on psychosocial measures and in these domains may be more valid observers (27). This means that if one chooses an externally administered subjective
measure, in addition to making the usual evaluation of its reliability and validity,
one has to take into account who is doing the testing. Further, one must be consistent.
It is not appropriate to have the physician do the measuring at one time, the psychologist at another time, and the social worker or family member at another time.
Likewise, one must not adapt haphazardly a test designed for patient self-administration to the externally administered format and vice versa. One interesting study
came to grief in part because a tool designed for patient self-administration was used
with a follow-up design that allowed an external observer to attempt to recover
missing data by phoning the patient, reading the questionnaire over the telephone,
and estimating a result (41).

There is another property of the quality of life measure, related to subjectivity
and self-administration, which contributes greatly to its cross-cultural validity. That

is, it is designed to use patients as their own internal controls. It can be used without norms. With this approach, the critical quality of life value is not the score a patient provides, but rather the change in that patient's score over time. In other words, when making comparisons of groups of patients, the central issue is not whether the overall score in one group is better than the other, but rather whether the change in scores observed over time is different in each group. In relatively homogenous populations it is probably reasonable to look at differences in raw score, but many of the problems associated with comparing people of different social, economic, and cultural milieus are circumvented when change in score within patients becomes the focus of the examination. However, to employ this approach, timing of the initial quality of life assessment is critical. Insofar as is possible, this first assessment must be done at the same time in the natural history of the investigation and treatment of the disease in every patient. Otherwise the baseline against which all comparisons are made will be inconsistent and the trial less evaluatable.

Quality of Life is Time-Variable

A third important property the quality of life parameter is that it is variable over time. In that sense it is like a measure of blood sugar or tumor size. It is sharply different from the cancer clinical trial measures we use which record response, disease-free survival, and survival. Survival and disease-free survival curves are monotonically decreasing. Studies which select these as primary outcome measures derive a single data point from each patient entered in the study. That data point is only acquired when the patient either dies or fails therapy. Thus it is entirely possible to enter a patient into a study, lose all track of him for 15 years, and recover all the survival data, without compromise, by having the patient walk into the clinic alive after that long interval. This is not the case with quality of life data, which because of its fluctuating nature is not recoverable once lost. Thus meticulous follow-up, and careful attention to the timing of measurement and consistency of measurement across treatments, becomes important.

Further, resources must be available to achieve the timely collection of data which is otherwise irretrievable. One trial, which compared continuous with intermittent treatment for an advanced malignant disease, was seriously flawed by the fact that quality of life was measured on a reasonably regular basis for those on continuous treatment, but was not measured consistently in those patients on the intermittent therapy arm when they were off therapy (42). Further, a lumped average score was used. As the authors themselves point out, the result they got was contrary to their expectation. The data lost could not be recovered.

Quality of Life is Subjective

The subjective nature of the quality of life measure is a source of some unease among investigators. Those of us raised in the Western basic science milieu tend to view medicine, at least in its research and development components, in Flexnerian terms, as a science amenable to the objectivity incumbent upon the Scientific Method. Since this model has as its basis a dispassionate molecular or biochemical understanding of disease, we believe that we will be distracted from our course by less precisely measurable concerns. What we have to keep in mind is that the heterogeneity of our patient populations and our inability to identify, let alone control, all variables that influence disease progression have forced us to accept broader statistical tolerances in clinical medicine than would reassure most basic scientists. We have difficulty probing our patients, so critical measurements are often significantly inaccurate (43). Most important, in clinical medicine the ultimate observer of the experiment is not a dispassionate third party, but a most intimately involved patient. Further, there is increasing evidence that there are real links between basic physiologic function and the broader psychosocial issues which are encompassed in the quality of life paradigm. To a certain extent, what the psychosocial measure may lack in precision it may compensate in relevance.

The goal of treatment is to make the manifest effects of an illness go away. In a sense the quality of life measure represents the final common pathway of all the physiological, psychological, and social inputs into the therapeutic process. Appropriate, rigorously designed and evaluated quality of life instruments can be used in carefully designed studies to provide objective representations of what we have until recently viewed as essentially intangible subjective processes.

TACTICS FOR CONDUCTING QUALITY OF LIFE TRIALS

Following are some general tactics for the conduct of quality of life trials.

1. Choose a study in which you expect substantial differences in quality of life outcome. To conduct a study in which you expect only subtle differences will likely prove frustrating and counterproductive.

2. The ideal study measures quality of life and overall survival in addition to other clinical parameters, which may include disease-free survival as well as specific physiologic data.

3. In calculating the number of patients required, a quality of life study may not necessarily increase the patient requirement. In fact, since each patient contributes repeated measures of the same variables over time, you may need no more patients than are required for estimation of survival or disease-free survival. (It is a well-known fact that repeated measures designs have an increased power to detect between group differences) (44).

4. Use quality of life instruments that are both reliable and valid. It is hoped that the World Health Organization Index, currently under development, will provide a reasonable standard. Do not re-invent the wheel.

5. Define precisely when the initial quality of life measurement is to be done, and by whom. This serves as the key measurement against which subsequent results are compared.

6. Repeat the quality of life measurement at intervals frequent enough to track treatment and the natural history of the disease. Do not confound your study by measuring some patients when they are sick and other patients when you expect them to be well. Where possible, it is best to measure quality of life with the same pattern of measurement in each treatment arm.

7. The period of accurate recall for a psychologic variable reflecting feeling states is somewhere between 2 and 4 weeks (45). It reflects an average of the time in question with some emphasis on either major events or more recent experiences. To emphasize the effect of an intervention, do the test shortly after. To minimize that effect, and possibly better sample the overall progression of the disease, do the

test before the next treatment event. Whatever your choice, be consistent across treatment arms.

8. Follow all patients until the natural endpoint of their disease is reached or until all influence of treatment is likely to have passed. Failure to do so may create biases related to "up-front" treatments.

9. Do not analyze your data solely by simple averaging. Techniques such as time series analysis and multivariate ANOVA (analysis of variance) take into account the pattern of quality of life response and reveal more of the social and biological effects of therapy.

10. In addition to looking at overall quality of life outcome, it is reasonable to evaluate each of the component factors. However, one must be modest with extrapolations.

The quality of life paradigm is new. It offers the potential for both patients and caregivers to use the same currency for evaluating the effectiveness of treatment. Over the past 10 years we have progressed from serious doubts about whether the concept is definable, to a broadly accepted definition, an understanding of the properties of the paradigm, and a framework for doing meaningful studies. We must be cautious lest our enthusiasm outpace our rigor.

REFERENCES

1. Sugimachi K, Maekawa S, Koga Y, Ueo H, Inokuchi K. The quality of life is sustained after operation for carcinoma of the esophagus. *Surg Gynecol Obstet* 1986;162:544–546.
2. Wortman PM, Yeaton WH. Cumulating quality of life results in controlled trials of coronary artery bypass graft surgery. *Controlled Clin Trials* 1985;6:289–305.
3. Oakley JR, Jagelman DG, Fazio VW, Lavery IC, Weakley FL, Easley K, Farmer RG. Complications and quality of life after ileorectal anastomosis for ulcerative colitis. Scientific Papers, Department of Colorectal Surgery, Department of Biostatistics, and Department of Gastroenterology, The Cleveland Clinic Foundation, Cleveland, Ohio, 1985;149:23–30.
4. Karnofsky DA, Burchenal JH. The clinical evaluation of chemotherapeutic agents in cancer. In: Maclead CM, ed. *Evaluation of chemotherapeutic agents*. Columbia University Press, 1947.
5. Yates JW, Chalmer B, McKegney FP. Evaluation of patients with advanced cancer using the Karnofsky Performance status. *Cancer*, 1980;45:2220–2224.
6. New York Heart Association. *Diseases of the heart and blood vessels: Nomenclature and criteria for diagnoses*, 6th ed., 1964.
7. Priestman TJ, Baum M. Evaluation of quality of life in patients receiving treatment for advanced breast cancer. *Lancet* 1976;1:899–901.
8. Ware JE. Conceptualizing disease impact and treatment outcomes. *Cancer* 1984;53:2316–2323.
9. Calman KC. Quality of life in cancer patients—An hypothesis. *J Med Ethics* 1984;10:124–127.
10. Kleinman A. Culture, the quality of life and cancer pain: Anthropological and cross-cultural perspectives. In: Ventrafridda V, ed. *Assessment of quality of life and cancer treatment*. Excerpta Medica International Congress Series 702, 1986;43–50.
11. Dimsdale JE. A perspective on type A behavior and coronary disease (editorial). *N Engl J Med* 1988;318:110.
12. Levy SM, Herberman RB, Maluish AM, Schlien B, Lippman M. Prognostic risk assessment in primary breast cancer by behavioral and immunological parameters. *Health Psychol* 1985;4(2):99–113.
13. McNeil B, Weichselbaum R, Pauker S. Tradeoffs, between quality and quantity of life in laryngeal cancer, Special Article, Speech and Survival. *N Engl J Med* 1981;305(17):983–987.
14. Torrance GW. Utility approach to measuring health-related quality of life. *J Chronic Dis* 1987;40:593–600.
15. Wood S, Williams JI. Reintegration to normal living as a proxy to quality of life. *J Chronic Dis* 1987;40:491–499.
16. Spitzer WO, Dobson AJ, Hall J, Chesterman E, Levi J, Shepherd R, Battista RN, Catchlove BR. Measuring the quality of life in cancer patients: A concise Q/L index for use by physicians. *J Chronic Dis* 1981;34:585–597.
17. Powell V, Powell C. Quality of life measurement. *J Med Ethics* 1987;13:222–223.

18. Andrews K, Stewart J. He can but does he? *Rheumatol Rehab* 1979;18:43–48.
19. Channer KS, et al. Failure of a negative exercise test to reassure patients with chest pain. *Q J Med* 1987;63:315–322.
20. Wood C. Are happy people healthier? Discussion paper. *J R Soc Med* 1987;80:354–356.
21. Schipper H, Levitt M. Measuring quality of life: Risks and benefits. *Cancer Treat Rep* 1985;69:1115–1125.
22. Schipper H, Clinch J. Assessment of treatment in cancer in measuring health: A practical approach. In: Teeling Smith G, ed. *Health: A practical approach.* New York: Wiley, 1988;109–155.
23. Padilla GV, Presant G, Grant MM, Metter G, Lipsett J, Heide F. Quality of life index for patients with cancer. *Res Nurs Health* 1983;6:117–126.
24. Schipper H, Clinch J, MacMurray A, Levitt M. Measuring the quality of life of cancer patients: The functional living index—Cancer: Development and validation. *J Clin Oncol* 1984;2(5).
25. Morris JN, Suissa S, Sherwood S, Wright SM, Greer D. Last days: A study of the quality of life of terminally ill cancer patients. *J Chronic Dis* 1986;39:47–61.
26. Presant BA. Quality of life in cancer patients: Who measures what? *Am J Clin Oncol*: Cancer Clinical Trials 1984;7:571–573.
27. Stam HJ, Challis GB. Ratings of cancer chemotherapy toxicity by oncologists, nurses, and pharmacists. *J Pain Symptom Manag* 1989;4:7–12.
28. Lasry JM, Margolese RG, Poisson R, et al. Depression and body image following mastectomy and lumpectomy. *J Chronic Dis* 1987;40:529–534.
29. Mor V. Cancer patients' quality of life over the disease course: Lessons from the real world. *J Chronic Dis* 1987;40:535–544.
30. Morris JN, Sherwood S. Quality of life of cancer patients at different stages in the disease trajectory. *J Chronic Dis* 1987;40:545–553.
31. Aaronson NK, Bullinger M, Ahmedzai S. A modular approach to quality of life assessment in cancer clinical trials. *Recent Results Cancer Res* 1988;111:231–249.
32. Fishman B, Loscalzo M. Cognitive–behavioral intervention in cancer pain management: Principles in application. In: Payne R, Foley KM, eds. *Medical clinics of North America.* Philadelphia: W. B. Sanders, 1987.
33. Ventafridda V, DeConno F, DiTrapani P, Gallico S, Guarise G, Rigamonto G, Tamburini M. A new method of pain quantification based on a weekly self-descriptive record of the intensity and duration of pain. In: Bonica JH, et al. *Advances in pain research and therapy.* New York: Raven Press, 1983;5:891–895.
34. Kaasa S, Mastekaasa A, Stokke I, Naess S. Validation of a quality of life questionnaire for use in clinical trials for treatment of patients with inoperable lung cancer. *Eur J Clin Oncol* 1988;24:691–701.
35. Sugarbaker PH, Barofsky I, Rosenberg SA, Gianola FJ. Quality of life assessment of patients in extremity sarcoma clinical trials. *Surgery* 1982;91:17–23.
36. Churchill DN, Morgan J, Torrance GW. Quality of life in end-stage renal disease. *Peritoneal Dialysis Bulletin* 1984;21–23.
37. Pezim ME, Nicholls RJ. Quality of life after restorative proctocolectomy with pelvic ileal reservoir. *Br J Surg* 1985;72:31–33.
38. Wiklund I, Lundvall K, Swedberg K. Assessment of quality of life in clinical trials (Editorial). *Acta Med Scand* 1986;220:1–3.
39. Gough IR, Furnival CM, Schilder L. Assessment of the quality of life of patients with advanced cancer. *Eur J Cancer Clin Oncol* 1983;19:1161–1165.
40. Selby PJ, Chapman JAW, Etazadi-Amoli J. The development of a method for assessing the quality of life of cancer patients. *Br J Cancer* 1984;50:13–22.
41. Ganz PA, Haskell CM, Figlin RA, LaSoto N, Siau J. Estimating the quality of life in a clinical trial of patients with metastatic lung cancer using the Karnofsky performance status and the functional living index-cancer. *Cancer* 1988;61:849–856.
42. Coates A, Gebski V, Stat M, et al. Improving the quality of life during chemotherapy for advanced breast cancer. *N Engl J Med* 1987;1490–1495.
43. Warr D, McKinney S, Tannock I. Influence of measurement, error on assessment of response to anticancer chemotherapy: Proposal for new criteria of tumor response. *J Clin Oncol* 1984;2:1040–1046.
44. Kirk RE. Experimental design: Procedures for the behavioral sciences. Belmont, California: Brooks/Cole Publishing Company, 1968.
45. Nunnally JC. *Psychometric theory.* New York: McGraw-Hill, 1967.

Quality of Life Assessments in Clinical Trials, edited by B. Spilker. Raven Press, Ltd. New York © 1990.

3

The Hierarchy of Patient Outcomes

James F. Fries and Patricia W. Spitz

Department of Medicine, Stanford University School of Medicine, Stanford, California 94305

"Quality of life" is a term at once pejorative and vague. The term as often used offers hope and meaning but lacks focus and precision. In the context of clinical studies, we have a restricted concept of quality of life in mind. We do not mean happiness, satisfaction, living standard, climate, or environment. Rather, we are speaking of health-oriented quality of life: those aspects that might be affected positively or negatively in clinical studies and the clinical situation.

The World Health Organization (WHO) definition of health is "not merely the absence of disease, but complete physical, psychological, and social well-being" (1). This broad and inclusive definition goes far beyond the medical model, which seeks only cure and palliation of disease. Essentially, it is this World Health Organization definition of health which encompasses our restricted definition of "quality of life." It is this increased breadth of mission which distinguishes quality of life studies from traditional clinical trials.

The purpose of this chapter is first to present a hierarchical framework into which specific individual instruments may fit, and second to describe the Health Assessment Questionnaire (HAQ) as an excellent example of a set of instruments designed to assess such a framework. We wish to emphasize that a hierarchical perspective allows the investigator flexibility in choice of instruments for particular purposes and is of critical general importance.

QUALITY OF LIFE, HEALTH STATUS, AND PATIENT OUTCOME

The terms "quality of life," "health status," and "patient outcome" as generally used have overlapping meanings. As noted, quality of life has a restricted meaning close to the WHO definition of health. Health status is a measure of that quality at a particular point in time. Patient outcome usually refers to a final health status measurement after the passage of time and the application of treatment. In the future, patient outcome will be increasingly described by a cumulative series of health status measurements.

It is highly desirable to represent any of these terms by a single number. Thus, in clinical studies, one could conclude that the quality of life (or patient outcome) with treatment A was 86, whereas with treatment B it was 93, hence treatment B was to be preferred. Unfortunately, there are major obstacles to calculation of a single index number that can serve as a primary dependent variable in clinical studies.

Such an index would require, for example, face validity, reliability, and sensitivity in a clinical study situation.

There are two ways to develop a single index number. First, it can be obtained directly. For example, one could use an analog scale question with an appropriate stem which asks the subject to make a mark which represents, broadly considered, their health status at the moment. Such a simplistic approach can in fact be useful for validating more sophisticated approaches, but experience with such scales has shown them to be very insensitive and to fail to identify the specific positive and negative inputs that are included in the global judgment.

The second approach is to calculate a single index number indirectly, by combining numbers from different scales representing different facets of health status. Good measurement characteristics and sensitivity might be obtained by such an approach, but it involves an indefensible series of major value judgments by the investigator in the implicit or explicit weighting systems which must, of necessity, be employed. Detailed discussion of techniques for assigning weights and utilities is beyond the scope of this chapter, but, in summary, the value judgments required are known to differ substantially among individuals, in the same individual at different periods of life, and between patients sick with a particular problem and those without the problem (2,3).

Therefore, if attempts to develop single variable indexes are attempted, a clear exposition of techniques used to combine the component data are required. Not only should the required value judgments be defended as thoroughly as possible, but the index itself must be conceptually complete. All of the elements that make up the composite quality of life, health status, or patient outcome must be included. Completeness is crucial, since otherwise an uncounted outcome can under some circumstances dominate a particular situation. One cannot use just economic variables, or just physical ones. All relevant dimensions must be defined and measured.

THE DIMENSIONS OF HEALTH OUTCOMES

Implicit in the concept of patient outcome assessment is a shift from reliance on measures of medical process (such as antibody to DNA, erythrocyte sedimentation rate, latex fixation titer, or even joint space narrowing or periarticular erosions on X-ray), toward those elements that are of direct importance to the patient (4). These are readily identified. Multiple surveys of patients or public, prompted or open-ended, have yielded similar answers, although the rank order of importance varies from survey to survey and situation to situation (5–7). Patients desire to be alive as long as possible; to function normally; to be free of pain and other physical, psychological, or social symptoms; to be free of iatrogenic problems from the treatment regimen; and to remain solvent. These five dimensions (death, disability, discomfort, drug side effects, and dollar cost) define patient outcome (8). The dimensions must be considered mutually exclusive and collectively exhaustive. That is, the terms must be defined broadly so that any specific aspect of patient outcome may be categorized under one or another heading.

These primary outcome dimensions separate rather naturally into subdimensions (9). Economic impact consists of direct medical costs and the indirect costs due to effects on productivity. Iatrogenic effects may be due to medication or to surgery. Discomfort may be physical or psychological. Disability can involve fine movements

PROTOTYPE INDIVIDUAL PATIENT OUTCOME

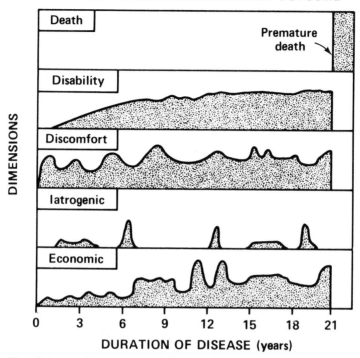

FIG. 1. The Five Primary Dimensions of Patient Outcome. In this example, the health outcomes of a patient with rheumatoid arthritis are graphed over time. Over 21 years of illness, the patient suffers economic distress; iatrogenic difficulties; symptomatic physical, psychological, and social distress; becomes progressively disabled; and dies prematurely.

of the upper extremity or locomotor activities of the lower extremity. Death can be broken down by specific cause and quantitated in terms of expected time to death.

The subdimensions can in turn be considered comprised of different components. The components in turn may be developed from particular questions and specific variables. Thus, a hierarchy may be developed which is conceptually complete and which provides a location in the framework for all possible measures relevant to outcome (Figs. 1 and 2).

PRACTICAL USE OF THE HIERARCHY OF OUTCOMES

Uniform agreement on specific assessment instruments and on assessment techniques that are suitable in all medical situations is unlikely. In particular situations, strong arguments can be made for using one instrument instead of another and for obtaining information by questionnaire, by physician interview, by telephone, by performance testing, or by other techniques. Indeed, uniform agreement is probably undesirable, since such agreement might stifle the growth of the field, discourage development of improved techniques, and ignore the particular strengths of those instruments not selected. General agreement on hierarchy, however, is not only possible, it has already been implicitly accomplished to a considerable extent.

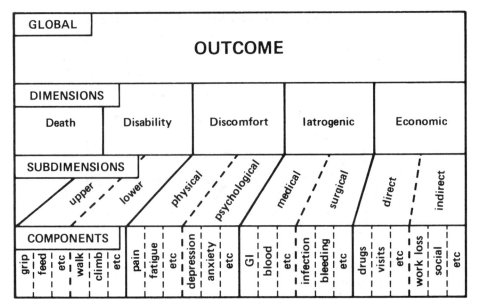

FIG. 2. The Hierarchy of Patient Outcome.

There are at least seven advantages to employing an outcome hierarchy. First, a hierarchy allows a variety of assessment techniques to be mixed as appropriate to the particular situation. Although it is crucial to measure disability, in most cases when quality of life is assessed it is much less important which of the available reliable and valid instruments is chosen. Second, it allows elaboration in specific areas where detailed and specific assessment is required for a particular task.

Third, the hierarchy provides a perspective on the role of a particular instrument. If one is particularly interested in, for example, patient satisfaction, this area can be readily conceived as a component of psychological discomfort and its position in the hierarchy identified. One can avoid exaggeration of the importance of such a measure by noting its level in the hierarchy and its distance from the primary desires expressed by patients.

Fourth, the hierarchy provides a minimum number of summary indexes at the level of dimensions. One cannot determine if treatment A is better than treatment B by individually analyzing 100 different dependent variables; some level of aggregation is essential. Although the value judgment problem involved in determining a single index variable may be insurmountable, the lesser value judgments required to develop indexes for individual outcome dimensions are more defensible.

Fifth, the hierarchy makes assumptions explicit. The upper levels of the hierarchy flow so naturally from patient desires that it is difficult to defend major changes in structure, but if an investigator desires to alter the explicit assumptions and present a different hierarchy, such a change may be argued on its merits.

Sixth, a structure, even loosely conceived, encourages longitudinal study and cumulative assessment of treatment impact. Long-term studies must maintain some degree of constancy between measures made in different years of the study, and the framework assists in this requirement (Fig. 2).

Finally, the hierarchy emphasizes and encourages completeness of assessment. Consider the necessity for such completeness with common examples. Total hip replacement cannot be completely assessed without consideration of operative and perioperative mortality, the cost of the procedure and the source of those funds, the cost savings and side effect benefits of decreased medication requirements, the lessening of pain, and any changes in function that result. Coronary artery bypass surgery cannot be fully evaluated without counting both short-term and long-term death rates, the costs of one procedure versus another, the changes in pain and the duration of that effect, improvement or loss of function, and change in future medication requirements. Treatment with antihypertensives cannot be completely assessed without counting all effects on morbidity and mortality, costs of alternative treatments, and presence of impotence or other side reactions.

Consideration of five outcome dimensions provides a revealing way to compare alternative treatment regimens. The number of dimensions is small enough to be judged reasonably and large enough to allow identification of specific areas of clear superiority of one treatment over another.

Overall judgment of the superiority of a particular regimen may be made at three levels. First, one treatment might be superior over all five dimensions. Thus, a decision in its favor would be "value-independent" since any set of relative value judgments between the different dimensions would yield the same conclusions. Secondly, utility judgments relating the relative importance of the various dimensions can be developed. Typically, such value judgments will have wide confidence limits reflecting differing individual values and differences depending on the clinical situation of the respondent. Utilizing the 95% confidence limits is a conservative way to handle this problem. Thus, one treatment might be superior to the other using any set of value judgments that are within the 95% confidence limits of a formal survey of value trade-offs. For example, a small increase in cost and in side effects might be more than offset by major changes in longevity, disability, and symptom level using "any reasonable" value system.

Finally, if neither of these tests yields a clearly superior agent, combination of dimensions may be accomplished using standard utility theory constructs and the *mean* value trade-offs of a representative population. This test will be more sensitive to differences between regimens, but the results may not apply given the value systems of particular reasonable individuals. Such situations should be clearly identified as value-dependent so that a reviewer may recalculate results using alternative value systems.

THE CONCEPT OF CUMULATIVE OUTCOME

Chronic illness must be measured chronically. As noted, health status generally refers to a patient's status at a particular point in the course of illness and outcome to the most recent (or end of study) health status measurement.

Figure 1 shows the typical course of a patient with rheumatoid arthritis. Death occurs 4 to 12 years prematurely on average, disability increases through the disease course, pain and symptomatology vary at different points, side effects occur irregularly, and costs are generally progressive but are influenced strongly by particular events along the way. A health status measurement represents a vertical slice at a particular point in time. Conventional outcome assessment represents the most recent of such measurements.

Obviously, a concept of cumulative outcome is far superior because the outcome actually desired by the patient is inversely related to the area under all of the curves rather than just to the value at some specific point in time. A treatment that reduces the area under the curve, even if the condition later returns to a similar point, represents a health benefit.

Cumulative outcome represents the most sensitive measure of the effect of a treatment in chronic illness (9). For example, it is relatively easy to demonstrate that intramuscular gold therapy in rheumatoid arthritis will decrease the area under the disability and pain curves, although viewed from a cross-sectional analysis many years later, this effect may not be ascertainable. Sequential and accurate health status measurements at regular intervals allow calculation of the approximate area under the curve. With this technique, the relevant dependent variables are measured in disability years, discomfort years, side-effect–index units recorded cumulatively, lifetime medical costs, and time to death as represented by life table determinations. The most sophisticated quality of life studies will utilize such measures.

It may be argued that happenings late in a disease course should be weighted less than those occurring earlier; that distant events should be "discounted." Such adjustment is usual in economic projections. Although such adjustment is unlikely to make a difference very often in comparisons of two treatments, we recommend that cumulative outcome results be presented with discounting a 0% per year, 6% per year, and 12% per year.

THE HEALTH ASSESSMENT QUESTIONNAIRE

The Health Assessment Questionnaire (HAQ) was designed with this hierarchical model in mind. The hierarchy was developed first, then the specific instruments for each dimension were developed and validated. The measurement technique has been validated for self-assessment by questionnaire, and Health Assessment Questionnaire instruments have been validated for use by mail, in the office, by telephone, by paraprofessional, and by physician (8). These instruments were designed to be efficient, were structured for time available during office medical visits, and were intended to be compatible with high return rates when administered by mail. Initial development of the Health Assessment Questionnaire was under the auspices of the Stanford Arthritis Center funded by the National Institutes of Health, and it has been subsequently widely used by many investigators including ARAMIS (American Rheumatism Association Medical Information System), the National Health and Nutrition Survey (NHANES I follow-up), and other projects.

The instrument was designed for use in all illnesses rather than only rheumatic disease and was designed to allow supplementation by additional measures for particular studies. The impact of illness varies markedly among different diseases, thus the instrument allows comparison of the impact of such disparate processes. For example, in osteoarthritis, pain is dominant; in rheumatoid arthritis, disability; and in cancer, death.

The Health Assessment Questionnaire was developed by parsing questions and components from a variety of instruments previously used for similar purposes. Correlation matrices were constructed which allowed elimination of variables redundant to other variables or inconsistent with the dimension consisting of the mean of all remaining variables. It has been validated in over 30 studies, revised as required, and now has been administered over 100,000 times in various national and international settings.

Development of the instrument continues. The disability section was constructed first and has received the widest attention and the most frequent use. It can be completed by a patient in less than 5 minutes and scored in less than 1 minute. It measures disability over the past week by asking a total of 20 questions in 8 categories of function: dressing, arising, eating, walking, hygiene, reach, grip, and activities. There are at least two component questions in each of these categories which are representative of the universe of functional activities. Scoring is patterned after the American Rheumatism Association (ARA) functional classes: normal, adequate, limited, or unable (10). For each component question the level of difficulty is scored from zero to three, with zero equal to no difficulty and three equal to unable to do. The highest component score in each category determines the score for the category unless aids of assistance are required. Dependence on equipment or physical assistance adjusts a lower category score to two (with much difficulty or limited). Category scores are averaged to give the Disability Index, a continuous scale ranging from zero to three.

Extensive research activity on the pain dimension resulted in a return to absolute simplicity. Attempts to elaborate pain activity by part of the body involved, times during the day which were painful, and severity of pain in different body parts failed to yield indexes that outperformed a simple analog scale (11–13). Returning to the basic principle that symptomatology is what the patient says it is, discomfort is measured by a double-anchored visual analog scale. It is scored from zero (no discomfort) to three (severe discomfort).

Iatrogenic events are measured separately, including both self-report and audit of hospital records and death certificates. Weights have been established for different side effects after rating by physicians, patients, and health professionals. Two indexes are developed: an index of fatal side effects and an index of nonfatal side effects. Standardized rules are used to attribute particular events to particular therapies. The nonfatal side effect index includes all side effects reported, with hospitalizations factored in.

Economic impact is assessed both as direct costs and indirect costs. Costs are measured in terms of units of service required rather than charges or costs actually paid, allowing automatic adjustment for inflation and for different pricing structures in different regions. Standard costs for each service are developed every 2 years from multiple sources, averaged, and applied to computations which cumulate such variables as doctor visits, hospital days, and medication costs into a direct cost figure, and productivity losses into an indirect cost figure.

The fact of death is ascertained regularly by protocol and an audit is made of all deaths, including death certificate and clinical information, in order to identify cause of death and to allow attribution to specific therapy when appropriate.

The disability section of the Health Assessment Questionnaire has undergone repeated testing and revision and the psychometric properties of the scale have been, and continue to be, evaluated (8,14). The disability scale is reliable. Two week test re-test reliability was assessed on 37 rheumatoid arthritis and osteoarthritis patients who were enrolled in the Arthritis Self-Management courses given by the Stanford Arthritis Center. There were no significant differences for the Disability Index using Student's paired t-test (D = 0.04, t = .78, df = 36). Spearman's rho was 0.87. Strong correlations were also reported by other groups. Pincus et al. modified the

Health Assessment Questionnaire to use only one question in each of the eight categories and added questions on satisfaction and change in activities and reported on the reliability properties of the disability scale (15). The correlation for 1 month test re-test on 28 rheumatoid arthritis patients was 0.78. Goeppinger et al. in their study of the use of the Health Assessment Questionnaire disability scale in a rural, low education population, reported a 1 week test re-test of 0.95 on 30 rheumatoid arthritis patients and 0.93 on 30 osteoarthritis patients (16).

Correlational analysis of intercomponent and component-index were reported on the initial scale (8). After the scale was revised, correlational analysis was again performed. Pearson's correlations on the categories and Disability Index ranged from 0.71 for Eating to 0.80 for Hygiene and for Reach on a sample of 348 rheumatoid arthritis patients. Internal consistency of individual questions with the appropriate category was evaluated by alpha reliability coefficients for each of the eight categories of 170 rheumatic disease patients (12). The coefficients were all high, ranging from 0.71 for the Reach category to 0.89 for Eating. Similarly, high correlations were obtained on 60 rheumatoid arthritis and osteoarthritis rural Virginia patients using Cronbach's alpha and interitem correlations (16).

Principal component analysis of the 15 original questions identified two components (11). The first explained 65% of the variance and the second, which had positive loadings on lower extremity activities involving large movements and negative loadings on upper extremity small movements, explained another 10% of the variance.

The initial validation studies were designed to assess the feasibility of the self-administered format and to test whether the scale actually measured functional ability (8). The comparison of patient-completed questionnaire responses with interview on a sample of 20 rheumatoid arthritis patients indicated that similar results were obtained using either format. Spearman's rho for the Disability Index was 0.85. On another sample of 25 rheumatoid arthritis patients, questionnaire responses were compared to activity performance. Spearman's rho was 0.88. Cathey et al. compared the performance of five standardized work tasks using work simulator machinery with the patient-reported Disability Index in 26 rheumatoid arthritis patients (17). Correlations between the total work score and the Index was 0.765.

Validation studies have been replicated, primarily in rheumatoid arthritis and osteoarthritis patients, usually following modifications or translations (18–21). Results have been consistent. Kirwan et al. reported a correlation of 0.92 between self-administered questionnaires and rheumatologist interview on 33 British rheumatoid arthritis patients (18). Self-reported disability correlated well with interview in the Netherlands ($r = 0.94$, $N = 38$) and in Austria ($r = 0.86$, $N = 46$) (19,20). Sullivan et al. completed home performance evaluations on 64 patients with rheumatoid arthritis, osteoarthritis, and gout (21). The mean difference between reported and observed disability was 0.18 (CI $-.8$, 1.2) and the correlation was 0.83. Our initial studies and those reported subsequently provided evidence that the disability scale is measuring what it purports to measure and that patient self-reports are a valid measure of disability.

Both convergent validity (agreement with another measure of the same attribute) and discriminate validity (weaker agreement with measures of different attributes) were examined in a study comparing the Health Assessment Questionnaire disability and pain scales with the Arthritis Impact Measurement Scale (AIMS) from the Boston University Multipurpose Arthritis Center (11). There was strong agreement between the two questionnaires. Spearman's rho was 0.91 for the disability-related scales; for the pain-related scales Spearman's rho was 0.64. In a combined factor analysis of the AIMS and HAQ scales, the factor loadings for physical disability and pain were quite close between measures: physical, 0.88 (AIMS) and 0.85 (HAQ); and pain, 0.87 (AIMS) and 0.84 (HAQ).

On the other hand, and fitting the hierarchical model, interdimensional correlations of HAQ disability and HAQ pain (rho = 0.30), AIMS pain (rho = 0.39), and AIMS psychological (rho = 0.23) were weak. Disability was also weakly correlated with the Beck Depression Inventory ($r = 0.37$) and the Hamilton Interviewer Rating Scale ($r = 0.24$) on 107 rheumatoid arthritis patients (22). Thus, disability, as measured by the Health Assessment Questionnaire, is an attribute distinct from pain or psychological distress.

The Disability Index is able to differentiate across patients. In a cross-sectional analysis, the Disability Index increased in morning stiffness, the number of involved joints, and latex positivity (14). Average Disability Index scores differ by diagnosis. The mean Disability Index was higher for rheumatoid arthritis (1.2) and progressive systemic sclerosis (0.92) than for osteoarthritis (0.4–0.6) and systemic lupus erythematosus (SLE) (0.66), supporting the conventional wisdom that osteoarthritis and systemic lupus erythematosus are less disabling diseases (14,23–25). Average disability in fibromyalgia is similar to that of systemic sclerosis, 0.9 (17).

Since the Health Assessment Questionnaire was designed, in part, to evaluate interventions, a useful disability measure must also be sensitive and able to detect clinically important changes in function among and within patients. Liang et al. showed a change in disability in a study of 50 osteoarthritis patients who had hip or knee replacements (26). Bombardier et al. used the Health Assessment Questionnaire in a 6-month multicenter clinical trial of auranofin and placebo (27). Their results showed statistically ($p < .01$) and clinically significant changes in function between the experimental group of 154 patients (change = $-.31$, SEM = .04) and the control group of 149 patients (change = $-.17$, SEM = .05). The magnitude of the differences in disability changes between the two groups was similar to the differences for the changes in clinical variables: number of swollen joints, number of tender joints, pain, and grip strength. The results of this randomized clinical trial demonstrate that the disability scale is able to detect meaningful changes in function.

In a study of risk factors for hospitalization and surgery, the Disability Index predicted an increase in admissions ($p < .01$) (28). The partial odds ratio for those with a Disability Index in the highest quartile was 9.4 for surgery and 27.2 for joint replacement. These analyses were adjusted for age, sex, and disease characteristics. The Disability Index is also a predictor of mortality. Wolfe et al. reported a relative risk for mortality of 1.77 (95% CI: 1.02–3.06) for each unit increase in the Disability Index (29). They also found that the initial Disability Index was associated with increased utilization of both inpatient and outpatient services.

The Health Assessment Questionnaire has been in wide and increasing use both in research and clinical practice in many areas as noted above. It is proven sensitive to measuring the change in disability in a clinical study and the progression of disability with age in national probability samples (NHANES) (27,30). It is currently being modified for use in AIDS populations.

The Health Assessment Questionnaire is often supplemented for specific clinical projects, and such use is encouraged. We have been unhappy with available tools for efficient assessment of psychological impacts although these are measured to a substantial degree by other parts of the Health Assessment Questionnaire. The disability section, as generally used, does not adequately pick up problems with the organs of special sense and adaptations including questions on eyesight and hearing have been developed. The Health Assessment Questionnaire lacks questions on social networking and patient satisfaction, and when information on these outcomes is desired, supplementation is required. We have no present plans to develop instruments in these areas but continue to regularly survey available instruments as appropriate supplements to the Health Assessment Questionnaire.

CONCLUSIONS

The quality of life can be measured accurately and validly. It can be related to the value systems of the patient and the public. The outcome hierarchy makes dimensions and components comprehensible and provides both perspective and focus. A treatment which does not affect at least one major dimension positively is unlikely to be a major contribution. Individual instruments may be judged on their ability to most optimally perform specific tasks. Far more importantly, the concept of an outcome hierarchy allows harmony among the many investigators seeking to improve this field and helps avoid self-serving arguments for particular instruments. The need for quality-of-life studies is increasingly perceived but is not yet dominant in health assessment. The combined efforts of the many investigative groups, working in concert, are required to persuade the unpersuaded of the merits and importance of this approach.

ACKNOWLEDGMENT

This work was supported in part by a grant from The National Institutes of Health to ARAMIS (AM21393).

REFERENCES

1. World Health Organization. The first ten years of the World Health Organization. Geneva: WHO, 1958.
2. Sox HC, Blatt MA, Higgin MC, Marton KI. *Medical decision making.* London: Butterworths, 1988.
3. Moskowitz AJ, Kuipers B, Kassirer JP. Academia and clinic: Dealing with uncertainty, risks, and tradeoffs in clinical decisions: A cognitive science approach. *Ann Intern Med* 1988;108:435–449.
4. Fries JF. Toward an understanding of patient outcome measurement. *Arthritis Rheum* 1983;26:697–704.
5. White KL. Improved medical care: Statistics and the health service system. *Public Health Rep* 1967;82:847–854.
6. Lorig K, Cox T, Cuevas Y, Kraines RG, Britton MC. Converging and diverging beliefs about arthritis: Caucasian patients, Spanish-speaking patients and physicians. *J Rheumatol* 1984;11:76–79.
7. Potts M, Mazzuca S, Brandt K. Views of patients and physicians regarding the importance of various aspects of arthritis treatment. Correlations with health status and patient satisfaction. *Patient Educ Couns* 1986;8:125–134.
8. Fries JF, Spitz PW, Kraines RG, Holman HR. Measurement of patient outcome in arthritis. *Arthritis Rheum* 1980;23:137–145.
9. Fries JF. The assessment of disability: From first to future principles. *Br J Rheumatol* 1983;22(suppl):48–58.
10. Steinbrocker O, Trager CH, Betterman RC. Therapeutic criteria in rheumatoid arthritis. *JAMA* 1949;140:659–662.
11. Brown JH, Kazis LE, Spitz PW, Gertman PM, Fries JF, Meenan RF. The dimensions of health

outcomes: A cross-validated examination of health status measurement. *Am J Public Health* 1984;74:159–161.

12. Langley GB, Sheppeard H. Problems associated with pain measurement in arthritis: Comparison of the visual analogue and verbal rating scales. *Clin Exp Rheumatol* 1984;2:231–234.

13. Anderson KO, Bradley LA, McDaniel LK, et al. The assessment of pain in rheumatoid arthritis: Disease differentiation and temporal stability of a behavioral observation method. *J Rheumatol* 1987;14:700–704.

14. Fries JF, Spitz PW, Young DY. The dimensions of health outcomes: The Health Assessment Questionnaire, disability, and pain scales. *J Rheumatol* 1982;9:789–793.

15. Pincus T, Summey JA, Soraci SA, et al. Assessment of patient satisfaction in activities of daily living using a modified Stanford Health Assessment Questionnaire. *Arthritis Rheum* 1983;26:1346–1353.

16. Goeppinger J, Doyle M, Murdock B, et al. Self-administered function measures: The impossible dream? *Arthritis Rheum* 1985;28:S145 (abstract).

17. Cathey MA, Wolfe F, Kleinheksal SM. Functional ability and work status in patients with fibromyalgia. *Arthritis Care Res* 1988;1:85–98.

18. Kirwan JR, Reeback JS. Stanford Health Assessment Questionnaire modified to assess disability in British patients with rheumatoid arthritis. *Br J Rheumatol* 1986;25:206–209.

19. Siegert CEH, Vleming LV, VBan-Denbroucke JP, Cats A. Measurement of disability in Dutch rheumatoid arthritis patients. *Clin Rheumatol* 1984;3:305–309.

20. Singer F, Kolarz G, Mayrhofer F, Scherak O, Thumb N. The use of questionnaires in the evaluation of the functional capacity in rheumatoid arthritis. *Clin Rheumatol* 1982;1:251–261.

21. Sullivan FM, Eagers RC, Lynch K, Barber JH. Assessment of disability caused by rheumatic diseases in general practice. *Ann Rheum Dis* 1987;46:598–600.

22. Peck JR, Ward JR, Smith TW, et al. Convergent/discriminant validity of the HAQ disability index in rheumatoid arthritis using a multitrait-multimethod matrix. *Arthritis Rheum* 1987;30:S193 (abstract).

23. Wolfe F, Kleinheksel SM, Spitz PW, Lubeck DP, Fries JF, Young DY, Mitchell DM, Roth SH. A multi-center study of hospitalization in rheumatoid arthritis: Frequency, medical-surgical admissions, and charges. *Arthritis Rheum* 1986;29:614–619.

24. Poole J, Steen V. The use of the Health Assessment Questionnaire (HAQ) to determine physical disability in systemic sclerosis. *Arthritis Rheum* 1986;29:S152 (abstract).

25. Hochberg MC, Sutton JD. Physical disability and psychosocial dysfunction in systemic lupus erythematosus (SLE). *J Rheumatol* 1988;15:959–964.

26. Liang MH, Larson MG, Cullen KE, Schwartz JA. Comparative measurement efficiency and sensitivity of five health status instruments for arthritis research. *Arthritis Rheum* 1985;28:542–547.

27. Bombardier C, Ware J, Russell IJ, et al. Auranofin therapy and quality of life in patients with arthritis, results of a multicenter trial. *Am J Med* 1986;81:565–578.

28. Nevitt MC, Yelin EH, Henke CJ, et al. Risk factors for hospitalization and surgery in patients with rheumatoid arthritis: Implications for capitated medical payment. *Ann Intern Med* 1986;105:421–428.

29. Wolfe F, Kleinheksel SM, Cathey MA, et al. The clinical value of the HAQ disability index in patients with rheumatoid arthritis. *J Rheumatol* (*in press*).

30. Foley DJ, Branch LG, Madans JH, et al. Dysfunctioning among NHANESI survivors. In Cornoli-Huntley JC, Huntley R, Feldman JJ, ed. *Health status and well-being of the elderly.* New York: Oxford University Press (*in press*).

Quality of Life Assessments in Clinical Trials, edited by B. Spilker. Raven Press, Ltd. New York © 1990.

4

Measurements in Clinical Trials:

Choosing the Appropriate Approach

* Gordon H. Guyatt and
† Roman Jaeschke

* Department of Clinical Epidemiology and Biostatistics, and † Department of Internal Medicine, McMaster University Health Sciences Centre, Hamilton, Ontario L8N 3Z5, Canada

During the last decade, the importance of measuring aspects of health status related to patients' function and subjective experience has become increasingly recognized. The methods available for measuring how patients feel and how they function have become more sophisticated. The term "quality of life" has appeared as a label for the measurement of physical and emotional (as opposed to biochemical and physiological) function (1). Of course, quality of life is influenced by many factors other than one's health (including one's income, job satisfaction, and social opportunities). What health researchers are interested in is "health-related quality of life." Another appropriate term might be "perceived health status." For the sake of brevity and because of its widespread use, in the present discussion the term "quality of life" will be used to refer to the wide variety of subjective experiences (such as symptoms, physical function, and emotional function) that are related to health.

A host of quality of life indexes have been recently developed to measure complex domains like emotional and social function, well-being, disability, and overall health status. Readers of clinical journals note clinical trials in which quality of life is the primary outcome (2–4). The areas examined include the impact of a disease or condition on quality of life (5,6), the profile of dysfunction in a particular population (7), or the relation between quality of life and prognosis (8). For clinicians, one crucial arena for quality of life measurement is determining the impact of medical interventions on how patients feel and function.

The purpose of this chapter is to review the possible approaches to measurement of quality of life in clinical studies and to consider their relative merits. The present discussion, which is built on the previous contributions of authors in this area (1,9–14), focuses on the empirical performance of quality of life measures in clinical trials, rather than the theoretical framework on which the measures are based. A summary of the strengths and weaknesses of quality of life measures is presented in Table 1.

Before applying any quality of life instrument in a clinical study, one needs to address several issues. First, the purposes for which an instrument is used must be clearly stated. Second, the instrument to be used must have certain attributes, which

TABLE 1. *Taxonomy of measures of health related quality of life in clinical trials*

Approach	Strengths	Weaknesses
Generic Instruments:		
Health profile	Single instrument Established reliability and validity Detects differential effects on different aspects of health status Comparison across interventions, conditions possible	May not focus adequately on area of interest May not be responsive
Utility measurement	Single number representing quality of life Cost-utility analysis possible	Difficulty determining utility values Doesn't allow examination of effect on different aspects of quality of life May not be responsive
Specific Instruments:		
Disease-specific Population specific Function specific Condition or Problem specific	Clinically sensible May be more responsive	Doesn't allow across-condition comparisons May be limited in terms of populations and interventions

will determine its usefulness for a specific goal. Third, with the above in mind, one needs to determine the general category of quality of life instrument required, from which a suitable questionnaire can be chosen. The following discussion will examine these issues.

POTENTIAL PURPOSES OF QUALITY OF LIFE MEASUREMENT INSTRUMENTS

The potential applications of quality of life measures can be divided into three broad categories: discrimination, prediction, and evaluation.

Discriminative Index

A discriminative index is used to distinguish between individuals or groups with respect to an underlying dimension when no external criterion or "gold standard" is available for validating these measures. Intelligence tests, for example, are used to distinguish among children's learning abilities. The Minnesota Multiphasic Personality Inventory was developed in order to distinguish those with emotional and psychological disorders from the general population (15). Use of an index from this category in a clinical study is illustrated by the following example: If one has a group of patients with myocardial infarction and they are to be divided into those with good or poor quality of life (with a view, for example, to intervene in the latter group), a discriminative index is required.

Predictive Index

When a gold standard is available, a predictive index is used to classify individuals into a set of predefined measurement categories either at the time of initial measurement or some time in the future. This gold standard is subsequently used to determine whether individuals have been classified correctly. Although there is no gold standard available for measurement of quality of life, a predictive instrument can still be used in this area. Let us assume that some investigators have developed a quality of life instrument that is believed to be definitive, but takes over an hour to administer. Because an hour is a long interview, it is desirable to have a shorter version. One might choose a subsample of questions from the original and examine the performance of the new, shorter instrument, using the original as a gold standard.

Evaluative Index

An evaluative index is used to measure the magnitude of longitudinal change in an individual or group. The development of evaluative instruments has provided the main focus for those interested in measurement of quality of life in clinical trials. Such instruments are needed for quantitating the treatment benefit in clinical studies, and for measuring quality-adjusted life years in cost-utility analyses.

NECESSARY ATTRIBUTES OF A QUALITY OF LIFE MEASUREMENT INSTRUMENT

Before proceeding to a more detailed discussion of the approaches to quality of life measurement in clinical studies, it is necessary to briefly review the attributes inherent in any useful instrument. There are three essential attributes: reproducibility, validity, and responsiveness.

Reproducibility

A measure is reproducible insofar as it yields the same results when repeated in stable subjects. Reproducibility is best measured by repeated administration of an instrument to subjects whose status has not changed.

Validity

Validity or accuracy is a necessary property of any useful test or instrument: the instrument must be measuring what it is supposed to measure (16–18). Establishing accuracy is relatively easy if there is a criterion or gold standard to which the new instrument can be compared. However, there is no gold standard for quality of life measurement. As a result, the validity of quality of life measures is established by specifying the domain or dimension one wishes to measure, and the expected relations between that domain or dimension and other variables. Thus, one assembles empirical evidence to support the inference that a particular instrument is measuring what it is supposed to measure. Many questionnaires used in clinical trials rely on face validity: intuitively, the questions appear to relate to aspects of quality of life.

Unfortunately, it is difficult to be certain of what the results of such ad hoc instruments mean. For example, questionnaires asking patients if their function improved after a rehabilitation program may be measuring satisfaction with the program process, rather than quality of life. The validity of a questionnaire must be established before it can be applied as a meaningful outcome measure in clinical studies.

Responsiveness

Investigators may want to detect any clinically important changes in quality of life, even if those changes are small. Responsiveness (or sensitivity to change) refers to the instrument's ability to detect clinically important change. An instrument's responsiveness is determined by two properties (19). First, to be responsive it should be reproducible. Second, it must register changes in score when subjects' quality of life improves or deteriorates; this property can be called changeability. If an instrument's responsiveness is unproved and a controlled study in which the instrument is used is negative, there remain two interpretations. First, the treatment does not work; second, the instrument is not responsive. Thus, when beginning a study, it is desirable to use a questionnaire that has proved responsive in previous related investigations.

All quality of life measures, irrespective of the approach used, must be reproducible, valid, and responsive to be useful as outcome measures in clinical studies.

APPROACHES TO MEASURING QUALITY OF LIFE IN CLINICAL STUDIES: TAXONOMY OF MEASURES OF QUALITY OF LIFE

Generic Instruments

Generic instruments are designed to sample the complete spectrum of function, disability, and distress that is relevant to quality of life. In doing so, generic instruments are applicable to a wide variety of populations. Generic instruments can be divided into two major classes: health profiles, and utility measures.

Health Profiles

Health profiles are single instruments that measure different aspects of quality of life. Health profiles share a common scoring system, and can be aggregated into a small number of scores and sometimes into a single score (in which case, it may be referred to as an index). As generic measures, they are designed for use in a wide variety of conditions. For example, one of the most popular health profiles, the Sickness Impact Profile (SIP) (20) contains 12 "categories" that can be aggregated into two dimensions and five independent categories, and also into a single overall score. The Sickness Impact Profile has been used in studies of cardiac rehabilitation (21), total hip joint arthroplasty (22), and treatment of back pain (4). In addition to the Sickness Impact Profile, there are a number of other health profiles available: the Nottingham Health Profile (23), the McMaster Health Index Questionnaire (24), and a collection of related instruments developed by the RAND Corporation for their health-insurance study (25).

Although each health profile attempts to measure all important aspects of quality of life, they may slice the quality of life pie quite differently. For example, the McMaster Health Index Questionnaire follows the World Health Organization approach and identifies three dimensions: physical, emotional, and social. The Sickness Impact Profile includes a physical dimension (with categories of ambulation, mobility, and body care and movement), a psychosocial dimension (with categories including social interaction and emotional behavior), and five independent categories including eating, work, home management, sleep and rest, and recreations and pastimes.

Health profiles offer a number of advantages to the clinical investigator. Their reproducibility and validity have been established, often in a variety of populations. Using them for discriminative purposes, one can examine and establish areas of dysfunction affecting a particular population. For example, Prigatano et al. (5), using the Sickness Impact Profile, showed that patients with mild hypoxemia and chronic obstructive pulmonary disease were most severely affected in the areas of sleep, social interaction, employment, recreation, and pastime activities, whereas the degree of physical limitations was generally minimal. Identification of these areas of dysfunction may guide investigators constructing disease-specific instruments and target the potential therapeutic intervention at the areas of greatest impact on the quality of life. Health profiles, used as evaluative instruments, allow determination of the effects of the intervention on different aspects of quality of life without necessitating the use of multiple instruments (and thus saving both the investigator's and the patient's time). Because they are designed for a wide variety of conditions, one can potentially compare the effects on quality of life of different interventions in different diseases. Profiles which provide for a single score can be used in a cost-effectiveness analysis, in which the cost of an intervention in dollars is related to its outcome in natural units. For example, one could examine the incremental cost necessary to produce a five-point improvement in score on the Sickness Impact Profile.

Health profiles also have limitations. They may not focus adequately on the aspects of quality of life of specific interest to the investigator. For example, we recently encountered an investigator interested in measuring the effects of anti-arrhythmic therapy on quality of life. None of the 136 items in the Sickness Impact Profile relate directly to symptoms that may be ameliorated by anti-arrhythmic therapy: palpitations, presyncope, and syncope. Inadequate focus on the quality of life issues of a specific study is likely to result in an unresponsive instrument which may miss small but still clinically important changes in quality of life (26,27). On the other hand, when the intervention is likely to have an impact on aspects of quality of life included in a health profile, responsiveness may be adequate. For example, at least some of the Sickness Impact Profile dimensions have detected differences between intervention and control groups in randomized trials of cardiac rehabilitation (21), and amputation versus limb-sparing surgery in soft tissue sarcoma (28).

A final limitation of health profiles is that if they do not yield a single score that is preferentially weighted they cannot be used in cost-utility analysis. This issue is discussed further in the following section.

Utility Measurement

Utility measures of quality of life are derived from economic and decision theory. Quality of life is measured holistically as a single number along a continuum from death (0.0) to full health (1.0). Use of utility measures in clinical studies requires serial measurement of the utility of the patient's quality of life throughout the study.

There are two fundamental approaches to utility measurement in clinical studies. One is to ask patients a number of questions about their function. On the basis of their responses, patients are classified into one of a number of categories. Each category has a utility value associated with it, the utility having been established in previous ratings by another group (such as a random sample of the general population). This approach characterizes a widely used instrument called the Quality of Well-Being Scale (10,11,16).

The second approach is to ask patients to make a single rating which takes into account all aspects of their quality of life (12). There are many ways this rating can be made. The standard gamble asks subjects to choose between their own health state and a gamble in which they may die immediately or achieve full health for the remainder of their lives. Using the standard gamble, patients' utility or quality of life is determined by the choices they make as the probabilities of immediate death or full health are varied. The standard gamble has the advantage of fulfilling the fundamental axioms of utility theory as developed by von Neumann and Morgenstern (12). A more simple and more widely used technique is the time trade-off in which subjects are asked about the number of years in their present health state they would be willing to trade for a shorter life span in full health (12). A major advantage of utility measurement is its amenability to cost-utility analysis. In cost-utility analysis the cost of an intervention is related to the number of quality-adjusted life-years (QALYs) gained through application of the intervention. For example, it has been estimated (though not on the basis of data from clinical studies in which utilities were measured) that the cost per QALY gained is $4,500 for neonatal intensive care for 1,000 to 1,499 gram neonates and $54,000 for hospital hemodialysis (both figures in 1983 dollars) (12). Such comparisons provide a basis for allocation of scarce resources among health-care programs. Results from the utility approach may thus be of particular interest to program evaluators and health-policy decision makers.

Utility measurement also has limitations. Utilities can vary depending on how they are obtained, raising questions of the validity of any single measurement (29,30). Differences between scores obtained from standard gamble versus time trade-off methods are, however, seldom dramatic. Utilities do not allow the investigator to determine what aspects of quality of life are responsible for changes in utility. On the other hand, subjects provide a holistic rating taking both treatment and side effects into account. Finally, utilities at least potentially share the disadvantage of health profiles in that they may not be responsive to small, but still clinically important, changes.

However, utility measurement has proved responsive in at least two randomized clinical studies. Using the Quality of Well-Being Scale, Toevs, Kaplan, and Atkins showed that a program designed to improve compliance with an exercise program in chronic airflow limitation could improve quality of life. The cost-utility analysis showed that the cost of the program was $24,256 for each additional well-year (or QALY) gained (3). In a double-blind, randomized study of auranofin versus placebo in rheumatoid arthritis, both the Quality of Well-Being Scale and a measure based on both the time trade-off and standard gamble technique proved highly responsive (indeed, more so than traditional measures such as the number of tender or swollen joints) (31). This latter study allowed direct comparison between various measures of quality of life, and thus provides a model for the sort of study which will allow determination of the optimal methods for measuring quality of life in clinical studies.

Specific Instruments

An alternative approach to quality of life measurement is to focus on aspects of health status that are specific to the area of primary interest (18). The rationale for this approach lies in the increased responsiveness that may result from including only important aspects of quality of life which are relevant to the patients being studied. The instrument may even focus on problems that are specific to the individual patient (32).

The instrument may be specific to the disease (instruments for chronic lung disease, or for rheumatoid arthritis); specific to a population of patients (instruments designed to measure the quality of life of the frail elderly, who are afflicted with a wide variety of different diseases); specific to a certain function (questionnaires that examine emotional or sexual function); or they may be specific to a given condition or problem (such as pain) which may be caused by a variety of underlying pathologies. Within a single condition, the questionnaire may differ depending on the intervention. For example, whereas success of a disease modifying agent in rheumatoid arthritis should result in improved quality of life by enabling a patient to increase performance of physically stressful activities of daily living, occupational therapy may achieve improved quality of life by encouraging family members to take over activities formerly accomplished with difficulty by the patient. Appropriate disease-specific quality of life outcome measures should reflect this difference.

In addition to the likelihood of improved responsiveness, specific measures have the advantage of relating closely to areas routinely explored by the physician. For example, a disease-specific measure of quality of life in chronic lung disease focuses on dyspnea in day-to-day activities, fatigue, and areas of emotional dysfunction including frustration and impatience (32). Specific measures may therefore appear clinically sensible to the physician.

Disease-specific measures have been developed for many conditions, including cardiovascular disease (33), chronic lung disease (32,34), arthritis (35,36), and cancer (37,38). Specific instruments can be constructed to reflect the "single state" (how tired have you been: very tired, somewhat tired, full of energy) or a "transition" (how has your tiredness been: better, the same, worse) (39). Morbidity, including events such as recurrent myocardial infarction, can be integrated into specific measures (33). One may use disease-specific instruments for discriminative purposes: for example, determining the extent to which a primary symptom (dyspnea, for example) is related to the magnitude of physiological abnormality (for example, exercise capacity) (40). Disease-specific instruments can be applied for evaluative purposes to establish the impact of an intervention on a specific area of dysfunction and hence aid in elucidating the mechanisms of drug action (41).

Disease-specific instruments have proved useful in clinical studies (2,32,33). Guidelines for constructing specific measures are available (18,39, Chapter 5).

The disadvantages of specific measures are that they are (deliberately) not comprehensive, and cannot be used to compare across conditions or, at times, even across programs. Determining whether specific measures increase responsiveness and clinical credibility sufficient to warrant their use will require head-to-head comparisons of different approaches in the setting of randomized controlled studies (31).

Use of Multiple Quality of Life Measures in Clinical Studies

Clinical investigators are not restricted to using a single instrument in their studies. Much remains to be learned about optimal ways of measuring quality of life, and investigators may wish to see how different instruments perform. Aside from this sort of inquiry (which focuses on the instruments, rather than the intervention), an investigator may conclude that a single instrument will not yield all the relevant information. For example, utility and disease-specific measures contribute different sorts of data, and an investigator may want to use one of each.

Another, somewhat different way of using multiple instruments is to administer a battery of specific instruments. One example of a clinical study in which a battery of instruments was used to measure multiple aspects of quality of life was a double-blind, randomized trial of three antihypertensive agents in primary hypertension (42). The investigators identified five dimensions of health they were measuring: the sense of well-being and satisfaction with life, the physical state, the emotional state, intellectual functioning, the ability to perform in social roles, and the degree of satisfaction from those roles. Even within these five dimensions, additional components were identified. For example, separate measurements of sleep and sexual function were made. Patients taking one of the three drugs under investigation, captopril, scored better on measures of general well-being, work performance, and life satisfaction. The lesson for the clinician is clearly important: one can have an impact on not only the length, but also the quality of the patient's life according to the choice of antihypertensive agent.

This approach, although comprehensive, has limitations. First, investigators must find a valid, responsive instrument for every attribute they wish to measure. Second, it is possible (indeed likely) that only some of the instruments chosen will show differences between the treatments under investigation. Unless one of the instruments is designated as the primary measure of outcome before the study starts, different results in different measures may make interpretation difficult. The greater the number of instruments used, the greater the probability that one or more will favor one treatment or the other, even if the treatments' true effectiveness is identical. Thus, the alpha error (the probability of finding an apparent difference between treatments when in fact their outcomes do not differ) increases with each new instrument used. Although this problem may be dealt with through statistical adjustment for the number of instruments used, such adjustment is seldom made (43).

If only a small proportion of the instruments used favor an intervention (or if some measures favor the experimental treatment and other instruments favor the control), the clinician may be unsure how to interpret the results. For example, in a controlled study in which patients with recent myocardial infarction were randomized to receive standard care, an exercise program, or a counseling program, Mayou and colleagues (44) rated many variables. These included work (change in physical activity, satisfaction, and time of return), leisure (change in physical activity and satisfaction, intensity, and exercise for health), marriage (change in protectiveness, discussion, and family), sex (change in frequency and satisfaction), satisfaction with outcome, compliance with advice, quality of leisure and work, psychiatric symptoms, cardiac symptoms, and general health. For almost all of these variables, there was no difference between the three groups. However, patients were more satisfied with exercise than with the other two regimens, families in the advice group were less protective, and the advice group had a greater number of work hours and frequency of sexual intercourse at follow-up after 18 months. We agree with Mayou's interpretation of the results: the study did *not* support the effectiveness of rehabilitation in improving quality of life. However, program advocates might argue that if even some of the ratings favored treatment, the intervention is worthwhile. The use of multiple instruments opens the door to such potential controversy.

A third problem sometimes found in the battery approach arises if only one component or dimension of an instrument is used. The validity of using only one section of an instrument is questionable.

A final limitation of using a battery of instruments is that it gives no indication of the relative importance of various areas of dysfunction to the patient. For example, had Croog et al. (42) found that one antihypertensive agent disturbed sleep whereas another had an adverse impact on sexual function, their approach would not have allowed determination of which drug had a greater net adverse impact on patients' lives.

CONCLUSIONS

Choosing the appropriate approach to the use of a quality of life measure will determine the accuracy and validity of the conclusions obtained. Defining the precise goal of the study and determining the relative merits of existing instruments should be done before questionnaires are chosen. A large number of "proven" instruments which may fulfill investigators' goals exist, and the guidelines for construction of new, specific instruments are available.

REFERENCES

1. Bergner M. Measurement of health status. *Med Care* 1985;23:696–704.
2. Guyatt GH, Townsend M, Pugsley SO, et al. Bronchodilators in chronic airflow limitation, effects on airway function, exercise capacity and quality of life. *Am Rev Respir Dis* 1987;135:1069–1074.
3. Toevs CD, Kaplan RM, Atkins CJ. The costs and effects of behaviourial programs in chronic obstructive pulmonary disease. *Med Care* 1984;22:1088–1100.
4. Deyo RA, Diehl AK, Rosenthal M. How many days of bed rest for acute low back pain? A randomized clinical trial. *N Engl J Med* 1986;315:1064–1070.
5. Prigatano GP, Wright EC, Levin D. Quality of life and its predictors in patients with mild hypoxemia and chronic obstructive pulmonary disease. *Arch Intern Med* 1984;144:1613–1619.
6. Guyatt GH, Townsend M, Berman LB, Pugsley SO. Quality of life in patients with chronic airflow limitation. *Br J Dis Chest* 1987;81:45–54.
7. Nelson E, Conger B, Douglass R, et al. Functional health status levels of primary care patients. *JAMA* 1983;249:3331–3338.
8. Siegrist J. Impaired quality of life as a risk factor in cardiovascular disease. *J Chron Dis* 1987;40:571–578.
9. Fletcher AE, Hunt BM, Bulpitt CJ. Evaluation of quality of life in clinical trials of cardiovascular disease. *J Chron Dis* 1987;40:557–566.
10. Kaplan RM. *Quality of life measurement: Measurement strategies in health psychology.* 1985;115–146.
11. Kaplan RM, Bush JW. Health-related quality of life measurement for evaluation research and policy analysis. *Health Psychol* 1982;1:61–80.
12. Torrance GW. Measurement of health state utilities for economic appraisal. *J Health Econom* 1986;5:1–30.

13. Spitzer WO. State of science 1986: Quality of life and functional status as target variables for research. *J Chron Dis* 1987;40:465–471.
14. Deyo RA. Measuring functional outcomes in therapeutic trials for chronic disease. *Controlled Clin Trials* 1984;5:223–240.
15. Hathaway S, McKinley C. *Minnesota multiphasic personality inventory*. New York Psychological Corporation, 1951.
16. Kaplan RM, Bush JW, Berry CC. Health status: Types of validity and the index of well-being. *Health Serv Res* 1976;11:478–507.
17. Kirshner B, Guyatt GH. A methodologic framework for assessing health indices. *J Chron Dis* 1985;38:27–36.
18. Guyatt GH, Bombardier C, Tugwell PX. Measuring disease-specific quality of life in clinical trials. *CMAJ* 1986;134:889–895.
19. Guyatt GH, Walter S, Norman G. Measuring change over time: Assessing the usefulness of evaluative instruments. *J Chron Dis* 1987;40:171–178.
20. Bergner M, Bobbitt RA, Carter WB, Gilson BS. The Sickness Impact Profile: Development and final revision of a health status measure. *Med Care* 1981;19:787–805.
21. Ott CR, Sivarajan ES, Newton KM, et al. A controlled randomized study of early cardiac rehabilitation: The Sickness Impact Profile as an assessment tool. *Heart Lung* 1983;12:162–170.
22. Liang MH, Larson MG, Cullen KE, Schwartz JA. Comparative measurement efficiency and sensitivity of five health status instruments for arthritis research. *Arthritis Rheum* 1985;28:542–547.
23. Hunt SM, McKenna SP, McEwen J, Backett EM, Williams J, Papp E. A quantitative approach to perceived health status: A validation study. *J Epidemiol Comm Health* 1980;34:281–286.
24. Sackett DL, Chambers LW, MacPherson AS, Goldsmith CH, McAuley RG. The development and application of indices of health: General methods and a summary of results. *AJPH* 1977;67:423–428.
25. Ware JE, Brook RH, Davies-Avery A, et al. *Conceptualization and measurement of health for adults in the health insurance study*: Volume 1, *Model of health and methodology*. Santa Monica, CA: Rand Corporation, May 1980.
26. MacKenzie CR, Charlson ME, Digioia D, Kelley K. Can the Sickness Impact Profile measure change? An example of scale assessment. *J Chron Dis* 1986;39:429–438.
27. Deyo RA, Centor RM. Assessing the responsiveness of functional scales to clinical change: An analogy to diagnostic test performance. *J Chron Dis* 1986;39:897–906.
28. Sugarbaker PH, Barofsky I, Rosenberg SA, Gianola FJ. Quality of life assessment of patients in extremity sarcoma clinical trials. *Surgery* 1982;91:17–23.
29. Sutherland HJ, Dunn V, Boyd NF. Measurement of values for states of health with linear analog scales. *Med Decis Making* 1983;3:477–487.
30. Llewellyn-Thomas H, Sutherland HJ, Tibshirani R, et al. The measurement of patients' values in medicine. *Med Decis Making* 1982;2:449–462.
31. Bombardier C, Ware J, Russel IJ. Auranofin therapy and quality of life in patients with rheumatoid arthritis; Results of a multicenter trial. *Am J Med* 1986;81:565–578.
32. Guyatt GH, Berman LB, Townsend M, Pugsley SO, Chambers LW. A measure of quality of life for clinical trials in chronic lung disease. *Thorax* 1987;42:773–778.
33. Olsson G, Lubsen J, Van Es G, Rehnqvist N. Quality of life after myocardial infarction: Effect of long term metoprolol on mortality and morbidity. *Br Med J* 1986;292:1491–1493.
34. Mahler DA, Weinberg DH, Wells CK, Feinstein AR. The Measurement of dyspnea. Contents, interobserver agreement, and physiologic correlates of two new clinical indexes. *Chest* 1984;85:751–758.
35. Meenan RF, Anderson JJ, Kazis LE, et al. Outcome assessment in clinical trials. *Arthritis Rheum* 1984;27:1344–1352.
36. Fries JF, Spitz P, Kraines RG, Holman HR. Measurement of patient outcome in arthritis. *Arthritis Rheum* 1980;23:137–145.
37. Spitzer WO, Dobson AJ, Hall J, et al. Measuring the quality of life of cancer patients. *J Chron Dis* 1981;34:585–597.
38. Schipper H, Clinch J, McMurray A, Levitt M. Measuring the quality of life of cancer patients: The functional living index—Cancer: Development and validation. *J Clin Oncol* 1984;2:472–483.
39. MacKenzie CR, Charlson ME. Standards for the use of ordinal scales in clinical trials. *Br Med J* 1986;292:40–43.
40. Mahler DA, Rosiello RA, Harver A, Lentine T, McGovern JF, Daubenspeck JA. Comparison of clinical dyspnea ratings and psychophysical measurements of respiratory sensation in obstructive airway disease. *Am Rev Respir Dis* 1987;135:1229–1233.
41. Jaeschke R, Guyatt GH, Singer J. Using quality of life measures to elucidate mechanisms of drug action (*submitted*).
42. Croog SH, Levine S, Testa MA, et al. The effects of antihypertensive therapy on the quality of life. *N Engl J Med* 1986;314:1657–1664.
43. Pocock SJ, Hughes MD, Lee RJ. Statistical problems in the reporting of clinical trials. *N Engl J Med* 1987;317:426–432.
44. Mayou R, MacMahon D, Seight P, Florencio MJ. Early rehabilitation after myocardial infarction. *Lancet* 1981;2:1399–1401.

Quality of Life Assessments in Clinical Trials, edited by B. Spilker. Raven Press, Ltd. New York © 1990.

5

How to Develop and Validate a New Quality of Life Instrument

*Roman Jaeschke
and †Gordon H. Guyatt

†Department of Clinical Epidemiology and Biostatistics, and * Department
of Internal Medicine, McMaster University Health Sciences Centre,
Hamilton, Ontario L8N 3Z5, Canada

Despite the existence of a variety of quality of life instruments, there are instances where investigators wish to develop and validate new measures. Given that we have a profusion of well-validated generic health profiles(including the Sickness Impact Profile, the Nottingham Health Profile, the McMaster Health Index Questionnaire, and the Duke-UNC Health Profile [1–3]), and utility measures (including time trade-off, standard gamble, and the Quality of Well-Being Scale [4–7]), a compelling case must be made to justify the development of new general measures. If a specific instrument is required, questionnaires are available for patients with cancer (8–10), heart disease (11), joint diseases (12–15), and chronic lung disease (16). However, there are a wide variety of conditions for which specific instruments have not been developed, and investigators working in these unexplored areas may, for a number of reasons, require a quality of life measure.

Because adequate generic instruments are available, this chapter focuses on instruments that are specific to a disease, population, function, or particular problem (see Chapter 4). Our goal is to present a methodological framework for the development and assessment of quality of life measures. A conceptual approach to the instrument construction and validation is first described; in the second part of the chapter some specific issues are further developed.

Instruments used in clinical practice and research have three basic purposes: to discriminate among individuals along a continuum of health, illness, or disability; to predict outcome or prognosis; and to evaluate within-person change over time. Thus, the potential applications of quality of life measures can be divided into three broad categories: discrimination, prediction, and evaluation (17).

PURPOSE-SPECIFIC INSTRUMENT: IMPLICATIONS FOR THE
DEVELOPMENT OF AN INDEX

The requirements for optimizing one of the functions—discrimination, prediction, or evaluation—may actually impede the others. As a result, constructing and validating an index for one of these purposes does not necessarily insure that it can be used for the remaining ones.

The following steps are involved in constructing an index or questionnaire to evaluate quality of life:

1. Select the item pool
2. Reduce the number of items
3. Choose response options
4. Determine reproducibility
5. Determine validity
6. Determine responsiveness

A summary of the major issues in construction of an index for each of these steps is listed according to the purpose of the instrument in Table 1. In the following discussion, some of the points which are summarized in Table 1 will be highlighted. Because a gold standard or criterion measure (that is, an instrument that provides a definitive or universally accepted standard) for measurement of quality of life is seldom, if ever, available, we will focus on discriminative and evaluative criteria.

Item Selection and Item Reduction

When constructing a questionnaire, the first task is to collect a set of items that might plausibly be included in the final instrument. Items should be performed by virtually all subjects in order to discriminate among patients. For example, if one wishes to assess functional recovery after myocardial infarction, jogging will not be a particularly useful item if as many as 50% of the population did not jog before their myocardial infarction. On the other hand, if patients who previously jogged regularly consider it important to resume this activity, it may be crucial for an investigator wishing to examine the impact of a drug for post-myocardial infarction patients to include the item in a quality of life measure.

The number of items established in the first step must generally be reduced to a smaller number to improve the efficiency of the index. If the entire instrument is designed to discriminate among people, each individual question must have this discriminative ability. Therefore, questions to which most or all respondents give similar or identical answers are of no use. An evaluative instrument, on the other hand, must identify and delete items that are not responsive to change with an effective intervention. In both cases, pretesting may be necessary for optimal item reduction. An investigator interested in discriminating among subjects could administer the questionnaire to subjects at one point in time and delete items to which only a portion of the subjects provided adequate responses, or which were answered in a uniform manner by most subjects. An investigator developing an evaluative instrument could administer the questionnaire before and after an intervention of known effectiveness and delete items that failed to demonstrate adequate change.

Reproducibility

In much of the health measurement literature the words reproducibility, reliability, and precision are used synonymously. Reproducibility can be measured by the serial administration of a test to a group of subjects believed to be stable. However, dif-

TABLE 1. *Major issues in index construction and validation*

	Discriminative criteria	Predictive criteria	Evaluative criteria
Item selection	Tap important components of the domain Universal applicability to respondents Stability over time	Statistical association with criterion measure	Tap areas related to change in health status Responsiveness to clinically significant change
Item scaling	Short response sets that facilitate uniform interpretation	Response sets that maximize correlations with the criterion measure	Response sets with sufficient gradations to register change
Item reduction	Internal scaling or consistency Comprehensiveness and reduction of random error vs. respondent burden	Power to predict vs. respondent burden	Resonsiveness vs. respondent burden
Reliability	Large and stable intersubject variation: correlation between replicate measures	Stable inter- and intrasubject variation: chance corrected agreement between replicate measures	Stable intrasubject variation: insignificant variation between replicate measures
Validity	Cross-sectional construct validity relationship between index and external measures at a single point in time	Criterion validity: agreement with criterion measure	Longitudinal construct validity: relationship between changes in index and external measures over time
Responsiveness	Not relevant	Not relevant	Power of the test to detect a clinically important difference

TABLE 2. *Measuring change over time*

Instrument A	Time 1	Time 2	Intervention	Time 3	Difference score	Exercise test result
Subject 1	8	9		15	+6	Much improved
Subject 2	9	8		15	+7	Much improved
Subject 3	8	9		15	+6	Much improved
Subject 4	9	8		15	+7	Much improved
Subject 5	8	9		8	−1	Unchanged
Subject 6	9	8		9	+1	Unchanged
Subject 7	8	9		8	−1	Unchanged
Subject 8	9	8		9	+1	Unchanged

Instrument B	Time 1	Time 2	Intervention	Time 3	Difference score	Exercise test result
Subject 1	5	5		5	0	Much improved
Subject 2	9	9		9	0	Much improved
Subject 3	13	13		13	0	Much improved
Subject 4	17	17		17	0	Much improved
Subject 5	5	5		5	0	Unchanged
Subject 6	9	9		9	0	Unchanged
Subject 7	13	13		13	0	Unchanged
Subject 8	17	17		17	0	Unchanged

ferent aspects of reproducibility are relevant for discriminative and evaluative instruments.

To discriminate among subjects, the difference observed between individuals must be reproducible over two or more points in time. The reproducibility of a discriminative instrument is directly proportional to the magnitude of the variation or variance between subjects, and inversely proportional to the variability within subjects. Reproducibility can be quantitated by a Pearson's correlation coefficient. For an evaluative instrument, the only requirement is that replicate measurements on each individual remain stable over time, that is, the magnitude of the within-person variance is small. Small changes in the within-person variation may result in a low Pearson's correlation coefficient. This would not impair the usefulness of an evaluative instrument, provided this degree of within-person variation remained insignificant from both a statistical and a clinical standpoint.

To illustrate this point consider Table 2, which presents hypothetical data from repeated administration to stable subjects of two quality of life instruments and subsequent administration of the same instruments after intervention (18). Both questionnaires yield a single score on a scale from 0 to 20. Prior to using these instruments in a clinical study, an investigator decides to measure their reliability. He selects a group of eight patients, and administers both tests to them at time 1, obtaining results shown in Table 2. One can see already that it is unlikely that instrument A will be able to discriminate among subjects according to the underlying functional status. This does not trouble our investigator, who is only interested in measuring within-subject change over time. To test the instrument reliability, he recalls the eight subjects 1 week later and asks them to once again complete both questionnaires. The results are shown in the second column of Table 2.

Using the results, our scientist calculates the intraclass correlation coefficients for both questionnaires. Instrument A yields an intraclass correlation coefficient of 0, instrument B of 1. If he followed conventional wisdom, the investigator would toss out instrument A at this point, and proceed with confidence using instrument B. But let us assume he is a stubborn chap, and goes ahead with his clinical study using both questionnaires as measures of outcome. In addition, he applies a third measure, exercise capacity, as an additional outcome variable. His patients are randomized, half receiving active treatment and half placebo, and then are followed over time.

When the experiment is completed, the scientist breaks the code and finds that subjects 1 through 4 were randomized to active treatment and subjects 5 through 8 to placebo. He is delighted to discover that dramatic improvement in exercise capacity has occurred in subjects exposed to the experimental treatment. The questionnaire results intrigue him. Although questionnaire B appears to show no difference as a result of treatment, questionnaire A indicates a statistically significant difference between treatment and control groups that is consistent with the results of exercise testing. Our investigator concludes that instrument B is not a useful measure of functional status in patients with chronic lung disease. Instrument A, despite apparently atrocious reliability, turns out to be well suited for the purpose for which is was designed.

What has gone wrong? With conventional use of the correlation coefficient, reliability depends on a magnitude of the variance attributable to between-subjects' differences. For instrument B, this was extremely large, for instrument A, zero. However, because the investigator was able to use change scores to measure outcome, the size of the between-subject difference was not relevant to the usefulness of the questionnaires.

In order to be useful, a discriminative index must have a large and stable between-subject variation. For evaluative indexes, small within-subject variance in stable subjects and a large change in score when functional status improves or deteriorates are the factors of importance (18).

Validity

Criterion validity refers to the extent to which a measuring instrument produces the same results as a gold standard, or criterion measure, and thus is applicable only to predictive instruments. The main method for establishing that discriminative or evaluative instruments are measuring what they are supposed to measure (that is, that they are valid) is called construct validity. Construct validity is concerned with the extent to which a particular measure relates to other measures in a manner consistent with theoretical hypotheses concerning the concepts (or constructs) being measured. To demonstrate the construct validity of a discriminative quality of life instrument for patients with heart failure, an investigator may want to show that patients with poorer exercise capacity at formal exercise testing score lower in aspects of the new index that relate to physical function, and that global ratings of quality of life by the patient, relatives, and health workers bear a close relation to the results of the new index.

For an evaluative instrument measuring quality of life in patients with heart failure, an investigator may want to use the same physiological and global rating methods to validate the index, but between-subject differences at a single point in time would not be examined. Rather, it would be important to show that with an intervention, longitudinal within-subject changes in index scores bear the expected relation to changes in the other variables measured.

Responsiveness

Although demonstration of reproducibility and validity is sufficient to conclude that an instrument is useful for discriminative purposes, an evaluative instrument's responsiveness must be assessed before it can be used confidently as an outcome measure in a clinical study. The issue of responsiveness concerns the power of the index to detect a difference when one is present, and has direct implications for the sample size needed in studies using the instrument as a primary measure of outcome (18).

DEVELOPING DISEASE-SPECIFIC MEASURES OF QUALITY OF LIFE

It is clear from the previous discussion that an investigator organizing a clinical study of a new intervention would choose an instrument meeting evaluative criteria for measurement of quality of life. The investigator may find that an adequate disease-specific instrument is not available. Under these circumstances, a new questionnaire must be constructed. The following discussion expands on the principles outlined above, and describes an approach to the development of disease-specific quality of life measures.

Item Selection

Items selected for a disease-specific quality of life measure must be important to patients with the condition or illness, and should be derived from patients' statements about how the illness affects their lives. One could inquire about areas of physical and emotional dysfunction, inconvenience, and limitation. A problem with such direct questioning is that patients spontaneously recall only a small proportion of their total areas of dysfunction, and much of what is omitted is important. Therefore, one must provide a comprehensive series of probes that cover all possible areas of dysfunction to insure all important items are included. The nature of these probes depends on the level of detail required: questions can be general (chest pain with activity), more specific (chest pain with household chores), or even focused on specific activities (chest pain while cutting the lawn).

Probes must be gathered from a number of sources. These generally include the specific literature on the problems encountered by patients in the area under investigation, the general quality of life measurement literature, suggestions of clinicians (including physicians and nurse specialists) with experience in the area under investigation, and the experience of particularly articulate and/or disabled patients.

Item Reduction

Including all possible items gathered from a search in the final questionnaire would probably be neither efficient nor feasible. Therefore, criteria are needed to reduce the number of items to a questionnaire that can be readily administered (e.g., 10 to

20 minutes). The Item Selection Questionnaire which contains all possible areas of dysfunction generated from the initial search should be administered to patients representative of those who will be included in the subsequent clinical study. Patients are initially asked to volunteer problems resulting from their illness. If the volunteered items are not already part of the Item Selection Questionnaire, new items are added. When all spontaneous items have been elicited, respondents are asked each of the items on the questionnaire not already mentioned. Finally, they are asked to rate the importance of each problem item using a five-point Likert scale (extremely important, quite important, moderately important, somewhat important, not very important).

The frequency of each item is identified as a problem and the importance attached to each item clearly reflects the significance of that item to patients and constitutes appropriate criteria for retaining items in the final questionnaire. However, there are many ways in which the frequency and importance criteria can be combined. Although a number of more sophisticated alternatives such as factor analysis or principle component analysis are favored by some investigators, a simple and reasonable approach is to multiply the frequency of each item by its mean importance. This frequency-importance product is one criterion for item reduction. Another criterion is the potential responsiveness of the items to the drug which is going to be tested. If an item is unlikely to improve with the drug, there is no point in including it in the final questionnaire.

Questionnaire Format

If the questionnaire content overlaps with that established instruments, wording can be borrowed from these measures. For content areas with no overlap, guides are available for constructing questions (19).

Response options refer to the categories or scales that are available for responding to questionnaire items. For example, one can ask whether the subject has difficulty climbing stairs; two response options, yes and no, are available. If the questionnaire asks about the degree of difficulty, a wide variety of response options are available.

To insure questionnaire responsiveness, one must be able to detect small changes on each item if these changes occur. Asking about the presence or absence of difficulty climbing stairs (limiting the subject to two response options) is inappropriate; it would not detect the effect of an intervention that reduced, but did not eliminate difficulty climbing stairs. More suitable response options include visual analog scales (lines, usually 100 mm in length, anchored by the extremes of the item being measured, on which subjects make a mark representing their status), or Likert scales with multiple options (e.g., excellent, good, moderate, poor, very poor). Both methods have their proponents, but evidence for a rational choice between them is not available. Available data suggest that selection of a visual analog scale or a Likert scale with 7 to 10 response options is reasonable. The choice of a five-point Likert scale in the item reduction process is presented as a rough estimate of the relative importance of the items, but is not for constructing an instrument responsive to small, clinically important differences.

In the traditional approach to questionnaire administration, previous answers are unavailable to study subjects on the grounds that bias (for example, a tendency to repeat the same score even if change has occurred) is avoided. However, showing subjects their previous responses has been shown to decrease variability in stable subjects without attenuating changes in the questionnaire score associated with response to treatment (20). Thus, we believe that evaluative questionnaires should be administered with previous responses available to subjects.

Reproducibility and Responsiveness

We previously outlined why a traditional method of assessing instrument reliability, the correlation coefficient, is inappropriate for evaluative instruments. The usefulness of an evaluative instrument depends on its responsiveness, that is, its ability to detect clinically important changes even if these changes are small. Instrument responsiveness is proportional to the change in score that constitutes a clinically important difference (this can be considered the "signal" the instrument is trying to detect). It is inversely proportional to the variability in score in stable subjects (this can be thought of as "noise" that makes the signal difficult to detect). The ratio of the minimal clinically important difference (or, if unavailable, of the change produced by a treatment of known benefit) to the within-subject variability in stable patients is directly related to sample size requirements and can be used as an index of an instrument's responsiveness (18).

Ideally, two separate studies should generate the data needed to determine instrument responsiveness, the first examining the variability in stable subjects and the other examining whether the questionnaire score changes when real change has taken place. In the study designed to examine variability in stable subjects, a questionnaire is administered repeatedly to a group of subjects fulfilling eligibility criteria for the planned clinical study who are deemed stable by other criteria. The interval between administrations, the total number of administrations, and the interval between first and final administration should duplicate what is planned for the clinical study in which the instrument will be used. The data from this study should yield an estimate of the variability in stable subjects.

In the second study, designed to evaluate whether questionnaire score changes when real change occurs, the instrument is administered to subjects before and after application of an intervention of known efficacy. Either the same sample or a new group of patients can be used, but all should fulfill eligibility criteria for the subsequent study. Ideally, the instrument will not only demonstrate improvement in quality of life, but the improvement will be large in relation to the variability among stable subjects. When there is no convenient therapy of known benefit, the situation becomes more difficult; one solution is to administer the questionnaire serially to subjects in whom spontaneous improvement or deterioration is anticipated.

The ratio between the change seen in subjects in the second study to the variability in stable subjects seen in the first study provides an estimate of instrument responsiveness. The larger the differences in questionnaire score in subjects who really change (the signal), the greater the responsiveness; the larger the differences in questionnaire score in really stable subjects (noise), the less the responsiveness.

In the above discussion the nominator and denominator of the sensitivity equation were derived from two different studies on two different populations. It may be argued that another way of assessing responsiveness is to take the changeability and variability component from the same group of treated subjects. This approach should be more conservative, as the variability observed in the treatment response will have two components. One relates to the variability of a given variable under stable conditions. The other relates to the variability of the treatment effect. The combination of these two components should result in increased variability comparing to any single one (unless intervention decreases or removes variability observed in a steady-state; this is quite unlikely). Again, the ratio of the change produced by a treatment of known benefit to the between-subject variability in the change of score among the same group is directly related to sample size requirements and can be used as an index of an instrument's responsiveness.

Validity

As outlined previously, because evaluative instruments primarily measure change, construct validity must be established by examining correlations between change in the instrument under study versus changes in other variables. The process of validation is far stronger if investigators predict how the instrument will behave (if it really measures what it is supposed to measure) prior to collecting the data. For example, one might expect substantial correlations between changes in score on the new disease-specific instrument and changes in score on previously validated methods, such as the time trade-off and Quality of Well-Being Scale. Much lower correlations might be expected between, for example, changes in exercise capacity and changes in emotional function. These relations can be examined if other measures are applied, along with the new questionnaire, in the reproducibility and responsiveness studies.

PRACTICAL ISSUES FOR THE INVESTIGATOR

Although these recommendations describe an ideal approach, they will rarely be achieved in every detail. Having used the appropriate techniques to develop an instrument, an investigator may want to embark on a clinical study without initially establishing the reproducibility, responsiveness, or validity of a new instrument. The justification for this approach is a practical one: full elucidation of the properties of the questionnaire may result in unacceptable delay in commencing the study.

A solution to this dilemma is to use results of the study to examine the properties of the instrument. For example, results from study patients who remain stable by other criteria (such as global ratings of physical and emotional function) can be compared to results of those who improve or deteriorate by these same criteria. If a variety of other measures are applied to the patients along with the new measure, the results of the study can also be used to validate the instrument. Such validation may be important for convincing government agencies of the scientific credibility of the results.

Entering the clinical study without prior demonstration of responsiveness or validity does have dangers. For example, if no effect of the intervention is found, two interpretations remain: either the intervention did not work, or the instrument was insufficiently responsive to detect a treatment effect that was, in fact, present. This problem emphasizes the desirability of demonstrating instrument responsiveness prior to commencing studies of treatment effectiveness.

Another crucial issue is the quality of questionnaire administration. Avoiding systematic bias and random error in questionnaire administration may be even more important than choosing the best questionnaire. Workshops for training research staff in questionnaire administration are vital. These workshops need to be given a high profile, and the importance of optimal questionnaire administration must be stressed. Monitoring research staff performance following the training is also necessary if high-quality data collection is to be insured. One strategy is to require research staff to tape all interviewers. A random sample of these interviews can then be reviewed centrally, and research staff provided with feedback. Development of computerized administration holds promise as a method for avoiding the inconsistencies in administration associated with traditional self-administered questionnaires.

CONCLUSIONS

Different purposes for quality of life instruments dictate different approaches to instrument construction and testing. The approach to construction of disease-specific evaluative instruments for clinical studies can be used for a wide variety of chronic diseases. If scientifically rigorous approaches to questionnaire development, selection, and administration are used, the results will be valid and credible to government agencies and the scientific community.

REFERENCES

1. Bergner M, Bobbitt RA, Carter WB, Gilson BS. The Sickness Impact Profile: Development and final revision of a health status measure. *Med Care* 1981;19:787–805.
2. Hunt SM, McKenna SP, McEwen J, Backett EM, Williams J, Papp E. A quantitative approach to perceived health status: A validation study. *J Epidemiol Comm Health* 1980;34:281–286.
3. Sackett DL, Chambers LW, MacPherson AS, Goldsmith CH, McAuley RG. The development and application of indices of health: General methods and a summary of results. *AJPH* 1977;67:423–428.
4. Kaplan RM. Quality of life measurement. In: Karoly P, ed. *Measurement strategies in health psychology.* New York: Wiley-Interscience, 1985:115–146.
5. Kaplan RM, Bush JW. Health-related quality of life measurement for evaluation research and policy analysis. *Health Psychol* 1982;1:61–80.
6. Kaplan RM, Bush JW, Berry CC. Health status: Types of validity and the index of well-being. *Health Serv Res* 1976;11:478–507.
7. Torrance GW. Measurement of health state utilities for economic appraisal. *J Health Economics* 1986;5:1–30.
8. Spitzer WO, Dobson AJ, Hall J, et al. Measuring the quality of life of cancer patients. *J Chron Dis* 1981;34:585–597.
9. Preistman TJ, Baum M. Evaluation of quality of life in patients receiving treatment for advanced breast cancer. *Lancet* 1976;1:899–901.
10. Mor V, Laliberte L, Morris JN, et al. The Karnofsky performance status scale: An examination of its reliability and validity in a research setting. *Cancer* 1984;53:2002–2007.
11. Goldman L, Hashimoto D, Cook EF. Comparative reproducibility and validity of systems for assessing cardiovascular functional class: Advantages of a new specific activity scale. *Circulation* 1981;64:1227–1234.
12. Fries JF, Spitz PW, Young DY. The dimensions of health outcomes: The health assessment questionnaire, disability and pain scales. *J Rheumatol* 1982;5:789–793.
13. Meenan RF. The AIMS approach to health care measurement: Conceptual background and measurement properties. *J Rheumatol* 1982;5:794–797.
14. Helewa A, Goldsmith CH, Smythe HA, et al. Independent measurement of functional capacity in rheumatoid arthritis. *J Rheumatol* 1982;5:794–797.
15. Tugwell P, Bombardier C, Buchanan W, et al. The ability of the Mactar disability questionnaire to detect sensitivity to change in rheumatoid arthritis (abstr). *Clin Res* 1983;31:239.
16. Guyatt GH, Berman LB, Townsend M, Pugsley SO, Chambers LW. A measure of quality of life for clinical trials in chronic lung disease. *Thorax* 1987;42:773–778.

17. Kirshner B, Guyatt GH. A methodologic framework for assessing health indices. *J Chron Dis* 1985;38:27–36.
18. Guyatt G, Walter S, Norman G. Measuring change over time: Assessing the usefulness of evaluative instruments. *J Chron Dis* 1987;40:171–178.
19. Sudman S, Bradburn NM. *Asking questions: A practical guide to questionnaire design.* San Francisco: Jossey-Bass, 1982.
20. Guyatt GH, Berman LB, Townsend M, Taylor DW. Should study subjects see their previous responses? *J Chron Dis* 1985;38:1003–1007.

II

Standard Scales, Tests, and Approaches to Quality of Life Assessments

Quality of Life Assessments in Clinical Trials, edited by B. Spilker. Raven Press, Ltd. New York © 1990.

6

Economic Scales and Tests

*Henry G. Grabowski and †Ronald W. Hansen

*Department of Economics, Duke University, Durham, North Carolina 27706; †Simon Graduate School of Business Administration, University of Rochester, Rochester, New York 14627

Just as medical decision-makers must assess the merits of alternative therapeutic modalities, economists assess the merits of alternative allocations of resources. Health care decisions involve changes in both health outcomes and allocations of resources. It should not be surprising that there are areas of health care in which the decision process is of interest to and affected by both medical professionals and economists. The development of quality of life indices and their application is one area of mutual concern. This chapter focuses on those indices which are linked to economic concerns even though their application does not necessarily require economic training.

To place the economic measures of quality of life assessments in perspective, one should consider the types of issues which are of concern to economists. Generally economists are concerned with the allocation of resources to alternative ends or objectives. Resources are broadly defined to include not only natural resources, but also a wide variety of factors involved in the production of goods and services such as labor, capital equipment, knowledge, skills, and locational advantages. The objectives may be stated in terms of the production of goods and services but they ultimately involve the satisfaction of individual wants and desires.

When considering the production of goods and services, economists are often concerned with the efficiency of the production process, i.e., what is the least costly way of producing a given product or service? Economists also study consumer decision-making, frequently considering how individuals select varying combinations of goods and services to maximize their well-being. These two areas can be combined to address the question of how to allocate resources to the production of the set of goods and services that maximize consumer well-being or utility.

Although economists frequently use the terms "utility," "individual well-being," or "satisfaction," there is no consensus on how to measure these domains. We can often identify changes that increase or decrease individual satisfaction, but attempts to quantify the level of satisfaction is fraught with problems. Moreover, even if one is satisfied with a scale for a particular individual, it is not feasible to make interpersonal comparisons of utility. The question, "Has John reached a higher level of utility or satisfaction than Harry?" is not answerable from the perspective of normative economic theory.

Individuals can increase their utility by exchanging goods and services in the marketplace at prices expressed in monetary units such as dollars. We can compare individuals' income or wealth in dollar terms, and increases or decreases in income or wealth can be translated into increases or decreases in the utility levels achievable by individuals. Even though the ultimate objective may be expressed as improving the well-being of individuals, dollar values are used for the analytical purpose of assessing programs.

Wherever possible, economists tend to measure goods and services in common dollar units. However, this is difficult to do for many health-related issues since there is no explicit market for states of health. One cannot directly buy relief from pain or elimination of heart disease; one can only purchase medical services or products which may cure or alleviate health problems. Given the absence of market prices, economists have devised various methods to value health states. We will consider three such measures and describe how they can be incorporated into clinical trials.

One should note a caveat that applies to many quality of life measures. For the purposes of many evaluations one is concerned with aggregate or average values, thus the empirical basis for estimation is a representative sample. However, when the question involves choices for a specific individual, in most instances the preferences and values of that individual should be given greater weight. Clearly, the basis for establishing values must be consistent with their eventual use.[1]

PRODUCTIVITY OR HUMAN CAPITAL MODELS

The two major financial costs of disease are treatment costs and the loss in productivity during the course of the disease or subsequent disability. The productivity effects of death and disability have been incorporated in cost-benefit studies of health programs and in a variety of projects affecting public safety such as highway improvements and flood control projects.[2] In some applications, market-based productivity changes have been the sole measure of the value of programs affecting death and disability.

One way of viewing this approach is to consider it as valuing individuals only for their productivity, much as one might value investment in industrial equipment. Loss of human capital, whether in the form of death or diminished capacity, reduces the ability of the economy to produce, much like the destruction or impairment of capital equipment. However, such a narrow valuation of humans does not accord with values expressed in other contexts. Most defenders of the measure do not argue that productivity is the only measure of the value placed on changes in an individual's well-being. They will generally claim that it is an important portion of the value and that it should be adjusted to reflect other less well-defined and measured values. Although "quality of life" certainly implies more than lost workplace activity, work remains one of the major human activities, and the impact of disease on work will be reflected in other aspects of an individual's life condition. Loss in income may seriously impact the other dimensions of life, including effects on one's family.

---

[1] Where resources are provided through public sources and trade-offs are involved in their application to alternative programs, the issue of how to value the preferences of different individuals with stakes in the decision process must be explicitly faced by the decision maker (9).

[2] A review undertaken by the Office of Technology Assessment (10) provides numerous examples of such approaches in the health area.

A practical reason for the reliance on lost productivity or human capital approaches is the ease with which these changes in human conditions can be translated into dollar values for inclusion in cost-benefit studies. Their status is further enhanced by their use in civil court cases as the basis for the economic losses suffered in death and disability cases. Despite the theoretical shortcomings, they are often an acceptable measure that can be an important component of cost-benefit analyses tied to clinical trials.

The methodology for calculating lost productivity is at once both straightforward and potentially complex. The complexity is a function of the disease/disability and the occupation of the individual. Some very simple cases will be examined here, then complexities will be introduced.

The easiest case to consider is an acute illness which before its appearance has no effect on the patient's ability to perform his occupational activities. At a definable point the disease incidence begins, therapy is administered, and following a recuperation period the patient is restored to his/her predisease state with no subsequent impact on the ability to perform occupational activities. In this event all the productivity effects are measurable within the period from disease onset to recovery.

When examining lost productivity, one should be careful to separate productivity from salary and wages. One of the basic premises of microeconomics is that in a well-functioning labor market, the employer pays the worker an amount that equals his/her marginal productivity. Hence the compensation of the employee equals the value of the employee's productivity. Compensation includes more than gross salary since the employer typically provides vacation pay, retirement (including employer's social security contribution), and health and disability insurance. Thus, should an individual be unable to work, the lost productivity is the full compensation, not just the net wage received by the employee.

Sick pay is often provided by employers, and the income actually lost by the employee during the illness may be minimal. If one is concerned only with the employee perspective, then the effect of illness on income will be reduced or possibly eliminated by sick pay or disability compensation. From a broader perspective, however, there is a loss equal to the employee's reduced productivity. If the employer is self-insured for sick pay or disability, then the lack of productivity, although not representing an income loss to the employee, will be a direct loss to the employer. Insurance merely affects the distribution of the loss.[3]

In the simple case just constructed, information should be obtained on the extent of work loss over the duration of the illness and recovery period. Since the ability to return to work may be occupationally related, occupational information should be obtained. To translate the work days lost into a measure of lost productivity, one requires an estimate of daily compensation, i.e., wages plus benefits.

It may be possible to obtain wage information from the individuals in a clinical trial, but this poses several problems. First is the issue of data confidentiality. Most individuals are reluctant to share specific information about their income and if participation in the clinical trials is voluntary, mandatory salary information may deter some individuals from participating. Second, if the objective of the economic portion of the study is to measure the impact on a general population, then the use

---

[3] However, if the availability of insurance causes the worker to remain away from work beyond the period of full recovery, this is a productivity loss due to adverse insurance incentive effects. It is inappropriate to include this in the lost productivity associated with the illness, although these effects may be difficult to separate in actual practice.

of age and occupationally adjusted national average compensation information may be preferable. By using the income information from the study participants, one is in effect estimating general income levels from a sample which is small compared to other bases for income estimation.

The estimation process becomes more complex if the disease has produced a long-term impact on the individual's productivity. Individuals with the particular disability may be working at less than full normal capacity and may not be restored to full health. If one is analyzing two different treatments, in addition to determining work days lost, one needs to assess the level of productivity. For example, an individual whose normal occupation requires great manual dexterity may, as a result of arthritis, seek employment in an occupation requiring less dexterity. They may be fully employed but at a job which is less productive than the one for which they were originally trained, or the individual may remain in the same occupation but be less productive. Measuring days of work lost will not capture these reductions in productivity. The methods for measuring lost productivity through job switching will depend on the manner in which one expects the loss to manifest itself. The researcher may be required to collect information on job history with particular emphasis on job changes occasioned by the disease.

Many individuals are not members of the market labor force but are nevertheless productive in household or other activities. This producitivity may also be impaired by disease or disability and the value of this lost productivity should be calculated. Since there is no specific market wage, alternative methods for valuing this productivity must be used. Since many of these activities are replicated in the marketplace, researchers have valued them by utilizing the rates charged for cleaning services, meal preparation, child care, etc. The average daily economic value of homemaker services is comparable to the average marketplace compensation for females according to some recent studies.[4] During the clinical investigation, information on the change in activities should be obtained and then later analyzed to see how sensitive the evaluation of the program is to variations in the methods of valuing time in nonmarket activities.

In collecting activity data, one may be able to specify particular days during which individuals not in the market labor force are unable to perform their normal activities. What is often the case, however, is that these individuals continue with some but not all of their daily activities. For example, the housewife may continue to perform some of her activities but the remainder are either postponed, performed by other family members, or hired out. An analysis of the extent of lost productivity requires follow-up interviews.

For productivity effects that occur over lengthy periods of time, it is appropriate to adjust future values by a "discount rate." This reflects the time preference of individuals for present over future economic benefits, as well as the fact that economic resources can be productively invested for future gains. These factors provide the basis for a positive rate of interest in market economies. Although discounting is employed in economic analyses involving multiple time periods, no general consensus exists as to the specific discount or market interest rate that should be employed in cost-benefit analysis of health programs (1). In the absence of consen-

---

[4] See the analysis of homemaker time valuation by the Institute of Life Insurance (11). Further information on the allocation of time to homemaker services and their valuation in the market is provided in references (12), (13), and (14).

sus, many researchers use a range of plausible values and then perform a sensitivity analysis on how the discount rate parameter influences the results. Sensitivity analyses are appropriately employed for all parameters subject to uncertainty and measurement error.[5]

The productivity or human capital approach to valuing the effect of disease on the quality of life admittedly captures only a portion of the effect on quality of life. It measures health and quality of life as though they are a unit of production, not something of intrinsic value. By its construction it values the health of high earners more than of low wage earners, a feature which many find objectionable. This may have program implications since some diseases are more prevalent among individuals in their high income working years, whereas other conditions are more prevalent among individuals who have retired from the labor force.

Despite these shortcomings, productivity effects may prove to be a useful proxy for quality of life effects in certain circumstances. For example, productivity may be useful when one is focusing on a homogenous group of patients and where job market performance is an important component of well-being. Furthermore, it is often easier to collect data on this measure than on some of the theoretically preferable alternatives discussed below. For these reasons, the human capital model has gained a fair degree of usage in the benefit-cost studies as well as in the tort litigation process.

THE WILLINGNESS TO PAY CONCEPT

In assessing the value of goods and services to individuals, economists often employ the concept of willingness to pay. The act of market exchange is an expression of the willingness of individuals to give up some goods or services in exchange for other goods and services. In most instances money acts as a medium of exchange, breaking the direct link between items sold and items purchased in exchange.

To assess the value of different health states or quality of life, it is natural to determine the values in the manner in which the marketplace determines other values, i.e., by the willingness to pay for improved health or quality of life. As noted earlier there are no explicit markets for health, so one must uncover ways to calculate willingness to pay. The approaches taken can be divided into questionnaire-based and revealed preference-based methods.

Questionnaire-Based Models

Questionnaire-based willingness to pay approaches basically attempt to have the respondent estimate the value placed on different health states or quality of life. Designing a willingness to pay survey demands considerations similar to those of other survey research, including the quality of life measures discussed in greater detail in other chapters. One must be concerned with validity and reliability as well as ease of administration (2–4). The questions may ask for direct responses for the

---

[5] One special group worth noting in this context is the case of children. For this group, the human capital approach focuses on how the economic present value of expected lifetime earnings is affected by long-term illness or disability. Given the long term horizons and the greater uncertainty involving these economic calculations, a sensitivity analysis with respect to the discount factor and other economic parameters is generally undertaken as an integral part of the analysis.

items to be valued, use some forms of paired comparisons, or seek to value the specific attributes of the item or state, and aggregate to produce a value for the total. Specific issues arising when dollar values are involved in a health survey should be addressed.

In most instances the survey questions elicit a response for willingness to pay for an improvement or to prevent a worsening of health status. In such instances respondents' evaluations will be affected by their income or assets. In other words, we should expect on average that wealthy individuals will be willing to pay a larger dollar amount for a given improvement than will a poor individual (though the percentage of income or wealth may be similar). Thus the willingness to pay approach, like the human capital productivity approach, is also influenced by an individual's income.

An alternative formulation reverses the question to ask how large a payment would be required for the individual to willingly accept a reduction in health state or to forego an improvement. Since the response is not bounded by the individual's current assets, the values are likely to be larger and there is a presumption that there would be less of an income effect, though it is probably not eliminated.

A problem in many questionnaire-based measures is that the opinions are being solicited about hypothetical situations which may be far removed from the experience of the respondent. A healthy individual may have great difficulty imagining how his life would change were he partially paralyzed and hence have a hard time assessing his willingness to pay to avoid this condition. If the payment is hypothetical, i.e., he will not be charged based on his answer, his answer may be quite different than if he actually has to pay. There is also a problem of the respondent's giving an answer which he thinks the interviewer wants, particularly in personal interview situations using hypothetical payments.

In evaluating disease states in a clinical situation, the respondents have either experienced the health states being evaluated or have given more thought to the potential impact of these states. However, there is another source of bias produced by their status as a patient. They may believe that their answers to the questions may affect the amount they have to pay or the type of therapy they receive. Care should be taken in the study design to minimize these potential sources of bias.

The standard gamble approach has been employed to construct health indices (5). As explained in Chapter 7, this approach confronts the respondent with a choice between a certain event and a gamble that will result in either a better or worse state than the certain event. By determining the probability level at which individuals are indifferent between the gamble and the certain state, the relative value assigned to each state can be estimated. Many of the supporters of this approach see the development of a utility index in nonmonetary terms as a principal advantage. However, it is a disadvantage that one cannot then directly compare benefits and costs.

By including a dollar value as part of one of the health states, it is possible to translate the gamble approach into estimated dollar values for death or disease risks. For example, one can choose between perfect health or a gamble which, if won, results in $10,000 plus retained perfect health and, if lost, results in partial paralysis. The probability of winning which makes the respondent indifferent between accepting the gamble or the certainty of perfect health can be used to construct the respondent's assessment of the cost of paralysis. The rationale for this opinion-based method is similar to the revealed preference model discussed below.

Revealed Preference Models

One of the difficulties with opinion-based willingness to pay models is that they usually measure what individuals state they would be willing to pay rather than what individuals do in fact pay. Several attempts have been made to develop willingness to pay measures based on actual behavior affecting health or quality of life. However, since there is not a direct market for health, this must be inferred from other actions.

Individuals make many decisions that involve risks of death and/or disability. These decisions include job choice, purchase of safety equipment, recreational activities, and diet. In these decisions they trade off potential changes in health states for other attributes such as income or pleasure. By observing the choices people make which involve risk of death or disability, one may be able to calculate the value individuals place on their health. The basic premise behind revealed preference-based models is that the observed choices reflect the individual's relative valuation of health and other attributes, given the expected outcome probabilities.

There are many variations of revealed preference-based models but most are based on the following. An individual chooses between two activities, A and B, which differ in two dimensions, income (or some surrogate) and risk of death or disability. Individuals who accept the higher risk activity have revealed a willingness to face a higher probability of death/disability in return for an increase in income. For example, these individuals may choose an activity which exposes them to a 1 in 1,000 higher probability of death but offers a $2,000 higher income. These individuals value the 1 in 1,000 risk of death at a maximum value of $2,000. In some studies, linearity is assumed such that the implied "value of life" is $2 million.

Studies of this nature are relatively recent but have sparked a lot of controversy. Some assert that it is wrong for individuals to place a monetary value on their lives or health. One could argue on ethical grounds the merits of this position, but the empirical observations suggest that people do in fact risk life and limb for other objectives, including monetary rewards. A somewhat more neutral phrasing recognizes that death appears to be inevitable and that the question is one of changing the time of death rather than saving a life in perpetuity. Whereas most of the original work in this area was expressed as valuing a life, more recent work has focused on valuing a life-year (6,7).[6]

Even among individuals who are willing to accept the basic design of these studies, there are questions about the validity of the results. One source of concern is the extent to which the choices are being made by fully informed individuals. Are the probabilities of death or disabilities known to the individuals making the choice? To the extent that individuals act on incorrect estimates but the researcher uses true probabilities, the empirical estimates will be in error. For many occupations this difference may be substantial, however for others the risks may be well-known. Those who accept risky jobs (e.g., coal mining) may also have a constrained choice set due to both limited mobility and limited information.

There is some evidence that individuals have difficulty dealing with low probability, high value events (8). The difference between a 1 in a million and a 1 in 10 million chance is a 10 to 1 ratio, but both may be essentially zero to the average

---

[6] One of the interesting by-products from recent analyses of the value of a life-year is that they provide evidence on the implicit discount rate that individuals use in making life cycle decisions. For example, this revealed discount rate was found to be between 10 and 12% in the Moore-Viscusi analysis (7).

individual. Yet the risk faced in some occupations on a weekly or monthly basis are of this order of magnitude. Individuals, particularly healthy persons, may be myopic in dealing with questions concerning their own death.[7] The "it won't happen to me" phenomenon calls into question the rational choice-making assumptions of these revealed preference models.

The existing revealed preference studies for valuing life-years or quality of life have produced a relatively wide range of estimates.[8] These studies have also focused much more on mortality than on injury or morbidity effects. It is probably too soon to use the results of a single study as the definitive estimate. However, despite the criticism of the existing risk assessment/revealed preference models, they are a promising line of research. Most studies have been conducted using labor force data and the results are often intended to be used as inputs to assessments involving death and disease outcomes. These existing estimates may be used to value therapeutic choices, but the clinical setting offers some interesting possibilities for extending this research. Choices that individuals make regarding their own therapy in the face of different estimated outcomes can be used to derive relative values. Whether these can be expressed in dollar terms depends on the nature of the choices available.

SUMMARY

The productivity/human capital approach has been the most frequently employed of the economic models used in quality of life assessments in clinical studies. Data on the work activities of the patients can be gathered to assess the lost productivity in a variety of disease and treatment combinations. The major problem with this measure is that it does not address quality of life per se, but rather the ability to perform workplace activities.

Willingness to pay models have the virtue (or vice) of attempting to value changes in health states or quality of life from the same perspective used to determine individual values for other goods and services. The methods for obtaining willingness to pay estimates are problematic. Opinion-based estimates suffer from several potential sources of bias. Revealed preference models treat individuals as though they make well-informed choices in decisions involving risk of death and disability. This assumption may be far from the truth in some of the situations studied. These models have been developed relatively recently and with further work may produce very valuable results. Not only may they provide values to use in assessing clinical outcomes, but it may be possible to construct clinical trials which will advance our understanding of individuals' willingness to pay for changes in quality of life.

---

[7] The low utilization rate for automobile seat belts, despite their high potential for effectiveness in preventing many potential deaths and serious injuries, can be explained in part on such grounds (15).

[8] For a review of recent studies, see the analysis by Viscusi and Moore (16). One major reason for the difference in estimated values across studies is the different sample populations employed. Those studies that focus on more risky occupations generally have found lower values of life. This reflects a self-selection process in job market choice. In particular, individuals who choose jobs with above average risks generally have a greater preference for assuming risk in exchange for monetary compensation. Hence estimates based on their behavior cannot be utilized as representative of the general population without some adjustments.

REFERENCES

1. Warner KE, Luce BR. *Cost benefit effectiveness analysis in health care*. Ann Arbor, Michigan: Health Administration Press, 1982.
2. Kaplan RM, Bush JW, Berry C. Health status: Types of validity and the index of well-being. *Health Serv Res* 1976;11:478–507.
3. Brooks RG. *The development and construction of health status measures: An overview of the literature*. Lund: The Swedish Institute for Health Economics, 1986.
4. Read JL, Quinn RJ, Hoefer MA. Measuring overall health: An evaluation of three important approaches. In: Lohr KN, Ware JE, Jr., eds. *Advances in health assessment conference proceedings, J Chronic Dis, Special Issue,* 1987;40(Suppl. 1):7S–21S.
5. Torrance GW, Measurement of health state utilities for economic appraisal: A review. *J Health Econom* 1986;5:1–30.
6. Thaler R, Rosen S, The value of saving a life: Evidence from the labor market. In: Terleckyj NE, ed. *Household Production and Consumption*. New York: National Bureau of Economic Research, 1976;265–302.
7. Moore MJ, Viscusi WK. The quantity adjusted value of life. *Economic Inquiry* 1988;26:369–388.
8. Kunreuther H. Limited knowledge and insurance protection. *Public Policy* 1976;24:229–261.
9. Williams A. Measuring quality of life. In: Teeling Smith GS, ed. *Health economics: Prospects for the future*. London:Office of Health Economics, 1987;200–210.
10. Office of Technology Assessment of the U.S. Congress. *The implications of cost-effectiveness analyses of medical technology, background paper 1. Methodological issues and literature review*. Washington, D.C.: Government Printing Office, 1980.
11. Institute of Life Insurance. *Do you know what a homemaker is worth?* 1978.
12. Gauger WH, Walker KE. *The dollar value of household work*, Information Bulletin 60. Ithaca, NY:Cornell University, 1980.
13. Mushkin SJ, Landefeld JS. *Non-health sector costs of illness*, report A7. Washington, D.C.:Public Services Laboratory, Georgetown University, 1980.
14. Juster FT, Stafford FP. *Time goods and well being*. Ann Arbor, Michigan:University of Michigan, 1985.
15. Arnould RJ, Grabowski HG. Auto safety regulation: An analysis of market failure. *Bell J Econom* 1981;12:27–48.
16. Viscusi WK, Moore M. *Compensation mechanisms for job risks: Wages workers' compensation and product liability*, Princeton University Press, 1990.

Quality of Life Assessments in Clinical
Trials, edited by B. Spilker. Raven
Press, Ltd. New York © 1990.

7

Integrating Economic Evaluations and Quality of Life Assessments

David Feeny, Roberta Labelle, and
George W. Torrance

*Department of Clinical Epidemiology and Biostatistics, Centre for Health
Economics and Policy Analysis, McMaster University, Hamilton, Ontario,
L8N 3Z5 Canada*

The essence of economic evaluation is a comparison of the costs and consequences of different health care programs. There are a variety of meaningful ways to measure consequences. During the past two decades quality of life measures have been developed which provide a new and relevant approach to assessing the consequences of the use of health care resources.

The strategies and implications of combining traditional methods of economic evaluation with the newer techniques for quality of life assessment are examined here.[1] The major forms of economic evaluation are briefly described; a taxonomy for quality of life assessment measures is presented, then practical and conceptual considerations of combining these methods are discussed. Finally, the advantages and disadvantages of incorporating economic and quality of life outcome measures concurrently in clinical trials are briefly considered.

MAJOR STUDY DESIGNS FOR ECONOMIC EVALUATION OF HEALTH CARE SERVICES

Economic evaluation relies on the estimation of the dollar costs of providing alternative forms of health care services, such as surgical versus medical therapy for the same condition or one drug regimen versus another. The dollar (or pecuniary in economists' jargon) costs include direct costs (items such as professional fees, drugs, hospitalization, diagnostic tests) and indirect costs (earnings of patient forgone as a result of treatment). The basic study designs for three major forms of economic evaluation are summarized in Table 1. In each case the costs of treatment are compared to the outcomes of treatment. In cost-effectiveness analysis, outcomes are measured in natural units of clinical effects. These units are typically the ones employed in clinical studies. They may be as narrow as millimeters of mercury for reductions in blood pressure or as broad as life-years gained for reductions in mor-

---

[1] For a review of the methods of economic evaluation, see Chapter 6 by Grabowski and Hansen. The issues discussed in this paper are also considered in works by Feeny (1) and Feeny and Torrance (2).

TABLE 1. *Major study designs for economic evaluations*

Type of analysis	Compares	To
Cost-effectiveness	$ Value of resources used up	Clinical effects produced
Cost-utility	$ Value of resources used up	Quality of life produced by the clinical effects
Cost-benefit	$ Value of resources used up	$ Value of resources saved or created

Based on Drummond et al., ref. 8.

tality. The key feature of the cost-effectiveness analysis design is that the analyst need not assign a dollar value to the outcome. The analyst can also continue to rely on standard clinical measures.

In cost-utility analysis, the measure of clinical effects is adjusted to reflect the quality of life of the outcome. In this approach, life-years are converted into quality-adjusted life-years (methods for estimating the quality adjustment will be discussed below). As in cost-effectiveness analysis, the analyst is not required to place a dollar value on the outcome. Unlike that approach, however, cost-utility analysis does explicitly incorporate quality of life information in the results.

In cost-benefit analysis, costs and consequences are all expressed in pecuniary terms. This technique was first applied to the evaluation of public expenditures in water resource development. In the context of health care, however, most analysts have found cost-benefit analysis to be less satisfactory than cost-effectiveness analysis or cost-utility analysis for several reasons. In particular, many analysts are uncomfortable with ethical judgments that appear to accompany assigning dollar values to people's lives and their suffering. The result has been that cost-effectiveness analysis studies have become the dominant study design in health care evaluation.[2]

The focus in the health care evaluation literature on cost-effectiveness analysis has, in concert with the growth in the breadth of outcome measures for clinical studies, shifted toward comparing pecuniary and quality of life outcome measures. The trend reflects several factors. First, as health care interventions are increasingly focused less on reducing mortality and more on reducing morbidity and improving

---

[2] When cost-benefit analysis was first applied to the evaluation of health care services, estimates of the benefits of the delay of premature mortality were obtained by computing the present value of the lifetime earnings of survivors. This was labeled the human-capital approach. It has the advantage of providing a relatively straightforward procedure for estimating the benefits of reductions in mortality. It is not, however, consistent with the economic theory on which cost-benefit analysis is based. Conceptually the proper measure of the benefits of mortality reductions would be the patients' willingness to pay for reductions in their risk of premature mortality. Although some studies have asked respondents this question in hypothetical situations, the method does not appear to provide reliable and valid data for several reasons. First, patients are often poorly informed about the risk and reductions in risk that treatment will produce, therefore their answers are likely to be affected by any of their misperceptions of the clinical information on risks or the effectiveness of treatment. Their answers are also likely to be affected by what they have been told by their health care provider. Second, willingness to pay also depends on income, and like the human-capital approach, is therefore not free of the potential to overrepresent the preferences of the economically advantaged. (Because of this problem, many investigators also collect information on the ability to pay of respondents.) Third, individuals may be motivated to misrepresent their willingness to pay. For example, some may underestimate the value because of a concern that at a later date they may be expected to actually pay. Others may overstate their willingness in order to influence the priority assigned to their condition. These and other difficulties with inferring preferences from willingness to pay led some investigators to attempt to measure preferences directly, and in turn led to the development of cost-utility analysis.

quality of life, it has become more important to measure these outcomes directly and accurately. Second, clinical managers and third-party payers have become increasingly interested in the evaluation of new and existing treatment alternatives and have demanded evidence on costs and effects both in pecuniary and nonpecuniary terms.

TAXONOMY OF QUALITY OF LIFE MEASURES

A wide variety of quality of life measures have emerged. Such a diversity is both inevitable and appropriate since quality of life is a broad, multidimensional concept. Different measures may tap different domains of quality of life. Investigators also have a variety of objectives and thus may require a battery of instruments for different questions and situations. In the discussion that follows the focus is on the measurement of health-related quality of life. A variety of other factors including socioeconomic status also influence overall quality of life. In the context of clinical studies, however, the implicit assumption is that these other factors may be ignored for the purpose of comparing the quality of life impact among alternative treatments, thus justifying the development of instruments focused on health-related quality of life.

There are a number of ways to classify quality to life measures. One classification scheme is presented in Table 2 (see also Chapter 5). Specific instruments are developed for application in particular clinical situations. Typically these measures are tailored to the quality of life burden of the disease (or health problem) and its treatment. By including only those elements that are most important in the specific clinical situation, these measures can be constructed to include a wide range of effects (such as physical function, emotional function, and characteristics that are of special concern to individual patients) without imposing a large burden on respondents. These measures usually have also been constructed to maximize their responsiveness to change. A good example of a specific instrument is the Chronic Respiratory Disease Questionnaire developed by Guyatt (3).

Generic instruments are applicable across diverse populations. These measures typically span a number of dimensions of health-related quality of life, including physical function, social and emotional function, pain, self-care, and other activities. It is useful to distinguish at least two major subcategories of generic instruments: health profiles and utility measures. Health profiles provide separate scores for a number of categories or dimensions of health status or quality of life. The profile may or may not allow for aggregation into a single summary score. The Sickness

TABLE 2. *Taxonomy of quality of life assessment measures*

Category	Examples
I. Specific instruments	Chronic respiratory questionnaire
	Arthritis categorical scale
	Arthritis impact measurement set
II. Generic instruments	
A. Health profiles	Sickness impact profile
	General health rating index, RAND
B. Utility measures	Standard gamble
	Time trade-off

From Guyatt et al., ref. 16, with permission.

Impact Profile (4) is a good example of a health profile measure which allows for a single summary score.

Utility measures share some characteristics with health profiles and specific instruments. Like health profiles, utility measures are widely applicable. Utility instruments give scores on a very generalizable 0 (death) to 1 (perfect health) scale, thus facilitating broad comparisons of the effects of multiple health care programs. The design of utility measures for specific applications, however, allows the analyst to incorporate, as with specific instruments, items of particular importance or relevance in that setting. Utility instruments also typically include physical function, sensory function, emotional function, cognitive function, pain, and self-care. A good example of the application of utility analysis to the measurement of health-related quality of life is found in the evaluation of neonatal intensive care (5). The approach has also been applied in a major clinical trial designed to investigate the quality of life impact of a new oral gold compound for the treatment of arthritis (6).

The utility approach has an advantage relative to the specific approach in that the patient globally assesses the net effect of the treatment on his/her quality of life. Thus the patient's response summarizes his/her evaluation both of the positive treatment effects and the negative side effects. With specific instruments, these are measured separately and the analyst has little or no information on the patient's trade-offs among the therapeutic improvements and treatment side effects. The same point applies to health-profile instruments for which no single summary score is available.

THE UTILITY MEASUREMENT OF HEALTH STATES

Utility, a concept used in economics and decision analysis, refers to the level of satisfaction or enjoyment experienced by the consumer of the good or service. Because many investigators are unfamiliar with the utility approach to assessing quality of life, a brief review is provided. In general, economists do not attempt to measure utility (the preferences of consumers for various consumption alternatives) directly.[3] In the context of the analysis of behavior in most market settings, preferences may be inferred from the behavior of consumers. As a result, the discipline of economics has a well-developed set of statistical tools for the analysis of data drawn from experience, but a much less extensive set of tools for the direct measurement of utility.

The standard practice of inferring preferences for health states from health care expenditures is flawed for several reasons, however. First, the standard analysis assumes that consumers are well-informed. Thus to make reliable inferences of health-state utilities from the expenditures of consumers, one should be confident that consumers are well aware of the efficacy and effectiveness of the treatment alternatives and their consequences, and are making well-informed choices on the basis of their preferences. Many analysts find this assumption in the context of health care to be highly questionable. Instead it is assumed that consumers seek the advice of an expert, a health care professional, when considering the available health care technologies, their effects, and the best treatment plan for them. Accordingly, the actual expenditures reflect not only the preferences of the patient but the advice of the professional. Second, in most settings (at least within developed countries), patients have access to some form of third-party payment (health insurance) and do

---

[3] The direct measurement of utility is, however, a routine practice in the discipline of decision analysis.

TABLE 3. *Example of health-state description*

Able to see, hear, and speak normally for age.
Requires the help of another person to walk or get around; and requires mechanical equipment.
Occasionally fretful, angry, irritable, anxious, depressed, or suffering "night terrors."
Learns and remembers school work normally for age.
Eats, bathes, dresses, and uses toilet normally for age.
Free of pain and discomfort.
Able to have children with a healthy spouse.

From Feeny et al., ref. 17, with permission.

not bear fully the monetary cost of their treatment. Because of this cost sharing, it is again unlikely that preferences may reliably be inferred from health care expenditures.

These considerations have led some investigators to search for methods for the direct measurement of the utility of various health states. A small family of reliable measurement approaches has been developed.

The practical steps of the approach will be briefly outlined here; more detailed descriptions can be found in works by Torrance (7) and Drummond et al. (8). Typically a number of health-state scenarios are described, perhaps including the patient's subjectively defined current health state. These scenarios cover many dimensions, including physical function, sensory function, cognitive function, emotional well-being, pain, self-care, and any special features of the disease or its treatment (an example is provided in Table 3). Subjects are then asked to rank the health states, often with the assistance of a visual analog scale marked from 0 to 100 known as a feeling thermometer (Fig. 1). Scores on the feeling thermometer give the investigator a firm indication of the ordinal rankings of the health states (various treatment outcomes) and some information on the intensity of those preferences. The feeling thermometer would appear to give interval-scale values, but evidence to date indicates that although it does provide a good indication of ordinal rankings, it does not directly provide cardinal utility scores.

The measurement of cardinal scores for the utility of health states is performed using one of two techniques: standard gamble or time trade-off.[4] In the standard gamble approach, the subject is offered a choice between two alternatives: living in the health state in choice B with certainty or taking a gamble on treatment, choice A, with an uncertain outcome (Fig. 2). The most straightforward approach to measurement is to suggest that treatment A leads to perfect health with probability p and immediate death with probability $(1 - p)$.[5]

---

[4] Utility scores are cardinal in that they possess interval-scale properties. That is, the distance from 0.2 to 0.4 is the same as the distance from 0.4 to 0.6. The scores are not cardinal in the sense of a ratio scale; that is, 0.2 is not twice as good as 0.1. These interval-scale cardinal utilities should not be confused with the ratio-scale cardinal utilities of the utilitarian approach common among nineteenth century economists. For more on this distinction, see Ellsberg.

[5] It is not necessary to offer perfect health and death as the alternatives in choice A for each standard gamble. The standard gamble requires that the health state in choice B be a state that is ranked intermediately; that is, the outcomes in choice A include one state that is better than the one in B and one that is worse. (Clearly it is important that the ordinal rankings of the health states be established before standard gamble questions are posed.) If it is undesirable to offer death as an option in the standard gamble because it upsets respondents or because it is not a relevant outcome in the clinical situation, for instance, another state (one for which the utility score is low) can be substituted for death in choice A. The utility of the state in choice B may then be computed with respect to this state. Its utility in turn is determined separately by performing a standard gamble which includes death, thus providing the information to anchor B on the 0.0 (death) to 1.0 (perfect health) scale.

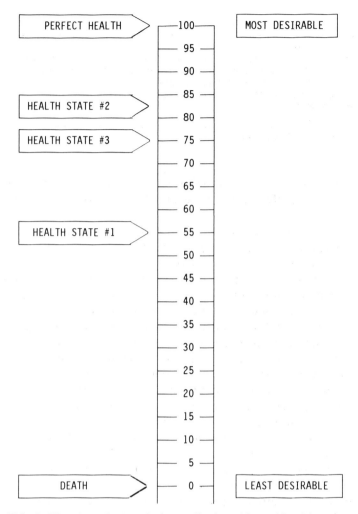

FIG. 1. Visual analog scale for ordinal ranking of health states.

The probability p is then varied until the subject is indifferent between choices A and B. The lower the indifference probability, the greater the risk of death the subject is willing to consider, and thus the lower the utility of the health state described under choice B. The utility scale is defined with 1.0 as perfect health and 0.0 as death.[6]

Because some respondents have had difficulty understanding probabilities, an al-

---

[6] If the standard gamble includes perfect health and death as the outcomes under choice A, and remembering that perfect health = 1.0 and death = 0.0, the indifference probability is then a cardinal score of the utility of the health state in choice B. The indifference means that the expected utility of A equals the expected utility of B. (Expected utility is the utility of an outcome times its probability.) The expected utility of A is p (1.0) + (1 − p) (0.0) which equals p. (In general, if O_1 and O_2 are the outcomes of the lottery, choice A, and O_3 is the sure thing, the outcome in choice B, then the utility of O_3 equals p times the utility of O_1 plus (1 − p) times the utility of O_2.) The standard gamble approach to measuring health state utilities is based directly on the analysis of decision making under uncertainty developed by von Neumann and Morgenstern (10). The axioms upon which von Neumann-Morgenstern functions are based insure that scores have interval-scale properties. These axioms, although closely related to the usual axioms of economic theory, are somewhat more restrictive (see for instance Baumol, and Luce and Raiffa [11, 12]).

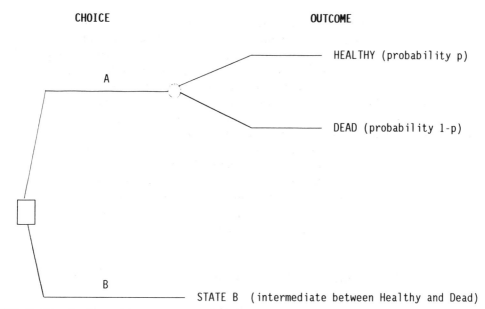

FIG. 2. Standard gamble approach for eliciting utility values. Modified from Torrance, ref. 7, p. 20.

ternative technique, time trade-off, has been developed (Fig. 3). In this technique the subject is offered a choice of living for t years in perfect health or t years in some alternative health state that is less desirable (and the one for which the analyst wants the utility score). Obviously the subject will choose perfect health. The interviewer then reduces the period of perfect health, x, until the subject is indifferent between the shorter period in perfect health and the longer period in the less desirable state. The utility value of that state then equals x/t.[7]

Standard gamble, time trade-off, and variations on these techniques provide reliable and valid methods for eliciting scores for health-state utilities. The prior use

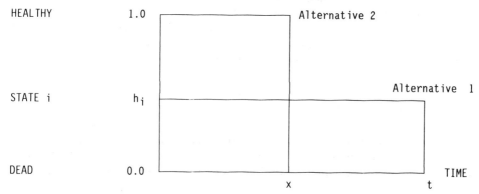

FIG. 3. Time trade-off approach for eliciting utility values. Modified from Torrance, ref. 7, p. 23.

---

[7] Although the scores derived from time trade-off provide a measure of the utility for a health state, they are not identical to those obtained using standard gamble. Conceptually this difference, though not quantitatively large (see Torrance [13]), is expected. In addition to tapping the subject's preferences for

of the feeling thermometer appears to help respondents consider and report their preferences for the health states being evaluated. The health states to be evaluated may include states the respondent has experienced, is now experiencing, or has never experienced (hypothetical states). In this regard, the utility approach differs from other quality of life measures. The utility approach, when it includes hypothetical states, allows the investigator to obtain important information from all patients on how they think they would feel if they experienced some of the infrequent outcomes. Evidence to date shows that evaluations by persons experiencing the state and by others for whom the state is hypothetical usually do not differ substantially (13) and (14). If there is a systematic difference it is that persons experiencing the state rate it marginally higher than those who have not experienced it, but this is not yet conclusive. Thus the quality of life of rare or infrequent outcomes may be assessed along with that of the frequent outcomes by combining actual and hypothetical states in the set of outcomes being evaluated.

COMBINING PECUNIARY AND QUALITY OF LIFE EVAULATIONS

The basic approach in cost-effectiveness analysis is to compare the pecuniary cost of treatment to its outcome, measured in broadly defined (e.g., life-years) or narrowly defined (e.g., kilograms of weight loss) natural units. These comparisons are potentially useful for management decisions for individual patients, clinical departments, hospitals, and systems of health care delivery. (In practice, cost-effectiveness studies are seldom used for individual patient management.)

The choice of outcome measure with which to compare data on cost depends on the objectives of the evaluation exercise. If the focus is on resource allocation among alternatives aimed at the same clinical problem, the outcome measure can be narrow. This approach often has the advantage of clinical sensibility in that health care professionals can readily understand and appreciate how outcomes are measured. Thus a comparison of the cost per kilogram of weight loss among alternative treatment programs is likely to be meaningful to clinicians. Similarly, comparing the cost per change score in a specific quality of life instrument among alternative therapies for the same disorder could be clinically sensible.

Thus, the assessment of alternative drug regimens for the control of chronic respiratory disease could be displayed in terms of a set of cost-effectiveness ratios of dollars per change in the Chronic Respiratory Questionnaire score for each drug regimen. Because the measure of quality of life is specific to a particular disease in this case, the cost-effectiveness ratio would be relevant only for comparisons among alternatives for the treatment of chronic respiratory disease, and would not allow for broader comparison, say at the level of resource allocation among clinical departments or within a health care system. Although the cost-effectiveness ratio using specific instruments as an outcome measure may be meaningful to clinicians, its narrow generalizability limits its usefulness to third-party payers, regulatory officials, and others.

---

the health state and its duration, the standard gamble score also reflects the subject's attitudes toward risk (the subject's risk preferences). Time trade-off scores do not reflect these risk attitudes. Furthermore, the standard gamble technique has the conceptual advantage in that it is based directly on the von Neumann-Morgenstern theory (10) and does not require additional assumptions about the structure of preferences.

Given that specific quality of life instruments have been developed only recently, it is not surprising that few, if any, studies combining dollar cost with these quality of life measures have appeared in the literature. One can speculate, however, that given the increasing popularity of the specific measures, such studies will be forthcoming.

Broader comparisons can be made by combining pecuniary measures with more generalizable or generic health profile measures of quality of life, such as the Sickness Impact Profile and others, that provide for a single global score. Given the wide applicability of these instruments, comparisons of cost-effectiveness of seemingly different programs, measured, for instance, as dollars per change in the Sickness Impact Profile score, could be made. Such comparisons come closer to the broadly formulated cost-effectiveness analysis in which cost per life-year gained is compared among a wide variety of alternative health care programs. The advantage in generalizability may, however, come at a cost of clinical sensibility. Clinicians may not readily understand changes in quality of life as measured on such scales. Thus the results of such a cost-effective evaluation may be useful for clinical managers, hospital administrators, and third-party payers, but they may not be especially meaningful to health care providers. Again, although such cost-effectiveness studies are infrequent in the literature, given the increasing popularity of health-profile measures among investigators, one can expect to see such studies in the future.

The use of specific and health profile measures in cost-effectiveness analysis will not, however, always be appropriate. The meaningfulness of cost-effectiveness analysis depends on comparing costs to a relevant and comprehensive measure of outcome or consequences. For specific and health profile instruments that do not provide a single score, the meaningfulness of cost-effectiveness analyses which utilize such measures is dubious. For instruments for which single summary scores are available, the cost-effectiveness analysis is more meaningful, but may still fall short of the potential available in cost-utility analysis in which mortality and morbidity effects may be combined.

Combining utility measures of quality of life with pecuniary measures of cost converts cost-effectiveness analysis into cost-utility analysis. The outcome is a comparison of the cost to the gain in utility, expressed as quality-adjusted life-years. At the pragmatic level the approach shares the advantages and disadvantages of combining pecuniary and health profile measures; the procedure facilitates broad comparisons but comes at the expense of attenuated clinical sensibility.

At a more fundamental methodological level, however, cost-utility analysis has an important advantage with respect to cost-effectiveness studies which employ health profile or specific quality of life measures. Both the family of economic evaluation approaches and the utility approach to the measurement of health-related quality of life are based on the same underlying economic theory.[8] The assumptions

---

[8] Economic analysis is, in general, based on the assumption that a person's preference ordering may be represented as an ordinal utility function (15). Informally, the axioms required for this type of analysis state that consumers have a complete and transitive ordering of preferences over all possible bundles of goods and services, that within the feasible choice set they will select the bundle that is most preferred by them, and that more is better than less. These axioms allow the analyst to represent preferences as an ordinal utility function and in turn legitimate the interpretation of the pecuniary evaluation of the value of resources used in producing health care services. The von Neumann-Morgenstern utility function approach for decision making under uncertainty (10) expands the set of axioms so that preferences may be represented by a utility function with interval-scale properties. The assumptions underlying these utility functions are therefore consistent with the assumptions underlying standard demand analysis in economic theory, the theory upon which the pecuniary evaluations are based.

TABLE 4. *Comparative cost-utility results for selected programs*

Program[a] [reference]	Reported cost/QALY[b] gained in U.S. dollars (year)	Adjusted[c] cost/QALY[b] gained in U.S. dollars
PKU screening[d] [Bush et al. (1973)]	<0 (1970)	<0
Postpartum anti-D[d] [Torrance and Zipursky (1977)]	<0 (1977)	<0
Antepartum anti-D [Torrance and Zipursky (1984)]	1,220 (1983)	1,220
Coronary artery bypass surgery for left main coronary artery disease [Weinstein (1981)]	3,500 (1981)	4,200
Neonatal intensive care, 1,000–1,499 g [Boyle et al. (1983)]	2,800 (1978)	4,500
T4 (thyroid) screening [Epstein et al. (1981)]	3,600 (1977)	6,300
Treatment of severe hypertension (diastolic ≥ 105 mm Hg) in males age 40 [Stason and Weinstein (1977)]	4,850 (1976)	9,400
Treatment of mild hypertension (diastolic 95–104 mm Hg) in males age 40 [Stason and Weinstein (1977)]	9,880 (1976)	19,100
Estrogen therapy for postmenopausal symptoms in women without a prior hysterectomy [Weinstein (1980)]	18,160 (1979)	27,000
Neonatal intensive care, 500–999 g [Boyle et al. (1983)]	19,600 (1978)	31,800
Coronary artery bypass surgery for single vessel disease with moderately severe angina [Weinstein (1981)]	30,000 (1981)	36,300
School tuberculin testing program [Bush et al. (1972)]	13,000 (1968)	43,700
Continuous ambulatory peritoneal dialysis [Churchill et al. (1984)]	35,100 (1980)	47,100
Hospital hemodialysis [Churchill et al. (1984)]	40,200 (1980)	54,000

[a] These studies use similar, but not identical methods. Generally, costs are net health care costs; however, discount rates and preference weights are not completely consistent. Differences in methods should be considered when comparing the relative cost-utility. For details, see original sources. Table taken from Torrance (1986), ref. 7.

[b] QALY denotes quality-adjusted life-year.

[c] Adjusted to 1983 dollars according to the U.S. Consumer Price Index for Medical Care for all urban consumers. Source: U.S. Bureau of Labor Statistics, Monthly Labor Review.

[d] The cost per QALY gained is negative because the pecuniary benefits of the intervention exceed the pecuniary costs, so that the net benefits are positive, or the net costs are negative.

From Torrance, ref. 7, with permission.

made in both approaches are consistent, and they are explicit. The analyst knows precisely what is being assumed about the structure of human preferences.

Although few studies have combined pecuniary measures with quality of life outcome measures based on the specific or health profile measures, a number of studies have employed cost-utility analysis. The results of several are summarized in Table 4. Given the growing use of cost-utility analysis, it is likely that investigators using this approach will have a broad range of evaluations of health care interventions with which to compare their results. For some purposes, such as influencing third-party payers or regulatory officials, this is potentially an advantage.

It makes sense to combine economic evaluations and quality of life measures in cost-effectiveness and cost-utility studies. Cost estimates summarize important, but incomplete, information on treatment alternatives. Quality of life is frequently the most important outcome. Thus cost-effectiveness ratios which reflect both sets of information provide a more complete assessment of the implications of treatment options. Specific, health profile, and utility measures of health-related quality of life can all be appropriate for use in such cost-effectiveness studies. The utility approach has the advantages of generalizability, the ability to combine mortality and morbidity effects, and inherent compatibility with pecuniary evaluations.

COMBINING PECUNIARY AND QUALITY OF LIFE MEASURES IN CLINICAL TRIALS

If both pecuniary evaluations and quality of life assessments of a particular drug or health care program are considered to be relevant and important, must they be done concurrently? Need they be incorporated in a clinical trial? There are a number of advantages to performing the evaluations together in the context of a prospective and rigorous clinical trial.

First, a quality-of-life measure may be included in a clinical trial because it is a relevant outcome measure. Second, data collected from studies with blinding as to outcome and appropriate baseline measurement are, in general, more reliable and valid. Third, there are important logistical advantages to collecting data on the costs of treatment, especially patient-borne costs, as part of an ongoing clinical study. For instance, the gathering of data on costs can be combined with the periodic administration of quality of life instruments. In the common situations in which recall is unreliable, such prospective data collection can be especially important. Fourth, data on clinical efficacy and/or effectiveness derived from well-designed randomized clinical trials are more reliable and precise. The results of the cost estimates are therefore combined with higher quality data on clinical effects; no matter how precise the cost estimates in an economic evaluation, the results of a cost-effectiveness analysis, cost-utility analysis, or cost-benefit analysis can be no better than clinical data on effectiveness. Finally, by combining clinical, economic, and quality of life investigations into a single study, all of the results are promptly available to affect clinical and health care policy.

These potential advantages are accompanied by disadvantages, however. First, already complex clinical evaluations are made more complex by adding additional measurement instruments. Furthermore, some clinical investigators will have little experience with or understanding of these instruments. Second, if the results of the clinical evaluation indicate that the new drug is not efficacious, the pecuniary evaluation may be redundant. Third, some clinicians who are consumers of such studies will find the pecuniary and quality of life information to be foreign, thus reducing the acceptability of the results. Finally, the generalizability of the results of a pecuniary evaluation conducted within a clinical trial is an important issue. Even management trials are not fully representative of ordinary clinical practice. For instance, trials typically include special compliance-enhancing strategies that increase both the costs of the care being provided and, potentially, the effectiveness of that care. There is no reason to believe that the percent increase in costs and percent increase in effectiveness will be roughly equal so that the cost-effectiveness ratio is left unbiased.

TABLE 5. *The advantages and disadvantages of incorporating economic evaluations and quality-of-life assessments in clinical trials*

A. Advantages
  1. Relevance of quality of life as an outcome measure
  2. Logistical advantages
  3. Quality of data on efficacy and/or effectiveness
  4. Timeliness of comprehensive results

B. Disadvantages
  1. Additional complexity
  2. Potential redundancy
  3. Acceptability of study results
  4. Generalizability of economic evaluations based on data obtained during a trial

Based on Drummond and Stoddart, ref. 15.

The advantages and disadvantages of including quality of life and economic evaluation components in clinical trials will vary with the questions being asked, stage of development of the drug or clinical intervention, and other factors specific to the clinical study. The discussion is summarized in Table 5.[9]

CONCLUSIONS

Pecuniary and quality of life evaluations complement each other by adding important information about the consequences of various health care interventions. Economic evaluation provides a framework for comparing the costs of care to its effects measured in both pecuniary and nonpecuniary terms. Quality of life measures provide crucial information on the outcomes of the clinical intervention. In this way, the use of quality of life assessment conforms to an underlying premise in the health and social sciences that health care is provided to improve the welfare of patients and, indirectly, their families. More traditional pecuniary measures, and the more recently developed quality of life measures, provide a means for quantification of these goals. Such studies provide clinicians with information that is useful in their decisions concerning patient management. The studies also provide third-party payers, regulatory authorities, and others with important information on the costs and consequences of various uses of scarce health care resources, now more comprehensively with the inclusion of quality of life measurement.

The combination of pecuniary, specific, and health profile quality of life measurement is still in its infancy. Although more fully developed, cost-utility analysis is only two decades old. Quality of life measurement is rapidly evolving at the conceptual, methodological, and pragmatic levels. It is very likely, however, that the incorporation of pecuniary measures, quality of life measures, and combinations of the two approaches will become increasingly common. Cost-utility analysis is ideally suited for these purposes.

ACKNOWLEDGMENT

The authors wish to thank William Furlong, Gordon Guyatt, Bert Spilker, and Marie Townsend for helpful comments on an earlier draft of the chapter.

---

[9] For a more detailed discussion of the issues, see Drummond and Stoddard (15).

REFERENCES

1. Feeny D. Can we use quality-of-life measures for economic evaluations? *Quality of Life and Cardiovascular Care* (Winter, 1988) 4, no. 4:185–190.
2. Feeny D, Torrance GW. Incorporating utility-based quality-of-life assessment measures in clinical trials: Two examples. *Med Care* 1989;27, no. 3 (suppl.):S190–S204.
3. Guyatt G, Townsend M, Pugsley SO, Keller JL, Short HD, Taylor DW, Newhouse MT. Bronchodilators in chronic air-flow limitation: Effects on airway function, exercise capacity, and quality of life. *Am Rev Resp Dis* 1987;135:1069–1074.
4. Bergner M, Bobbitt RA, Carter WB, Gilson BS. The Sickness Impact Profile: Development and final revision of a health status measure. *Med Care* 1981;19:787–805.
5. Boyle MH, Torrance GW, Sinclair JC, Horwood SP. Economic evaluation of neonatal intensive care of very low-birthweight infants. *N Engl J Med* 1983;308:1330–1337.
6. Bombardier C, Ware J, Russell IJ, Larson M, Chalmers A, Read JL. Auranofin therapy and quality of life in patients with rheumatoid arthritis: Results of a multicenter trial. *Am J Med* 1986;81:565–578.
7. Torrance GW. Measurement of health state utilities for economic appraisal: A review article. *J Health Econom* 1986;5:1–30.
8. Drummond MF, Stoddart GL, Torrance GW. *Methods for the economic evaluation of health care programmes.* Oxford:Oxford University Press, 1987.
9. Ellsberg D. Classic and current notions of "Measurable utility." *Econ J* 1954;64:528–556.
10. von Neumann J, Morgenstern O. *Theory of games and economic behaviour,* 1st ed., 2nd ed. Princeton, NJ:Princeton University Press, 1944;1947.
11. Baumol WJ. *Economic theory and operations analysis.* New York:W.W. Norton, 1965.
12. Luce RD, Raiffa H. *Games and decisions: Introduction and critical survey.* New York:John Wiley & Sons, 1957.
13. Torrance GW. Social preferences for health states. An empirical evaluation of three measurement techniques. *Socio-Economic Plan Sci* 1976;10:129–136.
14. Wolfson AD, Sinclair AJ, Bombardier C, McGeer A. Preference measurement for functional status in stroke patients: Inter-rater and inter-technique comparisons. In: Kane R, Kane R, eds. *Values and long-term care.* Lexington, Mass. DC Heath, 1982;191–214.
15. Drummond MF, Stoddart GL. Economic analysis and clinical trials. *Controlled Clin Trials* 1984;5:115–128.
16. Guyatt GH, van Zanten SJOV, Feeny D, Patrick D. Measuring quality of life in clinical trials: A taxonomy and review. *Can Med Assoc J* 1989;40:1441–1448.
17. Feeny D, Barr RD, Furlong W, Torrance G, Rosenbaum P, Weitzman S, Horsman J. Economic evaluation of treatment for childhood cancer: Costs, benefits, and the quality of life (*unpublished manuscript*), 1988.

Quality of Life Assessments in Clinical Trials, edited by B. Spilker. Raven Press, Ltd. New York © 1990.

8

Social Interaction Tests and Scales

*Edward Guadagnoli and †Vincent Mor

Department of Community Health; †Center for Gerontology and Health Care Research; Brown University, Providence, Rhode Island 02912

Of the domains selected to represent the concept of quality of life as defined in this book, social interaction or social participation is the least well conceptualized. Our inability to fine-tune its operational definition makes the development of valid, reliable measurement scales a formidable task. The practical use of this concept as a measure of quality of life in clinical trials depends on a definition that encompasses features of an individual's functioning that realistically can be influenced by the medical treatment or intervention under study. Conceptualizations and/or measures that include, for instance, the documentation of one's marital status are not relevant potential outcomes for medical clinical trials. Rarely, if ever, would a change in patients' marital status be an outcome of interest. The proper use of quality of life measures depends on the basic assumption that we expect the intervention under study to differentially influence health-related quality of life across intervention levels. Unfortunately, many potential measures of social interaction suffer from the inclusion of items that are not relevant to the assessment of health status or quality of life and are, therefore, not viable outcomes of interest for assessment of a medical intervention.

In this chapter we attempt to provide a definition for social interaction within the context of health-related quality of life, and we review several scales that might be used to measure or assess this concept. Given the practical considerations of clinical trials research (1), we selected for review brief measures that do not require administration by an expert (e.g., physician, social worker, or psychologist). For each measure selected we identify its underlying construct, if any, the population for which it was developed, and we describe its psychometric properties, scoring, analysis, and interpretation. We do not review single-item measures of social interaction.

SOCIAL INTERACTION

Social interaction is a component of the broader concept, social well-being. Donald and Ware (2) suggest that social well-being comprises social contact (social interaction) and social resource dimensions. Social interaction encompasses the activities of an individual and his/her involvement with others, whereas social resources relate to the resources or reserves available to an individual (2). If we accept this broad definition of social well-being, the concept is not appropriate for use in clinical trials designs since improved social resource availability is not likely to be an intended outcome of a medical intervention. However, an assessment of patients' activities with others and in social situations is a potential outcome of interest.

Few measures have been designed to measure social interaction specifically. This construct is typically included as part of a more comprehensive health status battery (e.g., the Sickness Impact Profile [3]) or as a component of a social health or well-being scale (e.g., the RAND Social Health Battery [2]).

Social interactions occur within several domains: family, social (friends), community, and work. Independent social interaction scales that measure each of these domains are rare. In fact, expectations that social interaction items will cluster statistically by role domain have not been met (2). Typically, a total interaction score comprising responses to items spanning each of these domains is calculated. A problem arises when this approach is used because all individuals may not be able to respond to all items in the overall scale (e.g., items dealing with employment).

Another potential problem in the measurement of social interaction is that individuals' preferences for interaction with others differ. It is a safe assumption that maximum physical or emotional functioning is valued by all individuals, but individuals' preferences for the quantity and quality of social interaction is more variable, making measurement of this concept problematic. Research suggests that the concept of quality of social interactions may not be an independent construct since individuals' responses are highly correlated with measures that assess well-being (2,4,5). The solution typically has been to assess the quantity of social interactions and to operate under the assumption that more social interaction is better. Ware (5) argues that assessment of the quantity of social interactions should be a health outcome measure because society values social functioning.

Social interaction is sometimes confused with the concept of social support. Although social interaction can be a component of social support, the terms are not synonymous. Social support is more broadly defined and is used rarely, if ever, as an outcome measure in research designs. It is "the emotional, instrumental, and financial aid that is obtained from one's social network" (6). The role of social support is postulated as either a buffer effect, providing protection from the negative influences of stress, or as a main effect, enhancing health or well-being without reference to the level of stress (7). In research designs, social support measures are typically independent variables included as potential correlates of physical and mental health indicators.

SOCIAL INTERACTION SCALES AS OUTCOME MEASURES

The use of social interaction instruments as outcome measures in clinical trials research may not be appropriate, even when other components of health-related quality of life are included. The selection of any outcome measure should be dictated by the expectation that the intervention will effect it. Social interaction measures should be included in the design of trials that involve interventions expected to impact one's willingness or ability to deal with others. For example, one might include a social interaction measure in a trial comparing the efficacy of treatments whose aim is to relieve physical deformation (burns, dermatology problems, etc.). In addition to providing physical relief, such treatments are also likely to be judged successful if they are associated with an increase in social activity over the treatment course. Similarly when an intervention's side effects are expected to affect patients' body image, social interaction data may provide the information necessary to choose between two (or more) otherwise efficacious treatments. Often, clinical trial results suggest little or no difference between nonsurgical, antineoplasm therapies. Nonetheless, patients report that side effects such as hair and weight loss affect their willingness to interact socially with others. In addition to direct measures of the side effects themselves, social interaction data can also be a useful indicator of a treatment's utility.

The inclusion of these measures can extend to research designs that do not directly involve medical interventions. For instance, investigators who conducted the Health Insurance Experiment (8) initially included social health as a component of their overall model of health, and therefore assessed social interaction as an outcome measure in their study of the influence of health care financing mechanisms on health status. Other "social experiments" such as the National Hospice Study (9) and the National Long-Term Care Channeling Demonstration (10) have included social interaction as an outcome measure with the assumption that improved community functioning will enhance individuals' physical capacity to deal with others.

TESTS AND SCALES

Once the decision to measure social interaction is made, an instrument must be selected. Given the practical constraints of conducting clinical trials research (1), particularly patient and staff burden, brief instruments are desired. Instruments that require expert raters are typically avoided because of increased time and expense requirements. Furthermore, satisfactory social interaction instruments should contain items that apply to all members of the population under study. Analytic, missing data, and measurement standardization problems arise when all items cannot be answered by all respondents (2). Seven instruments designed to measure social interaction are describe below.

Health Insurance Experiment Social Battery

Following an extensive review of the literature (11), investigators at RAND generated an 11-item social well-being scale for use in the Health Insurance Experiment (8). The RAND Social Health Battery was intended for use with the general population, although for the Health Insurance Experiment, individuals aged 14 to 61 comprised the population of interest. As indicated above, RAND's social well-being model incorporated two dimensions, social interaction and social ties. Their operational definition of social well-being included "interpersonal interactions (e.g., visits with friends) and activities indicative of social participation (e.g., memberships in clubs)" (2, p. 132). All but one of the 11 items dealt with the behavioral aspects of social activity. The remaining item was a subjective evaluation of one's ability to get along with others.

From the original 11-item scale, five items met internal and external consistency criteria established by the investigators for the construction of two multi-item scales. Both of these scales, Social Contacts and Group Participation, relate directly to the concept of social interaction. The Social Contacts scale comprises three items documenting visits with friends or relatives, home visits by friends, and visits to homes of friends. Potential responses are not identical across items. Items are rated along six or seven category ordinal scales. The Group Participation scale comprises two items detailing the number of voluntary group memberships and level of group activity. Based on item analyses, an item-response recoding scheme has been generated for each item. The battery, original item responses, and recoding scheme are included in Donald and Ware (2).

Due to variance differences within each scale, Donald and Ware (2) suggest standardizing items to a mean of zero and a standard deviation of one prior to summing to obtain scale scores. A high Social Contacts score is defined as "home visits by friends two or three times a month or more; visits with friends and relatives and visits to homes of friends once a week or more" (2, p. 106). The absence of visits indicates a low score on this scale. Five or more group memberships and very active group participation indicate high Group Participation, whereas no memberships define a low score.

Both scales appear to be homogenous and consistent. Internal consistency coefficients calculated across all Health Insurance Experiment data collection sites were .72 for the Social Contacts scale and .84 for the Group Participation scale (2). One year stability coefficients for the Social Contacts and Group Participation scales were .55 and .68, respectively (2).

The very low correlation between these measures ($r = .05$) suggests that these scales measure different components of social well-being. Correlations with other health measures, positive well-being, emotional ties, and current health, although statistically significant, were low (.04 to .19). This suggests that these measures are not redundant with other health dimensions. Correlations with functional or physical measures of health, however, were not reported. We expect correlations between functional status measures and social interaction scales to be higher than those reported for well-being, emotional ties, and current health. Finally, Donald and Ware (2) examined the influence of socially desirable response set on each of these scales. Adjusting for socially desirable response set did not result in changes among relationships between the two social interaction scales and other measures of health.

The RAND scale was not developed from data collected from patient samples. However, the Social Contacts scale should be amenable for use by patients. Assuming that measuring frequency of contact is of value to the assessment of the intervention of interest, one can expect variability in patient responses if this measure is used. We feel that measuring Group Participation is less likely to be of use in clinical trials research and suggest employing this scale in the design only if group membership and participation can be linked meaningfully to the goals or effects of the intervention.

The data describing the development and interpretation of these scales are perhaps the most extensive available for any individual scale. We refer the reader to the RAND series, *Conceptualization and Measurement of Health for Adults in the Health Insurance Study,* for further social well-being item- and scale-level descriptions and for similar information on other health component measures.

The Sickness Impact Profile

The Sickness Impact Profile (3) is a behaviorally based measure of health status (3,12). It contains 136 items that deal with 12 areas of dysfunction. The instrument does not appear to be based on a formal model of health. In addition to generating items from a review of the literature, the instrument's developers acquired the original Sickness Impact Profile item pool by asking individuals involved in sickness episodes to generate items. Among the 12 Sickness Impact Profile categories are a 20-item Social Interaction scale (e.g., "I am doing fewer social activities with groups of people") and an 8-item Recreation and Pastimes scale (e.g., "I am going out for entertainment less"). In addition to social activity items, the Social Interaction scale also contains items dealing with the quality of contact with others.

The Sickness Impact Profile was specifically designed as a health care outcome measure. It was "developed to provide a measure of perceived health status that is sensitive enough to detect changes or differences in health status that occur over time or between groups" (3, p. 787). Interview and self-administration have worked well with patients. Mail-administered Sickness Impact Profiles, however, have not yielded data comparable to the other forms of administration (3).

Respondents indicate whether an item describes their status today and is related to their health. Each item endorsed is assigned a standardized weight and items are summed to create scale and total scores. In addition to individual category scores and a total score, Physical and Psychosocial dimension scores can be calculated. The latter scores are not independent of individual category scores. Scores can range from 0 to 100, with higher scores indicating poorer health (13).

Much of the published work describing the final version of the Sickness Impact Profile has not involved discussion of the instrument's individual scales. Earlier studies describing scale level results from prior versions of the Sickness Impact Profile are available, however (12,14). The overall Sickness Impact Profile is reported to be internally consistent (Chronbach's alpha > .90), stable (24-hour reproducibility coefficient ≥ .50), and valid as demonstrated by the results of construct, convergent, and discriminant validity studies with other health status measures. Items comprising each category were confirmed using a cluster analysis procedure (3).

Like the RAND Social Health Battery, the Sickness Impact Profile has undergone extensive instrument development work. Item content suggests that both the Social Interaction scale and the Recreation and Pastimes scale are potential measures for clinical trial research designs that require social interaction outcome measures. However, further investigation dealing specifically with the validity of these scales as social interaction measures appears necessary.

The Psychosocial Adjustment to Illness Scale

Seven dimensions of psychosocial adjustment underlie the construction of this 46-item instrument (15). The domains selected were deemed most germane to psychosocial adjustment to medical illness. Among the seven areas assessed are two that relate to social interaction: Extended Family Relationships (four items) and Social Environment (six items). Within the framework of typical family interactions, the Extended Family Relationships scale assessess, "negative impact of the illness upon communication, quality of relationships, interest in interacting with family, and other variables reflective of this life domain" (15, p. 78). Social Environment "reflects the patient's current social and leisure time activities, as well as the degree to which the patient has suffered impairment or constriction of these activities as a result of the current illness and/or its sequelae" (15, pp. 78–79). Items in this category focus on both interest and behavior. Respondents rate Psychosocial Adjustment to Illness Scale (PAIS) items relative to "the past thirty days including today."

The PAIS was initially designed as a semistructured interview. A self-report version (PAIS-SR) has been developed in the interest of feasibility and cost-effectiveness (16). Characteristics of the instrument described here refer to the semistructured interview version of the instrument. In acknowledgment of the fact that the effects of illnesses vary, the instrument's authors have decided to establish illness-specific norms for the PAIS and PAIS-SR (15). Normative data exist for lung cancer patients', renal dialysis patients', acute burn patients', and essential hypertensive patients' responses to the PAIS. PAIS-SR norms are available for cardiac bypass patients and for a sample of multisite cancer patients. Items are scored on an ordinal scale from 0 to 3. Values associated with each response vary by item. Poorer adjustment is associated with higher scale scores.

Reported internal consistency coefficients (Chronbach's alpha) for the Extended Family Relationships scale and the Social Environment scale are variable. Assessed with respect to the dialysis, lung cancer, and cardiac sample, coefficient alphas ranged from .78 to .90 for Social Environment. Alphas for the Extended Family Relationships scale were lower, .62 and .66, with a very low .12 in the lung cancer sample.

Correlations among the social interaction domains of the PAIS are moderately high (r = .51 among lung cancer patients and r = .53 among Hodgkins disease patients [15]), suggesting that each domain may not be a unique component of psychosocial adjustment to illness.

Kaplan De-Nour (17), in a study of chronic hemodialysis patients' psychosocial adjustment, observed that patients' Social Environment scores were among the scores indicating the poorest adjustment, although patients reported little or no Extended Family Relationship adjustment problems. Scale scores do not appear to be redundant with measures assessing psychological functioning. Correlations of the Extended Family Relationships scale and the Social Environment scale with psychological measures were lower than correlations between PAIS scales tapping psychological content and these measures (15). Derogatis (15) tested the predictive ability of the PAIS by examining differences between patients screened positive and negative for lung cancer. Patients screened positive scored higher on the Social Environment scale. Extended Family Relationships scores did not differ between groups.

Compared to the RAND Social Health Battery and the Sickness Impact Profile, the PAIS has undergone less instrument development work. The work performed thus far is impressive, however. The idea of establishing PAIS scale norms for separate illnesses should help researchers in the selection of social interaction scales. When selecting a potential scale for a clinical trials investigation, a researcher would be able to establish whether acceptable variability in scores has been observed for the particular illness of interest. In addition, scale scores would be available for comparison following data collection. The high correlations reported between Social Environment and Extended Family Relationship suggest that the use of both scales in a clinical trial design may not be necessary.

The Framingham Disability Study Social Disability Scales

The Framingham Disability Study Social Disability Scales (18) were devised in order to assess the need status of elders so that policy makers providing social services to the elderly can make information-based decisions. The instrument's authors use the term disability "to describe aberrations in the normal performance of the individual" (18, p. 1,202). Their conceptualization of disability comprises four categories; physical, emotional, mental, and social. Social interaction is assessed within the social domain along with four other activities associated with independent living.

The Framingham Disability Study social disability measure is a self-report instrument containing an eight-item social interaction scale. The instrument contains items that assess both social activities (e.g., "About how often do you talk with friends or relatives on the telephone?") and social activities evaluation (e.g., "Would you say you see as much of your relatives as you would like?"). Intermediate scales measuring each of these concepts are constructed and then combined through a complex computer algorithm to summarize an individual's functioning (19). Based on the results of this algorithm, respondents' social interaction is then described as need met, no apparent problem; need met, potential problem; uncertain need met, potential problem; and need unmet, current problem (18). Few elders in the essentially white, upper-class Framingham cohort reported unmet social interaction need or potential unmet social interaction need (3%). Unmet need did not vary as a function of age or sex (18).

An interesting feature of this index is that is takes into account not only respondents' social interaction behaviors, but also their satisfaction with these behaviors. This feature is shared to some degree by the Sickness Impact Profile and the Psychosocial Adjustment to Illness Scale. In addition to assessing strictly objective criteria, the respondent also indicates his/her satisfaction with or preference for activity with others. A potential drawback is the lack of knowledge regarding the index's performance in a patient sample and the lack of available psychometric data. More importantly, however, is the inclusion of an item indicating respondents' employment status. The inclusion of this item in an instrument to assess the elderly is surprising. The usefulness of an instrument containing this type of question is apparent only when employment status is somehow associated with the intention of an intervention or the population assessed.

Ad Hoc Social Interaction Measures

The most common approach to social interaction assessment is to generate a small number of items thought to relate to the concept and use the sum total of their individual scores as the outcome measure. Items are typically behavior-based and item content often does not relate to a predefined underlying concept of social interaction. Psychometric data on which to assess the usefulness of these measures is often absent.

From interview data collected on 707 newly diagnosed patients participating in the Brown University Cancer and Aging Study (20), Willey and Silliman (21) constructed a three-item social activity scale. Individual items dealt with frequency of visits (telephone or in person) with relatives, friends, and others. Patients indicated visit frequency as none, little, some, or considerable. This measure cannot be described as totally behavioral since patients' responses actually indicated their perception of the frequency of visits, rather than the actual number of visits. A social activity score arose from the sum of these items. The scale's internal consistency was rather high (Chronbach's alpha = .84). Total scores ranged from 3 to 12, with higher scores indicating greater social activity. From the total score, Willey and Silliman established a social activity indicator (high versus low). Patients reporting low social activity scored between 3 to 6 unless they reported "considerable" activity for any one item. The latter patients composed the high social activity group along with patients scoring greater than 6. Willey and Silliman (21) reported that 20% of the lung, breast, and colorectal cancer patients comprising the sample reported low social activity. A greater proportion of older patients, low income patients, and patients without children within a half hour's drive of their home composed the low social activity group. Low social activity patients also reported more pain, functional impairment, and more time in bed during the 2 weeks prior to interview.

Two similar measures are the sociability subcomponent of Bradburn's (22) Social Participation Scale used in his study of psychological well-being, and House et al.'s (23) Social Relationships and Activity Scale. Both are three-item scales. Bradburn's (22) respondents reported how many times they met with relatives, got together with friends, and chatted with friends over the telephone. Bradburn (22) found sociability to be positively related to socioeconomic status (SES) (gamma = .29) and to postive affect (controlling for the influence of SES).Respondents' social participation and negative affect were not related. Little is known about the properties of House et al.'s (23) scale, however, further investigation may prove useful given the content of the scale. Items measure involvement in formal and informal organizations, active social activities, and passive and solitary activities (4).

SUMMARY AND CONCLUSIONS

Compared to other components of quality of life, social interaction is the least well-conceptualized. This construct does not relate solely to the individual assessed. Unlike physical and mental health, social interaction can be considered at least partially external to an individual's quality of life or health status (2). Difficulty dealing with this concept is exemplified by Ware and Donald's (2) revision of their health status model following analysis of their social health data. In deciding that social function should be considered external to an individual's health status (i.e., as an independent variable rather than an outcome variable), they concluded that this model "explains empirical results better than one that includes social function as an integral component of individual health" (2, p. 6).

We have taken the view here that social interaction is a potential outcome measure in clinical trials designs. The most important decision one makes in this regard is that social interaction is in fact an outcome measure of interest. Unless social interaction can be considered as influenced, directly or indirectly, by the intervention under study, the concept should not be measured. We feel this rule should be followed when any quality of life domain is considered for assessment.

We selected brief self-report measures for review. Several (the Sickness Impact Profile, and the Psychosocial Adjustment to Illness Scale) were developed specifically for use in patient populations. Scales contained in these measures and in the RAND Social Health Battery hold the most promise as social interaction measures. An impressive amount of instrument development work exists for these measures. The ad hoc measures described, although simple to administer, are less useful because we know little about their underlying constructs and about what actually is being measured. Other social interaction measures exist, however, we tried to select scales that assess features of social functioning appropriate to medical interventions and to all potential patients assessed. For example, we excluded from consideration social interaction measures whose content relates to issues such as marital satisfaction and employability. More extensive reviews of social health measures in general are presented in McDowell and Newell (24) and Mangen and Peterson (25).

FUTURE RESEARCH

The highest priority in this area should be to establish a consensus as to the definition of social interaction. Once this is done the adequacy of existing measures can be assessed and the development of new measures can proceed effectively. We feel the major conceptual issue to be addressed is the orientation of the definition. Should the concept be wholly defined in behavioral terms? If frequency of contacts are measured, should they be measured from the perspective of patient initiation, initiation by others, or of both? Finally, what role does interest or desire to participate in social interactions play in this conceptualization? Answers to these questions should bring us closer to a more solid formalization of this concept and will provide the framework for the development and assessment of measurement instruments.

ACKNOWLEDGMENT

This research was supported in part by National Cancer Institute grants CA44100, CA41020, and CA46331.

REFERENCES

1. Yancik R, Yates JW. Quality of life assessment of cancer patients: Conceptual and methodological challenges and constraints. *Cancer Bull* 1986;38:217–222.
2. Donald CA, Ware JE. *The quantification of social contacts and resources.* Santa Monica, CA:RAND, 1982.
3. Bergner M, Bobbit RA, Carter WB, Gilson BS. The Sickness Impact Profile: Development and final revision of a health status measure. *Med Care* 1981;19:787–805.
4. Orth-Gomer K, Unden A. The measurement of social support in population surveys. *Soc Sci Med* 1987;24:83–94.
5. Ware JE. The assessment of health status. In: Aiken LH, Mechanic D, eds. *Applications of social science to clinical medicine and health policy.* New Brunswick, NJ:Rutgers University Press, 1986;204–228.
6. Berkman L. Assessing the physical health effects of social networks and social support. *Ann Rev Pub Health* 1984;5:413–432.
7. Cohen S, Syme SL. Issues in the study and application of social support. In:Cohen S, Syme SL, eds. *Social support and health.* Orlando, FL:Academic Press, 1985;3–22.
8. Brook RB, Ware JE, Rogers WH, et al. Does free care improve adults' health? Results from a randomized controlled trial. *N Engl J Med* 1983;309:1426–1434.
9. Mor V, Greer OS, Kastenbaum R, eds. *The hospice experiment.* Baltimore:Johns Hopkins University Press, 1988.
10. Carcagno GJ, Kemper P. The evaluation of the national long term care demonstration: An overview of the channeling demonstration and its evaluation. *Health Serv Res* 1988;23:1–22.
11. Donald CA, Ware JE, Brook RH, Davies-Avery A. *Conceptualization and measurement of health for adults in the health insurance study: Vol. 4, Social Health.* Santa Monica, CA:RAND, 1978.
12. Bergner M, Bobbitt RA, Pollard WE, Martin DP, Gilson BS. The Sickness Impact Profile: Validation of a health status measure. *Med Care* 1976;14:57–67.
13. Read JL, Quinn RJ, Hoefer MA. Measuring overall health: An evaluation of three important approaches. *J Chron Dis* 1987;40:7S–21S.

14. Pollard WE, Bobbitt RA, Bergner M, Gilson BS. The Sickness Impact Profile: Reliability of a health status measure. *Med Care* 1976;14:146.
15. Derogatis LR. The psychological adjustment to illness scale (PAIS). *J Psychosom Res* 1986;30:77–91.
16. Derogatis LR, Lopez M. *Psychological adjustment to illness scale (PAIS & PAIS-SR): Scoring procedures & administration manual-I.* Baltimore:Clinical Psychometric Research, 1983.
17. Kaplan De-Nour AK. Psychological adjustment to illness scale (PAIS): A study of chronic hemodialysis patients. *J Psychosom Res* 1982;26:11–22.
18. Branch LG, Jette AM. The Framingham disability study: Social disability among the aging. *Am J Public Health* 1981;71:1202–1210.
19. Branch LG. *Vulnerable elders. Gerontological monographs No. 6.* Washington, D.C.:Gerontological Society, 1980.
20. Mor V, Guadagnoli E, Silliman RA, et al. Influence of old age, performance status, medical and psychological factors on cancer patient management. In: Yancik R, Yates JW, eds. *Cancer in the elderly: Approaches to early detection and treatment.* New York: Springer, 1989.
21. Willey C, Silliman RA. The impact of disease upon the social support experience of cancer patients. *J Psychosoc Oncol* 1990 (*in press*).
22. Bradburn NM. *The structure of psychological well-being.* Chicago:Aldine, 1969.
23. House JS, Robbins C, Metzner HL. The association of social relationships and activities with mortality: Prospective evidence from the Tecumseh community. *Am J Epidem* 1982;116:123–140.
24. McDowell I, Newell C. *Measuring health: A guide to rating scales and questionnaires.* New York:Oxford University Press, 1987.
25. Mangen DJ, Peterson W, eds. *Research instruments in social gerontology.* Minneapolis:University of Minnesota Press, 1982.

Quality of Life Assessments in Clinical Trials, edited by B. Spilker. Raven Press, Ltd. New York, 1990.

9

Psychological Tests and Scales

Sally A. Shumaker, Roger T. Anderson, and Susan M. Czajkowski

National Heart, Lung, and Blood Institute, National Institutes of Health, Bethesda, Maryland 20892

It is generally accepted that quality of life is an important criterion for assessing the effectiveness of most medical treatments. Quality of life research is now at a stage in which behavioral scientists are frequently called on to provide the most appropriate and psychometrically sophisticated measures of quality of life for a broad range of populations and circumstances. The current demand for reasonable quality of life assessments in clinical trials presents behavioral scientists with a unique opportunity to demonstrate the important links between human behavior and overall health status. However, with this opportunity comes the necessity of carefully assessing and evaluating conceptual models and research tools.

In this chapter, issues relevant to quality of life measures for particular clinical studies are considered. The properties of various psychological instruments currently used in quality of life research are discussed with a focus on a battery (i.e., multiple, distinct instruments) approach to quality of life assessment.

First a presentation of one model of quality of life, distinguishing between properties of the concept and factors that may influence quality of life, is presented. In addition, several general issues that may affect the choice of instruments for a particular battery are discussed. Then important properties used to determine the value of a particular instrument are considered, and these properties are applied to psychologically based measures used in quality of life research. Several specific studies are presented as examples of how psychologically based batteries have been applied to quality of life research. The chapter concludes with suggestions for future research in the area of battery-based quality of life assessments.

A MODEL OF QUALITY OF LIFE

Definition

Regardless of how quality of life is measured in a specific study, it is critical that a clear model of the construct is used. Although quality of life has been measured for several decades, consensus among investigators regarding an exact definition and measure has not been achieved. Quality of life has been conceptualized in a variety of ways and there is disagreement regarding what constitutes quality of life versus what influences it. Not surprisingly, measures of quality of life are highly variant and range from single items of such factors as employment status, to multidimensional scales. For the purposes of this chapter, a broad model of quality of life is provided. It is derived from the early economic indicator research (1), the more recent health-based research of quality of life (2,3), and the author's experiences with patients who have heart disease (4).

Quality of life is defined as individuals' overall satisfaction with life and their general sense of personal well-being. Six dimensions that determine quality of life are proposed. The first four dimensions—cognitive, social, physical, and emotional functioning—are usually associated with quality of life. A fifth dimension, personal productivity, refers to the degree to which an individual is able to contribute to society. This encompasses employment status (a frequent proxy for quality of life), but is intended to encourage a broader consideration of what constitutes "contributing to society" (e.g., actively pursuing a rewarding hobby or craft, homemaking, cooking, gardening, and volunteer work). The sixth dimension is intimacy, which includes sexual functioning as well as the expression and receipt of a broad range of behaviors that underlie feelings of intimate involvement with others (4).

Methodological Issues

A number of instruments have been developed to assess each of these six dimensions of quality of life. Several general issues influence the choice of a particular instrument for a specific quality of life dimension. First, each dimension of quality of life can be measured, to varying degrees, from either a subjective or objective perspective. Furthermore, researchers can measure either functional status alone, or functional status along with satisfaction. Finally, the selected comparison group should be reflected in the measures. For example, does one compare the group studied to the general population, the patient population from which the sample is drawn, or both?

The six dimensions composing quality of life in the model are influenced by a broad range of factors. It is important to maintain a conceptual distinction between these moderating factors and quality of life. The moderating factors can be divided into three categories: contextual (e.g., settings, economic structure, and sociocultural factors); interpersonal (e.g., social support, stress, economic strain); and intrapersonal (e.g., coping skills, personality variables, physical health and symptoms).

The actual quality of life-related goals of a study often vary considerably and may include the following: (a) using quality of life as baseline data to predict morbidity and mortality; (b) assessing the effects of treatment on overall quality of life or on specific dimensions of quality of life in more detail; (c) where treatment is unlikely to influence quality of life, establishing detailed quality of life normative data on a particular population; (d) assessing patterns of a quality of life component over time; and (e) assessing the components and moderators of quality of life most amenable to interventions with a more process-oriented approach. Each of these goals will lead to a different selection of appropriate instruments in a battery-based study of quality of life.

A variety of instruments and methods are used to assess quality of life. Some instruments yield a single overall score with separate subscores for various dimensions of quality of life. Other instruments yield a single score with implied dimensions that cannot be identified with separate scores. Another approach is to use a single instrument to assess a single component of quality of life (e.g., physical functioning). Finally, batteries of separate instruments are used to assess each dimension of quality of life, and this approach yields separate scores for each dimension that cannot be summed. Based on the model discussed above as well as the methodological concerns considered, the authors' bias is to use a battery approach where the instruments selected for any given clinical trial correspond to the dimensions of quality of life most likely to be *either positively or negatively* affected by treatment, and to use the best available instruments to assess each of these dimensions. A major drawback to this approach is the possibility that investigators will select those dimensions of quality of life to be most positively affected by the treatment under study. More likely, investigators may inadvertently overlook an aspect of quality of life affected by treatment. Thus, use of a battery approach requires a thorough understanding of the population under study, the clinical course of the untreated disease, and all potential effects of the intervention(s) (5).

Although the dimensions of quality of life are not limited to psychological constructs (e.g., physical functioning), this chapter focuses on the psychological constructs relevant to quality of life. Before considering these, however, the criteria used to judge the comparative research value of various instruments are reviewed.

CRITICAL PROPERTIES OF RESEARCH INSTRUMENTS

To be useful in clinical trials, psychological tests must represent objective and standardized measures of a sample of an individual's behavior, and be of diagnostic. or predictive value. The first criterion essentially means that the test meets the logical requirements of scientific pursuit; the second concerns the actual content of the instrument in terms of the number and nature of the items, and their usefulness in evaluating the desired behavior or trait in specified situations. In practice these are overlapping properties, and although they make up the basis of what is referred to as the psychometric properties of the test, they are identical to the implicit assumptions of the scientific method of investigation.

Dimensions on Which to Evaluate Psychological Measures

Objectivity and Standardization

A cardinal aim in most scientific endeavors is that observations should be free of subjective judgment. In psychological testing, the clinician must be assured that an individual will theoretically obtain the same score regardless of who is administering, scoring, or interpreting the data. Methods to objectively interpret a test score will depend on the type of assessment instrument used and the specific research goals. A raw score for a social or psychological construct generally has no inherent meaning, and the use of norms established for a specific instrument with regard to a specific population is required. Thus, for example, an individual's test score is meaningful by its location on a continuum of performance representative of an appropriate control sample, or diagnostic standard. In some situations the individual case is a legitimate unit of analysis, and a total score will be interesting in its own right. For example, comparison of pre- and postintervention scores of anxiety may provide useful information on recovery independent of the magnitude of deviation from the norm; other examples include tests employing self-description responses like self-concept or self-evaluations.

The above examples are functions in psychological assessment for controlling extraneous variables from contaminating scientific observation. A related function of standardization is to insure that scores obtained by different persons are comparable. Having physicians or assistants trained in proper administration and evaluation of psychological assessment is a requisite step in this process.

Adequacy of the Test

Whether a test has utility as a diagnostic or predictive indicator of behavior depends on proper construction of the test, as well as careful selection of a test suitable to the behavior under consideration. Psychometric evaluation of an assessment instrument begins with questions regarding its reliability and validity.

Reliability

Reliability refers to the consistency of measurement, and is usually determined by the extent that a score has repeatability between identical or equivalent tests. Conceptually, a test score contains a "true-score" component and an "error" component; to the extent that random error is large, a test score will be unstable and cannot be depended on to make inferences regarding the impact of a treatment. There are three basic ways to evaluate the reliability of a given test.

Internal consistency reliability is the most frequently used estimate of test reliability. Multiple responses are obtained in most behavioral assessments which are then summed or reduced to a single index. An implicit assumption in this approach is that the individual items measure the same thing, or that the items are consistent with each other. To the extent that this is true, a test can be held to measure the same attribute across subjects and time. Operationally, the higher the correlations of the items within the test, the higher is their multiple correlation with the single factor they measure in common. Thus, a measure of internal consistency is the average degree of association among the items on a test.

Test re-test reliability is the correlation between scores obtained by the same person on two separate occasions; the error variance corresponds to the random fluctuations of performance between the two observations. This interpretation is complicated by the fact that changes may have occurred during the time interval itself. Thus, low test re-test reliability does not necessarily reflect the psychometric properties of the test. For example, the stability coefficients for the trait anxiety scale (State-Trait Anxiety Inventory) range from .65 to .86, although its internal consistency has been reported to be in the .90s (6).

This issue brings up a potential difficulty in behavioral assessment that is similar to dietary intake studies. Since some behavioral attributes may lack temporal stability, the usefulness of point prevalence estimates of the attribute is threatened. The researcher is compelled to show whether it is reasonable to expect that any changes in the behavioral attribute due to treatment can be detected, and whether data on duration and frequency are useful. Toward this end, the temporal stability of the behavior measured by each instrument to be included in the clinical study should be examined. It must be decided whether strategies are needed to increase reliability (e.g., increasing the number of estimates, or using group estimates), or to use alternative assessment instruments (e.g., the Depression Adjective Check List [7], and the Beck Depression Inventory [8]) that are more sensitive to daily fluctuations in mood.

Equivalent-forms reliability refers to the agreement between an individual's score on two or more tests designed to measure the same attribute. It insures that scores obtained on two administrations are independent and measures the temporal stability of responses to the items between both tests. Important sources of error variance in this type of reliability assessment include fluctuations in time (e.g., intervening events and practice effects), and in the composition of the forms (e.g., number, content, order, range, and difficulty of items).

Validity

Demonstrating reliability in measurement is essentially proving the existence of a stable, or generalizable concept. However, reliability says nothing about the nature of that concept; thus, a set of items may yield a repeatable score that may be invalid indicators of the construct under study. Validity is defined as the extent to which an instrument measures what it was intended to measure. Establishing validity in measures is achieved by the extent of agreement between the measure and a designated standard or "criterion." Some authors argue that validity is more important than reliability. However, both forms of errors can seriously influence the correctness of inference, and therefore should be viewed as equally important qualities. Both must be maximized in the selection or development of an instrument. Although it is true that validity in measurement is necessary to interpret what a test score means conceptually, it can be shown statistically that small decrements in reliability can result in large decrements in validity. The following kinds of evidence are generally used to infer validity of measurement.

Content validity is the extent that a test samples a representative range of the behavior under study. In interpreting content validity, questions regarding item sufficiency in the proposed testing situations and patient sample should be carefully addressed. For example, the range of items needed to adequately assess Activities of Daily Living functioning in arthritic patients would be too gross for application to many coronary heart disease samples; and some depression questionnaires sample mainly one or two aspects of depression, e.g., subjective (8) and somatic complaints (9). A clear idea of what aspects of the behavioral attribute are of interest to the study is essential to judge the degree of content validity for a particular assessment instrument.

Construct validity refers to evidence that a measured construct behaves in a manner consistent with its referent theoretical or logical properties. Construct validity is established through a series of tests and observations demonstrating that the variable as measured: (a) does not vary with measures of related but different constructs (discriminant validity); (b) does vary with related and similar constructs (convergent validity); (c) taps the measures of the construct intended; and (d) is not dominated by irrelevant factors (10). This process is used to increase confidence that an observed effect pertains to the variable of interest. In quality of life research, one of the largest problems in establishing construct validity is the lack of agreement over the operational definition of quality of life as well as differences in population characteristics and the disease-specific criteria used in many measures.

Predictive validity is the degree to which a test can predict how well an individual will do in a future situation. Predictive validity is determined by the degree of correspondence between the assessment instrument and the specific criterion used for future performance.

All validation reports for assessment instruments should describe the conditions under which the validation was conducted, including population demographics and the range of skills or attributes in the sample. It is crucial that these be considered before employing an instrument. *No test is inherently "valid"; rather a test is valid with regard to a specific purpose, range, and sample.*

Selecting a Method to Measure Psychological Aspects of Quality of Life

Unless patients under study are frail or otherwise unable to easily complete a written questionnaire, a self-report is usually the method of choice for psychological assessments in clinical trials. Some advantages of self-report include cost-efficiency relative to other behavioral assessment techniques, easy scoring, applicability to a wide range of populations, and the ability to gather data on multiple dimensions of quality of life. For diagnostic purposes, self-report questionnaires may be employed during the early stages of assessment (e.g., screening), but do not provide the detailed information necessary to apply diagnostic labels. (The reader is referred to the American Psychiatric Association classification system, DSM-III, for further information on this point.)

PSYCHOLOGICAL MEASURES IN QUALITY OF LIFE RESEARCH

Psychological assessment in quality of life research may employ two strategies: index or battery. The merits of each approach, along with examples, are discussed below.

Indices

Indices are inventories that provide a single number to characterize a set of item responses by a simple cumulative score (11). Assumptions in this approach are that an individual or group with a high index score has more of the measured property than those with a lower index score.

Two psychological indices are the Psychological General Well-Being Index (12) and the General Health Questionnaire (13). Both were developed as multidimensional measures of affective and emotional states that reflect well-being. Another prominent instrument in this area is the Mental Health Inventory developed for RAND's Health Insurance Experiment (14). Also of interest are indices of general health which have significant item clusters on social and psychological functioning. Nonindex general health instruments also exist which include components of psychological and social functioning. One example is the Sickness Impact Profile, developed by Bergner and associates (15).

The General Health Questionnaire

The General Health Questionnaire (13) is a self-administered questionnaire designed to measure acute or episodic changes in a subject's usual psychological functions, and does not attempt to measure duration of disturbance. Anxious and depressive moods and associated somatic manifestations which may be indicative of nonpsychotic psychiatric disorders are emphasized. The General Health Questionnaire is intended as a screen for use in general population surveys, primary care settings, and medical outpatients. Its format includes a time-frame of "past few weeks," with four response categories in a gradient of "less than usual" to "much more than usual." Several versions of the General Health Questionnaire have been developed. The most commonly used are a main 60-item version on general health, somatic symptoms (e.g., cardiovascular, neuromuscular, and gastrointestinal functioning), sleep behavior, personal and interpersonal behavior, and subjective feelings of distress; a 30-item version developed to reduce the influence of organic impairment by removal of somatic indicators which could select subjects with only medical illness, and measures personal and interpersonal functioning and subjective distress (16); and a 28-item factor analyzed version with the four subscales "somatic symptoms," "anxiety and insomnia," "social dysfunction," and "severe depression" (17). A cutoff score for case identification in the different versions has not been established and has varied over the years.

Reliability of the General Health Questionnaire is high: test re-test reliability is $R = 0.90$ for general practice patients, $R = 0.75$ for psychiatric patients who self-reported no change in symptoms between administrations, and $R = 0.51$ for psychiatric patients who were rated by their physicians as unchanged (18). Estimates of internal consistency by the split-half method are above 0.90 (19). The General Health Questionnaire is highly correlated with a standardized psychiatric interview (13), as well as with other screening tests (20). Sensitivity and specificity with the Standardized Psychiatric Interview using medical outpatient and general practice samples in English-speaking countries are 96% and 88% for the 60-item version when a cutting point of 12 is used (21); 91% and 87% for the 30-item version using a cutting point of 5 (20), and 94% and 73% for the scaled version based on a cutoff score of 5. The General Health Questionnaire was not significantly correlated with cognitive impairment, indicating good discrimination from neurological-associated impairment (22).

The General Health Questionnaire is a well-validated scale and appears to be a good measure of recent onset of anxiety and depression; however, it lacks sensitivity for long-standing impairments like intermittent depression and conditions lasting longer than six months. The dominant affect in the depression factor is dysphoric mood, and for anxiety it is nervousness and strain. The range of content and psychometric development of this instrument is more extensive than other scales of psychological impairment; particularly unique is the isolation of depression and anxiety in the 28-item scaled version. Although the General Health Questionnaire has not been used previously for quality of life research, with its focus on change in psychological state and impairment in normal functioning it appears to be a good choice among existing instruments. In view of the overlap in self-reports of symptoms of anxiety and depression (23) in most measures of psychological disturbance, the General Health Questionnaire may be preferred since it allows each factor to be compared relative to the other, and gives total scores indicating severity of general psychological distress.

Profiles

As the term is commonly used today, profiles refer to instruments that include several independent dimensions of a construct, and yield subscale scores for each content area. Although there are no psychological profiles developed specifically for quality of life, a widely used instrument is the Profile of Mood States.

The Profile of Mood States

The Profile of Mood States (24) is designed to assess mood states and transient changes in mood. Six identifiable moods or affective states are measured: tension-anxiety; depression-dejection; anger-hostility; vigor-activity; fatigue-inertia; and confusion-bewilderment. The scales for these mood states were determined by factor analysis results in several studies. The Profile of Mood States is self-administered, and contains 65 adjectives relating to mood states during the past week, which are scored on a 5-point scale from 0 (not at all) to 4 (extremely). The time reference may be eliminated to measure mood traits. A score for each factor is produced by simply adding responses. A summary measure of total distress can also be obtained by summing all scores.

In the normative samples consisting of male college students, male psychiatric outpatients, and male patients at a university hospital outpatient clinic, all the internal consistency coefficients of Profile of Mood States factors were found to be near 0.90. Without the intervention of treatment, test re-test coefficients in a sample accepted for psychiatric treatment ranged from $R = 0.65$ for vigor to $R = 0.74$ for depression for a median time of 20 days. Correlations of scores following 6 weeks of treatment were much lower. In addition to factorial validity for the six Profile of Mood States factors, predictive and concurrent validities were established for Profile of Mood States in several studies (24). In the normative samples the Profile of Mood States factors were found to be moderately to highly correlated with three clinically derived distress scales on somatization, anxiety, and depression. Discriminative validities of the separate factors are not strong, especially anxiety (tension) and depression where the intercorrelations ranged from $R = 0.56$ to 0.77. Of the 26 intercorrelations reported among the five factors, the median coefficient is $R = 0.60$. Validity data are not presented in the manual for the total measure of distress score; studies in cancer patients have found moderate correlations of the total measure of distress with degree of physical impairment, extent of disease, and pain, suggesting its usefulness as an overall distress measure.

Overall the evidence from large standardization samples suggests that the Profile of Mood States is a valid and reliable descriptive tool for assessing mood states in both psychiatric and nonpsychiatric populations. Despite its being developed to address several specific moods, however, the moderate to high intercorrelations among factor scores suggest that the Profile of Mood States may be better suited to measuring general mood disturbance. Studies have shown that the strongest associations between Profile of Mood States factor scores and extent of disease or prognostic factors have been for vigor and fatigue, and there is very little association with factors relevant to emotional distress. It is not clear to what extent disease affects emotional distress measured by the Profile of Mood States, but it is concluded that this instrument is a reasonably good measure of general mood disturbance in a wide range of populations, and may be a valuable test to include in a psychological quality of life battery.

Scales

The following instruments were designed to measure a distinct psychological trait or property, and have been widely used in psychological research. In quality of life research, they may be selectively combined with other instruments to form a psychologically based quality of life battery.

Depression

There are several self-rating depression scales commonly used in the clinical setting. The most prominent are the Beck Depression Inventory (25), the Zung Self-Rating Depression Scale (9), and the Center for Epidemiological Studies of Depression (26).

Beck Depression Inventory

The Beck Depression Inventory (25) is a 21-item test designed to measure the severity or depth of depression "today." It does not attempt to identify chronic depression. As a general measure of depressive symptomology, the Beck Depression Inventory emphasizes cognitive and affective aspects of depression; behavioral and somatic features of depression contribute 33% to the total score (27). Perhaps reflecting its intended use in psychiatric patients, item composition was based on clinical experience rather than selected from other scales. The Beck Depression Inventory contains 94 multiple-choice questions grouped into 21 categories; a shorter 13-category version, and self-administered and oral interview versions are available. Severity is measured in terms of frequency, change from usual functioning, and perceived severity of distress. The Beck Depression Inventory yields a single score based on simple cumulation of the highest values circled for each item. The scores range from 0 to 63. Several cutting points have been used to determine severity and caseness, but they have not been established; a score of 17 has been used to separate none versus moderate depression. This instrument was initially designed as a screen of depressive symptomology for use with psychiatric samples, but it has shown applicability in medical inpatients (28,29), general practice (30), outpatients enrolled in a clinical trial (31), and college students (32,33).

The Beck Depression Inventory has demonstrated high reliability with split-half reliability of $R = 0.93$ (25), and coefficient alpha estimations reported to range from .79 to .91 (34). Since it is intended to measure transient or acute changes in severity of depressive symptoms, measures of temporal stability (test re-test) are not indicated. However, high test re-test reliability has been reported for this measure for up to 3 months (35). Convergent validity has been established through correlations with other self-report depression scales: $R = 0.64$ with the Zung Self-Rating Depression Scale (36), $R = 0.66$ with the Depression Adjective Checklist (37), and $R = 0.70$ with the Symptom Check List-90 (38). Criterion validity has been established with correlation of $R = 0.75$ to 0.80 with psychiatrists' ratings of depression using the Hamilton Rating Scale for Depression (39,40) and remained significantly correlated at 6 months follow-up, and $R = 0.77$ was reported with same day psychiatric ratings (32). Using a cutting point of 17 to detect none versus moderate depression, sensitivity was 76% and specificity was 77% (25). Like any of the self-rating depression inventories, the Beck Depression Inventory has been found to be highly correlated with self-report measurements of anxiety (27,38) and general psychopathology (42,23). Carroll (27) found that the highest correlations between Beck Depression Inventory scores and the Hamilton Rating Scale for Depression are for low and moderate severity depression.

It is concluded that the Beck Depression Inventory is a reliable and valid self-report of acute depressive moods of moderate severity. Since the total score reflects transient symptoms, it is an inadequate indicator of clinical depression. Information on how well it measures stable depression is limited.

Zung Self-Rating Depression Scale

Like the Beck Depression Inventory, the Zung Self-Rating Depression Scale (9) was designed as a quantitative measure of depressive symptomology. However, it emphasizes more somatic and behavioral components (50% of total score) than most other self-rating scales. The scale is self-administered, and contains 20 items covering affective, psychological, and somatic features of depression. Severity is determined solely by frequency of symptoms, with "the past week" timeframe. The patient indicates the frequency with which a depressive symptom is experienced, ranging from "none or a little" to "most of the time." The range of scores is 20 to 80, with a cutting point of 50 to distinguish mildly depressed persons from normals, 60 for presence of moderate depression, and 70 for presence of severe depression (42). The Self-Rating Depression Scale has received widespread clinical and research use in monitoring changes in symptomology during treatment in a variety of populations, including psychiatric, medical, and mildly depressed and normal college students (43).

Estimates of internal consistency of the Self-Rating Depression Scale have been reported to be $R = 0.73$ for split-half (44), and interitem correlations have been around $R = 0.80$ (45). Because this scale is intended to measure acute or transient depressive mood symptomology, test re-test estimates are not applicable. The validity has been extensively documented in Hedlund and Vieweg (43), and the evidence presented is largely for clinical populations. This instrument has been shown to be moderately correlated with the Minnesota Multiphasic Personality Inventory-Depression scale, ranging from $R = 0.50$ to 0.70 in clinically depressed or psychiatric samples; highly correlated with other self-rated depression scales such as the Beck Depression Inventory and the Depression Adjective Check List; and moderately correlated with physician ratings of depression (27). Carroll and his colleagues (27) found that the Self-Rating Depression Scale measures of severity were only moderately correlated with an interview-based assessment; this may result from the exclusive reliance in the scale on frequency of symptoms. It appears to be acceptable as a screening instrument, but not as an independent measure of clinical depression (a claim made by Zung for the scale). Sensitivity of the Self-Rating Depression Scale to distinguish among mild, moderate, and severely depressed patients is inadequate, and does not reach the level reported for the Beck Depression Inventory. Similar to other self-report inventories, the Self-Rating Depression Scale is moderately correlated with symptoms of other dimensions of psychopathology and lacks sufficient specificity to be used as an indicator of clinical depression.

Center for Epidemiologic Studies-Depression Scale

The Center for Epidemiologic Studies-Depression Scale (26) is a self-report measure of depressive symptomology, and is intended for use in identifying high risk groups in epidemiological studies. It contains 20 items drawn from other self-report scales (largely from the Beck Depression Scale, Zung Self-Rating Depression Scale, Depression Adjective Check List, and the Minnesota Multiphasic Personality Inventory Depression Scale which assess the frequency and duration of symptoms associated with depression in the preceding week. Similar to the Beck Depression Inventory, subjective and behavioral aspects of depression are emphasized; factors include cognitive, affective, behavioral, somatic symptoms, and positive affect. Response categories range from "rarely or none" to "most or all of the time," and are based on a stated time range of "less than 1 day" to "5–7 days." Scores are weighted by frequency and summed across all items. They range from 0 to 60, and a cutting point of 16 is commonly used to discriminate cases from noncases.

The Center for Epidemiologic Studies-Depression Scale has been shown to have high internal consistency, with alpha coefficients reported to be .85 in a community sample, and .90 in a patient sample (26). It is highly correlated with several self-report depression scales (e.g., Symptom Check List-90 and Depression Adjective Check List), and with psychiatrists' ratings of depression across psychiatric groups of varying depressive illness severity (44). Sensitivity in detecting depression identified by a clinical scale was 99%, using 16 as a cutting point (26), and fell to 64% when cases were identified by clinical interview in a community setting (46). Specificity has ranged from 56% to 96%, being highest for case detection based on clinical interview and self-reports (46,47). Like the other two self-rated depression scales reviewed here, the Center for Epidemiological Studies-Depression Scale has problems with specificity; Orme et al. (45) found moderate correlations between the scale and anxiety, self-esteem, and trait anxiety. It offers several unique features, including an excellent item format which can indicate how many days over the week symptoms persisted, brevity for large-scale epidemiological studies, an emphasis on case detection rather than severity, and high sensitivity for acute depression.

Anxiety

Self-report measures provide information regarding cognitive components of anxiety, and for medical patient surveys involve either surveys of general acute anxiety reactions (states) and anxiety traits. Major scales used in the research are the State-Trait Anxiety Inventory (discussed below) (6), the Multiple Adjective Checklist for state and trait anxiety, the Taylor Manifest Anxiety Scale, and the Institute of Personality and Ability Testing (IPAT) Anxiety scale which measures trait anxiety.

Spielberger State-Trait Anxiety Inventory

The Spielberger State-Trait Anxiety Inventory (STAI) (6) is the most widely used anxiety scale. Spielberger and his colleagues developed the STAI between 1964 and 1970, when the initial version was published, and published a revised version in 1983 as FORM Y. Items were taken from the Taylor Manifest Anxiety Scale, the Welsh Anxiety Scale, and the IPAT Anxiety Scale, and tested using different college student samples. Items for state-anxiety were selected for their ability to discriminate between stress and nonstress conditions; trait anxiety items were chosen for their stability over time. The State-Anxiety Scale (STAI FORM Y-1) consists of 20 statements on a 4-point scale covering apprehension, tension, nervousness, and worry which evaluate how the subject feels "at this moment." The Trait-Anxiety (STAI FORM Y-2) consists of 20 statements on a 4-point scale pertaining to how the subject generally feels. Both scales were designed to contain an anxiety present and anxiety absent factor. The State-Trait Anxiety Inventory was designed for high school and college students, and adults. To score the 20 responses for each scale are summed. High scores are interpreted as indicating more state or trait anxiety, and can be compared with normative data provided in the test manual. Alpha coefficients of internal consistency for the state anxiety scale range from 0.86 to 0.95, and for the trait anxiety scale range from 0.89 to 0.91. Median test re-test correlations for the trait scale ranged from $R = 0.65$ to 0.86. Since state anxiety is by definition unstable, test re-test estimates are not informative. Validation studies of Form Y indicate that discrimination between state and trait anxiety was achieved, yielding two separate factors (48). Convergent validity of the State-Trait Anxiety Inventory is established by high correlations with other self-report scales of emotional disturbance (e.g., Minnesota Multiphasic Personality Inventory). Correlations between this trait-anxiety scale and other trait anxiety scales range from $R = 0.52$ to 0.80. The state-anxiety scale discriminates between military recruits beginning a stressful training program and high school students, and detects anxiety induced by stressful experimental conditions in college students (6). Both trait and state anxiety scales showed moderate correlations with medical symptom indices which indicates a possible organic bias; however, data on specificity and sensitivity are not provided by Spielberger. The State-Trait Anxiety Inventory is as good a self-report measure as can be found for measuring anxiety. However, the following shortcomings in measuring anxiety should be considered: in the State-Trait Anxiety Inventory there is high correlation between state and trait anxiety and there is high correlation between trait anxiety and related but independent psychological disturbance (e.g., depression). These problems suggest that at least trait anxiety is a more general measure of psychological distress than intended by its authors. The evidence for validity of the state-anxiety scale is stronger, and shows discrimination among levels of severity.

METHODOLOGICAL PROBLEMS WITH THE BATTERY APPROACH TO QUALITY OF LIFE ASSESSMENT

Studies that use batteries to assess quality of life are described here to illustrate some of the benefits and problems of this approach. First considered are several methodological flaws that are not limited to studies which employ a battery approach, but which severely weaken research in the quality of life area in general. Then, methodological problems unique to the battery approach are presented.

General Methodological Problems

Many studies on quality of life in the cardiovascular disease area contain methodological flaws that qualify or invalidate their findings regarding the effects of various cardiovascular disease treatments on quality of life. The most serious of these problems are: lack of double-blinding in clinical trials of cardiovascular therapies; lack of placebo control groups; use of inappropriate controls or reference groups; use of retrospective self-report data rather than inclusion of pretreatment data; and lack of standardized, well-validated, and reliable measures of quality of life.

An illustration of the problems inherent in the use of a single rather than double-blind design can be found in the two prospective, multicenter, randomized, clinical trials comparing the effects of several hypertensive medications (captopril versus methyldopa or oxprenolol) on quality of life (49). In these trials, quality of life was operationalized as complaint rate, activity index, and depression. Patients taking captopril had a significantly lower symptom complaint rate than those taking methyldopa; however, the study was single-blind, and a number of questionnaires had to be discarded due to evidence that physicians helped their patients to complete the instruments. The possibility that systematic bias may be introduced when a study is not double-blind severely limits the ability to draw conclusions regarding the effects of a treatment on quality of life.

Many studies comparing the effectiveness of various cardiovascular therapies on quality of life lack placebo control groups or use inappropriate controls. Examples include Hill et al. (49), mentioned above, and Croog et al. (50), a randomized clinical trial that also compared the effects of several hypertensive medications on quality of life. Both studies used placebo periods prior to the active treatment phases of the study, but did not include a placebo group during the active treatment phase due to ethical considerations. The use of a placebo control group is important because it allows an assessment of the extent to which treatment effects occur due to the treatment itself, versus nonspecific factors such as expectations of treatment success.

Problems in interpreting data also occur when inappropriate control or reference groups are used for comparison purposes. Siegrist et al. (51) compared hypertensive patients who were being treated with those who refused treatment across several quality of life dimensions, including physical symptoms, mental alertness, emotional well-being, and work-role performance. The two groups are not comparable since individuals who refuse hypertensive treatment probably differ in many respects from those who adopt and maintain a treatment regimen. Similarly, Wiklund et al. (52) compared the quality of life of 177 men at 1 year following a myocardial infarction with that of a random sample of 175 healthy men used as a reference group. The post-myocardial infarction group reported significantly more symptoms and emotional disturbances, and differed from the healthy controls in type of leisure activity. Again, the reference group used differed from the post-myocardial infarction group in ways other than the presence of cardiovascular disease (e.g., lifestyle factors predictive of cardiovascular disease and psychosocial factors).

Interventions often include nonspecific components, such as increases in social support, that are not included in a control group. For example, Patel and Marmot (53) randomly assigned hypertensive subjects to a program involving weekly relaxation and stress management sessions, or to receive health-education leaflets concerning smoking and diet. The weekly relaxation sessions involved an increase in social support available to participants, but not to those in the control group. Therefore, the significant differences between the two groups found on the quality of life measures may have resulted from the greater support received by those assigned to the group. Naismith et al. (54) have similar interpretive problems in their study comparing the quality of life of post-myocardial infarction patients who received intensive psychological counseling versus information materials on risk factor reduction.

Lack of pretreatment data makes it impossible to compare patients' quality of life following a treatment or event to their prior level of quality of life. LaMendola and Pellegrini (55) interviewed coronary artery bypass graft (CABG) patients 6 months to 4 years following surgery. In addition to the lack of comparability in terms of amount of time following surgery (which was not controlled for in the analyses), quality of life was assessed following surgery only, and therefore it was impossible to compare the patients' postsurgical quality of life to their presurgical state in order to discuss how patients' quality of life changed over time. Similar problems occurred for Flynn and Frantz (56) and for Raft et al. (57) in their studies of quality of life following coronary artery bypass graft sugery.

Finally, a common problem with many studies on quality of life is the use of measures that are not well-validated or reliable. Often, instruments used to measure quality of life components such as employment status or social functioning consist of a single item or a series of items that are created specifically for the study. Furthermore, attempts are rarely made to assess the reliabilities of scales used (see earlier discussion). Use of a single item to assess a quality of life domain such as employment status is inadequate to reliably capture the complexity of an individual's employment situation. The use of sets of items that have inadequate internal consistency (and are thus insensitive measures of quality of life) can also impede the identification of important differences. More serious still, in terms of threats to internal validity, is the use of subjective open-ended items, rated post hoc, as measures of specific quality of life dimensions.

Examples of the use of interview data to rate patients' quality of life include two studies of quality of life following a myocardial infarction (58,59). In both of these studies, patients were interviewed about such quality of life dimensions as work, leisure, sexual activity level, family and social life, emotional state, and work status. Mayou et al. (58) used consensus ratings of change in activity and satisfaction based on the interview data, but failed to specify how these consensus ratings were determined. Although these are extreme examples of the use of ad hoc measures in quality of life research, few studies use measures that have been validated, have adequate reliability, and are sensitive enough to reliably distinguish quality of life changes due to treatment. Given the homogeneity of most clinical trial populations, the psychometric properties of instruments are particularly important.

Problems Specific to a Battery Approach to Quality of Life Measurement

A characteristic of many quality of life studies that is especially problematic when a battery approach is employed is the use of small sample sizes. Sample sizes of 20 to 30 patients are not unusual in the quality of life literature. Although a small sample may provide preliminary information about quality of life or be useful for relatively simple, exploratory analyses, the use of multiple quality of life measures and the resulting use of multivariate analytical procedures require relatively large sample sizes. Even when univariate procedures are employed, sample sizes of 30 or less may not provide the power necessary for testing specific hypotheses. An example of this problem is Gundle et al.'s study (60), in which a number of predictor variables, including pre-operative symptoms, Type A behavior, and pre-operative employment status, were used to predict several quality of life variables (such as sexual functioning and postoperative work status) using a sample of 30 coronary artery bypass graft surgery patients.

Even when sample sizes are adequate, reliable and valid measures are used, and the study is generally well-designed, several problems can occur that are unique to a battery approach. One such problem is the use of univariate statistical techniques to analyze multiple measures of quality of life. An example of this is the Jenkins et al. (61) prospective, observational study assessing quality of life in 318 coronary artery bypass graft surgery patients who were interviewed before and 6 months following surgery. Quality of life was assessed across a broad range of dimensions, including cognitive, physical, social, emotional, and sexual functioning. Results showed improvement on many of the quality of life dimensions, especially for reports of angina, anxiety, depression, and sleep problems. However, no attempt was made to control for the increased chance of a Type I error, since a large number of measures were used (e.g., 11 scales were used to assess the psychological functioning components). The use of paired *t*-tests for such a large number of comparisons is inappropriate; instead, a multivariate approach, or at least the use of multiple comparison procedures that minimize Type I error (e.g., multiple range statistics) are advisable when a battery of quality of life measures are used.

Another study that employed a comprehensive, multidimensional quality of life assessment with standardized, well-validated measures is the Croog et al. (50) clinical trial which compared the effects of three hypertensive medications on the quality of life of 626 hypertensive men. Quality of life was defined as emotional well-being (including anxiety, depression, and vitality), physical symptoms, sexual functioning, cognitive functioning, work performance and satisfaction, and social participation. Quality of life was measured prior to a 4-week placebo period and at 4, 8 and 24 weeks into active treatment. Multivariate procedures were used, and when univariate tests were performed on the basis of an overall significant multivariate statistic, multiple range procedures were employed to minimize Type I error. Results showed that patients taking captopril had significantly more favorable scores on the quality of life measures than those on methyldopa or propranolol.

The Croog et al. (50) clinical trial is an example of a generally well-designed study that uses a battery approach to assess quality of life. The use of a double-blind, randomized design, well-validated measures of multiple quality of life dimensions, the large number of patients studied, and the use of multivariate statistical analyses are positive features of this study. Methodological flaws include the lack of a placebo period during the active treatment phase (although a placebo period was used prior to treatment). Additionally, questions have been raised about the type and dosages of drugs used in the study (i.e., the two drugs being compared to captopril have well-documented side effects).

Several major issues raised by the Croog et al. study are unique to a battery approach. First, although quality of life was assessed at multiple times (prior to placebo, following the 4-week placebo period, after 8 weeks of treatment, and after 24 weeks of treatment), the only statistical comparisons reported are changes from the pretreatment (postplacebo) measure to that administered at 24 weeks of therapy. This approach does not allow an assessment of patterns across time. However, an analysis of change across time is particularly difficult when multiple measures are used. Complex statistical techniques such as multivariate repeated measures analyses of variance are required, and problems occur when data are missing for some measurement periods. The handling of missing data is a controversial issue in quality of life research in general, particularly when attrition is due to death or major morbidity. It is extremely problematic with multivariate repeated measures designs, however, since equal sample sizes are needed at each measurement period.

Another issue raised by the Croog et al. study is the decision to assess quality of life comprehensively, with inclusion of measures that cover a broad range of quality of life domains, versus inclusion of only those domains that are relevant to the treatments or diseases under study. The former approach, adopted by Croog et al., is a more general quality of life measurement strategy whereas the latter is more disease- and treatment-specific. The use of a general measurement strategy may be more desirable when the effects of the treatment or disease on quality of life are largely unknown (for example, when quality of life is being assessed for a new drug or category of drugs or for one whose effects are not well-documented). However, when quality of life components that are not clearly linked to a specific treatment are included in a battery, they may simply add unnecessary complexity to the design and analysis. For example, it is not clear why any of the hypertension medications used in the Croog et al. study would affect neuropsychological functioning. It may therefore be preferable to use disease-specific quality of life measures, with clearly stated hypothesized relationships between these measures and the treatments or disease processes under study.

SUMMARY AND CONCLUSIONS

A battery-based approach to quality of life assessment in clinical trials requires careful consideration of: (a) the dimensions of quality of life most relevant to the clinical trial, (b) the best available instruments for the dimensions of quality of life to be measured, and (c) the analytical techniques required in multiple measure studies. In this chapter the basis for evaluating instruments that tap the psychologically oriented quality of life dimensions are considered and the psychometric properties of a few of the more frequently used psychological measures are described. The presentation is not an exhaustive review of psychological measures. Rather, it provides a guide to the criteria that should be used in instrument selection when a battery approach is desired to evaluate quality of life.

There are currently available instruments that assess each of the six dimensions of quality of life; however, they vary considerably with respect to the psychometric properties reviewed in this chapter. Furthermore, most of the available instruments were not designed to reliably discriminate between treatment effects in the homogenous populations that are frequently sampled in clinical trials. (This latter point is also true of the indices specifically developed for quality of life assessment.)

Most "dimensions" of quality of life are composed of several components, each of which would require a separate instrument to evaluate. For example, emotional or affective functioning might include anxiety and depression (the most common constructs assessed) as well as variables such as hostility, anger, or happiness. Cognitive functioning can be assessed with a broad range of instruments that examine factors such as short- or long-term memory, visual reproduction, facial recognition, laterality, or confusion. Thus, in selecting instruments for a quality of life battery, the relevant aspects of each quality of life dimension must be considered. For example, if a treatment may affect cognitive functioning, then the investigator must determine what specific aspects of cognitive functioning are most likely to be influenced by treatment, because a full neuropsychological battery could easily take up to 4 hours for each patient to complete.

A battery approach to quality of life assessment of psychological well-being has the potential of providing rich data on this inherently multidimensional concept. Furthermore, a reliable measure of each dimension of quality of life recognizes the variable impact that any treatment has on various aspects of an individual's functioning and also allows for targeted interventions. Although, there are instruments available to assess the various quality of life dimensions, a battery approach has its drawbacks. In most clinical trials a separate instrument for each dimension of quality of life is impractical in terms of patient burden, staff time, and data analysis. Thus, a carefully selected subset of instruments are recommended for quality of life assessments of psychological well-being.

REFERENCES

1. Andrews FM, Withey SB. *Social indicators of well-being: Americans' perceptions of life quality.* New York: Plenum, 1976.
2. Wenger NK, Mattson ME, Furberg CD, Elinson J, eds. *Assessment of quality of life in clinical trials of cardiovascular therapies.* Washington, D.C.: LeJacq, 1984.
3. Katz S, guest ed. The Portugal conference: Measuring quality of life and functional status in clinical and epidemiological research. *J Chronic Dis* 1987;40(6), special issue.
4. Shumaker SA. Quality of life research in NHLBI-sponsored trials. In: Shumaker SA, Furberg C, eds. Research on quality of life and cardiovascular disease. Special issue, *Am J Prev Med (in press).*
5. Kaplan R, Stewart A. Pros and cons of single versus multi-outcome quality of life assessments. In: Shumaker SA, Furberg C, eds. Research on quality of life and cardiovascular disease. Special issue, *Am J Prev Med (in press).*
6. Spielberger CD. *Manual for the State-Trait Anxiety Inventory (Form Y).* Palo Alto, CA: Consulting Psychologists Press, 1983.
7. Lubin B. *Manual for the Depression Adjective Checklists.* San Diego, CA: Education and Industrial Testing Service, 1967.
8. Gallagher D, Nies G, Thompson L. Reliability of the Beck Depression Inventory with older adults. *J Consult Clin Psychol* 1974;50:152–153.
9. Zung WW. A self-rating depression scale. *Arch Gen Psychiatry* 1970;12:63–70.
10. Cook TD, Campbell DT. *Quasi-experimentation: Design & analysis issues for field settings,* Boston: Houghton Mifflin, 1976.
11. Babbie ER. *Survey research methods.* Belmont, CA: Wadsworth, 1973.
12. Dupuy J. The Psychological General Well-being (PGWB) Scale. In: Wenger N, Mattson M, Furberg C, Elinson J, eds. *Assessment of quality of life in clinical trials of cardiovascular therapies.* pp. 170–199. Washington, D.C.: Le Jacq, 1984.
13. Goldberg D. Manual of the general health questionnaire. Windsor, England: NFER Publishing, 1979.
14. Ware JE, Johnston S, Davies-Avery A, Brook R. *Conceptualization and measurement of health status for adults in the Health Insurance Study: Vol. III, mental health.* Santa Monica, CA: Rand Corporation (R-1987/3-HEW), 1979.
15. Bergner M, Bobbitt RA, Carter WB, et al. The Sickness Impact Profile: Development and final revision of a health status measure. *Med Care* 1981;19:787–805.
16. Cleary PD, Goldberg ID, Kessler LG, Nycz GR. Screening for mental disorder among primary care patients. *Arch Gen Psychiatry* 1982;39:837–840.

17. Goldberg DP, Hillier V. A scaled version of the General Health Questionnaire. *Psychol Med* 1979;9:139–145.
18. Goldberg DP, Cooper B, Eastwood MR, et al. A standardized psychiatric interview for use in community surveys. *Br J Prev Soc Med* 1970;24:18–23.
19. Goldberg D, Rickels K, Downing R, et al. A comparison of two psychiatric screening tests. *Br J Psychiatry* 1976;129:61–67.
20. Goldberg DP. The detection of psychiatric illness by questionnaire. London: Oxford University Press, 1972.
21. Goldberg DP, Blackwell B. Psychiatric illness in general practice: A detailed study using a new method of case identification. *Br Med J* 1970;2:439–443.
22. DePaulo JR, Folstein M, Gordon B. Psychiatric screening on a neurological ward. *Psychol Med* 1980;10:125–132.
23. Gotlib IH. Depression and general psychopathology in university students. *J Abnorm Psychol* 1984;1:19–30.
24. McNair DM, Lorr M, Droppleman LF. *EITS Manual for the Profile of Mood States*. San Diego, CA: Educational Testing Service, 1971.
25. Beck AT, Ward CH, Mendelson M, et al. An inventory for measuring depression. *Arch Gen Psychiatry* 1961;4:561–571.
26. Radloff LS. The CES-D scale: A self-report depression scale for research in the general population. *Appl Psychol Measurement* 1977;1:385–401.
27. Carroll BJ, Fielding JM, Blashki TG. Depression rating scales: A critical review. *Archives of General Psychiatry*, 1973;28:361–366.
28. Schwab JJ, Bialow M, Brown JM, Holzer CE. Diagnosing depression in medical inpatients. *Ann Intern Med* 1967;67:695–707.
29. Carney RM, Rich MW, Telvede A, et al. Major depressive disorder in coronary artery disease. *Am J Cardiol* 1987;60:1273–1275.
30. Salkind MR. Beck Depression Inventory in general practice. *J R Coll Gen Pract* 1969;18:267–271.
31. The Cardiac Arrhythmia Pilot Study (CAPS) Investigators: Recruitment and baseline description of patients in the Cardiac Arrhythmia Pilot Study. *Am J Cardiol* 1988;61:704–713.
32. Bumberry WO, Oliver JM, McClue JN. Validation of the Beck Depression Inventory in a university population using psychiatric estimate as the criterion. *J Consult Clin Psychol* 1978;48:150–155.
33. Tanaka-Matsumi J, Kameoka V. Reliabilities and concurrent validities of popular self-report measures of depression, anxiety, and social desirability. *J Consult Clin Psychol* 1986;54(3):328–333.
34. Gallagher D, Nies G, Thompson LW. Reliability of the Beck Depression Inventory with older adults. *J Consult Clin Psychol* 1961;50:152–153.
35. Strober M, Green J, Carlson G. Utility of the Beck Depression Inventory with psychiatrically hospitalized adolescents. *J Consult Clin Psychol* 1981;49:482–483.
36. Marcella A, Sanborn K, Kameoka V. Cross validation of self-report measures of depression among normal populations of Japanese, Chinese, and Caucasian ancestry. *J Clin Psychol* 1975;31:281–286.
37. Lubin B. Adjective checklists for measurement of depression. *Arch Gen Psychiatry* 1965;12:57–62.
38. Dinning WD, Evans RG. Discriminant and convergent validity of the SCL-90 in psychiatric inpatients. *J Pers Assess* 1977;41:304–310.
39. Hamilton M. A rating scale for depression. *J Neurol Neurosurg Psychiatry* 1960;23:55–62.
40. Hammen CL. Depression in college students: Beyond the Beck Depression Inventory. *J Consult Clin Psychol* 1977;48:126–128.
41. Meites K, Lovallo W, Pishkin V. A comparison of four scales for anxiety, depression, and neuroticism. *J Clin Psychol* 1980;36:427–432.
42. Zung WW. *The measurement of depression*. Cincinnati: Merrell-National Laboratories, 1974.
43. Hedlund JL, Vieweg BW. The Zung Self-Rating Depression Scale: A comprehensive review. *J Oper Psychiatry* 1979;10(1):51–63.
44. Weissman MM, Sholomskas D, Pottenger M, et al. Assessing depressive symptoms in five psychiatric populations: A validation study. *Am J Epidemiol* 1977;106:203–214.
45. Orme JG. Factorial and discriminant validity of the Center for Epidemiologic Studies of Depression. *J Clin Psychol* 1986;42(1):28–33.
46. Myers JK, Weissman MM. Use of a self-report symptom scale to detect depression in a community sample. *Am J Psychiatry* 1980;137:1081–1084.
47. Husaini BA, Neff JA, Harrington JB, et al. Depression in rural communities: Validating the CES-D scale. *J Community Psychol* 1980;8:20–27.
48. Vagg PR, Spielberger CD, O'Hearn TP. Is the State-Trait Anxiety Inventory multidimensional? *Pers Indiv Diff* 1980;1:207–214.
49. Hill JF, Bulpitt CJ, Fletcher AE. Angiotensin converting enzyme inhibitors and quality of life: The European trial. *J Hypert* 1985;3 (Suppl. 2):S91–S94.
50. Croog SH, Levine S, Testa MA, Brown B, Bulpitt CJ, Jenkins CD, Klerman GL, Williams GH. The effects of antihypertensive therapy on the quality of life. *NEJM* 1986;314:1657–1664.

51. Siegrist J, Matschinger H, Motz W. Untreated hypertensives and their quality of life. *J Hypert* 1987;5 (Suppl. 1):S15–S20.
52. Wiklund I, Sanne H, Vedin A, Wilhelmsson C. Psychosocial outcome one year after a first myocardial infarction. *J Psychosom Res* 1984;28:309–321.
53. Patel C, Marmot MG. Stress management, blood pressure and quality of life. *J Hypert* 1987;5 (Suppl. 1):S21–S28.
54. Naismith LD, Robinson JF, Shaw GB, MacIntyre MM. Psychological rehabilitation after myocardial infarction. *Br Med J* 1979;1:439–442.
55. LaMendola W, Pellegrini R. Quality of life and coronary artery bypass surgery patients. *Soc Sci Med* 1979;13A:457–461.
56. Flynn MK, Frantz R. Coronary artery bypass surgery: Quality of life during early convalescence. *Heart Lung* 1987;16:159–167.
57. Raft D, McKee DC, Popio KA, Haggerty JJ. Life adaptation after percutaneous transluminal coronary angioplasty and coronary artery bypass grafting. *Am J Cardiol* 1985;56:395–398.
58. Mayou R, Foster A, Williamson B. Psychosocial adjustment in patients one year after myocardial infarction. *J Psychosom Res* 1978;22:447–453.
59. Trelawny-Ross C, Russell O. Social and psychological responses to myocardial infarction: Multiple determinants of outcome at six months. *J Psychosom Med* 1987;31:125–130.
60. Gundle MD, Reeves BR, Tate S, Raft D, McLaurin L. Psychosocial outcome after coronary artery surgery. *Am J Psychiatry* 1980;137:1591–1594.
61. Jenkins CD, Stanton B, Savageau JA, Denlinger P, Klein MD. Coronary artery bypass surgery: Physical, psychological, social and economic outcomes six months later. *JAMA* 1983;250:782–788.

Quality of Life Assessments in Clinical Trials, edited by B. Spilker. Raven Press, Ltd. New York, 1990.

10

Functional Disability Scales

William D. Spector

National Center for Health Services Research, Rockville, Maryland 20857

The periodic assessment of physical disabilities has become an integral part of the standard medical evaluation of elders, supplementing the diagnosis, history, laboratory tests, and physical examination. Goals of treatment for chronic diseases include measures that go beyond notions of cure and survival, to more sensitive measures of progress which relate to overall functioning. Interventions for chronic diseases are applied at any point along the disease-impairment-disability-handicap continuum (1,2). Increasingly, clinicians and researchers need reliable and validated measures of functional disability to measure clinical progress, evaluate programs, and establish appropriate eligibility criteria for social and insurance programs (3–5).

Considered here are a small number of functional disability scales for which reliability and validity have been studied and which have gained some acceptance in the clinical and health services research field. The scales included vary greatly in terms of the scope of their use and the extensiveness of the validation work that has been published.

Most of the scales discussed are not new. To a large extent this is because many of the newer scales have not been extensively evaluated. The chapter includes a discussion of the Pfeffer Functional Activities Questionnaire, which is relatively new (less than 10 years old) compared with the other scales which are as much as 40 years old. Although the newer scale has not gained large acceptance, the conceptual basis of the scale and the relatively extensive research on reliability and validity make it worthy of inclusion.

Functional disability measures can be grouped into generic and disease-specific scales. This chapter is concerned with generic measures including activities of daily living, instrumental activities of daily living, and mobility. The disease-specific scales are discussed elsewhere in this book. Multidimensional scales that include functional disability items as one dimension are also not discussed here. A number of articles present a more comprehensive review of disability measures (6–9). The reader may refer to these reviews for descriptions of other instruments.

This chapter focuses mainly on four scales and variations of these scales: the Index of Activities of Daily Living (10), the Barthel Index (11), the Instrumental Activities of Daily Living Scale (12), and the Functional Activities Questionnaire (13). Scales that combine instrumental activities of daily living and activities of daily living measures are also reviewed but mainly with the intent to discuss methodological issues.

DEFINING DISABILITY AND IMPAIRMENT

In this chapter we define terms following the World Health Organization's International Classification of Impairments, Disabilities, and Handicaps. Using this approach, *impairments* are defined as abnormalities of body structure and appearance and organ or system function, resulting from any cause. These include mental impairments and loss of limbs, and limitations in range of motion, for example. *Disabilities* are defined as "restrictions or lack of ability to perform an activity in a manner or within the range considered normal for a human being." Impairments relate to performance of an organ or mechanism; disability relates to the performance of an activity by an individual. A person may be mentally impaired, have restricted range of motion, or be missing an arm, but not show any disabilities because he or she can carry out all basic activities independently. In another example, limitations in eye function, referred to as visual impairment, may result in an inability to dress or wash oneself, which are examples of disabilities.

The disability definition used here contrasts with the broader definition that is often used in literature on disability associated with persons under 65 years of age. There disability usually refers to specifc tasks associated with roles in society. Disability from this point of view includes concepts such as work disability (14–16). This broader definition overlaps with the World Health Organization definition of *handicap*, "a disadvantage for a given individual resulting from an impairment or a disability, that limits or prevents the fulfillment of a role that is normal for that individual." Some researchers distinguish between work disability and disability in community living (17). To clarify this distinction, the term *functional disability* is used in this chapter to refer to the narrower definition of disability which includes only activities related to community living (activities of daily living and instrumental activities of daily living), but not limitations in work roles.

Many of the scales that have been developed are based on unifying concepts other than disability, such as self-care, for example. Consequently they include measures other than disabilities. When this occurs note is made of it in our discussion, so constructs can be clarified.

METHODOLOGICAL CONSIDERATIONS

Kirshner and Guyatt (18) have suggested a framewrok for evaluating health indices. They divide scale development into six aspects: selection of item pool, item scaling, item reduction, reliability, validity, and responsiveness. A seventh aspect, the purpose of the scale, they treat as an overriding factor that affects all other aspects of the scale. This framework was used as a guide to compare and contrast the disability scales discussed in this chapter.

The description of each scale is divided into six sections: description, purpose and use, scale structure, reliability, validity, and responsiveness. The quality of research on disability scales for each of these topics varies. When results for a specific topic are sparse, general methodological concerns are discussed. The discussion of responsiveness is almost totally conceptual, because few studies are available that provide change information on standardized scales. This chapter reviews the two activities of daily living scales separately, discusses the Instrumental Activities of Daily Living Scale, and concludes with a brief discussion of scales that involve both activities of daily living and instrumental activities of daily living measures.

ACTIVITIES OF DAILY LIVING SCALES: KATZ SCALE OF ACTIVITIES OF DAILY LIVING AND THE BARTHEL INDEX

Descriptions

The Katz Activities of Daily Living scale is based on six functions: bathing, dressing, going to the toilet, transferring (bed to chair), continence, and feeding. The scale includes basic self-care activities. One of the items, transfer, may be classified as a measure of mobility; incontinence may be classified as an impairment. The items in the scale and their respective definitions are conceptually based to reflect the organized locomotor and neurologic aspects of basic activities necessary for survival independent of cultural and social forces. In studies of recovery from chronic disease, the order of recovery using the Katz scale is similar to the progression of functional development of a child (10).

Each activity is divided into three levels, but these levels can be combined so that each activity can be dichotomized to independence and dependence. Patients who are independent do the activity without human assistance, but they may use a prosthesis. Human assistance includes supervision as well as hands-on help.

Using the dichotomies, an ordered unidimensional aggregate scale can be constructed. The aggregate scale consists of eight levels designated by the letters A to G, plus "other." The levels of disability are as follows: independent in all six functions; dependent in one function; dependent in bathing plus one other; dependent in bathing, dressing, plus one other; dependent in bathing, dressing, toileting, plus one other; dependent in bathing, dressing, toileting, transferring, plus one other; dependent in all six functions; and other. Other includes all patterns that do not fit into the above categories. Persons with these patterns are less disabled than those classified in the G category, but more disabled than those classified in A or B. The scale is sometimes scored by counting the number of dysfunctions, thereby eliminating the "other" category. This approach relies heavily on the Guttman properties of the scale, which may vary depending on the specific implementation of the scale.

The scale was designed to be administered as an assessment completed by a clinician, but use by nonclinicians with knowledge of gerontology has been reported (10). Information is derived from direct observation of residents, discussion with the primary caregiver, and from medical records. For demented residents, information is derived from the primary caregiver and medical records only. The final score is based on judgment of the assessor after reviewing information from all sources.

The Katz scale is a measure of performance. Some scales, such as the Barthel Index, measure ability. The advantage to measuring performance is that it measures a real situation, whereas the second approach often assesses a hypothetical situation (i.e., if a person were to consider doing this activity, would he be able to do it?). Psychological and personality characteristics of the individual may confound an assessment based on a hypothetical situation. The disadvantage is that the performance measure is influenced by motivation and environmental factors that may enable or inhibit a person from doing a set of activities on his/her own. It therefore crosses the dimensions of social roles and activities as well as physical problems. Performance measures may better reflect the need for services, however. One approach used in some large surveys has been to ask about performance, but also determine if the lack of performance is due to a disability or health problem.

The Barthel Index includes 15 items: drinking, feeding, dressing upper body, dressing lower body, donning brace or prosthesis, grooming, washing and bathing, bladder control, bowel control, chair transfers, toilet transfers, tub/shower transfers, walking on level for 50 yards, climbing one flight of stairs, and maneuvering a wheel chair. The first nine activities may be classified as self-care items, whereas the next six items are measures of mobility (11).

The Barthel Index includes a much more comprehensive assessment of mobility than the Katz scale. The Barthel Index has incontinence separated into bowel and bladder incontinence and provides more detail for dressing by distinguishing between upper body and lower body limitations, whereas the Katz scale combines them. Each item in the Barthel Index is valued on three levels: can do by oneself, can do with the help of someone else, and cannot do at all. In contrast to the Katz scale, these items are measures of ability ("can do") and not performance ("do"). Arbitrary weights ranging from 0 to 15 are used to create an aggregate score. A score of 0 represents total dependence and a score of 100 represents total independence.

Purpose and Use

The Katz Activities of Daily Living (ADL) scale was developed as an evaluative tool to study the results of treatment and prognosis in the elderly and chronically ill, but it has been used for a number of purposes both as originally designed or in modified forms. The Katz scale was developed at the Benjamin Rose Hospital, a chronic care hospital, and early studies using the scale studied recovery from stroke, fracture of the hip, and rheumatoid arthritis (19–21). More recent studies have used the Katz scale in nursing homes (22–25). For these populations the scale discriminates well, providing a good distribution of disability levels with few elders that are not disabled based on the scale and few elders that are totally disabled on all items. For nursing home residents, a useful modification to improve discrimination was made by Spector et al. (26) in which the final category was divided into those who were dependent in 5 ADLs plus needed some human help with feeding and those who were dependent in 5 ADLs plus needed total help with feeding (resident does not participate or was fed intravenously or with tubes).

The scale has also been used in studies of elders in the community. For this population the scale does not discriminate well. Branch et al. (27), using a Katz Activities of Daily Living scale modified for personal interview rather than assessment (with only four items), found 7.6% dependent based on the scale. Adding grooming and walking across a small room increased the frequency to 15.9%.

The Katz scale has also been used to measure functional deterioration as a health status measure to evaluate effectiveness in major health services experiments. In the "Continued Care Study," the effectiveness of regular home visits by a public health nurse after discharge from a rehabilitation hospital was evaluated. In the "Chance for Change" study, the effectiveness of home visits by health assistants working with an interdisciplinary team after discharge from an acute hospital was evaluated (28,29).

The Barthel Index was developed in a chronic hospital setting (11) and has become the instrument of choice for rehabilitation studies. In contrast to the Katz scale, it has not been adopted for studying disabled elders in the community. The scale has been used to monitor progress for severely disabled persons in comprehensive medical rehabilitation centers (30). Studies of stroke have shown a correlation between admission and discharge scores on the Barthel Index and discharge location and recovery. A higher likelihood of recovery was found for those with an admission score of 21 or greater and discharge scores of 41 or greater. A high proportion of those attaining a score of 61 or more returned home (31). Studies of functional change from stroke rehabilitation using the Barthel Index have demonstrated that the motor persistence score and half-hour recall are the strongest psychological predictors of recovery (32). Urinary incontinence, arm motor deficit, sitting balance, hemianopia, and age were found to be the greatest physical predictors of recovery (33).

Scale Structure of the Katz Activities of Daily Living Scale and the Barthel Index

The Katz scale is a semi-Guttman scale. A Guttman scale orders items with one pattern by degree of severity. For example, if a person is dependent in feeding, he would also be dependent in bathing, dressing, toileting, transferring, and continence, for example. In the 1963 paper, 86% of persons were represented by the strict hierarchy.

Other researchers have presented coefficients of reproducibility (CR) and scalability (CS) for the Katz Activities of Daily Living scale. The coefficient of reproducibility, the percent of total possible errors that are not made by using the strict pattern, is reported with analyses of ordered scales. It is a measure of both reliability and reproducibility. The original article by Guttman sets a standard of .90 or greater for a reliable and reproducible scale (34). A second measure, the coefficient of scalability, measures the amout of improvement over the minimum coefficient of reproducibility. A minimum CR greater than 0 occurs when there are persons on the extremes of the scale (i.e., totally dependent or totally independent). A minimum standard for the coefficient of scalability is .60. Kane and Kane (7) report studies at the Hebrew Rehabilitation Center for the Aged that found coefficients of reproducibility of greater than .94 for samples of home care recipients and a sheltered home sample. Spector et al. (24) looked at a nursing home population, and report a coefficient of reproducibility of .95 and a coefficient of scalability of .86. Researchers in Sweden report CS's above .70 with patients in acute care settings (35–37).

The Katz scale is a semi-Guttman scale because it does not use the order of items strictly as determined by the Guttman analysis, but includes levels defined, for example, as dependency in one activity of daily living, or dependency in bathing + one activity of daily living. Although the scale exceeds all scaling standards for a Guttman scale, the researchers were not willing to consider all nonhierarchical patterns as error. Therefore a number of patterns were combined in the scale and were not all placed into the "other" category, which is the closest category the researchers have to represent error. The patterns that were grouped together were treated as representing equivalent degrees of disability.

Although the hierarchical properties of the activities of daily living measure have been reported by Katz, it is important for users to test the scalability of their own data to determine if their particular implementation of the measure meets the standards derived from these other experiences. Differences in sample populations and modifications of the scales such as a different reference period, adding (e.g., grooming) or replacing items (e.g., walking for transferring), or variations in definitions (e.g., including cutting meat in eating dependency) may alter the scale properties and the ordered relationship of items.

The Barthel Index is not an ordered scale. Aggregation is based on a weighting scheme and as such does not guarantee that there is a uniform underlying dimension as is implied with the Katz scale. Interpretation of the Barthel Index is more difficult as a result, because it is not certain that a lower score on the Barthel, for example, implies more disability, unless one is confident that the arbitrary weights are correct. Secondly, the same score may result from a number of different profiles. If there is concern over loss of specific profile information when an aggregate scale is used, individual item scores may be retained and used to supplement the aggregate scores for completeness of information.

Reliability

Reliability is the proportion of the true variance to the total variance. There are three basic reliability measures: interperson reliability (consistency of scoring between different individuals), test re-test reliability (consistency of scoring over a short period of time when subjects have not changed), and internal reliability, the correlation of individual items to the total score. Internal reliability is usually measured with Chronbach's alpha (38). The coefficient of reproducibility is also a measure of reliability for ordered scales. Published reports of reliability using the Katz and Barthel instruments are not extensive, however.

The coefficient of reproducibility as discussed above is a measure of the internal consistency of an ordered measure. These results have been discussed above for the Katz scale. Katz et al. (10) report an interperson reliability of .95 or better after training. Spector et al. (24) report a similar experience. Test re-test reliability has not been reported.

The Barthel Index has been shown to have both high test re-test reliability and interperson reliability. Granger, Albrecht, and Hamilton (30) report test re-test reliability of .89 and interperson reliability of .95. High internal reliability has also been found in studies at the Hebrew Rehabilitiation Center for the Aged (alpha scores of between .953 and .965) (7). Shiner et al. (39) report high interperson reliability and test re-test reliability with stroke patients both at the individual item level and the aggregate level, comparing results from observers and administrators and among observers and among administrators. Individual Spearman's rho correlations ranged from .71 to 1.00. Interperson reliabilities ranged from .75 to 1.00. The lowest correlations were found for wash and bathe and grooming. Overall pearson R correlations for the aggregate scores were .99 or higher. Mean scores were almost identical for each group. The Chronbach alpha for each item was .98 or higher. Results comparing a personal interview with a telephone interview resulted in a mean score by telephone of 85.9 compared with 86.6, and correlations ranging from .70 to 1.00. For proxies, correlations ranged from .85 to 1.00. The authors emphasize that these results are dependent on highly trained interviewers. They advise that telephone interviews should not be given to patients who may score differently on verbal responses versus performance.

Sensitivity to Setting

There is concern that the measurement of disability used in a clinical trial may be sensitive to the study's setting. Few comparisons have been made on the same persons over a short period of time in different settings (e.g., hospital versus nursing home, hospital versus home). Depending on how the measures are defined, the sensitivity to setting may differ. Katz et al. (10) warn that the Katz scale is sensitive to environmental artifacts. In both hospitals and nursing homes, organizational rules often established because of concerns for safety and cost may affect the score on dressing, transferring, toileting, or bathing. Because the scale is based on actual performance, not ability, the Katz scale is particularly sensitive. The Barthel Index, which is an ability measure, should be less sensitive. The differential availability of prosthetic devices also may affect the disability score in alternative settings. Comparisons of assessments in the hospital and in the home over a short period with a modified index of activities of daily living have found more severe disability measured in the home. Presumably this results from the unavailability of many mechanical devices in the home (40,41). In some circumstances, Katz et al. (10) recommend that ability as well as performance may need to be assessed to determine the impact of environmental artifacts on the disability score. One approach is to ask the resident to simulate the activity.

Validity

Three measures of validity are usually determined: criterion validity, content validity, and construct validity. Criterion validity refers to the extent that the same results as a gold standard are produced. Content validity refers to the judgment that the items included in the scale are representative of the domain measured. Construct validity refers to the variation explained by other constructs or tests. A fourth aspect of validity, sometimes included with construct validity, is the ability to predict. Kane (42) argues that the ability of a scale to predict who will get medical problems is the ultimate test of a scale.

There are no gold standards for disability measures. Therefore, validity testing for these scales is limited to content and construct validations. With respect to content validity, the Katz scale includes measures of basic self-care. All measures would be classified as disability measures except incontinence, an impairment. However, in general, incontinence fits the hierarchy, and with incontinence included, the scale exceeds standards for scalability.

Some research has suggested that incontinence should not be included in the scale, but treated separately. Jagger, Clarke, and Davies (43), with questions similar to those in the Katz scale and using principal component analysis, identified two components, physical activities and incontinence of feces and urine. Nevertheless, inclusion of incontinence for a population of nursing home residents improves discrimination. One solution may be to present the information with two scores for each person: a physical activities score and a continence score.

With respect to construct validity of the Katz scale, Katz et al. (44) report moderate correlations for the index of activities of daily living with measures of range of motion, intelligence, and orientation. Jackson et al. (25), using the Katz scale, showed a positive relationship between more disability and the proportion of nursing home residents with at least one disruptive behavior.

The Katz scale has been shown to have predictive validity also. Other studies have demonstrated a positive relationship between activities of daily living dependency level and mortality among nursing home residents. These studies also showed a relationship between the Katz scale and discharge status (26,45). Spector et al. (26) found the relationship weakened as length of stay increased.

The Barthel Index includes measures of self-care and mobility, as well as continence. Jette (46,47), in two articles examining the correlations of a number of self-care, instrumental, and basic activities of daily living, identified five dimensions. The dimensions varied slightly in the two studies. At issue was the combination of mobility transfers from chair to bed, and items such as attending meetings and driving a car. If transferring and mobility are combined as in the second study, the Barthel may be viewed as a two-dimensional scale including mobility and personal care items. Incontinence was not included in either of the Jette studies.

A number of construct validity results have been reported for the Barthel Index. The scale is highly correlated with both the Katz scale and the Kenny Self-Care Evaluation (48), and the Pulses Profile (30). For patients in a comprehensive stroke program, the admission Barthel score discriminated between those who died and those who survived (mean score of 6.2 versus 41.9) (31). Other studies have found similar results (49,50). The scale also predicts the likelihood of discharge home. Those with an admission score of 20 or less were much less likely to return home than those with a discharge score of more than 20. Those with a discharge score of 60 or less were less likely to be discharged home than those with a discharge score of more than 60 (31,51).

For chronically ill persons living alone, the Barthel score was highly correlated with the number of personal care tasks performed independently. Low correlations were found for household tasks such as light housework and cooking meals, but no relationships were found for instrumental activities such as shopping, laundry, and heavy housecleaning. The Barthel Index was also shown to be negatively correlated with psychological measures and age. Those with more disability were less likely to make decisions easily, had decreased ability to fulfill usual roles, and were more likely to be disoriented or depressed. Those with more disability were likely to be older (52).

Using a modified activities of daily living index (17 items that are similar to the Barthel Index), Sheikh et al. (40) compared scores on the activities of daily living scale with the number of neurological deficits, a measure of the extent of cerebral lesions. Those scoring high on activities of daily living had a high number of neurological deficits, and those scoring low had a low number of neurological deficits ($R = .376$). A sensitivity of .70 and a specificity of .87 were found.

The Katz scale and the Barthel Index administered on the same patients produce a high degree of agreement. A Barthel score of between 0 and 49 is comparable to a Katz F or G, a Barthel score of between 50 and 79 is comparable to a D or E, a score of 80 to 99 on the Barthel is comparable to a B or C, and a score of 100 on the Barthel is comparable to an A on the Katz. The Kappa Coefficient of Agreement was .77. The Kappa Coefficient adjusts for random chance of agreement. A score greater than .75 represents excellent agreement (48,53).

Responsiveness of the Instruments to Medical Treatments

The study of functional change is in its infancy, with few published results that may serve as standards for comparison studies. To a large extent this is because change results are very sensitive to the exact formulation of the scale. Studies of change generally have used idiosyncratic versions of the original scales or are not population based. Consequently they are not reported here. Instead, some important methodological issues are reviewed.

For a scale to be useful for clinical studies and health services evaluations, it must be sufficiently responsible to change to detect clinically important changes. A study may show no effect on functional disability levels because the measure is not sensitive enough as well as because the intervention is not effective. This is an important concern.

Scales may be made more sensitive by increasing the number of levels of severity. However, increase in the number of levels of an item is accompanied by reduced reliability. In addition, these distinctions need to be clinically meaningful. Although the ability to distinguish between measurement error and true change is important, disability studies generally have not made appropriate corrections for attenuation when evaluating correlations with change measures (54).

INSTRUMENTAL ACTIVITIES OF DAILY LIVING

Instrumental activities of daily living scales include activities that concern a person's ability to adapt to the environment. The activities include items such as shopping, use of transportation, meal preparation, and housework. Independence on these scales demonstrates an ability to live independently in the community. Residents in specialized housing may be able to maintain independence, although they are dependent in some of the items if services are provided in these settings. The scales are generally not appropriate for residents in nursing homes or other institutions, but discriminate well in continuing care community environments which generally include an assisted living level of care. Norms for residents in different settings have not been established.

In general instrumental activities of daily living measures are recommended to supplement activities of daily living as part of a geriatric assessment for a population of elders, expanding the number of disabilities that can be identified. Its use as a clinical tool in an institutional environment is limited, but may be useful in discharge planning from a hospital (3–5).

The Lawton Instrumental Activities of Daily Living Scale and the Older Americans Resources and Services Instrument

In the Lawton scale, the instrumental activities of daily living (12) include eight items: ability to telephone, shopping, food preparation, housekeeping, laundry, transportation, medications, and ability to handle finances. All eight items are used for women but only five are used for men as food preparation, housekeeping, and laundry are eliminated. The scale measures performance in contrast to ability. Instrumental activities of daily living questions incorporated into multidimensional instruments use modifications of the Lawton scale using all items for men, but question if the inability is due to a disability or health problem (e.g., 1982 and 1984 National Long-Term Care Surveys). The Duke Older Americans Resources and Services instrument asks all questions of both men and women but asks about ability, not performance (55).

The Pfeffer Functional Activity Questionnaire

The Pfeffer Functional Activities Questionnaire, a 10-item scale, expands on the Lawton Instrumental Activities of Daily Living Scale by including measures more directly tapping cognition: tracks current events; pays attention to, understands, and discusses plot of television programs, books, or magazines; remembers appointments, medicines, or other things; and plays skilled games or hobbies. The scale has items similar to the Lawton scale: shopping, simple financial activities, and meal preparation. In addition there is a more difficult financial activity than in the Lawton scale, and a preparation of tea or coffee item. Activities such as use of the telephone, housekeeping, or laundry are not included.

The scale is administered by a nonprofessional. Each item is divided into six levels: someone has recently taken over the activity; requires advice or assistance; does without assistance or advice but more difficult than used to; does without difficulty or advice; never did, and would find it difficult to start now; and never did, but can do if had to. The first four levels are scaled from 0 to 3 and the last two levels are scored 1 and 0, respectively.

Purpose and Use of Instrumental Activities of Daily Living Scales

Lawton (56) indicates that the Instrumental Activities of Daily Living Scale was intended to identify independence on tasks instrumental to an independent life. It is recommended for use as a guide to help identify the optimum living situation for an elderly person. The instrumental activities of daily living are viewed as a set of activities on a continuum of complexity between physical self-maintenance on activities of daily living and effectance behaviors: recreational and creative behaviors. Although a number of studies have used instrumental activities of daily living items, generally the Lawton scale has been modified and the ordered relationship of the items has been ignored.

The Functional Activity Questionnaire was designed to sample activities more complex than those on the Lawton scale, but which are universal. It was envisioned for use in retirement communities with the intent to tap mild dementia (13). It has not received wide acceptance, but its conceptual basis and psychometric properties suggest increased use in the future.

Scaling Instrumental Activities of Daily Living Scales

The Lawton Instrumental Activities of Daily Living Scale is a Guttman scale. The CR for the Instrumental Activities of Daily Living Scale is reported as .96 for men and .93 for women in the original article (12). The scale orders from the most dependent in the following order: unable to use telephone, takes care of all shopping needs, plans and prepares and serves adequate meals independently, maintains light housework independently, does all laundry, travels by car or public transportation, takes medications with correct dosage at right time, and manages all financial tasks except major purchases or banking.

The Pfeffer scale aggregates six levels for each of the 10 items by using arbitrary weights: dependent = 3, requires assistance = 2, has difficulty = 1, never did and would have difficulty = 1, did not do, but could do now = 0. Concern about arbitrary weights has been addressed above.

Reliability of Instrumental Activities of Daily Living Scales

For the Lawton scale, the high coefficients of reproducibility indicate strong internal reliability. Interperson reliability results show a correlation of .85 between total scores for two social workers who scored the same persons. Test re-test reliability results have not been published (13).

For the Pfeffer scale, internal reliability is strong with correlations among individual items on the Functional Activities Questionnaire and total score ranging from .81 to .90. Interrater reliability of a neurologist and nurse was high (Tau B = .802). Test re-test reliability results are not available (13).

Validity of Instrumental Activities of Daily Living Scales

For the Lawton scale, correlations with activities of daily living, mental status, physical health (based on history, physical findings, and laboratory tests), and a behavior and adjustment scale have been reported. Correlations are .77, .74, .50, and .36, respectively (12).

The correlation between a modified Lawton scale (using weights) and the Pfeffer scale was reported as .72 (13). Comparisons of correlations of a modified Lawton scale and measures of social and cognitive function found the Pfeffer scale to be better correlated than the modified Lawton Instrumental Activities of Daily Living Scale. The largest differences were for correlations with estimates of residual deficit by neurologists ($-.83$ and $-.68$, respectively), and the mini mental state ($-.71$ and $-.55$, respectively). This is not surprising because of the larger number of activities in the Pfeffer scale that directly relate to cognition.

COMBINING ACTIVITIES OF DAILY LIVING AND INSTRUMENTAL ACTIVITIES OF DAILY LIVING

To further improve discrimination in healthy populations, an instrumental activities of daily living scale is often combined with an activities of daily living scale to broaden the definition of disability (4,57). The appropriate method for combining activities of daily living and instrumental activities of daily living items has not been thoroughly studied, however. Many researchers use simple aggregation approaches. Often an arbitrary number of activities of daily living and instrumental activities of daily living are combined by counting the total number of disabilities. For example, Jette and Branch (57) combine six activities with five instrumental activities in this manner. No evidence is provided that these items are a Guttman scale or why assigning a weight of one for each activity is appropriate. Nevertheless, scales of this type are interpreted as if more disabilities imply more severe disability.

A couple of scales that have received some interest in the research community that include both instrumental activities of daily living and activities of daily living items are the Rosow Scale and the Rapid Disability Scale. Rosow and Breslau (58) presented a Guttman scale which combines activities of daily living and instrumental activities of daily living items with more emphasis on instrumental activities of daily living. The scale had a CR of .91. The scale is rarely used in total, however, but some of the items have been incorporated in large surveys.

Linn and Linn (59) introduced a modified Rapid Disability Scale which includes detailed activities of daily living, a general instrumental activities of daily living item, and a number of impairments and psychological items. It is a multidimensional scale going beyond activities of daily living and instrumental activities of daily living, but uses a simple scoring system that would be difficult to justify. Reliability results are strong, but validity testing has not been extensive. The scale has been gaining in popularity.

Spector, Katz, et al. (60) analyzed the scalability of four activities of daily living (bathing, dressing, transferring, and feeding) with two instrumental activities of daily living (shopping and transportation). CR's from secondary analysis of data from three studies (Cleveland-GAO study, Georgia-Medicaid study, and the Homemaker-Day Care study) were all above .94. CS's were all above .74. Correlation analyses of individual items indicated that a strict hierarchical relationship between shopping and transportation was not apparent. A number of persons were dependent in shopping and bathing but independent in transportation, whereas another group was dependent only in transportation. Nevertheless, persons dependent in activities of daily living were also dependent in both instrumental activities of daily living; a number of persons were dependent in instrumental activities of daily living only. In the three data sets, few persons were dependent in activities of daily living only (less than 1% in the Georgia-Medicaid and Homemaker-Day Care study, and 2% in the GAO-Cleveland study). The authors suggested that the activities of daily living and instrumental activities of daily living could be combined into the following scale: independent in instrumental activities of daily living and activities of daily living; dependent in shopping or transportation; shopping and transportation; shopping, transportation, plus one activities of daily living; shopping, transportation, bathing, plus one activities of daily living; shopping, transportation, bathing, dressing, plus one activities of daily living; and six activities. For this scale, in the three studies, the frequency of the "other" category ranged from 2.2% to 4.8%.

Validation of the instrumental activities of daily living-activities of daily living hierarchy was based on the three aggregated categories: independent in instrumental activities of daily living and activities of daily living, dependent in instrumental activities of daily living only, and dependent in instrumental activities of daily living and activities of daily living. The level of disability was correlated with age. The independent proportion decreased with age, and the proportion dependent in instrumental activities of daily living only increased with age, as did the proportion dependent in both instrumental activities of daily living and activities of daily living. Those dependent in instrumental activities of daily living were more likely to die in a year than those independent, but were less likely to die than those dependent in both instrumental activities of daily living and activities of daily living. The proportion hospitalized in a year increased with level of disability.

SUMMARY

This chapter attempted to review a small number of functional disability scales, emphasizing scales that include one type of disability measure, either activities of daily living or instrumental activities of daily living. Disability scales that were part of multidimensional instruments including psychological and social dimensions were not reviewed. Selected scales that have received acceptance in the clinical and research arenas and have sufficient reliability and validity were reviewed in detail. These scales vary in terms of the quality and extent of their reliability and validity as well as the number of studies in which they are included. Important differences were highlighted and conceptual concerns were discussed.

In general, any of the scales discussed in detail would be worthy of strong consideration for inclusion in a clinical trial as well as other evaluation studies. No scale is best for all purposes, however. The scale should be chosen based on the specific purpose for its use.

Often, however, these scales are used in modified form for purposes that are broader than their original intent. For example, modifications of these scales have been used in large surveys like the National Medical Expenditure Survey and evaluations of community care demonstrations like the Channelling Demonstration. Also, eligibility criteria used for private long-term care insurance and federally funded home-based programs are typically based on modified measures of disability.

Appropriate evaluation and implementation of programs as well as interpretation of medical research studies depend on proper understanding of the measures that are applied. The properties of these measures should be carefully studied after implementation to insure that established relationships are replicated. This is particularly important if a scale is applied to a new population or if major modifications have been made. Researchers should be cautious about constructing new scales or using scales that have not been validated. They should be equally cautious about combining items in simplistic ways without doing appropriate scalability and validity analyses. The interpretation that a higher score (or lower score) implies more severe disability may be incorrect. Finally, researchers should be encouraged to publish reliability and validity results of scales used in evaluative and population studies to help further understanding of the usefulness of these instruments.

REFERENCES

1. Besdine RW. The educational utility of comprehensive functional assessment in the elderly. *J Am Geriatr Soc* 1983;31:651–656.
2. World Health Organization. *International classification of impairments, disabilities, and handicaps.* Geneva: World Health Organization, 1980.
3. Williams TF. Comprehensive assessment of frail elderly in relation to needs for long-term care. In: Calkins E, Davis PJ, Ford AB, eds. *The Practice of Geriatrics.* Philadelphia: W. B. Saunders, 1986.
4. Kane RL, Ouslander JG, Abrass IB. *Essentials of clinical geriatrics.* New York: McGraw Hill Book Co., 1984.
5. Rubenstein LZ, Abrass IB. Geriatric assessment. In: Exton-Smith AN, Weksler ME, eds. *Practical geriatric medicine.* Edinburgh: Churchill Livingstone, 1985.
6. Ernst M, Ernst NS. Functional capacity. In: Mangen DJ, Peterson WA, eds. *Health, program evaluation, and demography*, vol. 3. Minneapolis: University of Minnesota Press, 1984.
7. Kane RA, Kane RL. *Assessing the elderly.* Lexington, MA: DC Heath, 1981.
8. Deyo RA. Measuring functional outcomes in therapeutic trials for chronic disease. *Controlled Clin Trials* 1984;5:223–240.

9. Hedrick SC, Katz S, Stroud MW. Patient assessment in long-term care: Is there a common language? *Aged Care Serv Rev* 1981;2:1–19.

10. Katz S, Ford AB, Moskowitz RW, Jackson BA, Jaffe MW. Studies of illness in the aged. The Index of ADL: A standardized measure of biological and psychosocial function. *JAMA* 1963;185(12):914–919.

11. Mahoney FI, Barthel DW. Functional evaluation: The Barthel Index. *Md State Med J* 1965;14:61–65.

12. Lawton MP, Brody EM. Assessment of older people: Self-maintaining and instrumental activities of daily living. *The Gerontologist* 1969;9:179–186.

13. Pfeffer RI, Kurosaki MS, Harrah CH, Chance JM, Filos S. Measurement of functional activities in older adults in the community. *J Gerontol* 1982;37(3):323–329.

14. Luft H. *Poverty and health.* Cambridge, MA: Ballinger, 1978.

15. Nagi SZ. Some conceptual issues in disability and rehabilitation. In: Sussman MB, ed. *Sociology and rehabilitation*, 1965;100–113.

16. Wolfe BL. Measuring disability and health. *J Health Econom* 1984;3:187–193.

17. Nagi SZ. An epidemiology of disability among adults in the United States. *Milbank Memorial Fund Quarterly* 1976;54(4):439–467.

18. Kirshner B, Guyatt G. A methodological framework for assessing health indices. *J Chronic Dis* 1985;38(1):27–36.

19. Staff of the Benjamin Rose Hospital. Multidisciplinary studies of illness in aged persons: III. Prognostic indices in fracture of hip. *J Chronic Dis* 1960;11:445–455.

20. Katz S, Jackson BA, Jaffee MW, Littell AS, Turk CE. Multidisciplinary studies of illness in aged persons: VI. Comparison study of rehabilitated and nonrehabilitated patients with fracture of the hip. *J Chronic Dis* 1962;15:979–984.

21. Katz S, Vignos PJ, Moskowitz RW, Thompson HM, Sveck KH. Comprehensive outpatient care in rheumatoid arthritis: A controlled study. *JAMA* 1968;206:1249–1254.

22. Spector WD, Kapp MC, Tucker RJ, Sternberg J. Factors associated with presence of decubitus ulcers at admission to nursing homes. *The Gerontologist* 1988;28(6):830–834.

23. Sternberg J, Spector WD, Fretwell MD, Jackson ME, Drugovich ML. Use of psychoactive drugs in nursing homes: Prevalence and residents' characteristics. *J Geriatr Drug Therapy*, (*in press*).

24. Spector WD, Takada HA, Tucker RJ. Risk of physical functional change in nursing homes. Final report prepared for the National Center for Health Services Research, grant no. HS05625. Providence, RI: Center for Gerontology and Health Care Research, Brown University, 1989.

25. Jackson ME, Drugovich ML, Fretwell MD, Spector WD, Sternberg J, Rosenstein RB. Prevalence and correlates of disruptive behavior in the nursing home. *J Health Aging*, (*in press*).

26. Spector WD, Kapp MC, Eichorn, AM, Tucker RJ, Rosenstein RB, Katz S. Case-mix outcomes and resources use in nursing homes. Final report prepared for the Health Care Financing Administration HCFA, cooperative agreement no. 18-C-98719/1. Providence, RI: Center for Gerontology and Health Care Research, Brown University, 1988.

27. Branch LG, Katz S, Kniepmann K, Papsidero JA. A prospective study of functional status among community elders. *Am J Public Health* 1984;74(3):266–268.

28. Katz S, Ford AB, Downs TD, Adams M, Rusby DI. *Effects of continued care: A study of chronic illness in the home.* Washington, D.C.: U.S. Government Printing Office, 1972.

29. Papsidero JA, Katz S, Kroger MH, Akpom CA. *Chance for change.* East Lansing: Michigan State University Press, 1979.

30. Granger CV, Albrecht GL, Hamilton BB. Outcome of comprehensive medical rehabilitation: Measurement by pulses profile and the Barthel Index. *Arch Phys Med Rehabil* 1979;60:145–154.

31. Granger CV, Sherwood CC, Greer DS. Functional status measures in a comprehensive stroke care program. *Arch Phys Med Rehabil* 1977;58:555–561.

32. Novack TA, Haban G, Graham K, Satterfield WT. Prediction of stroke rehabilitation outcome from psychologic screening. *Arch Phys Med Rehabil* 1987;68:729–734.

33. Wade DT, Skilbeck CE, Hewer RL. Predicting Barthel ADL score at 6 months after an acute stroke. *Arch Phys Med Rehabil* 1983;64:24–28.

34. Guttman L. A basis for scaling qualitative data. *Am Sociolog Rev* 1944;9:139–150.

35. Brorrsson B, Asberg KH. Katz index of independence in ADL: Reliability and validity in short-term care. *Scand. J Rehabil Med* 16:125–132.

36. Asberg KH. Assessment of ADL in home care for elderly: Change in ADL and use of short-term hospital care. *Scand J Soc Med* 1986;14:105–111.

37. Asberg KH. Disability as a predictor of outcome for the elderly in a department of internal medicine. *Scand J Soc Med* 1987;15:261–265.

38. Chronbach LJ. Coefficient alpha in the internal structure of tests. *Psychometrika* 1951;16:297–334.

39. Shinar D, Gross CR, Bronstein KS, Licata-Gehr EE, Eden DT, Cabrera AR, Fishman IG, Roth AA, Barwick JA, Kunitz SC. Reliability of the activities of daily living scale and its use in telephone interview. *Arch Phys Med Rehabil* 1987;68:723–728.

40. Sheikh K, Smith DS, Meade TW, Goldenberg E, Brennan PJ, Kinsella G. Repeatability and validity

of a modified activities of daily living (ADL) index in studies of chronic disability. *Int Rehab Med* 1979;1:51–58.

41. Haworth RJ, Hollings EM. Are hospital assessments of daily living activities valid? *Int Rehab Med* 1979;1:59–62.
42. Kane RL. Commentary: Functional assessment questionnaire for geriatrics patients—or the clinical Swiss army knife. *J Chronic Dis* 40(Suppl. 1):95S–98S.
43. Jagger C, Clarke M, Davies RA. The elderly at home: Indices of disability. *J Epidemiol Community Health* 1986;40:139–142.
44. Katz S, Downs TD, Cash HR, Grotz RC. Progress in development of the index of ADL. *The Gerontologist* 1970;10:20–30.
45. Densen PM, Jones EW, McNitt BJ. An approach to the assessment of long term care. Final report, research grant No. HS-01162. Boston: Harvard Center for Community Health and Medical Care, 1976.
46. Jette AM. Functional status index: Reliability of a chronic disease evaluation instrument. *Arch Phys Med Rehabil* 1980;61:395–401.
47. Jette AM. Functional capacity evaluation: An empirical approach. *Arch Phys Med Rehabil* 1980;61:85–89.
48. Gresham GE, Phillips TF, Labi MLC. ADL status in stroke: Relative merits of three standard indexes. *Arch Phys Med Rehabil* 1980;61:355–358.
49. Wylie CM. Measuring end results of rehabilitation of patients with stroke. *Public Health Rep* 1967;82:893–898.
50. Carroll D. Disability in hemiplegia caused by cerebrovascular disease: Serial studies of 98 cases. *J Chronic Dis* 1962;15:179–188.
51. Granger CV, Greer DS. Functional status measurement and medical rehabilitation outcomes. *Arch Phys Med Rehabil* 1976;57:103–108.
52. Fortinsky RH, Granger CV, Seltzer GB. The use of functional assessment in understanding home care needs. *Med Care* 1981;19(5):489–497.
53. Sheikh K. Disability scales: Assessment of reliability. *Arch Phys Med Rehabil* 1986;67:245–249.
54. Lord FM. Elementary models for measuring change. In: Harris CW, ed. *Problems in measuring change*. Madison, Wisconsin: The University of Wisconsin Press, 1963;21–37.
55. Center for the Study of Aging and Human Development. *Multidimensional assessment: The OARS methodology*. Durham, NC: The Center for Study of Aging and Human Development, Duke University, 1978.
56. Lawton MP. Assessment, integration, and environments for older people. *The Gerontologist* 1970;10:38–46.
57. Jette AM, Branch LG. Impairment and disability in the aged. *J Chronic Dis* 1985;38(1):59–65.
58. Rosow I, Breslau N. A Guttman health scale for the aged. *J Gerontol* 1966;21:556–559.
59. Linn MW, Linn BS. The rapid disability rating scale—2. *J Am Geriatr Soc* 1982;30:378–382.
60. Spector WD, Katz S, Murphy JB, Fulton JP. The hierarchical relationship between activities of daily living and instrumental activities. *J Chronic Dis* 1987;40(6):481–489.

Quality of Life Assessments in Clinical
Trials, edited by B. Spilker. Raven
Press, Ltd. New York © 1990.

11

The General Health Policy Model:

An Integrated Approach

Robert M. Kaplan and John P. Anderson

*Division of Health Care Sciences, Department of Community and Family
Medicine, University of California, San Diego, La Jolla, California 92093*

QUALITY OF LIFE MEASUREMENT

Quality of life data are becoming increasingly important for evaluating the cost-utility
and cost-effectiveness of health care programs. Such analyses require the evaluation
of very different types of health care interventions using the same outcome unit.
This chapter highlights some of the strengths and weaknesses of general health outcome measures. The value of general versus disease-specific measures within clinical
populations is also addressed. In addition, we consider the boundaries of the quality
of life concept.

Why Measure Quality of Life?

The conceptualization and measurement of health status has interested scholars
for many decades. Following the Eisenhower administration, a President's Commission on National Goals identified health status measurement as an important
objective. In *The Affluent Society*, Galbraith described the need to measure the effect
of the health care system on "quality of life." Within the last decade, many groups
have attempted to define and measure health status (1–3). Before considering any
specific approach, it is worth noting that traditional indicators of "health" have well-
identified problems that need to be addressed before they can be considered part of
an adequate measure of "quality of life."

Mortality

Mortality remains the major outcome measure in many epidemiologic studies and
some clinical trials. Typically, mortality is expressed in a unit of time and the rates
are often age-adjusted. Case fatality rates express the proportion of persons who
died of a particular disease divided by the total number with the disease (including
those who die and those who live). Mortality rates have many benefits as health
outcome measures. They are "hard" data (despite some misclassification bias [4]),

and the meaning of the outcome is not difficult to comprehend. Despite their many advantages, mortality outcomes have some obvious limitations. Mortality rates consider only the dead and ignore the living. Many important treatments or programs might have little or no impact on mortality rates and many frequently occurring illnesses, such as arthritis, have relatively little impact on mortality. Thus, there has been an incentive to define and measure nonfatal outcomes.

Morbidity

The most common approach to health status assessment is to measure morbidity in terms of function or role performance. For example, morbidity estimates often include work days missed or bed disability days. Many different approaches to health status assessment using morbidity indicators have been introduced. These include, for example, the Sickness Impact Profile (5), which represents the effect of disease or disability on a variety of categories of behavioral function, and the RAND Health Status measures, which have separate categories for the effects of disease or health states on physical function, social function, and mental function. These measures are important quantitative expressions of health outcome. However, they do not integrate morbidity and mortality, although as each birth cohort ages, mortality cases accrue.

Death is a health outcome, and it is important that this outcome not be excluded from any expression of health status. For example, suppose we are evaluating the effect of program A, which integrates support and treatment, for randomly assigned groups of very ill, elderly, nursing home residents against the effect of program B, which offers no support or treatment. Let us suppose that program A maintains patients at a very low level of function throughout the year, but that in the comparison group (program B), the sickest 10% died. Looking just at the living in the follow-up, one finds program B patients to be healthier, since the sickest have been removed by death. By this standard, the program of no supportive treatment might be put forth as the better alternative. With a measure that combines morbidity and mortality the outcome will be very different, because mortality effects will reduce the overall health of program B to a very low level.

Behavioral Dysfunction

When Sullivan (6) reviewed the literature on health measurement more than 20 years ago, he emphasized the importance of behavioral outcomes. Behavioral indicators such as absenteeism, bed-disability days, and institutional confinement were identified as the most important consequences of disease and disability. Ability to perform activities at different ages could be compared to societal standards for these behaviors. Restrictions in usual activity were seen as *prima facie* evidence of deviation from well-being. Many other investigators have focused on point-in-time measures of dysfunction as measures of health (3,7,8).

Prognosis

The problem with measures of behavioral dysfunction is that they often neglect what will happen in the future. The spectrum of medical care ranges from public health, preventive medicine, and environmental control through diagnosis, to therapeutic intervention, convalescence, and rehabilitation. Many programs affect the probability of occurrence of future dysfunction (e.g., vaccines), rather than alter present functional status. In many aspects of preventive care, for example, the benefit of the treatment cannot be seen until many years after the intervention. A supportive family that instills proper health habits in its children, for example, may also promote better "health" in the future, yet the benefit may not be realized for years. The concept of health must consider not only the present ability to function, but also the probability of future changes in function. A person who is very functional and asymptomatic today may harbor a disease with a poor prognosis. Thus, many individuals are at high risk of dying from heart disease even though they are perfectly functional today. Should we call them "healthy"? We hold that the term "severity of illness" should take into consideration both dysfunction and prognosis (or probability of future dysfunction and mortality).

Many medical treatments may cause near-term dysfunction to prevent future dysfunction. For example, coronary artery bypass surgery causes severe dysfunction for a short period of time, yet the surgery is presumed to enhance function or decrease mortality at a later time. Patients may be incapacitated and restricted to coronary care units following myocardial infarction. Yet the treatment is designed to help them achieve better future outcomes. Pap smears and hysterectomies are performed in order to decrease the probability of future deaths due to cancer. Much of health care involves looking into the future to enhance outcomes over the life span. Therefore, it is essential to divide health into current and future components. We prefer the term "prognosis" to describe the probability of transition among health states over the course of time (9).

IS QUALITY OF LIFE DIFFERENT FROM HEALTH STATUS?

In the preceding sections, we have described some common elements in existing measures of health status. However, there is considerable variability in the definition of quality of life. Some authors define quality of life as health outcomes that are different from traditional health outcomes. Using these definitions, quality of life measures are typically limited to psychological and social attributes (10). By contrast, our definition of health-related quality of life focuses on the qualitative dimension of functioning. It also incorporates duration of stay in various health states. We will return to this definition later in the chapter; in the next section, however, we will review the value dimension, which is an important aspect of quality of life.

The Value Dimension

Scholars have debated the components of "health" for many centuries (11). Most concepts of morbidity involve three types of evidence: *clinical, subjective*, and *behavioral* (6). *Clinical* outcomes include clinical judgment, physical findings, laboratory tests, or results of invasive procedures. Clinical evidence is valuable if, and only if, it is clearly related to well-defined behavioral health outcomes. For example, significant abnormalities in certain blood proteins are of concern only if these deviations correlate with morbidity or early mortality. The burden of proof is on the scientist to demonstrate these associations.

Subjective evidence includes symptoms and complaints that are also very important in health care. Symptoms are a major correlate of health care utilization, but not all symptoms should be given equal weight because neither the type nor the number of symptoms necessarily depicts the severity of disease. For example, an adult with an acute 24-hour flu may have an enormous number of symptoms. Although these can include nausea, headache, cough, sneezing, aches and pains, vomiting, and diarrhea, it is not clear that this condition is more severe than the single symptom of a very severe headache.

Several factors need to be considered. First, we must determine the degree to which the symptoms limit functioning. Consider an individual with five symptoms—an itchy eye, runny nose, coughing, fatigue, and headache—but who still feels well enough to work and to perform all usual activities. Another person with the single symptom of a severe headache may be limited to bed and not move around. Would we want to call the person with five symptoms less well? Another dimension is the duration of the symptoms. A year in pain is certainly worse than a day in pain. The final, and perhaps the most often neglected, factor is the value or preference associated with different types of dysfunction.

Biomedical investigators often avoid reference to values or preferences because these constructs are considered not "scientific." However, the value dimension in health status is inescapable. Fishburn defined value as the quantification of the concept of worth, importance, or desirability (11). Ultimately, our judgments of the value of health states, and whether one level of functioning is "better" than another level of functioning, depend on subjective evaluations. If we advise individuals to change their diet to avoid heart disease, we inherently assume that the reduced probability of heart disease later in life is valued more than the immediate but enduring mild displeasure of dietary change. The phrase "quality of life" necessarily presumes a qualitative judgment.

As noted earlier, Sullivan emphasized *behavioral dysfunction* as the third type of evidence for morbidity. Behavioral dysfunction includes disruption in role performance, confinement to hospitals, or work loss.

SHOULD QUALITY OF LIFE BE LIMITED TO PSYCHOLOGICAL AND SOCIAL ATTRIBUTES?

Some authors use the term "quality of life" as a limited descriptor of psychological and social health (10). We believe that most psychological and social dimensions can be incorporated into a general health status measure. However, some concepts of social health are correlates of health outcomes rather than outcomes themselves. We have addressed these issues elsewhere (12–14) but will summarize them in the following sections.

Social Health

For nearly 35 years, physicians, psychologists, sociologists, and epidemiologists have been attempting to include social support and social function in a definition of health status. Despite relentless efforts, it has been difficult to meaningfully define social support as a component of health. The term "social health" was included in the World Health Organization definition of health that accompanied their charter document in 1948 (15). They defined health as, "a state of complete physical, mental, and social well-being and not merely the absence of infirmity." In identifying the dimensions of health, the World Health Organization neglected to provide any operational definitions. Thus, different investigators have taken different approaches in their attempts to capture physical, mental, and social dimensions. Since the publication of the World Health Organization statement, many investigators have tried to develop measures to operationalize the three components of health status. With surprising consistency, authors quote the World Health Organization definition and then present their methods for measuring the three components. So prevalent is the notion that health status must include these three components that many reviews now negatively evaluate any measure that does not conform to the World Health Organization definition. For example, Meenan (16) disapproved of several health measures because, "these approaches fall short of conceptualizing or measuring health in the World Health Organization sense of a physical, psychological, and social state" (p. 785).

With the command of the World Health Organization so plainly set forth, many investigators have struggled to develop their measures of social health. Yet there have been consistent problems. For example, Kane and Kane (17) devoted a substantial section of their monograph to describing problems in the quantification of social health. These problems included vague concepts, lack of norms, the interactive nature of variables, difficulty in construction of a continuum, and the subjective nature of social health.

Only Ware and colleagues have begun to question the meaning of social health (18,19). In one paper, Donald, Ware, and colleagues (19) reviewed 70 studies relevant to social health. From these they selected 11 studies for more detailed analysis. The great majority of these studies focused on what we now call social support. Yet, there were at least two separate components being assessed by the many investigators contributing to this literature. One component, was social contacts, or the performance of social role. The other component is social resources, which is more analogous to the concept of social support. This distinction is very important. Social contacts might include participation in work, attendance at school, and other aspects of functioning. Social resources are relevant to social life, friendships, and family relationships.

In a series of analyses, it has been demonstrated that social support may be a predictor for health outcomes (13,19), but the direction is not always clear. For example, Heitzmann and Kaplan (20) have demonstrated that social support may predict positive outcomes for women but negative outcomes for men. Social support is not an outcome that can serve as the target of health care. On the other hand, social functioning is a component of health status. Diseases and disabilities affect social function. Social function is a central component in the concept of quality of life.

Optimizing social health raises issues of social control and public policy. Considering the example of function, there is strong consensus that function is desirable. Thus, it seems reasonable to devote public resources to maximize the level of function and quality of life within a community. Optimized health status might be considered a common goal, as is national defense, a strong educational system, etc. Many current methods of health measurement do include a social functioning component. On the other hand, including social support in the definition of health status would imply that community resources should be used to obtain some defined level of social support. We might expect considerable public disagreement about what the social support objective might be. For example, would we want to develop a public policy that requires people to have friends?

Excluding social support from the definition of health makes policy analysis relatively straightforward. There is little disagreement about what levels of functioning are desirable (21,22). When people agree on what is desirable, the objective of health care can be directed toward achieving the desired states. A major issue is in defining a mix of programs that most efficiently and effectively achieve these objectives. Programs that enhance social support might be considered in this mix, but we believe that including social support in the definition of health only confuses the definition of these objectives.

Mental Health

The separate category for mental health in the World Health Organization definition prompted many investigators to develop separate measures of mental health functioning. Perhaps the best known effort in this area is the work by Ware and his associates (23). These investigators adapted Dupuy's (24) General Well-Being Index and administered it to large numbers of people as part of the RAND Health Insurance Experiment. Ware et al. (25) argue that the correlation between psychological distress and physical functioning is only .25 and suggested that this confirmed that mental health was a separate dimension. In addition, they offered comparisons between those with no physical limitations but with differences on items about psychological distress. For this high physically functioning group, those with higher scores on mental distress used three times as many mental health services as those low in distress.

The separate measurement of mental health remains a major issue in the conceptualization of general health status. Although our position is against the norm, we believe mental health can be conceptualized as a portion of general health status and that there is considerable disadvantage to attempting separate measurement and specification of mental function. We do understand that some investigators are interested in specific subcomponents of mental health, such as cognitive functioning. In these cases, more detailed measures might be considered additions to (but not replacements for) the general measures.

We argue that the World Health Organization conceptualization of health status promotes an artificial dichotomy between mental and physical function. In order to understand this argument, it is important to think about the impact of mental illness, anxiety, or poor social adjustment on functioning. Mental health affects longevity (26) and quality of life. In other words, the impact of mental health on general health status is expressed through its impact on life expectancy, functioning, and symptoms. However, many individuals with perfect physical functioning experience symptoms. For example, an individual experiencing anxiety at work might check a symptom describing anxiety. This anxiety might effect quality of life in a manner similar to a physical symptom such as shortness of breath. Severe anxieties, such as phobias, may disrupt role performance. Thus, individuals may be limited to their homes because they are afraid to go outside. Many individuals experience symptomatic depression that does not disrupt their activities of daily living. At the other extreme, anxiety and depression can be so severe that they result in hospitalization. Thus, the impact of the condition on functioning is very much the same as the impact of a physical malady.

As in physical health, the duration of mental health conditions must also be considered. For example, depression may last 3 days, 3 weeks, or 1 year. The total impact needs to be expressed as a function of its duration. More importantly, mental health status may effect differential transition among functional states over the course of time. The term "positive health" is used typically to describe some aspect of lifestyle or mental outlook that is associated with better future health. Or, people with positive health have lower probabilities of transition to poor health over the course of time. An individual who can cope with stress may seem no different from individuals without such coping skills. However, given certain epidemiologic linkages, they may have a higher probability of better functioning at future points in time.

Much of the confusion about mental health has been generated by a very refined technology for assessing mental states. Often, detailed questionnaire methods have been factor analyzed to describe different dimensions of mental health. Nevertheless, these very different levels of functioning may ultimately impact the general well-being. This may be analogous to the many available measures of blood chemistry. For example, indicators of kidney function (creatinine, BUN, etc.) may be identified as separate factors, yet the importance of these measures is their relationship to longevity and to function at particular points in time. We might not be concerned about elevated creatinine, for example, if these blood levels were not correlated with death or dysfunction due to kidney disease.

There are some justifications for not separating mental and physical function. The growing literature on psychoneuroimmunology (27) clearly demonstrates the intertwining nature of physical and mental health outcomes. In addition, experiments have demonstrated that general health status can be improved in medical patients even though physical functioning is unaffected. For example, patients with chronic obstructive pulmonary disease do not achieve changes in lung function following rehabilitation. However, they may reach higher levels of activity and reduced symptoms (28). The rehabilitation programs are not necessarily medical and may depend on physical or respiratory therapists. Indeed, the changes in outcome may result from improved attitude or from the enhanced ability to cope with symptoms. Ultimately, we are interested in patient function and quality of life. It may not matter if this is achieved through enhanced lung function or improved coping skills. The most important point is that all providers in health care are attempting to improve quality of life and extend the duration of life. It is valuable to allow mental health providers and physical health providers to compare the benefits of their services using a common unit.

Health-Related Quality of Life

The objectives of health care are twofold. First, health care and health policy should increase life expectancy. Second, the health care system should improve the quality of life during the years that people are alive. It is instructive to consider various measures in health care in light of these two objectives. Traditional biomedical indicators and diagnoses are important to us because they may be related to mortality or to quality of life. We prefer the term "health-related quality of life" to refer to the impact of health conditions on function. Thus, health-related quality of life may be independent of quality of life relevant to work setting, housing, air pollution, or similar factors (29).

Numerous quality of life measurement systems have evolved during the last 20 years. These systems are based primarily on two different conceptual approaches. The first approach grows out of the tradition of health status measurement. In the late 1960s and early 1970s, the National Center for Health Services Research funded several major projects to develop general measures of health status. Those projects resulted in the Sickness Impact Profile (SIP) (5), the Quality of Well-Being Scale (30,31), and the General Health Rating Index. The latter measure, originally developed at Southern Illinois University, was adapted by the RAND Corporation under Health and Human Service grants and has become known as the RAND Health Status Measure (8). These efforts usually involved extensive multidisciplinary collaboration between behavioral scientists and physicians. Most of the measures are focused on the impact of disease and disability on function and observable behaviors, such as performance of social role, ability to get around the community, and physical functioning. Some systems include separate components for the measurement of social and mental health. All were guided by the World Health Organization's definition of health status: "Health is a complete state of physical, mental, and social well-being and not merely absence of disease" (5).

The second conceptual approach is based on quality of life as something independent of health status. Some investigators now use traditional psychological measures and call them quality of life outcomes. For instance, Follick et al. (10) suggest that quality of life represents psychological status in addition to symptoms and mortality. Croog et al. (32) used a wide variety of outcome measures and collectively referred to them as "quality of life." These measures included the patients' subjective evaluation of well-being, physical symptoms, sexual function, work performance and satisfaction, emotional status, cognitive function, social participation, and life satisfaction. Yet mortality is not part of the concept. Other investigators, including Hunt and colleagues (33) regard quality of life as subjective appraisals of life satisfaction. In summary, a wide variety of different dimensions have all been described as quality of life. Although agreement is lacking on which dimensions should be considered the standard for assessing quality of life in research studies, recurrent themes in the methodologic literature can assist in the evaluation of existing instruments. As will be shown, our approach to quality of life measurement focuses on health-related outcomes of mortality, morbidity, symptoms, and prognosis. We believe that many definitions of quality of life are poorly operationalized. Before addressing our definition of health-related quality of life, it will also be important to clarify some economic terms that are often used in the same literature.

Cost-Utility Versus Cost-Benefit

The terms *"cost-utility," "cost-effectiveness,"* and *"cost-benefit"* are used inconsistently in the medical literature (34). Some economists have favored the assessment of *cost-benefit*. These approaches measure both program costs and treatment outcomes in dollar units. For example, treatment outcomes are evaluated in relation to changes in use of medical services and economic productivity. Treatments are cost-beneficial if the economic return exceeds treatment costs. Diabetic patients who are aggressively treated, for example, may need fewer medical services. The savings associated with decreased services might exceed treatment costs. As Kaplan and Davis (35) have argued, there is relatively little strong empirical evidence that patient education or behavioral treatments are actually cost-beneficial. In addition, as suggested by Russell (36), the requirement that health care treatments reduce costs may be unrealistic. Patients are willing to pay for improvements in health status just as they are willing to pay for other desirable goods and services. We do not treat cancer in order to save money. Instead, treatments are given in order to achieve better health outcomes.

Cost-effectiveness is an alternative approach in which the unit of outcome is a reflection of treatment effect. In recent years, cost-effectiveness has gained considerable attention. Some approaches emphasize simple, treatment-specific outcomes. For example, the cost per pound lost has been used as a measure of cost-effectiveness of weight loss programs (37). Public competitions, for example, achieve a lower cost-per-pound loss ratio than do traditional clinical interventions. The major difficulty with cost-effectiveness methodologies is that they do not allow for comparison across very different treatment interventions. For example, health care administrators often need to choose between investments in very different alternatives. They may need to decide between supporting liver transplantation for a few patients versus prenatal counseling for a large number of patients. For the same cost, they may achieve a large effect for a few people or a small effect for a large number of people. The treatment-specific outcomes used in cost-effectiveness studies do not permit these comparisons.

Cost-utility approaches use the expressed preference or utility of a treatment effect as the unit of outcome. As noted in World Health Organization documents (38), the goals of health care are to add years to life and to add life to years. In other words, health care is designed to make people live longer (increase the life expectancy) and to live a higher quality of life in the years prior to death. Cost-utility studies use outcome measures that combine mortality outcomes with quality of life measurements. The utilities are the expressed preferences for observable states of function on a continuum bounded by 0 for death to 1.0 for optimum function (39–41). In the next section, we outline a model that combines utilities with measures of mortality, morbidity, symptoms, and prognosis. The system can be used as either a health-related quality of life measure or an instrument in cost-utility analysis.

A COMPREHENSIVE SYSTEM—THE GENERAL HEALTH POLICY MODEL

Our approach is to express the benefits of medical care, behavioral intervention, or preventive programs in terms of well-years. Others have chosen to describe the same outcome as Quality-Adjusted Life-Years (QALY's) (42). Well-years integrate mortality and morbidity to express health status in terms of equivalents of well-years of life. If a cigarette smoker died of heart disease at age 50 and we would have expected him to live to age 75, it might be concluded that the disease cost him 25 life-years. If 100 cigarette smokers died at age 50 (and also had life expectancies of 75 years), we might conclude that 2,500 (100 men × 25 years) life-years had been lost.

Yet, death is not the only outcome of concern in heart disease. Many adults suffer myocardial infarctions that leave them somewhat disabled over a longer period of time. Although they are still alive, the quality of their lives has diminished. Our model permits all degrees of disability to be compared to one another. A disease that reduces the quality of life by one-half will take away .5 well-years over the course of 1 year. If it effects two people, it will take away 1.0 well-year (equal to 2 × .5) over a 1-year period. A medical treatment that improves the quality of life by .2 for each of five individuals will result in a production of 1 well-year if the benefit is maintained over a 1-year period. Using this system, it is possible to express the benefits of various programs by showing how many equivalents of well-years they produce (39–41). Yet, not all programs have equivalent costs. In periods of scarce resources, it is necessary to find the most efficient use of limited funds. Our approach provides a framework within which to make policy decisions that require selection from competing alternatives. Preventive services may in this way compete with traditional medical services for the scarce health care dollar. Performing such comparisons requires the use of a general health decision model. In the next section, the general model of health status assessment and benefit–cost-utility analysis will be presented.

The General Model

Building a Health Decision Model

The Health Decision Model grew out of substantive theories in economics, psychology, medicine, and public health. These theoretical linkages have been presented in several previous papers (43–45). Building a health decision model requires at least five distinct steps.

Step 1: Defining a function status classification. During the early phases of our work, a set of mutually exclusive and collectively exhaustive levels of functioning were defined. After an extensive, specialty-by-specialty review of medical reference works, we listed all of the ways that disease and injuries can affect behavior and role performance. Without considering etiology, it was possible to match a finite number of conditions to items appearing on standard health surveys, such as the Health Interview Survey (National Center for Health Statistics), the Survey of the Disabled (Social Security Administration), and several rehabilitation scales and on-going community surveys. These items fit conceptually into three scales representing related but distinct aspects of daily functioning: mobility, physical activity, and social activity. The mobility and physical activity scales have three levels, whereas social activity has five distinct levels. Table 1 shows the steps from the three scales. Several investigators have used this function status classification (or a modified version of it) as an outcome measure for health program evaluation (46,47). However, the development of a truly comprehensive health status indicator requires several more steps.

Step 2: Classifying symptoms and problems. There are many reasons a person may not be functioning at the optimum level. Subjective complaints are an important component of a general health measure because they relate dysfunction to a specific problem. Thus, in addition to function level classifications, an exhaustive list of symptoms and problems has been generated. Included in the list are 25 complexes of symptoms and problems representing all of the possible symptomatic complaints that might inhibit function. These symptoms and problems are shown in Table 2.

Step 3: Preference weights to integrate the Quality of Well-Being Scale. We now have described the three scales of function and 25 symptom/problem complexes.

TABLE 1. *Quality of Well-Being Scale elements and calculating formulas*

Step no.	Step definition	Weight
	Mobility Scale (MOB)	
5	No limitations for health reasons	−.000
4	Did not drive a car, health related (younger than 16); did not ride in a car as usual for age, and/or did not use public transportation, health related; or had or would have used more help than usual for age to use public transportation, nealth related	−.062
2	In hospital, health related	−.090
	Physical Activity Scale (PAC)	
4	No limitations for health reasons	−.000
3	In wheelchair, moved or controlled movement of wheelchair without help from someone else; or had trouble or did not try to lift, stoop, bend over, or use stairs or inclines, health related, and/or limped, used a cane, crutches or walker, health related; and/or had any other physical limitation in walking, or did not try to walk as far or as fast as others the same age are able, health related	−.060
1	In wheelchair, did not move or control the movement of wheelchair without help from someone else, or in bed, chair, or couch for most or all of the day, health related	−.077
	Social Activity Scale (SAC)	
5	No limitations for health reasons	−.000
4	Limited in other role activity, health related	−.061
3	Limited in major (primary) role activity, health related	−.061
2	Performed no major role activity, health related, but did perform self-care activities	−.061
1	Performed no major role activity, health related, and did not perform or had more help than usual in performance of one or more self-care activities, health related	−.106

Calculating Formulas:

Formula 1: Point-in-time Well-being score for an individual (W):

$$W = 1 + (CPXwt) + (MOBwt) + (PACwt) + (SACwt)$$

where wt is the preference-weighted measure for each factor and CPX is symptom/problem complex. For example, the W score for a person with the following description profile may be calculated for one day as follows:

QWB Element	Description	Weight
CPX-11	Cough, wheezing, or shortness of breath, with or without fever, chill, or aching all over	−.257
MOB-5	No limitations	−.000
PAC-1	In bed, chair, or couch for most or all of the day, health related	−.077
SAC-2	Performed no major role activity, health related, but did perform self-care activities	−.061

$$W = 1 + (-.257) + (-.000) + (-.077) + (-.061) = .605$$

Formula 2: General Health Policy Model Formula for Well-Years (WY) as an output measure:

$$WY = [\text{No. of persons} \times (CPXwt + MOBwt + PACwt + SACwt)] \times time$$

TABLE 2. *List of Quality of Well-Being Scale symptom/problem complexes (CPX) with calculating weights for QWB scale, version 6B*

CPX no.	CPX description	Weights
1	Death (not on respondent's card)	−.727
2	Loss of consciousness such as seizure (fits), fainting, or coma (out cold or knocked out)	−.407
3	Burn over large areas of face, body, arms, or legs	−.367
4	Pain, bleeding, itching, or discharge (drainage) from sexual organs—does not include normal menstrual (monthly) bleeding	−.349
5	Trouble learning, remembering, or thinking clearly	−.340
6	Any combination of one or more hands, feet, arms, or legs either missing, deformed (crooked), paralyzed (unable to move) or broken —includes wearing artificial limbs or braces	−.333
7	Pain, stiffness, weakness, numbness, or other discomfort in chest, stomach (including hernia or rupture), side, neck, back, hips, or any joints of hands, feet, arms or legs	−.299
8	Pain, burning, bleeding, itching, or other difficulty with rectum, bowel movements, or urination (passing water)	−.292
9	Sick or upset stomach, vomiting or loose bowel movements, with or without fever, chills, or aching all over	−.290
10	General tiredness, weakness, or weight loss	−.259
11	Cough, wheezing, or shortness of breath *with* or *without* fever, chills, or aching all over	−.257
12	Spells of feeling upset, being depressed, or of crying	−.257
13	Headache, or dizziness, or ringing in ears, or spells of feeling hot, or nervous, or shaky	−.244
14	Burning or itching rash on large areas of face, body, arms, or legs	−.240
15	Trouble talking, such as lisp, stuttering, hoarseness, or inability to speak	−.237
16	Pain or discomfort in one or both eyes (such as burning or itching) or any trouble seeing after correction	−.230
17	Overweight or underweight for age and height of skin defect of face, body, arms or legs, such as scars, pimples, warts, bruises, or changes in color	−.186
18	Pain in ear, tooth, jaw, throat, lips, tongue; missing or crooked permanent teeth—includes wearing bridges or false teeth; stuffy, runny nose; any trouble hearing—includes wearing a hearing aid	−.170
19	Taking medication or staying on a prescribed diet for health reasons	−.144
20	Wore eyeglasses or contact lenses	−.101
21	Breathing smog or unpleasant air	−.101
22	No symptoms or problem (not on respondent's card)	−.000
23	Standard symptom/problem (not on respondent's card)	−.257
24	Trouble sleeping	−.257
25	Intoxication	−.257
26	Problems with sexual interest or performance	−.257
27	Excessive worry or anxiety	−.257

* CPX 24-27 are assigned standard weights until empirical weights can be derived in new studies.

With these, all we can do is compare populations in terms of frequencies of each scale step (and, if necessary, symptom/problem complex). Although comparisons of frequencies are common in health services research, our system offers a strategy for integrating the frequencies into a single comprehensive expression. If our intent is to say which of these distributions is "better off" and which "worse," simple frequency distributions may not be able to help much. For example, is a group with 80 people able to travel and limited in their mobility and 5 restricted to their homes worse off than a group in which 85 can travel freely, but 10 are restricted to their homes? Obviously comparing frequency distributions is complex. Further, the example involves frequencies for only one scale. How can one make decisions when there are three scales and symptom/problem complexes to consider?

Another step is necessary to integrate the three scales and the symptom/problem complexes in a manner that will allow a single numerical expression to represent each combination of steps on the scales and symptom/problem complexes. The empirical means of accomplishing this is measured preferences for the health states. These might be regarded as "quality" judgments. As we noted earlier, the General Health Policy Model includes the impact of health conditions on the quality of life. This requires that the desirability of health situations be evaluated on a continuum from death to completely well. An evaluation such as this is a matter of utility or preference, thus combinations of behavioral dysfunction and symptom/problem complexes are scaled to represent degrees of relative importance.

Human judgment studies are used to determine weights for the different states. We have asked random samples of citizens from the community to evaluate the relative desirability of a good number of health conditions. Random sample surveys were conducted in the San Diego community during 2 consecutive years. The probability sample included 866 respondents ethnically representative of the population. When necessary, interviews were conducted in Spanish. From a listing of all possible combinations of the scale (mobility, physical activity, social activity, and symptom/problem complexes), we drew a stratified random sample of 343 case descriptions (items) and divided them into eight sets of computer-generated booklets. All respondents were assigned randomly to one of the eight booklets, creating eight subgroups of approximately 100 respondents each. In a series of studies, a mathematical model was developed to describe the consumer decision process. The validity of the model has been cross validated with an R of .94 (10). These weights, then, describe the relative desirability of all of the function states on a scale from 0 (for death) to 1.0 (for asymptomatic optimum function). Thus, a state with a weight of .50 is viewed by the members of the community as being about one-half as desirable as optimum function or about halfway between optimum function and death.

Some critics have expressed concern that community, rather than specific population weights are used. The advantage of community weights is that they are general (like the model) and do not bias policy analysis toward any interest group. More important, however, is that empirical studies consistently fail to show systematic differences between demographic groups (21), providers, students and administrators (20), and Americans versus British (48). Relevant to the general versus disease-specific issue, Balaban and colleagues (49) found that weights provided by rheumatoid arthritis patients are remarkably similar to those we obtained from members of the general population.

Using preference weights, one component of the general model of health is defined. This is the Quality of Well-Being Scale, which is the point-in-time component of the General Health Policy Model (50,51). The quality of well-being score for any individual can be obtained from preferences or "quality" judgments associated with his/her function level, adjusted for symptom or problem.

The example in Table 1 describes a person classified on the three scales of observable function and on a symptom/problem. The table shows the adjustments for each of these components. Using these, a weight of .605 is obtained. By including symptom/problem adjustments, the index becomes very sensitive to minor "top end" variations in health status. The adjustments for particular symptom/problems are shown in Table 2. For example, there are symptom/problem complexes for wearing eyeglasses, having a runny nose, or breathing polluted air. These symptom adjustments apply even if a person is in the top step in the other three scales. For example,

a person with a runny nose receives a score of .83 on the Quality of Well-Being
Scale when he is at the highest level of behavioral function (i.e., the top step on
each scale shown in Table 1). Thus, the index can make fine as well as gross distinctions.

Mathematically, the quality of well-being score may be expressed as:

$$W = \frac{1}{N} \sum_{l=1}^{L} W_\kappa N_\kappa$$

where

W = the symptom-standardized, time-specific quality of well-being score.
  l indexes the function levels $[l = 1, \ldots, L]$.
W_κ = the quality of well-being (weight, utility, relative desirability, social preference) for each function level, standardized (adjusted) for all possible symp-
  tom/problem complexes.
N_κ = the number of persons in each function level.
N = the total number of persons in the group, cohort, or population.

Thus, quality of well-being is simply an average of the relative desirability scores
assigned to a group of persons for a particular day or a defined interval of time.

Several studies attest to the reliability (21,52) and validity (51) of the Quality of
Well-Being Scale. For example, convergent evidence for validity is given by significant positive correlations with self-rated health and negative correlations with
age, number of chronic illnesses, symptoms, and physician visits. However, none
of these other indicators were able to make the fine discrimination between health
states which characterize the Quality of Well-Being Scale. These data support the
convergent and discriminant validity of the Scale (51).

Step 4: Estimate transitions among health states.   The Quality of Well-Being
Scale is the point-in-time component of the model. A comprehensive measure of
health status also requires an expression of prognosis or the probability of moving
between health states over time. People who are well now want to remain well.
Those who are at suboptimal levels want to become well, or at least not get worse.
A General Health Policy Model must consider both current functioning and probability of transition to other function levels over the course of time. When transition
is considered and documented in empirical studies, the consideration of a particular
diagnosis is no longer needed. We fear diseases because they affect our current
functioning or the probability that there will be a limitation in our functioning some
time in the future. A person at high risk for heart disease may be functioning very
well at present, but may have a high probability of transition to a lower level (or
death) in the future. Cancer would not be a concern if the disease did not affect
current functioning or the probability that functioning would be affected at some
future time.

When weights have been properly determined, health status can be expressed
precisely as the expected value (product) of the preferences associated with the states
of function at a point in time and the probabilities of transition to other states over
the remainder of the life-expectancy. Quality of well-being (W) is a static or time-
specific measure of function, whereas the well-life expectancy (E) also includes the
dynamic or prognostic dimension. The well-life expectancy is the product of quality

TABLE 3. *Illustrative computation of the well-life expectancy*

State	k	Y_k	W_x	$W_x Y_k$
Well	A	65.2	1.00	65.2
Non-bed disability	B	4.5	.59	2.7
Bed disability	C	1.9	.34	.6

Current Life Expectancy .... 71.6 life-years
Well-Life Expectancy ....68.5 well-years

From Kaplan and Bush, ref. 51

of well-being times the expected duration of stay in each function level over a standard life period. The equation for the well-life expectancy is

$$E = \sum W_\kappa Y_\kappa$$

where E is the symptom-standardized well-life expectancy in equivalents of completely well-years, and Y_κ is the expected duration of stay in each function level or case type estimated with an appropriate statistical (preferably stochastic) model.

A sample computation of the well-life expectancy is shown in Table 3. Suppose that a group of individuals was in a well state for 65.2 years, in a state of non-bed disability for 4.5 years, and in a state of bed disability for 1.9 years before their deaths at the average age of 71.6 calendar years. In order to make adjustments for the diminished quality of life they suffered in the disability states, the duration of stay in each state is multiplied by the preference associated with the state. Thus, the 4.5 years of non-bed disability become 2.7 equivalents of well-years when we adjust for the preferences associated with inhabiting that state. Overall, the well-life expectancy for this group is 68.5 years. In other words, disability has reduced the quality of their lives by an estimated 3.1 years.

Step 5: Estimating the benefit–cost-utility ratio. The San Diego Group has shown in a variety of publications how the concept of a well or weighted life expectancy can be used to evaluate the effectiveness of programs and health interventions. The output of a program has been described in a variety of publications as quality-adjusted life-years (43,53), well-years, equivalents of well-years, or discounted well-years (20,51,54). Weinstein (55,56) calls the same output Quality-Adjusted Life-Years (QALYs), and this has been adopted by the Congressional Office of Technology Assessment (57). It is worth noting that the quality-adjusted life-years terminology was originally introduced by Bush, Patrick, and Chen (43), but later abandoned because it has surplus meaning. The term "wellness" or "well-years" implies a more direct linkage to health conditions. Whatever the term, the number shows the output of a program in years of life adjusted by the quality of life which has been lost because of diseases or disability.

CONCLUSIONS

The term "quality of life" has been used inconsistently in the health services research literature. The definitions range from descriptions of functioning, to qualitative judgments of functioning, to measures typically unrelated to traditional health outcomes. In this chapter, we argue that "quality of life" is often poorly defined.

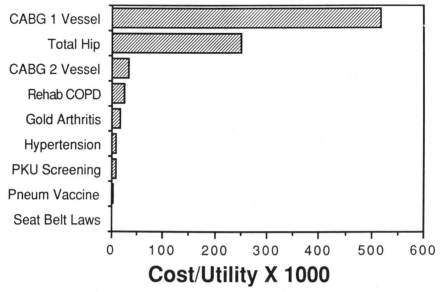

FIG. 1. Cost per quality-adjusted life-years for various programs, 1988 U.S. dollars. CABG, coronary artery bypass surgery; COPD, chronic obstruction pulmonary disease; PKU, phenylketonuria.

Several dimensions of quality of life emerge across different discussions. These include: mortality, functioning and role performance, symptoms, prognosis, and preference weights. We have proposed a system that combines these dimensions into a single number.

The objectives of health care include the extension of the life expectancy and the maximization of quality of life during years people are alive. In other words, health care should add years to life and also add life to years. All activities in the system should be evaluated by estimating their contribution toward these goals. The General Health Policy Model attempts to quantify the contributions from various providers and interventions so that the outcomes can be compared across very different interventions. These broad comparisons require an aggregate measure of health outcome. Profiles that have different dimensions for different components of outcome have little value for these comparisons. For example, many investigators suggest mental health outcomes cannot be evaluated using the same systems as used to measure physical health outcomes. However, we ultimately must make decisions about the comparative value of programs aimed at mental or physical health problems. Further, we must evaluate products that may have some benefits in one domain and side effects in another. A comprehensive system is required for these evaluations.

The General Health Policy Model has been used to evaluate outcomes in a variety of settings. Unfortunately, we will not have the opportunity to review each of these applications in detail. Suffice to say that different investigators have estimated the expected well-year benefits of competing interventions. Figure 1 summarizes many of these studies with adjustments to 1988 dollars. As the figure suggests, some interventions such as coronary artery bypass surgery for patients with ejection fractions less than 20% have been estimated to cost nearly one-half million dollars to produce the equivalent of a life-year. Traditional medical interventions in prevention, such as cholesterol and blood pressure reduction, may be much less expensive to produce the equivalent of a year of life. However, some nontraditional interventions including smoking cessation programs are even more cost-effective. Interestingly, our estimate suggests that the most cost-effective program has nothing to do with traditional health care: it involves passing laws that require the use of seat belts.

The use of the General Health Policy Model requires many heroic assumptions. The data for Fig. 1 come from a variety of different studies. In many of these cases, the health benefits were estimated using expert judgment. The accuracy of many of these estimates is unknown because they are based on judgments and not empirical studies. Furthermore, there are important assumptions in the application of the model that include the discount rate and the reliability of the estimate of treatment effectiveness. Despite these limitations, we believe the General Health Policy Model provides a unique new way of thinking about alternatives in health care. We hope to see more systematic experimental trials that employ structured measures such as the Quality of Well-Being Scale. As more data accumulate, we hope to provide a stronger database for comparing different alternatives in health care.

ACKNOWLEDGMENT

This work was supported by Grants no. RO1 HL 34732 and AR 33489 from the National Institutes of Health and Grant no. RO1 HS 05617 from the National Center for Health Services Research and Technology Assessment.

REFERENCES

1. Walker S, Rosser R, eds. *Quality of life: Assessment and applications.* London: WTP Press, 1988.
2. Wenger NK, Mattson ME, Furberg CD, Elinson J. *Assessment of quality of life in clinical trials of cardiovascular therapies.* New York: LaJacq, 1984.
3. Bergner M. Measurement of health status. *Med Care*, 1985;23:696–704.
4. National Institutes of Health. Epidemiology of Respiratory Diseases Task Force, Washington, D.C., U.S. Government Printing Office, NIH Publication, 1979;81:2019.
5. Bergner M, Bobbitt RA, Carter WB, Gilson BS. The sickness impact profile: Development and final revision of a health status measure. *Med Care* 1981;19:786–787.
6. Sullivan DF. Conceptual problems in developing an index of health. Office of Health Statistics, National Center for Health Statistics, Monograph Series II, No. 17, 1966.
7. Katz ST, Downs H, Cash H, Grotz R. Progress and development of an index of EDL. *Gerontologist*, 1970;10:20–30.
8. Stewart AL, Ware JE, Brook RH, Davies-Avery A. *Conceptualization and measurement of health for adults: Volume II, Physical health in terms of functioning.* Santa Monica: RAND, 1978.
9. Fanshel S, Bush JW. A health-status index and its applications to health-services outcomes. *Operations Research*, 1970;18:1021–1066.
10. Follick MJ, Gorkin L, Smith T, et al. Quality of life post-myocardial infarction: The effects of a transtelephonic coronary intervention system. *Health Psychology*, 1988;7:169–182.
11. Fishburn P. *Decision and value theory.* New York: Wiley, 1964.
12. Kaplan RM, Anderson JP. A general health policy model: Update and applications. *Health Services Research*, 1988;23:203–235.
13. Kaplan RM. Social support and social health: Is it time to rethink the WHO definition of health? In: Sarason IG, Sarason BR, eds. *Social support: Theory, research, and applications.* The Hague, Martinus Nijhoff, 1985c; 95–112.
14. Kaplan RM. Human preference measurement for health decisions and the evaluation of long-term care. In: Kane RL, Kane RA, eds. *Values and long-term care.* Lexington, MA: Lexington Books, 1982;157–188.
15. World Health Organization. Constitution of the World Health Organization. Geneva: WHO Basic Documents, 1948.

16. Meenan RF. AIMS approach to health status measurement: Conceptual background and measurement properties. *J Rheumat* 1982;9:785–788.
17. Kane RA, Kane RL. *Assessing the Elderly*. Boston: D.C. Heath, 1985.
18. Donald CA, Ware JE, Jr., Brook RH, Davies-Avery A. Conceptualization and measurement of health for adults in the health insurance study. *Social health (R-198714-HEW) (vol. IV)*. Santa Monica: RAND, 1980.
19. Ware JE, Jr, Donald CA. *Social well-being: Its meaning and measurement*. Santa Monica: RAND, 1980.
20. Heitzmann C, Kaplan RM. Interaction between sex and social support in the control of type II diabetes mellitus. *J Consult Clin Psychol* 1984;52(6):1087–1089.
21. Patrick DL, Bush JW, Chen MM. Methods for measuring levels of well-being for a health status index. *Health Serv Res* 1973b;8;228–245.
22. Kaplan RM, Bush JW, Berry CC. The reliability, stability, and generalizability of a health status index. *American Statistical Association, Proceedings of the Social Statistics Section*, 1978;704–709.
23. Ware JE, Jr., Johnston SA, Davies-Avery A, Brook RH. Conceptualization and measurement of health for adults. In: *The Health Insurance Study, Vol. III, Mental Health*. Santa Monica: RAND, 1979.
24. Dupuy H. Utility of the national center for health statistics general well-being schedule in the assessment of self-representation of subjective well-being and distress. *National Conference on Education in Alcohol, Drug Abuse, and Mental Health Programs*, Washington, D.C., 1974.
25. Ware JE, Jr., Manning WG, Duan N, et al. Health status and the use of outpatient mental health services. *Am Psychol* 1984;30:1090–1100.
26. Wells KB. *Depression as a tracer condition for the national study of medical care outcomes*. Santa Monica: RAND, 1985.
27. Biondi M, Pancheri P. Stress, personality, immunity and cancer: A challenge for psychosomatic medicine. In: Kaplan RM, Criqui MH, eds. *Behavioral epidemiology and disease prevention*. New York: Plenum, 1985;271–298.
28. Atkins CJ, Kaplan RM, Timms RM, Reinsch S, Lofback K. Behavioral programs for exercise compliance in chronic obstructive pulmonary disease. *J Consult Clin Psychol* 1984;52:591–603.
29. Rice RM. Organizational work and the overall quality of life. In: Oscamp S, ed. *Applied social psychology annual: Applications in organizational settings., Vol. 5*. Beverly Hills, CA: Sage, 1984;155–178.
30. Kaplan RM, Bush JW. Health-related quality of life measurement for evaluation research and policy analysis. *Health Psychol* 1982;1:61–80.
31. Bush JW. Relative preferences versus relative frequencies in health-related quality of life evaluations. In: Wenger NK, Mattson ME, Furberg CD, Elinson J, eds. *Assessment of quality of life in clinical trials of cardiovascular therapies*. New York: LaJacq 1984;118–139.
32. Croog SH, Levine S, Testa MA, Brown D, Bulpitt CJ, Jenkins CD, Klerman GL, Williams GH. The effects of anti-hypertensive therapy on quality of life. *New Engl J Med* 1986;314:1657–1664.
33. Hunt SM, McEwen J. The development of a subjective health indicator. *Sociol Health Illness*, 1983;2:231–245.
34. Doubilet P, Weinstein MC, McNeil BJ. Use and misuse of the term "cost-effectiveness" in medicine. *New Engl J Med* 1986;314:253–256.
35. Kaplan RM, Davis WK. Evaluating the costs and benefits of outpatient diabetes education and nutritional counseling. *Diabetes Care*, 1986;9:81–86.
36. Russell L. *Is prevention better than cure?* Washington, D.C.: The Brookings Institution, 1986.
37. Yates BT, DeMuth NM. Alternative funding and incentive mechanisms for health systems. In: Broskowski A, Marks E, Budman SH, eds. *Linking Health and Mental Health*. Beverly Hills, CA: Sage, 1981;77–99.
38. World Health Organization. *Health promotion: A discussion document on the concept and principles*. Copenhagen: WHO Regional Office for Europe, 1984.
39. Kaplan RM. Quantification of health outcomes for policy studies in behavioral epidemiology. In: Kaplan RM, Criqui MH, eds. *Behav Epidem Dis Prev*. New York: Plenum, 1985;31–54.
40. Kaplan RM. New health promotion indicators: The general health policy model. *Health Promotion*, 1988;3:35–49.
41. Kaplan RM, Anderson JP. The quality of well-being scale: Rationale for a single quality of life index. In: Walker S, Rosser R, eds. *Quality of life: Assessment and application*. London: MTP Press, 1987;51–77.
42. Weinstein MC, Stason WB. *Hypertension: A Policy Perspective*. Cambridge, MA: Harvard University Press, 1976.
43. Bush JW, Chen MM, Patrick DL. Cost-effectiveness using a health status index: Analysis of the New York State PKU screening program. In: Berg R, ed. *Health Status Index*. Chicago: Hospital Research and Educational Trust, 1973;172–208.
44. Chen MM, Bush JW, Patrick DL. Social indicators for health planning and policy analysis. *Policy Sciences* 1975;6:71–89.

45. Fanshel S, Bush JW. A health status index and its application to health-services outcomes. *Operations Research* 1970;18:1021–1066.

46. Reynolds WJ, Rushing WA, Miles DL. The validation of a function status index. *J Health Soc Behav* 1974;15:271.

47. Stewart AL, Ware JE, Jr., Brook RH, Davies-Avery, A. *Conceptualization and measurement of health for adults: Vol. 2, Physical health in terms of functioning.* Santa Monica: RAND, 1978.

48. Patrick D, Sittanpalam Y, Somerville S, et al. A cross-cultural comparison of health status values. *Am J Public Health* 1985;75(12):1402–1407.

49. Balaban DJ, Fagi PC, Goldfarb NI, Nettler S. Weights for scoring the quality of well-being instrument among rheumatoid arthritic. *Med Care* 1986;24(11):973–980.

50. Kaplan RM, Bush JW. Health-related quality of life measurement for evaluation research and policy analysis. *Health Psychol* 1982;1:61–80.

51. Kaplan RM, Bush JW, Berry CC. Health status: Types of validity for an index of well-being. *Health Serv Res* 1976;11:478–507.

52. Anderson JP, Kaplan RM, Berry CC, Bush JW, Rumbaut RG. Interday reliability of function assessment for a health status measure: The quality of well-being scale instrument. University of California at San Diego, (*unpublished*).

53. Bush JW, Fanshel S, Chen MM. Analysis of a tuberculin testing program using a health status index. *Social-Economic Planning Sciences* 1972;6:49–69.

54. Patrick DL, Bush JW, Chen MM. Toward an operational definition of health. *J Health Soc Behav* 1973a;14:6–23.

55. Weinstein MC, Feinberg H. *Clinical decision analysis.* Philadelphia: W.B. Saunders, 1980.

56. Weinstein MC, Stason WB. *Cost-effectiveness of coronary artery bypass surgery.* Harvard University: Center for Analysis of Health Practice, 1983.

57. Office of Technology Assessment, U.S. Congress. *A review of selected federal vaccine and immunization policies: Bases on case studies of pneumococcal vaccine.* Washington, D.C.: U.S. Government Printing Office, 1979.

III

Special Perspectives on Quality of Life Issues

Quality of Life Assessments in Clinical Trials, edited by B. Spilker. Raven Press, Ltd. New York © 1990.

12

An Ethical Perspective

Robert J. Levine

Yale University School of Medicine, New Haven, Connecticut 06510

One should not introduce new therapies into the practice of medicine without having first conducted appropriate research to establish their safety and efficacy. There is a broad social consensus that such research is required ethically; for some classes of therapies it is also required by law. What is not clear is whether the ethical obligation to conduct such research entails a requirement to assess the effects of a new therapy on quality of life. It is not because there are irreconcilable controversies in the field that we have this lack of clarity; rather it is because the controversial issues remain to be identified and controverted to the point that a broad social consensus begins to emerge.

It is against this backdrop that the ethical obligation to conduct quality of life assessments during the course of development of new therapies is considered. This begins with identification and discussion of the major ethical principles and norms that have become part of the broad social consensus in the fields of therapeutic innovation and medical therapy, focusing on those that are most germane to the problem at hand. It is proposed that if these principles and norms are applied consistently, there is an ethical obligation to conduct quality of life assessments in connection with some but not all projects designed to develop new therapies. This conclusion is presented in the form of the following guideline: In general, quality of life assessments are required when there are good reasons to predict that their results will yield information that will be of practical utility to doctors and patients making choices about whether to use the new therapy, and when the importance of such information justifies the costs and risks of developing it. The chapter ends with a discussion of criteria for determining the applicability of this guideline.

OBLIGATIONS TO CONDUCT RESEARCH

Before considering whether there is an ethical obligation to assess the effects on quality of life of new (or, for that matter, old) medical therapies, it is a good idea to reflect on an even more fundamental question: Is there an ethical obligation to do any biomedical research at all? Does society[1] have an obligation to conduct or

---

[1] The term "society" here follows the usage of the President's Commission (18, p. 4): "In speaking of society, the Commission uses the term in its broadest sense to mean the collective American community. The community is made up of individuals who are in turn members of many other, overlapping groups, both public and private: local, state, regional, and national units; professional and workplace organizations; religious, educational, and charitable institutions; and family, kinship, and ethnic groups. All these entities play a role in discharging societal obligations."

finance research having as its ultimate purpose the development of improved means to accomplish the purposes of the medical profession?

If society has such an obligation—and an argument why it does soon follows—it is not among the most pressing. To illustrate this point, Hans Jonas contrasts and compares the obligation to conduct biomedical research with some of the more fundamental obligations of society, such as protecting its members from harm and securing the conditions of its (the society's) preservation (1, p. 13). Such objectives necessarily have the highest priority. Unless society can, for example, secure the conditions of its preservation, it is impossible for its members to live meaningful lives in that they cannot live according to plans grounded in reasonable expectations regarding the consequences of their actions (2, p. 48ff.).

Biomedical research is usually directed not at preserving society but rather at improving it. Only in the most extreme circumstances could biomedical research be said to be directed toward preserving society. For example, if we were faced with an epidemic having the proportions of the Black Death of the Middle Ages but caused by an infectious agent refractory to all known curative or preventive measures, then biomedical research could play a role in preserving society. Society's obligation to conduct research designed to end such an epidemic would assume a very high priority indeed. In such circumstances, one could claim that there was a strict obligation to conduct biomedical research, the goal of which was to preserve society. Otherwise, the improvement of society through the conduct of biomedical research may be considered an ethically optional goal.

Jonas helps put the nature of this obligation in perspective (1, p. 14):

> Unless the present state [conditions of life in our society] is intolerable, the melioristic goal [of biomedical research] is in a sense gratuitous, and this is not only from the vantage point of the present. Our descendants have a right to be left an unplundered planet; they do not have a right to new miracle cures. We have sinned against them if by our doing we have destroyed their inheritance . . . not . . . if by the time they come around arthritis has not yet been conquered (unless by sheer neglect).

Ours is a society that has a commitment to progress. As citizens we expect more of society than the fundamental obligations discussed so far. We are committed to a vigorous and persistent effort to improve the conditions of life in our society. In the domain of our concern, we expect that through biomedical research we will continue to develop improved methods and modalities with which we can combat or prevent diseases and their attendant disability, pain, suffering, and premature death. Our perception of ourselves as a society committed to progress is reflected in the way we have shaped our society in the twentieth century. As a people we have charged our government with responsibility for conducting and supporting biomedical research and for encouraging and regulating such research in the private sector. To the extent that the government is charged with this responsibility and to the extent it has accepted this charge, one may say that the government has assumed on behalf of society an obligation to conduct biomedical research.

Government's acceptance of this charge is manifested in its creation and continued operation of agencies such as the National Institutes of Health and the National Science Foundation. It supports additional biomedical research outside its own agencies by means of grants and contracts. Further, it encourages biomedical research in the private sector by protecting economic incentives for the development of safe and effective new remedies. By accepting the charge of the people, by responding in these ways to their expectations, government has created a set of expectations regarding its future activities. As a people we rightfully expect that the government will continue to conduct, support, and encourage biomedical research. Failure to do so would be morally blameworthy in the sense that it is morally wrong not to honor one's commitments; one is bound to honor commitments in the absence of good reasons to do otherwise. Thus, in the ordinary course of events in our society, i.e., in the absence of crises that threaten the integrity of the society, our government can be regarded as having assumed an ethical obligation to conduct, support, and encourage biomedical research.

Regarding the obligations of other agents and agencies in our society, it seems clear that none have a strict obligation to conduct biomedical research unless they are voluntarily engaged in some activity that necessarily entails such an obligation. Included most conspicuously among such agents are those who wish to develop and market a new drug or device designed to cure, diagnose, or prevent human diseases or to alleviate their manifestations. Such persons are required ethically and legally to substantiate their claims of safety and efficacy for their new products through the conduct of what the Food, Drug, and Cosmetic Act calls "adequate and well-controlled" studies. Others may be bound ethically and legally to conduct biomedical research through accepting funds to conduct such research from either the government or private philanthropies. It can also be argued that in our society any person who wishes to make a public claim that something has an effect on the health of persons, has an ethical obligation to back up such a claim with appropriate evidence.

In our society there are no persons or agencies who have a strict ethical obligation to conduct biomedical research. Some, however, have assumed or may assume such an obligation through various sorts of commitments they have made. The government, for example, has accepted the mandate of society to conduct, support, and encourage biomedical research. Others, such as those who wish to introduce new therapies for diseases, assume an obligation to conduct research designed to demonstrate their safety and efficacy.

OBLIGATION TO ASSESS QUALITY OF LIFE

Does the acceptance of such an obligation entail or encompass an obligation to assess quality of life? Let us consider a more sharply focused question: When one's obligation to conduct biomedical research arises by virtue of one's intention to develop a new therapy, does one assume an obligation to assess its effects on the quality of life of patients for whom it will be prescribed or to whom it will be recommended?

In order to begin to answer this question it is necessary to reflect on the purpose of this class of biomedical research. There is a general consensus in our society that biomedical research cannot be justified unless it is designed sufficiently well so that there will be a reasonable expectation that it will accomplish its purpose. The National Commission for the Protection of Human Subjects of Biomedical and Behavioral Research (National Commission) articulated this consensus (3, p. 22): "Subjects should not be exposed to risk in research that is so inadequately designed that its stated purposes cannot be achieved."

In the field of therapeutic innovation, the central purpose is to develop therapies that will accomplish the goals of curing or preventing diseases or of ameliorating their manifestations. This purpose is related to the basic ethical principle of beneficence which, as interpreted by the National Commission, embodies two general rules: "Do no harm, and maximize possible benefits and minimize possible harms" (4, p. 6).

In the context of medical practice, considerations of beneficence are expressed in such familiar maxims as *primum non nocere* (first do no harm) and the Hippocratic Oath's "I will use treatment to help the sick according to my ability and judgment." In biomedical research, the leading ethical codes such as the World Medical Association's Declaration of Helsinki enjoin the physician-investigator not only to secure the well-being of individuals (research subjects and patients) but also to develop information that will form the basis of being better able to do so in the future (5, pp. 16–17). According to the Nuremberg Code, the risks of research must be justified by "the humanitarian importance of the problem to be solved by the experiment."[2]

Research in the field of therapeutic innovation has a tendency to focus on "outcome measures or endpoints which are considered objective in so far as they are based on external observation of the patient" (6, p. 115). In the field of oncology, for example, one measures how many patients have substantial reductions in the size of their tumors and how long these remissions last. Research on antihypertensive agents reflects a principal concern with the magnitude of reduction of diastolic blood pressure. In the course of these studies one also records and reports the adverse effects experienced by the patient-subjects.

Based on the results of such research, the physician may have reasonable confidence that a chemotherapeutic regimen is likely to reduce the size of a cancer or that an antihypertensive agent is likely to lower blood pressure. Such information is important, of course, but there is much more to medical practice than that. Patients do not consult physicians because they are offended by sphygmomanometer readings. They have a much broader view of what it means to secure their well-being now and in their personal futures. What they really want to know is this: "What is my life likely to be like if I take these drugs. What will I be able to do? How will I feel? And what if I don't?" These are, of course, questions about not only the quantity but also the quality of their lives.

Such questions lead us to a consideration of another basic ethical principle, respect for persons. This principle, as interpreted by the National Commission (4, pp. 4–5), also

> incorporates at least two basic ethical convictions: First, that individuals should be treated as autonomous agents, and second, that persons with diminished autonomy are entitled to protection. . . . An autonomous person is an individual capable of deliberation about personal goals and of acting under the direction of such deliberation. To respect autonomy is to give weight to autonomous persons' considered opinions and choices while refraining from obstructing their actions unless they are clearly detrimental to others. To show a lack of respect for an autonomous agent is to repudiate that person's considered judgments, to deny an individual the freedom to act on those considered judgments, or *to withhold information* necessary to make a considered judgment, when there are no compelling reasons to do so (emphasis supplied).

The most widely recognized instrumentality through which doctors show respect for the persons who are patients is informed consent. Informed consent, as envisioned in both law and ethics, includes (among other things) a presentation of information to the patient (5, p. 99ff.); the essential categories of information are

---

[2] The Declaration of Helsinki and the Nuremberg Code are reprinted in *Ethics and Regulation of Clinical Research* (5).

commonly referred to as "elements." The elements that are most germane to the present discussion are disclosure of (a) risks, (b) benefits, and (c) alternatives. Such disclosure must be in a language that the patient can understand, and it should convey meanings that are relevant to the patient's concerns. It should be responsive to questions such as those mentioned earlier: "What is my life likely to be like if I take these drugs? What will I be able to do? How will I feel? And what if I don't?"

Meaningful answers to such questions are often (not always) required by the patient to enable him or her to make considered judgments about therapies. Autonomous persons live according to life plans which reflect their personal conceptions of what it means to lead a good life. The usually unanticipated contingency of disease often forces persons to reconsider and reevaluate their life plans.[3] Faced with a disease that is almost certain to cause death within 5 years, for example, the patient may wish to reconsider a life plan that included graduate education. Similarly, the same patient might accept or reject therapy designed to postpone the fatal outcome based on an assessment of the expected effects of therapy on his or her life plan. The patient may decide, for example, that there is a better chance of completing and enjoying graduate school without repeated episodes of severe nausea and vomiting and frequent threats of bone marrow depression with all of its ramifications.

Concerns about a patient's life underlie the questions mentioned earlier, which can be restated, "If I take these medicines (or undergo that surgery) am I more or less likely to be able to live according to my life plan (to lead what I consider a good life) than if I pursue another course of therapy?" In order to show respect for autonomous persons who are patients, doctors must attempt to be responsive to such questions.

During the course of new therapy development, it is usually possible to foresee when such questions will be relevant after the new therapy is introduced into the practice of medicine (*infra*). Research that neglects to develop information upon which answers to such questions may be based, when the relevance of such questions can be foreseen, must be regarded as inadequate. Research must be designed sufficiently well that there will be a reasonable expectation that it will accomplish its purposes: (a) to develop therapies that will enhance the well-being of patients as such well-being is envisioned by particular patients, and (b) to develop information that will enable patients to make satisfactory choices regarding the use of such therapies.

Schipper and Clinch expressed in somewhat different terms a conclusion that is substantively the same (6, p. 116): "In the end, the carefully designed, well-conducted randomized clinical trial may provide statistical evidence of an outcome difference. However, the evidence is mathematical. It remains the obligation of the researcher to assure that the 'significance' has biological and human importance."

Let us consider briefly the obligations of "the researcher." The development of a new therapy is generally a complex enterprise involving the cooperation of multiple individuals and institutions. The responsibility for coordinating the activities of all of the participants resides with the individual or institution that intends to make a public claim regarding the safety and efficacy of the new therapy. In the case of drugs, devices, and other articles regulated by the Food and Drug Administration (FDA), the responsible agent is called the "sponsor," who requests of the FDA

---

[3] For an excellent discussion of the concept of "life plan," the central role it plays in living a meaningful life, and the interplay between sickness and life plans, see *Stories of Sickness* (2).

permission to make the public claim by filing a New Drug Application (NDA). It is the sponsor's obligation to see to it that all of the required activities are performed satisfactorily during the development of a new therapy. Therapeutic innovation in fields such as surgery in which there is no traditional way to identify an agent having responsibilities analogous to those of the sponsor may be problematic. There are likely to be fewer problems in such fields if some individual or institution regularly assumes the responsibilities of the sponsor. Drawing on the model provided by FDA-regulated activities, this author suggests that such responsibilities are or should be assumed by those who intend to make a public claim regarding the safety and efficacy of a new therapy.

CRITERIA FOR DETERMINING THE NEED FOR QUALITY OF LIFE ASSESSMENTS

As already noted, quality of life assessments are required only for some but not all new therapies. A guideline for determining when in the course of developing a new therapy there is a requirement for such assessments is proposed: In general, quality of life assessments are required when there are good reasons to predict that their results will yield information that will be of practical utility to doctors and patients making choices about whether to use the new therapy and when the importance of such information justifies the costs and risks of developing it.

The proposed guideline presents the obligation to conduct quality of life assessments in the form of a *prima facie* rule. A *prima facie* rule is ethically binding unless it is in conflict with other stronger rules or unless in a specific situation there is ethical justification for overriding the rule's requirements. In this case, the requirement for quality of life assessment does not apply if the importance of the anticipated information does not justify either the costs to the sponsor of the new therapy or the risks to the research subjects.

Under what circumstances might it be claimed that there are good reasons to predict that quality of life studies will yield information that will be of practical utility? Suggestive evidence is provided by a finding that the new therapy has an effect that is likely to impair quality of life. It may produce, for example, nausea, exercise intolerance, or dumping syndrome. To the extent that the patient must necessarily experience this effect for a long time, the need for quality of life assessment is increased proportionately. Patients with chronic diseases, for example, may have to receive the therapy for the rest of their lives or, for another example, the effects of a single intervention such as gastrectomy may be irreversible (7,8).

The criterion of "practical utility" is closely related to the concept of "material risk" in the law of informed consent. Legally, any risk of a proposed medical intervention that is "material" must be disclosed to the patient. In a leading informed consent case, *Canterbury v. Spence* (9), the court held: "A risk is thus material when a reasonable person, in what the physician knows or should know to be the patient's position, would be likely to attach significance to the risks or cluster of risks in deciding whether or not to forego the proposed therapy."[4] Thus a risk is "material" if information about it has practical utility in reaching a decision about whether to accept or reject a proposed therapy. The legal formulation does not

---

[4] For further discussion of the various standards for determining the materiality of risks, see *Ethics and Regulation of Clinical Research* ((5, pp. 103–105).

determine the ethical obligation to develop data about quality of life. It does, however, provide some perspective on the purpose of such information.

Terms such as "practical utility," "importance," and "justifies" do not have precise, inelastic meanings. Deciding what is important or justified in particular cases cannot be accomplished according to an ethical algorithm. As in most such matters, there is a need for informed and sensitive judgments.

Let us consider some examples of situations in which information about quality of life might have great practical utility. In these three examples quality of life considerations are likely to be very important; for many patients they will be more important than any other. These examples illustrate the types of situations in which the obligation to do quality of life assessments seems most compelling.

1. In the first example, therapy is to be administered to patients who feel well for the purpose of achieving a slight reduction in the probability of a serious morbid event in the distant future; this is exemplified by drug therapy of patients with mild essential hypertension (10).

2. In some cases, highly toxic chemotherapy may offer a small chance of remission to patients with highly resistant cancers, e.g., hypernephroma. This small chance notwithstanding, the average patient who accepts chemotherapy is likely to experience decreases in both quality and quantity of life (6,11).

3. In some cases, two therapies may yield the same results when expressed in such terms as overall survival or disease-free survival. However, there are substantial differences in the quality of life of patients who choose to receive these therapies. This situation is exemplified by the use of either radical mastectomy or simple mastectomy in the treatment of some patients with breast cancer (12).

According to Spilker (13, pp. 266–267) quality of life assessments are "generally not necessary . . . when a drug is life saving." Let us consider this criterion in some detail. When a drug or any other therapy is very likely to save a patient's life and to restore the patient promptly to his or her premorbid state of "normal living" (14), there is no requirement for quality of life evaluation. No reasonable patient would refuse an appendectomy for acute appendicitis or antibiotic therapy for meningococcal meningitis because he or she is unwilling to accept the transient detriments to quality of life expected of such therapeutic interventions.

There are, however, life-saving therapies that many reasonable people reject because they would find the quality of life during or following their administration unacceptable. Prominent examples include cardiopulmonary resuscitation, ventilators, and nasogastric tube feeding in certain patients who are near death (15). On similar grounds, many reasonable persons are likely to refuse to accept a totally implantable artificial heart at its current state of development (16).

What if a therapy is more likely than another to cure a lethal disease? We cannot assume that all or even most persons will opt for such a therapy if it is likely to create an important detriment to the quality of their lives. This is illustrated in the work of McNeil and colleagues who asked healthy volunteers to imagine that they had cancer of the larynx in order to determine how much longevity they would exchange for voice preservation (17). The volunteers were 37 middle and upper-management executives and 12 firefighters, each group averaging age 40. Using principles of expected utility theory to develop a method for sharpening decisions, they found that to avoid artificial speech the firefighters would trade off about 6% of their full life expectancy. Although executives would trade off more—an average of 17%—the difference was nonsignificant. "Although most subjects were willing to accept some decrease in long-term survival to maintain normal speech, virtually none would ever accept any decrease below 5 years."

Subjects were informed that with surgery 60% could expect to survive 3 years and with radiation, 30% to 40%. The subjects reacted as follows: If radiation offered only a 30% chance of survival for 3 years, practically none would decline surgery. By contrast, if the chance of survival for 3 years were 40%, 19% of the subjects would choose radiation therapy alone and 24% would choose radiation followed by delayed laryngectomy if necessary. The authors conclude "that treatment choices should be made on the basis of patients' attitudes toward the quality as well as the quantity of survival."

On the basis of the foregoing considerations it can be concluded that even if a therapy is designed to be life-saving, the need for quality of life assessment should be determined according to the criterion specified earlier, viz., when there are good reasons to predict that their results will yield information that will be of practical utility to doctors and patients making choices about therapies and when the importance of such information justifies the costs and risks of developing it.

Spilker proposes one additional criterion for determining the necessity for quality of life studies; that is, when a treatment is "extremely expensive" (13, p. 267). This proposition raises issues that have not been addressed so far in this chapter. These issues are related to the third of the three ethical principles identified by the National Commission, justice (4, pp. 8–10). Justice requires that the burdens and benefits of society be distributed fairly or equitably.

In March 1983, the President's Commission for the Study of Ethical Problems in Medicine and Biomedical and Behavioral Research (President's Commission) addressed the problems of equitable distribution of health services (benefits) in its report, *Securing Access to Health Care*. The Commission made these recommendations (18, pp. 4–5):

> The Commisssion concludes that society has an ethical obligation to ensure equitable access to health care for all. . . . Equitable access to health care requires that all citizens be able to secure an adequate level of health care without excessive burdens.

In its commentary on the latter recommendation, the President's Commission elaborated as follows:

> A determination of this level will take into account the *value* of various types of health care in relation to each other as well as the *value* of health care in relation to other important goods for which societal resources are needed. Consequently, changes in the availability of resources, in the effectiveness of a different forms of health care, or in society's priorities may result in a revision of what is considered "adequate" (emphasis added).

In recent years the costs of health care in the United States have been increasing at a rate that substantially exceeds inflation (19). Eventually, if they have not already, the costs of health care will become unacceptably high in that they will deny us the ability to finance "other important goods for which societal resources are needed."

In order to make informed choices in the public policy arena, decision makers must have access to relevant information regarding the expected consequences of their choices.[5] Relevant information about new medical modalities must take into

---

[5] This discussion addresses the need for information in the public policy arena because it is public

account effects on both quantity and quality of life for reasons already discussed. In choosing among alternative therapies designed to accomplish the same health objective, the prudent decision maker in the policy arena should generally select the one shown to be superior in cost-utility analysis; for example, the therapy which secures the largest number of quality-adjusted years of life expectancy for each dollar spent (20).

It is not suggested that cost-utility is the only relevant consideration in making policy decisions. There are many other factors that must be taken into account (18), a discussion of which is beyond the scope of this chapter. However, since information about quality of life will often be relevant to, and sometimes decisive in, making policy decisions regarding expensive new technologies, the cost of a new therapy should be taken into account when determining the necessity of quality of life assessments.

In cases in which the prime consideration is to develop data designed to facilitate decision making in the policy arena rather than in the context of the doctor-patient relationship, our guideline should be restated: In general, quality of life assessments are required when there are good reasons to predict that their results will yield information that will be of practical utility to decision makers in the policy arena in choosing whether to finance the new therapy and when the importance of such information justifies the costs and risks of developing it.

Further work is required to determine who should bear the responsibility of conducting and financing research having as its aim the enhancement of decision making in the policy arena. The grounds for assigning this responsibility to the sponsor of the new therapy are not as clear as they were for research designed to enhance decision making in the context of the treatment of individual patients.

ACKNOWLEDGMENT

The author is grateful to Harvey Schipper and Bert Spilker for their helpful criticisms of a draft of this chapter.

REFERENCES

1. Jonas H. Philosophical reflections on experimenting with human subjects. In: Freund PA, ed. *Experimentation with human subjects*. New York: George Braziller, 1970:1–31.
2. Brody H. *Stories of sickness*. New Haven and London: Yale University Press, 1987.
3. The National Commission for the Protection of Human Subjects of Biomedical and Behavioral Research. *Institutional review boards: Report and recommendations*. DHEW Publication No. (OS) 79–008, Washington, D.C., 1978.
4. The National Commission for the Protection of Human Subjects of Biomedical and Behavioral Research. *The Belmont Report: Ethical principles and guidelines for the protection of human subjects of research*. DHEW Publication No. (OS) 78–0012, Washington, D.C., 1978.
5. Levine RJ. *Ethics and regulation of clinical research*, 2nd ed. Baltimore: Urban & Schwarzenberg, 1986.
6. Schipper H, Clinch J. Assessment of treatment in cancer. In: Smith GT, ed. *Measuring health: A practical approach*. New York: John Wiley & Sons, 1988:109–155.

(governmental) officials who are responsible for distributing the benefits of society equitably. A consideration of the needs of others who require similar information is beyond the scope of this chapter. Such others include those who make decisions regarding hospital formularies, the scope of coverage by private insurance companies and health maintenance organizations, and the like.

7. Troidl H, Kusche J, Vestweber KH, et al. Quality of life: An important endpoint both in surgical practice and research. *J Chron Dis* 1987;40:523–528.
8. O'Young J, McPeek B: Quality of life variables in surgical trials. *J Chron Dis* 1987;40:513–522.
9. *Canterbury v. Spence*, 464 F 2d 72, CA DC 1972.
10. Fletcher AE, Hunt BM, Bulpitt CJ. Evaluation of quality of life in clinical trials of cardiovascular disease. *J Chron Dis* 1987;40:557–566.
11. Levine RJ. Uncertainty in clinical research. *Law, Medicine & Health Care* 1988;16:174–182.
12. Lasry JCM, Margolese RG, Poisson R, et al. Depression and body image following mastectomy and lumpectomy. *J Chron Dis* 1987;40:529–534.
13. Spilker B. *Guide to clinical interpretation of data.* New York: Raven Press, 1984.
14. Wood-Dauphinee S, Williams JI. Reintegration to normal living as a proxy to quality of life. *J Chron Dis* 1987;40:491–499.
15. President's Commission for the Study of Ethical Problems in Medicine and Biomedical and Behavioral Research. *Deciding to forego life-sustaining treatment: Ethical, medical and legal issues in treatment decisions.* U.S. Government Printing Office, Stock No. 040-000-00470-0, Washington, D.C., 1983.
16. The Working Group on Mechanical Circulatory Support of the National Heart, Lung and Blood Institute. *Artificial heart and assist devices: Directions, needs, costs, societal and ethical issues.* Bethesda, Maryland: National Heart, Lung and Blood Institute, 1985.
17. McNeil BJ, Weichselbaum R, Pauker SG. Speech and survival: Tradeoffs between quality and quantity of life in laryngeal cancer. *New Engl J Med* 1981;305:982–987.
18. President's Commission for the Study of Ethical Problems in Medicine and Biomedical and Behavioral Research. *Securing access to health care: The ethical implications of differences in the availability of health services.* U.S. Government Printing Office, Stock No. 0-401-553-QL3, Washington, D.C., 1983.
19. Ginzberg E. A hard look at cost containment. *N Engl J Med* 1987;316:1151–1154.
20. Drummond MF. Resource allocation decisions in health care: A role for quality of life assessments? *J Chron Dis* 1987;40:605–616.

Quality of Life Assessments in Clinical Trials, edited by B. Spilker. Raven Press, Ltd. New York © 1990.

13

Cultural Considerations

Stuart S. Campos and Thomas M. Johnson

Department of Anthropology, Southern Methodist University, Dallas, Texas 75275

The 1980s saw a rapid growth in the area of quality of life research. Studies encompassing a multitude of cultures currently are being conducted by developmental aid agencies, health care facilities, and university scholars, to name a few. These studies focus on issues having an impact on quality of life, such as overpopulation, poverty, disaster relief, urbanization, industrialization, migration, and immunization campaigns. Recently the *Journal of Social Indicators Research* was created, reflecting the increased interest in quality of life, and providing a common forum for all aspects of quality of life research.

Due to developing global interests in this area of research, the need for culturally sensitive methods to assess quality of life has never been greater. Researchers are increasingly asking whether a method used to assess quality of life in culture A can also be used in culture B. Although some researchers may desire a scale or similar instrument for global assessment of cultures, permitting comparison of the "nature" of one culture with another (or the views of an individual from one culture with someone from another), no such scale exists. In fact, given the multiplicity of variables or domains comprising a culture, that goal is unrealistic, both theoretically and methodologically.

This does not mean, however, that researchers should abandon attempts to include cultural variables in quality of life assessments. In fact, greater effort should be expended in considering cultural issues. Before culturally sensitive methods can be developed, however, the relationship between culture and quality of life must be understood. This chapter (a) introduces concepts necessary to understand the relationship between quality of life and culture, (b) discusses the advantages and disadvantages of different types of quality of life measures, and (c) proposes an approach that includes the cultural considerations essential when developing or modifying quality of life assessment instruments for effective use in multicultural settings.

ANTHROPOLOGICAL VIEWS OF CULTURE

The term "culture" is used as a scientific concept by all of the social sciences. There is still no single accepted definition of culture. In cultural anthropology, culture is generally defined as a shared conception and perception of reality that is socially transmitted to succeeding generations. Culture also includes norms that regulate behavior and result in distinctive roles that define "society" as the organization and

163

interaction of people. In short, culture includes learned and shared ways of interpreting the world and interacting in society, and thereby provides all individuals with ideas about what is good or bad, desirable or undesirable, valued or devalued, in life.

Each member of society occupies several different social roles. The sum total of these roles makes up an individual's status in society. An example of an individual's social roles may include husband, father, accountant, parishioner, and friend. In each role, individuals have expectations placed on them as to how to act toward others. Roles are prescribed by society, thus social interaction is based on a culture-specific consensus concerning the appropriateness of actions, ideals, or expectations of a person in a given status.

Contemporary societies are very diverse. That is to say, even though the members of a society share the same culture, they still may have radically different experiences and beliefs concerning quality of life. A society may appear to be an identifiable homogeneous group when viewed superficially from outside, yet when examined systematically from within, actually appears to be quite heterogenous. Such "plural" societies consist of smaller groups that are recognized as distinctive by members of the society. Examples of smaller groups are individuals with common occupation, wealth, religious affiliation, ethnic background, age, geographic location, and ideology. These groups sometimes are so distinctive in relation to the rest of society (e.g., cults, youth gangs, ethnic communities) that they are considered to be outside the larger group or society, although many of their views and values may be similar to the larger group.

Quality of life perceptions by any group or individual are to a large extent "culture bound." In other words, standards for evaluating quality of life vary dramatically from society to society or within a society depending on their particular culture. Unwary or unskilled researchers studying quality of life cross-culturally may be victims of "ethnocentrism"—the interpretation of the behavior of others in terms of one's own personal feelings, which likewise are powerfully shaped by cultural values. In terms of quality of life, ethnocentrism is the enemy of understanding. In order to assess quality of life in a culturally sensitive way, researchers must adopt the tenet of cultural relativism, the practice of analyzing beliefs in the context of the culture in which they belong. Cultural relativism would suggest that although there are values that are universally accorded recognition (such as food and shelter), there are no absolute standards of quality of life which can be indiscriminately applied to all cultures.

QUALITY OF LIFE ASSESSMENT

There are two approaches a researcher can use to assess quality of life: objective and subjective. The differences between the two are substantial, and choosing one over the other has important implications for the research conducted. Before one approach is chosen the researcher must be explicitly aware of the scope of the project and its goals for measuring quality of life. All research efforts are constrained by logistics and funding, but a project's goals should determine which approach to quality of life assessment is chosen.

Objective Approaches

The objective approach assumes that health, physical environment, income, housing, and other observable and quantifiable indicators are valid measures of quality of life and that there are absolute standards for assessing these variables which are used to determine or define quality of life. On the surface, an objective method for assessing quality of life seems logical. After all, there are dimensions of life that all people require and/or value, such as food, shelter, mobility, and good health.

Certainly there are minimal levels of nutrition compatible with life, and there are evaluation technologies (at the individual level, such as dietary intake logs, and at the group level, such as per capita food production) to assess nutritional levels as one facet of quality of life. In addition, it is possible to assess amount of square feet of living space per person, presence of running water and plumbing, and the like as measures of adequacy of shelter. It is also possible to determine the amount of migration through census data, case studies, and other techniques. Looking at job, income, and housing changes may be used to assess social mobility. There are also standard data sources for health care utilization, and surveys glean data about the type of health care available and/or accessible for given populations.

Many of these objective measures may be misleading, however. Stability and predictability of food supply may be far more important for quality of life than absolute per capita protein/caloric intake. Cultures vary widely in the type of housing that is available and desirable, and the extent to which privacy is a salient dimension of quality of life. In many parts of the world population density is very high, yet privacy is also high due to both the nature of housing construction and the norms of interaction within living spaces; conversely, in other cultures population density is low, yet normal patterns of interaction preclude privacy. For many people in other cultures, "privacy" is not even a meaningful concept. To be sure, running water and adequate sanitation have been associated with reduced morbidity and mortality around the world, yet the social consequences of, for example, closing centralized water wells and discouraging communal use of natural waterways for bathing or washing clothes may be perceived as reducing quality of life because of disrupted traditional patterns of social interaction. Although migration is now a ubiquitous feature of life in many cultures, and many may assume that migration is uniformly disruptive in quality of life terms, it is clear that forced migration is more deleterious than voluntary migration. Social mobility may also be used as a measure of quality of life, but upward social mobility may not be uniformly positive. Studies indicate that the first generation of upwardly mobile people suffers more adverse health consequences, and family disruption is common. On the other hand, so-called "blocked mobility," where a group may be relatively affluent by world standards but feels systematically excluded from opportunities for social and economic advancement, may perceive that their quality of life is suboptimal. The freedom to practice religion may be considered indicative of high quality of life, but religious pluralism or totalitarianism, particularly when it is associated with systematic social discrimination (such as in Northern Ireland) can have very adverse effects on quality of life.

Clearly, objective quality of life criteria such as nutrition, population density, housing, sanitation, migration, social mobility, and religious practices, will be different in different cultures because they are inextricably linked to less objective aspects of culture such as values, attitudes, and ideology. Without an understanding of the values and beliefs of a population, and of how those values and beliefs are manifested in individual people, the weighting and priority attached to any life area is arbitrary. Consequently any naive assertion as to the quality of life of a group or individual based on the above criteria alone is of questionable validity. Criteria such as income, health, food, and shelter as evaluated in one cultural context cannot necessarily be relied on to measure quality of life in another culture.

In the literature using objective approaches to quality of life assessment, there have been several problems involving disagreement about which indicators are relevant, and lack of understanding of the association between objective conditions of life and the subjective perception of these conditions (1). Inconsistencies occur between and even within studies. For example, in one study of the quality of life in different United States cities, little correlation exists among the variables used to assess the quality of life of these areas. Thus a city could score high in living conditions and low in measures such as racial discrimination, crime rate, and cost of living. "The failure to find highly correlated variables suggests that the measures employed are not addressing a common, underlying dimension of life experience" (1).

Finally, a number of studies have already demonstrated that objective conditions of life are only tenuously related to the subjective experience of quality of life (2–6). One such study indicates that people who are disabled because of an accident may report happiness levels which are surprisingly high and even comparable to people who are not disabled (7,8). Similarly, Campbell found that older blacks in the United States report higher levels of happiness than older whites despite their inferior objective living conditions (6). Further, it has been shown that women express a greater fear of violent assault compared to men despite the objective reality that men are more likely to be victims of violent assaults (9).

These studies and many others raise substantial doubt about the utility of objective quality of life indicators. Studies that use only objective quality of life *measures* simply project their own values and priorities onto their subjects, contributing little to understanding of quality of life *experience*. Stated another way, objective measures do not assess the *quality* of life, but rather the *quantity* of life.

Subjective Approaches

Subjective approaches attempt to assess people's qualitative *perceptions* of life experiences. Such approaches must consider more idiosyncratic evaluations on the part of people, and do not link quality of life to absolute or standard variables: they assess persons' feelings regarding quality of life. Subjective studies have identified a number of existential dimensions which seem to be linked to a high quality of life. Three are: (a) positive social relationships; (b) stability and conformity to a set of role expectations; and (c) disparity between expectations and achievements.

As an example of positive social relationships affecting quality of life, numerous studies have found that positive subjective descriptions of marital and familial relationships are the best predictors of high quality of life assessment (3,5,6,10). Conversely, people who are widowed, divorced, and separated express lower life satisfaction (11–14). As an example of the effect of stability of role expectations on quality of life, another study found that American women who were brought up earlier in this century, and therefore who have more traditional views, express levels of satisfaction with their roles as homemakers comparable to that of males in respect to their occupations. However, younger women whose socialization and role expectations differ from the older cohort express less satisfaction with housekeeping activities (15). A related study indicates that younger women who now are able to choose between homemaking roles and outside work are happier than those who feel that they have no choice (11). Still other studies have shown that level of life satisfaction is related to disparity between one's goals and achievements (16). To the extent that people are successful in achieving the goals *they set for themselves* at different life stages, they will more likely report higher quality of life.

Quality of Life Assessment in Medical Research

Quality of life assessment is now becoming more important in the evaluation of medical care, particularly since medical interventions increasingly are designed to help people cope with chronic health problems and diminished functional capacity, rather than simply to cure acute conditions and restore people to their prior level of functioning. This is also true in the case of mental health care where deinstitutionalization has placed many people with diminished adaptive capacity in community settings. In either case, it is clear that the presence or absence of *disease* (measurable biophysiological abnormality) is not as important in predicting quality of life as is *illness* (the subjective psychological and social distress caused by symptoms) (17). In fact, approximately 50% of patients with symptom complaints in primary health care settings have no demonstrable physical disease, and are often referred to as the "worried well" (18–21). Conversely, people with hypertension may have disease, yet have no subjective sense of being sick; in fact, the problem with treating hypertension is that in curing the disease (through use of medications), subjective quality of life often suffers because patients *feel* worse than when they were "diseased." Health care workers and quality of life researchers alike need to be aware of this distinction between objective (disease) and subjective (illness) dimensions of sickness.

In short, by utilizing *subjective* measures to assess quality of life, individual, social, and cultural factors are automatically included in the analysis, since individuals' subjective experiences result from complex interaction of variables at all three levels. Unfortunately, a review published in 1988 indicated that 41% of the quality of life studies analyzed used only objective measures, despite the fact that subjective measures have produced more consistent findings than did the objective measures (22). Although 41% may appear high, it represents an important increase in utilization of subjective measures, because a 1981 review in the same journal found that 87% of the studies used only objective assessment techniques (1).

CANTRIL SELF-ANCHORING STRIVING SCALE

The most accurate manner in which to assess quality of life is subjective because objective categories, which reflect bias on the part of the researcher, are not valid measures cross-culturally or between social groups. Ironically, as we have discussed above, measures which are purported to be "objective" are actually based on the subjective opinions of the researchers.

There is a great need, especially in medical research and practice, for a method

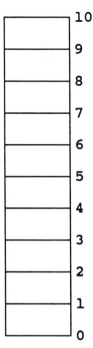

FIG. 1. Cantril Self-Anchoring Striving Scale.

to assess quality of life that collects comparable and quantifiable data without imposing culture-specific standards. Such a method must also have a high degree of flexibility, being adaptable for use in many different situations. A quality of life approach is needed which can be broadly applied in highly diverse areas of medicine. It is neccessary to measure a person's response and progress in therapy, whether treatment is psychological, pharmacological, somatic, or a combination of these.

The Cantril Self-Anchoring Striving Scale can be used as a quality of life assessment method that is most capable of fulfilling the above criteria. This scale is a simple, widely applicable method for tapping the unique "reality" of each individual, that has been translated into 26 different languages and found to have a reliability coefficient of .95 (12). It is extremely versatile, and can be used to assess global perceptions of quality of life. This scale can also be used to elicit subjective assessments of very specific aspects of life, such as housing, nutrition, health care, treatment outcomes, and the like.

The Cantril Self-Anchoring Striving Scale is based on a model of a ladder with 10 rungs (Fig. 1), with the top rung representing "the best possible _____" and the bottom representing "the worst possible _____" for the research subject or patient. To do a global quality of life assessment, the blank should be completed with general statements such as, "the best possible life for you," or "the most successful outcome for you." For assessment of more specific variables, the blanks should be completed with statements like "the best possible housing situation," "the best possible treatment outcome," or "the most satisfactory diet." The quality of life researcher simply asks patients to rate "where they are on the ladder currently" and "where they were [some period of time ago]," and may also choose to ask "where they think they will be [some period of time in the future]." Then the researcher simply asks, "What reasons do you have for putting yourself on [whatever rung]?'' In this ''self-anchoring'' approach, each individual defines quality of life based on his or her own assumptions, perceptions, aspirations, and values relative to the two extremes, or anchoring points. This self-defined continuum is then used as the measuring device. The scale can be used as either a pre-post or retrospective assessment of a clinical or community-level intervention.

In analyzing data from the Cantril Self-Anchoring Striving Scale, quantitative change scores can be computed to evaluate the impact of any interventions on quality of life. Mean quality of life levels can also be computed, although this is of less value. Qualitatively, it is then necessary to conduct content, cluster, or domain analysis of responses to the reasons people give for putting themselves on certain rungs of the ladder.

It must be stressed that the Cantril Self-Anchoring Striving Scale is a technique used to elicit information and a scale used to record and quantify it. It is not an index with a set of *a priori* criteria used to evaluate an individual. In order to utilize the scale, only one question needs be designed to elicit information on each quality of life issue to be assessed. The questions used to qualify the numerical responses from the scale are extremely important. It is not enough for clinicians to conduct research on a particular area—for example, aphasia—and devise questions. Open-ended questions must be used when asking patients to discuss why they gave their numerical responses (rungs on the ladder): only this type of question can elicit *patient* concerns about aphasia, which may be quite different from *clinician* concerns. One study found that when three groups (one of rehabilitation clinicians and two of aphasic patients) generated separate lists of situations in which communication problems occur, the patient groups' lists were much more similar to each other's than to the clinicians' list (23). Moreover, the clinicians vastly underestimated the patient's focus on social concerns. In addition, the patients generated more concrete situations, which are useful to quality of life research. This study suggests that previous quality of life measures that have relied solely on clinical judgment for determination of their content may inadequately represent patient, and therefore cultural, values.

The benefits of using quality of life as both a measurement and a rehabilitation tool in clinical therapy are enormous, as long as the patients' subjective assessments are considered. It is theoretically possible for a clinician-generated index that assesses an aphasic patient's quality of life to reflect a response to therapy, while an index using the Cantril Self-Anchoring Striving Scale may show a reduced or unimproved quality of life. This is because physicians typically rate quality of life improvement in aphasia based on ability to speak, whereas patients are more concerned with the perceived social benefits of being better able to speak.

CONCLUSION

It is strongly suggested that a subjective approach be used in any quality of life research project and, when applicable, that objective measures also be used. It is only through the use of a subjective measure of quality of life that a patient's implicit cultural and personal values can be included in the assessment. Objective measures are often purported to be cross-culturally valid, however, they are only valid in the most general sense. Objective measures do not account for subcultural differences in perceptions of quality of life. In addition, although a certain group shares the same culture, the individuals of the group still have widely varying personal beliefs and values. Thus, while an objective assessment instrument may be valuable for assessing general quality of life issues for the cultural group, it is unable to assess the feelings and concerns regarding quality of life for a particular patient. With the subjective Cantril Self-Anchoring Striving Scale approach described, it is possible to account both for the broader values of the group and also for the idiosyncratic concerns and values of the individual.

REFERENCES

1. Najman JM, Levine S. Evaluating the impact of medical care and technologies on the quality of life: A review and critique. *Soc Sci Med* 1981;15F:107–115.
2. Palmore E, Luikart C. Health and social factors related to life satisfaction. *J Health Soc Behav* 1972;13.
3. Bharadwaj L, Wilkening EA. The prediction of perceived well-being. *Soc Indicat Res* 1977;4.
4. Larson R. Thirty years of research on the subjective well-being of older Americans. *J Gerontol* 1978;31.
5. Wilkening EA, McGranahan D. Correlates of subjective well-being in Northern Wisconsin. *Soc Indicat Res* 1978;5.
6. Campbell A, Converse PE, Rodgers WL. *The quality of American life.* New York: Russell Sage, 1976.
7. Bulman RJ, Wortman CB. Attributions of blame and coping in the 'real world': Severe accident victims react to their lot. *J Pers Soc Psychol* 1977;35.
8. Brickman P, Coates D, Janoff-Bulman R. Lottery winners and accident victims: Is happiness relative? *J Pers Soc Psychol* 1978;36.
9. Mason R, Faulkenberry GD. Aspirations, achievements and life satisfaction. *Soc Indicat Res* 1978;5.
10. Weaver CN. Job satisfaction as a component of happiness among between males and females. *Personn Psychol* 1978;31.
11. Orden SR, Blackburn NM. Dimensions of marriage happiness. *Am J Sociol* 1968;173.
12. Bradburn NM, Caplovitz D. *Reports on happiness.* Chicago: Aldine, 1965.
13. Glenn ND. The contribution of marriage to the psychological well-being of males and females. *J Marr Fam* 1975;37.
14. Near JP, Rice RW, Hunt RG. Work and extra-work correlates of life and job satisfaction. *Acad Mgmt J* 1978;21.
15. Rodgers WL. Work status and the quality of life. *Soc Indicat Res* 1977;4.
16. Cantril H. *The patterns of human concerns.* New York: University Press, 1966.
17. Kleinman A, Eisenberg L, Good B. Culture, illness, and care: Clinical lessons from anthropologic and cross-cultural research. *Ann Int Med* 1978;88.
18. Hilkevitch A. Psychiatric disturbances in outpatients of a general medical outpatient clinic. *Intl J Neuropsych* 1965;1.
19. Lipsitt DR. Psychodynamic considerations of hypochondrias. *Psychother Psychosom* 1974;88.
20. Katon W, Ries R, Kleinman A. The prevalence of somatization in primary care. *Comp Psych* 1984;25.
21. Cummings NA. The dismantling of our health system: Strategies for survival of psychological practice. *Am Psych* 1968;41.
22. Hollandsworth JG. Evaluating the impact of medical treatment on the quality of life: A 5-year update. *Soc Sci Med* 1988;26.
23. Lomas J, Pickard L, Mohide A. Patient versus clinician item generation for quality-of-life measures. *Med Care* 1987;25.

Quality of Life Assessments in Clinical Trials, edited by B. Spilker. Raven Press, Ltd. New York, 1990.

14

A Marketing Perspective

Louis A. Morris*

Division of Drug Advertising and Labeling, Food and Drug Administration, Rockville, Maryland and Center for Marketing Policy Research, The American University, Washington, D.C. 20016

In the final analysis, for quality of life assessment to have any utility it must play a role in the politics of therapeutic selection. A purpose of quality of life assessment is to provide feedback to prescribers about health outcomes that are meaningful to the patient. In theory, if doctors understand the quality of life ramifications of the therapies they select, they can base their choice of treatment on factors that "really matter" to the patient.

Of course, what "really matters" to me may not "really matter" to you. The search for a single aggregate measure of quality of life that completely and accurately measures health status has been unsuccessful (1). Apparently, people conceptualize "health status" in a multidimensional fashion. Accurate classification of health status requires specification along a number of dimensions (2). There is some debate in the literature about the number of dimensions necessary to thoroughly evaluate health quality of life and what they should be called (3).

If therapies cannot be fully assessed along a single dimension but must be categorized along a constellation of dimensions, the choice of the "best" therapy requires a complex evaluation of each potential therapy's performance along a range of outcomes. As the number of relevant dimensions increases, so does the likelihood that any therapy will perform better along certain dimensions but worse on others. This evaluation, in turn, is based on the degree to which each of the dimensions is valued by the decision maker. The problem that arises is deciding which value system is to be used to evaluate and select a therapy. The ethical consensus is that to the fullest extent possible, the patient's value system, rather than the physician's, must be considered when judgments are made among therapies that pose quality of life trade-offs (4).

With therapies assessed only in terms of direct physiological outcomes, the physician, on rudimentary knowledge about the patient, was best trained to make complicated judgments about therapies. However, quality of life data add new dimensions with which therapies must be evaluated. Evaluation of these dimensions requires very personal knowledge about the patient's proclivities and values to insure an appropriate choice of treatment. Thus, the inclusion of quality of life information

---

* This is written in the author's capacity as a private citizen. No official support or endorsement by the Federal Food and Drug Administration is intended or should be inferred.

as part of a therapeutic evaluation necessitates greater knowledge and application of the patient's value system to therapeutic decision making.

The thesis of this chapter is that a marketing perspective on quality of life measurement can help us understand (a) how therapeutic selection can better incorporate the patient's values, and (b) ultimately, how therapies can be designed to better fit patients' needs and value systems. With these goals in mind, this chapter first reviews the modern concept of marketing. Second, it describes three ways in which quality of life measurement may be used in pharmaceutical marketing. Third, it describes how quality of life data can be built into the physician's decision-making process for pharmaceuticals in a way that reflects patient values for different quality of life outcomes.

THE MARKETING CONCEPT

Most people view marketing and selling as analogous concepts. In each case, the producer transfers goods and services for which the consumer pays an appropriate price. Over the years, however, the marketing concept has evolved and changed its focus away from the selling of commodities and toward the "exchange" process between two social units (5). Several important implications flow from this change in focus.

Rather than emphasizing goods and services, consumer needs are the nucleus of the marketing function. Rather than accrue profits through sales volume, modern marketers view consumer satisfaction as the route to repeat business, consumer loyalty, and ultimately to increased profits. Rather than viewing the selling function as a one-way flow of goods and services, marketing is accomplished through a two-way flow between producer and consumer. Not only are goods and services exchanged, but anything of value may be part of the marketing process.

To the extent that a product or service enhances the quality of life of an individual, one would assume that the individual would be motivated to seek to obtain that product compared to another product that does not improve quality of life outcomes to as great an extent. Problems can arise, however, in the exchange process that reduce ability to select the highest valued product for each patient.

First, product selection must be individualized for the patient. As discussed above, the multidimensional nature of quality of life measurement suggests that competing products have variable quality of life profiles which are differentially valued by patients. Therefore, individual products will have different patient groups who value each product. Selecting which patient groups are best suited for each product is difficult given the different quality of life profiles of the products and disparate patient value systems.

Second, even if a product has a distinct advantage over another when graded against an individual's value system, that product may not be perceived as such because communications about the product are inadequate or unclear. The transfer of information from a sender to a receiver is necessarily limited by shortcomings of human information processing. Therefore, simply learning and remembering relevant information about the product and the patient are difficult given the cluttered informational environment in which most clinicians operate.

Two marketing principles, market segmentation and product positioning, help facilitate mutually beneficial exchanges between producer and consumer. The first principle, marketing segmentation, is based on the premise that we can refine the exchange process by clustering consumers into homogeneous groups or market segments. Rather than mass market a therapy (i.e., develop one therapy and communications program suited for all potential consumers), we can create more carefully targeted therapies by grouping consumers into homogeneous markets (e.g., the elderly, middle age, children) and develop therapies more suited for their needs, plus more meaningful communications programs.

Market segmentation is a common practice in medical marketing when, for example, different dosage forms are used by pediatric and geriatric patients or when marketers create different advertising campaigns for family physicians and specialists. However, the "basis" or variable used to segment a market need not be a demographic category such as age or profession. Any variable that reliably measures a consumer trait or characteristic can be used as a market segmentation basis.

In recent years, considerable attention has been devoted to segmenting markets on the basis of primary and secondary traits (psychographics) (6), lifestyle and value orientation [the Values and Lifestyles (VALS) typology] (7), and motives for using particular products (benefit segmentation) (8). Thus, quality of life could be used to group patients into homogeneous segments. Patients with similar quality of life preferences for therapeutic outcomes could be viewed as representing distinct market segments. However, would quality of life serve as a meaningful basis for market segmentation and would such an orientation facilitate better exchanges between patient and provider (be it doctor and/or pharmaceutical company)? We will return to this issue later in this chapter.

The second principle, product positioning, is based on the premise that within a competitive marketing environment, each product must maintain a distinct image in the consumer's mind. The meaning that a consumer attributes to a product is based on the consumer's assessment of the product's attributes. Attributes may be physical descriptions of the product (e.g., a white-colored tablet), effects produced by the product (e.g., the drug causes drowsiness and decreases ability to drive a car), or symbolic elements (e.g., one must be quite sick to take such a serious medication).

Marketers can "position" their product by changing; (a) the product itself (e.g., the chemical structure, dosage form, packaging, or even the product's name), (b) the advertising, (c) the distribution system (e.g., through physicians' offices, hospitals, pharmacies), and (d) the pricing structure (price and quality are often assumed to be positively correlated). In addition, factors outside the marketer's control can influence the product image; for example, the press may publicize stories about the product's risks or benefits.

An important lesson from marketing is that product positioning must be clear and meaningful. Emphasizing too many attributes will lead to unclear positioning as consumers will have difficulty understanding how one product is different from its competitors. Marketers must choose which attributes to emphasize (so the product will be perceived as distinct from the other products in the class) and how to communicate those distinctions. A superior marketing position is obtained to the extent that a product is beneficial to the target market compared to competing products. Thus, choosing a product positioning (i.e., creating a theme that characterizes the product) is a function of: (a) assessing the competition to understand existing product positions and finding a unique "niche," and (b) understanding the needs and values of the target market to find a theme that will clearly emphasize the perceived benefits of the product for the target market.

In marketing pharmaceuticals, the drug decision maker and the drug user are different people. All things being equal, physicians will typically seek to select the therapy that will most benefit the patient. It is not clear how accurately physicians can make these judgments, especially when the perceived benefits are based on subjective perceptions of health status rather than physical response. Therefore, marketers need to be careful that the product benefits emphasized in product positioning are meaningful to the patient and that these benefits are understood and valued by the physician as well.

QUALITY OF LIFE AND MARKETING

With this primer on marketing as a background, one can see how quality of life measures would be appealing to marketers. Quality of life data hold the potential for translating physical and biological effects to psychological and behavioral effects that have special value to patients. In an age where "consumerism" in medicine is increasing, physicians are likely to be more responsive to claims made about a therapy's impact on patients' quality of life. Therapies that are perceived as "humanistic" are likely to be positively evaluated by patients and physicians (9).

However, quality of life data are new to marketing. Examining the evolution of this relationship, we only begin to see how marketing managers can use quality of life data. Following through with the logic presented above, it is possible to discern three ways in which marketers are currently using quality of life measurement or how they may use it in the future.

Category 1. A Better Product

During the early stages of use of quality of life data within any single product category, advertisers are able to make broad claims that their product has superior quality of life outcomes. For example, claims that Ridura (Smith, Kline, and Beckman's arthritis therapy) or Procardia (Pfizer's antianginal medicine) "improves quality of life" or that Transderm-Nitro (Ciba-Geigy's nitroglycerine patch) "helps angina patients get more out of life" suggest superiority of the product on some quality of life measure.

In this case, the marketer is capitalizing on the physician's interest in quality of life. The marketer may or may not have completed quality of life studies to make such a claim, as such a vague claim may be supported by clinical data relating to overall safety and effectiveness. It should be noted that recently the Food and Drug Administration objected to several of these claims because the marketer inferred the drug took some positive action in treating a disease, when the data indicated that the side effect profile for the medication did not cause an inhibition of functioning. Thus, the advertised drug did not "improve" quality of life, but merely reduced the probability that a negative influence of quality of life would occur.

Other action by the Food and Drug Administration suggests that marketers may need to qualify their claims more specifically in the future. For example, it recently objected to the claim that Tenex (A. H. Robbins' antihypertensive) was "patient friendly" and requested that additional information about dosage and side effects be added to clarify why the medicine was so "friendly." One may also assume that the usefulness of these broad quality of life claims is likely to decrease as competitors make similar claims. A once-differentiated product becomes undifferentiated as the competition catches up.

Category 2. A Different Product

Once quality of life claims become more common, marketers can utilize the wealth of information flowing from quality of life studies to differentiate their product along meaningful quality of life dimensions. The multidimensionality of quality of life measurement promises a vast number of new claims that can be made about individual products. Not only can new attributes be added to enhance the product's image, but the attributes chosen to be emphasized by the marketer may help physicians select products better suited for individual patients.

As discussed above, marketers can choose to emphasize individual quality of life scale outcomes where a particular product outperforms others. Thus, if a product performs better on a cognitive functioning scale than competing products but is no different or worse on other scales, the marketer would use cognitive functioning as a major positioning variable. Advertisements can be geared to emphasize cognitive functioning (e.g., a theme of "when alertness counts" might be used) and pictures of patients in tasks requiring alertness can be shown (e.g., an air traffic controller). A competitor whose product is outperformed on the cognitive functioning scale, but which performs better on a physical functioning scale, would logically emphasize this advantage when positioning their product. The advertisements for this product might emphasize physical performance (e.g., when "endurance" counts) and display pictures of patients in tasks or roles requiring physical stamina (e.g., a fireman). Not only would advertisements be geared to reinforce this positioning, but the name of the product, its distribution system, any collateral materials developed (e.g., patient educational materials, desk top media), public relations efforts, and more could all be directed to emphasize this theme.

Using quality of life data to position products is common in medical marketing. For example in the area of hypertension therapy, Hytrin (Abbott/Wellcome) is claimed to maintain physical, mental, and sexual performance; Prinivil (Merck) is promoted as letting active patients stay active; Trandate (Glaxo) is promoted as preserving vitality and exercise tolerance; and Capoten (Squibb) is promoted as contributing to the patient's feeling of well-being.

When selecting drug therapy, the physician must decide which product is best for each patient. Given an equivalence of medical and diagnostic criteria, the physician presumedly attempts to match the quality of life theme emphasized for the drug to the physician's perception of the importance of the theme to the individual patient. The extent to which quality of life data are used as part of the physician's evaluation criteria when selecting drug products is unclear, however. Studies of physician prescribing indicate that efficacy, side effects, and cost are the most important criteria influencing physicians' selection of drug products (10,11). However, these studies may be dated and the use of quality of life data in physicians' decisions regarding drug product selection has not been adequately addressed in the scientific literature (although they are probably well known to marketers through proprietary research).

As suggested above, there is reason to believe that physicians are becoming more interested in quality of life because of their desire to satisfy their patients. It is also likely that physicians perceive quality of life data as indicative of the physiological differences in drug effects that more meaningfully expresses the drug's influence on the patient's lifestyle and performance. Thus, quality of life may not be perceived as a unique contribution to drug effects assessment, but as a means of translating physiological effects to patient performance measures. From an advertising perspective, demonstrating the benefits of a product, as opposed to merely describing its advantages on lower order attributes, may more fully communicate the advantages of one product over another, especially if the benefits are not immediately perceived by the receiver of the message.

Another use of quality of life data which has immense importance to the pharmaceutical industry is its use in cost-benefit analyses. With the large increase in institutional purchasing and the increase in the number of formularies controlling product selection, pharmaceutical companies are increasingly being asked to justify their product's adoption to purchasing and approving boards. Cost figures are straightforward, but the benefits of a product are much more difficult to estimate.

Quality of life data have the potential to demonstrate direct benefits of a pharmaceutical product on patients' lives. Furthermore, unique contributions to quality of life from different products can help justify the outlay of higher payment levels by purchasing institutions. Thus, quality of life may help justify and support pharmaceutical pricing levels.

Category 3. A Basis for Segmentation

Using quality of life data to make claims for product superiority or to differentially position products are common uses of these data. However, even if the physician is aware of the advantages of different therapies, how is the physician to know which therapy an individual patient would prefer? There are three possible ways for the physician to make such a determination.

First, the physician could make a determination based on gross observations of the patient, scanning the chart for background data, and simple questions posed to the patient about hobbies, lifestyle, and preferred activities. Using this approach, the doctor makes broad assumptions based on gross characteristics of the patient. Thus, a physician may presume that cognitive functioning is important for a college professor whereas physical performance is important for a laborer. However, most quality of life variables are more specific, calling for distinctions between more precise sets of variables that may not be immediately evident to an observer. For example, the Sickness Impact Profile contains 12 subscales measuring factors such as home management, body care and movement, ambulation, recreation and pastimes, social interaction, and alertness (12). The Activities of Daily Living Scale and the Instrumental Activities of Daily Living Scale contain subscales representing bathing, dressing, feeding, shopping, housekeeping, and others (13). Gross observation of the patient and simple, indirect questions may not provide enough information for the physician to reach a valid conclusion. In addition, there is no guarantee that the physician's perceptions are representative of the patient's. A laborer may value cognitive functioning (alertness) more than physical stamina (ambulation), whereas a college professor may hold the opposite set of values.

A second way that the physician could integrate the quality of life preferences of the patient into clinical decision making is to question the patient in depth and solicit feedback along a number of critical dimensions. This is the optimum solution to the problem of how to build patient utilities into the process. Unfortunately, the prospect of soliciting and obtaining such precise feedback is likely to require enormous time and patience by the physician (14). There may be a large number of quality of life variables measured and the physician would have to discuss all quality of life outcomes, or at least the statistically significant ones, where therapies differed. The physician would have to guard against framing effects (15) and other sources of bias to insure that the patient's stated preferences were forthright and reflective of personal values. Finally, the complexity of the data confronting the patient may be overwhelming. In the face of this potential for information overload, the physician would have to either simplify the discussion (perhaps by summarizing or ignoring certain variables) which could prove biasing, or guard against confronting the patient with such a complex set of decisions that the patient abdicates his/her role in the decision-making process and leaves the therapy decision totally to the doctor. Thus, while in-depth discussion of quality of life trade-offs among different therapies is the preferred method of obtaining patient feedback, it may be difficult to implement in a straightforward manner.

A third possibility that may be used in conjunction with patient discussion, is to use quality of life data, along with other data, to segment patients into meaningful subgroups. Patients can be grouped on the basis of consistencies in the values they assign to various quality of life outcomes and the resultant groups may be described along various demographic, psychographic, lifestyle, and physician-patient interaction proclivities. Once the market segments are defined and described, both marketers and physicians would have a more precise categorical schema by which patients may be assigned to therapeutic options.

Operationally, the segmentational process would require at least two stages. First, quality of life outcomes would need to be related to patients' value states. Each important quality of life outcome may be traced through an association pathway to underlying values with the use of a "means-end" analysis (16). The means-end chain is produced through a qualitative interviewing technique called "laddering." Applying the laddering procedure to quality of life data, consumers would first be asked to provide the major "distinctions" they perceive among quality of life profiles from different competing drugs. These data can easily be obtained from clinical trials already completed. For example, after reviewing the quality of life outcomes from clinical trials of three antihypertensive drugs, patients may conclude that one difference between the drugs is that one drug seems to make patients "sleepy," other drugs lead to more "confusion," etc.

Next, subjects would be asked to provide their personal interpretation of the meaning (or "consequences") that would result from the distinctions they listed. For example, subjects would be asked, "What would it mean to you if a drug made you sleepy?" They might answer, "I couldn't drive in my car at night." Subjects would then be asked to provide the next higher order consequence: "What would it mean to you if you could not drive your car at night?" Each answer would become more personal and eventually underlying values would be derived through elicitation of these complicated and personalized linkages.

Once the laddering study was completed, a second larger study would be undertaken. The second study would involve using the quality of life distinctions, consequences, and values derived from the laddering study, along with other descriptive variables as input into a segmentation study. Subjects would be asked to rate the personal importance of each of these variables. Using clustering techniques, patients would be grouped into a series of empirically derived categories. Care would need to be exercised to insure that the derived clusters were psychometrically valid. Additionally, the derived clusters would need to be examined to be certain that they were theoretically meaningful and internally consistent. It may be necessary to use stepwise or hierarchical clustering techniques to insure that values serve as the primary clustering variables, with consequences and distinctions added to the procedure at a later time.

The important result from these analyses is the identification of a series of patient groups based on the values patients place upon distinctions in quality of life outcomes among competing therapies; the distinctions themselves, and the consequences of those distinctions. Once patients are assigned to these groups, a secondary analysis can be undertaken to describe each group. The descriptive data, gathered in the initial study, would include demographic, lifestyle, personality, and psychographic data (i.e., relevant activities, interests, and opinions). In addition, doctor-patient communication variables and information-seeking patterns could be added. Descriptive data are essential to learn the characteristics of each group so that at some later time individual patients can be placed into the appropriate category. In addition, simply identifying the relevant subgroups would provide guidance in understanding which, and how many, values underlie preferences about therapeutic outcomes.

Before such a segmentational study could be successfully implemented, several issues would need to be addressed. First, it is unclear if the segmentational basis for the study (patient values, therapeutic distinctions, and consequences) would cluster in a meaningful fashion that would allow their association with the quality of life profiles underlying different therapies. If, for example, the identified consequences clustered on dimensions that were uncorrelated with factors that made each therapy distinct and different, it would be impossible to link quality of life outcomes to specific drug therapies. On the other hand, even if patient values could not be meaningfully linked to quality of life profiles, the identification of a segmental pattern based on patient values may be of benefit in and of itself. For example, if risk aversion is identified as an independent segment, patients with this profile may opt for more conservative treatment whereas risk-taking patients may prefer aggressive treatment. In the long run, it may be possible for manufacturers to develop new treatments that match the preferred quality of life profiles of different patient segments. Being able to identify a distinct patient segment which may benefit from a drug may also help in the drug approval process.

A second issue that would need to be addressed is the ability of physicians to utilize any identified categorization system. One could make a case that doctors currently tailor their prescriptions to individual patients and that a segmentational strategy would reduce, rather than increase, the specificity of their treatment. However, the advantage offered by a value-based segmentational strategy is incremental to existing strategies based on diagnostic criteria. The advantage offered by quality of life data in general is to allow differentiation among competing brands within a therapeutic category where diagnostic criteria are fairly constant across patients. Thus, the segmentational strategy would serve as a guide to physicians at a lower level of decision making (i.e., the brand or product level) than basic choices of treatment (i.e., the therapeutic category).

To utilize a value-based segmentational strategy, an implementation system would need to be developed. Physicians would need to learn how to correctly assign patients to groups. It may be necessary to develop a short checklist to serve as an assignment guide. A brief questionnaire for physicians to administer to patients may also be necessary. Hatcher, Green, Levine, and Flagle (17) have demonstrated that "triaging" rules can be successfully established and followed to assign hypertensive patients to various health education interventions.

Would physicians use this type of system? Physicians would need to believe in the efficacy of such a system, so evaluation studies would be essential. Although some successes have been reported when patients are assigned to treatments based on their desires and coping skills, a recent review of the literature on matching patients on the basis of their "aptitude" to specific therapies indicates disappointing results (18). This review concentrated on psychological therapies for anxiety, depression, obesity, pain, and tobacco dependence, so it is unclear how drug treatments would be affected. It is likely that value-based segmentation would be more successful for some treatment categories than others.

In any event, physicians are apt to be quite skeptical. A marketing program directed to physicians would be essential to promote awareness of the system, address questions about its usefulness, and urge its trial. However, its ultimate success would be dependent on how much the developed system improved patient satisfaction with treatment.

PHYSICIAN DECISION MAKING

We have attempted to make a case that physicians could actively utilize quality of life data when making prescribing decisions. To more fully understand how quality of life data would influence this process, it is necessary to examine how physicians make prescribing decision.

The most common model of physician decision making assumes that a rational, thoughtful analysis is undertaken when physicians choose among therapeutic alternatives for the patient. An alternate model of physician decision making is also possible. In this second model, the physician uses a deliberate decision-making process when making a diagnosis, but once the diagnosis is made a drug is chosen out of habit. Under this latter model, there is little thought given to choosing a drug; rather, once the patient is characterized, the selection of therapy is a fait accompli. Under both the deliberative and habitual decision-making models, quality of life data can be conceived as playing a role in the physician's selection of therapy.

The Deliberative Model

Frequently the physician is faced with an atypical prescribing situation (e.g., the patient's illness is uncommon, there are extenuating circumstances making the preferred treatment contraindicated, or patient demographics (geriatrics, pediatrics) make the preferred treatment unadvisable. At times, the physician simply has not developed strong prescribing habits or the introduction of unique new treatments may force the physician to reevaluate preferred treatments. Under these circumstances the physician is forced to undertake a careful, deliberative decision-making process.

In these instances, once a diagnosis is made the physician must recall from memory a set of medicines that could serve as therapeutic options. If there is only one option available, the choice of treatment is easy. If there are multiple options, two steps are needed to make a selection.

First, the physician "edits" his/her knowledge base about the product class, the patient, and the illness to select the criteria that should be utilized to make the decision. For example, the effectiveness of treatment, the safety profile, and the price of the medication may be cited as the most important aspects of treatment to evaluate in order to make a choice. Due to informational processing limits, a relatively small number of selection criteria can be used. It should also be noted that the physician can utilize a combination of both abstract criteria (e.g., effectiveness and safety) and concrete criteria (e.g., price). To the fullest extent possible, performance levels are recalled for each of the brands in the active set of therapeutic alternatives for each of the relevant evaluation criteria.

Second, the physician reaches a decision by "evaluating" the brands on the selected criteria using a decision heuristic. Any number of heuristics are possible or several heuristics may be used in combination or in a sequential fashion. For example, the physician may rule out brands that are above a certain price level and weigh safety and efficacy equally to make a choice. Which heuristics are used is likely to be due to physician preferences and situational factors driving the decision.

In this deliberative process, quality of life data may play a role during both the "editing" and "evaluation" stages. During the editing stage, quality of life could be one of the variables chosen by the physician to select a treatment. In his/her own mind, the physician may phrase this criteria as the degree to which the drug "helps," "pleases," or "satisfies" the patient. Even if not chosen as a primary evaluation criteria, quality of life data may serve as a "signal" for physicians of how well a drug performs on other selected abstract criteria. For example, it may be difficult to judge the "effectiveness" level for each drug under evaluation. High scores on a quality of life subscale could allow the physician to infer a high effectiveness level.

Given information-processing limits, it is likely that the physician will be unable to recall a significant amount of information about a brand's performance. Effective advertising with frequent repetition may act as a reminder that would increase the likelihood that emphasized product attributes will be recalled. Thus, any advertising stressing quality of life should increase the recall of quality of life differences emphasized in the advertising. Furthermore, if the physician perceives quality of life as important, there is a greater likelihood that quality of life would be a salient product attribute retained in memory and "available" (i.e., retrieved) when decisions are made. It is also conceivable that effective advertising could convince physicians that quality of life is an important factor that should be utilized when making prescribing decisions. Thus, not only could advertising make quality of life more likely to be recalled, it could also increase the use of quality of life in the decision-making process.

Habitual Decision Making

Once a physician has made a thoughtful selection of treatment, it would be inefficient to go through the same process each time a treatment needs to be selected. Under an habitual decision-making process, the physician automatically chooses a favorite brand once he/she envisions the need for such a product. In this case, once the patient is properly categorized (e.g., placed in certain diagnostic categories or "labeled" as a certain type of patient), the selection of treatment is preordained. Thus, out of habit, a physician may prescribe the same first-line antihypertensive drug for each newly diagnosed hypertensive patient, all geriatric patients with angina may get the same drug, and all ulcer patients who smoke may be prescribed the same medication.

Under an habitual decision-making model, quality of life data would be used by physicians to characterize patients, rather than as a means of evaluating treatment. For example, the physician examining an active, vibrant elderly patient with hypertension could "label" the patient as such and choose a therapy that helps the patient maintain that lifestyle. All elderly patients characterized as "active and vibrant" would be prescribed the same medication.

Some form of deliberative decision-making process would have to occur prior to the establishment of habitual processing. Thus, advertising would first have to convince physicians that quality of life is an important evaluative factor and, secondly, that it can be used as an effective categorizing factor.

Quality of life has the potential to refine the physician's categorization processes, supplementing (not necessarily replacing) existing categorical processes. In essence, the physician's perception of the patient is expanded beyond biological (i.e., diagnosis) and demographic characteristics (e.g., age, gender) but is also made in terms of perceptions of the patient's lifestyle.

As discussed earlier in this chapter, a segmentational system that associates quality of life data with underlying values and provides descriptive data of correlated lifestyles helps to build the patient's preferences into the physician's categorical processing. Also, as suggested, any evaluation of the physician's use of a segmentational system must include measures of the physician's perceptions of the patient to understand how patients are "labeled" and characterized. It would be important to adjust segmentation models based on patient preferences to models that physicians could understand and utilize. Research may be needed to understand the physician's categorical processes and adjustments may need to be made in the physician's processing to align the physician's schema with a patient-based segmentation schema.

CONCLUSION

Quality of life data have helped pharmaceutical marketers to quantify their products along dimensions that are meaningful to the patient. In addition to justifying the benefits of different medication to institutional purchasers and decision makers, quality of life data bring the maker of pharmaceutical products into a more direct relationship with the patient. For quality of life to exert its most profound effects, however, data from quality of life studies need to be part of the decision-making process underlying therapeutic choice. We are just beginning to learn how to incorporate quality of life data into these decisions and much theoretical and empirical work lies ahead.

We have begun to see marketers utilize quality of life data to position their products. It is uncertain if such positioning is leading to therapeutic decisions that maximize patient preferences for obtaining therapeutic benefits and avoiding adverse effects. In the long run, however, there could be great payoffs in patient satisfaction and in medicine as a whole if we can find ways of building the patient's preferences for drug therapy directly into the physician's decision processes. By linking quality of life outcomes to patients' values we may develop ways of improving the exchange process between the doctor and patient as well as between the pharmaceutical company and patient. Much exciting research needs to be done.

REFERENCES

1. Bergner M. Measurement of health status. *Med Care* 1985;23:696–704.
2. Torrance GW. Measurement of health state utilities for economic appraisal. *J Health Econ* 1986;4:1–30.
3. Ware JE. Standards for validating health measures: Definition and content. *J Chron Dis* 1987;40:473–480.
4. Zarin DA, Pauker SG. Decision analysis as a basis for medical decision making: The tree of Hippocrates. *J Med Phil* 1984;9:181–213.
5. Kotler P. A generic concept of marketing. *J Marketing* 1972;36:46–54.
6. Wells WD. Psychographics: A critical review. *J Marketing Res* 1975;12:196–213.
7. Mitchell A. *The Nine American Lifestyles*. New York: The MacMillan Company, 1983.
8. Pernia J. The second generation of market segmentation studies: An audit of buying motivation. In: Wells W, ed. *Lifestyle and psychographics*. Chicago, IL: American Marketing Association, 1974;287–324.
9. Linn LS, DiMatteo MR, Cope DW, et al. Measuring physicians' humanistic attitudes, values and behaviors. *Med Care* 1987;25:504–515.
10. Lilja J. How physicians choose their drugs. *Soc Sci Med* 1976;10:363–365.
11. Miller RR. Prescribing habits of physicians (Parts I–III). *Drug Intel Clin Pharm* 1973;7:492–500.
12. Bergner M, Bobbitt RA, Carter WB, et al. The Sickness Impact Profile: Development and final revision of a health status measure. *Med Care* 1981;19:787–805.
13. Spector WD, Katz S, Murphy JB, et al. The hierarchical relationship between activities of daily living and instrumental activities of daily living. *J Chron Dis* 1981;40:481–489.
14. Earker SA, Sox HC. An assessment of patient preferences for therapeutic outcomes. *Med Dec Making* 1981;1:29–39.
15. McNeil BJ, Weichselboom R, Pauker SG. Fallacy of the five-year survival rate in lung cancer. *N Engl J Med* 1978;299:1397–1401.
16. Reynolds TJ, Gutman J. Laddering theory, method, analysis, and interpretation. *J Advertising Res* 1988;23:11–31.
17. Hatcher ME, Green LW, Levine DL, Flagle C. Validation of a decision model for triaging hypertensive patients to alternate health education interventions. *Soc Sci Med* 1986;22:813–819.
18. Dance KA, Neufeld RW. Aptitude-treatment interaction research in the clinical setting: A review of attempts to dispel the "patient uniformity" myth. *Psych Res* 1988;104:192–213.

Quality of Life Assessments in Clinical Trials, edited by B. Spilker. Raven Press, Ltd. New York © 1990.

15

An Industry Perspective

*Doug Henderson-James and †Bert Spilker

Glaxo, Inc., Research Triangle Park, North Carolina 27709; †Project Coordination, Burroughs Wellcome Co., Research Triangle Park, North Carolina 27709

The first major quality of life study on a pharmaceutical product published in *The New England Journal of Medicine* occurred in 1986 (1). Journal editors felt the subject was of sufficient importance to the medical community to make it that issue's lead article. This event sent a clear message to the entire drug industry about quality of life data. This message was confirmed by subsequent sales increases of the product described.

This chapter explores company, marketing, medical, and regulatory perspectives of quality of life issues. From a corporate view, the major quality of life issues are organizational and conceptual. The essential goals a marketing unit seeks from quality of life data are a strong marketing position and competitive advantage. Medical groups focus on defining a product profile that they hope will enhance clinical benefits for patients, and regulatory groups seek information that increases the chances of approval and acceptance for the company's products.

CORPORATE PERSPECTIVE

What Are the Corporate Issues?

From the corporate view, the two major issues relating to quality of life are why quality of life studies should be conducted and how the company's resources should be organized to conduct these studies most effectively.

Why Conduct Quality of Life Studies?

There are five general reasons for conducting quality of life studies. Each of these reasons has important commercial implications for the company and several reasons have important medical implications for physicians who prescribe drugs and for patients who take them. First, improved quality of life benefits over traditional therapies may assist regulatory strategies. For example, the data may increase the pressure within regulatory agencies in some countries for a drug to be approved more rapidly. In some cases a new drug or a new indication for a marketed drug may be approved based primarily or secondarily on quality of life data. These data may enable drugs to be differentiated which are otherwise similar in terms of conventional efficacy and safety parameters. Quality of life studies may also be used to modify and improve the labeling of a marketed drug.

The second reason for conducting quality of life studies is that they can assist in pricing products. Cost-benefit and cost-effectiveness studies are a subset of quality of life studies which focus on economic issues. These studies can be used to assist companies in setting prices for their products. Cost-benefit studies measure costs incurred and benefits derived by comparing alternative therapeutic regimens. Costs and benefits are both calculated using a single monetary value (i.e., dollars). If a company can demonstrate increased quality of life benefits to patients with a new drug, they may charge patients more than for existing drugs and still maintain the same or better cost to benefit relationship.

The third reason for a company to conduct quality of life studies is to provide its customers with complete product information. Advertising and other promotional vehicles as well as professional publications are important methods used to disseminate information to customers. The degree to which this effort is pursued depends on the company's culture and goals. Advances in life-prolonging technologies and increased public awareness of quality of life issues are focusing public attention on the risks as well as benefits of medicines. If an anticancer drug prolongs the life of a patient who is severely ill but reduces his or her quality of life, what is the medical, economic, or societal wisdom for its use? This major bioethical question is being discussed without adequate information about the effects of most drug regimens on quality of life. This inadequacy must be addressed by the pharmaceutical industry to protect the future of its drugs.

Fourth, quality of life considerations help determine which types of information are most useful to obtain for specific audiences (e.g., to get a drug on a formulary). This information can be used to design appropriate pre- or post-marketing studies to evaluate the drug.

Finally, in situations of therapeutic, or even generic, substitution, quality of life evaluations might be able to show differences that would help a company counter substitution practices. Differences might be as subtle as taste distinctions that lead to decreased patient compliance and to decreased medical benefits with generics.

How Should a Company Organize a Group to Address Quality of Life Issues?

Several questions should be answered before a company's resources are allocated to quality of life studies.

1. Which division or department should be responsible for conducting quality of life studies?
2. How should marketing and medical groups, the groups concerned with quality of life issues, interact?
3. Should quality of life activities be assigned to existing groups or should a new organizational structure be created?

The usual contenders for organizational control of quality of life studies are marketing and medical units. The traditional location of clinical studies suggests that a medical group is the more logical site for controlling quality of life studies. Medical groups determine the efficacy and safety of a product; however, the impetus for quality of life studies usually comes from marketing groups.

As the economics of health care delivery have changed and cost containment issues have become dominant, a more competitive marketplace has been created. Hospitals, health maintenance organizations, government programs, and some traditional insurance programs have established restricted formularies to control dispensing patterns. A restrictive formulary limits the number of drugs available for physicians to use for the same condition. Absence of a drug from a formulary limits its sale. Placement on many formularies requires additional information beyond the usual efficacy and safety data present on a drug. Quality of life information becomes an important marketing tool to help drugs enter formularies and thus enhance sales. An improved product profile, a positive cost-benefit profile, or both provide the competitive advantage that marketing constantly seeks. Such information lies within the domain of quality of life studies.

Quality of life studies require well-designed protocols, clear endpoints, and attention to study conduct. Both marketing and medical involvement are needed to assist a sponsor in the choice of (a) appropriate endpoints that will meet the study's objectives, (b) site selection, and (c) protocol design. Medical personnel must monitor the study and analyze the results. Although quality of life studies must be conducted by medical groups, those groups may be directed by or controlled by marketing interests, if not by marketing personnel.

Medical and marketing goals are not necessarily the same. To be successful, marketing must respond to the needs of its various audiences. It would like information about a drug that is individualized to specific customers (e.g., health maintenance organizations, state Medicaid programs). Medical groups want to define the profile of a drug that will be used by all of marketing's audiences.

Information developed independently of a specific customer's needs may make it much more difficult to convince that customer to use the drug. For example, marketing groups usually respond to specific needs of health marketing organizations, hospitals, and other providers whose decisions may be influenced by quality of life data. Quality of life studies that include sites of these provider groups will make the results of a study more compelling to those groups.

The allocation of human resources to quality of life studies depends on how clinical medicine is organized within the company and on how senior executives view the importance of quality of life studies. These studies may be best directed from medical groups responsible for all other phase 1 to 4 trials. If this approach is adopted, then a single medical advisor well versed in quality of life methodology should serve as a consultant to all medical groups conducting these studies. Alternatively, a separate group may be established within the medical unit to pursue the planning and initiation of quality of life studies. This group should have strong organizational ties to the other medical groups that conduct phase 1 to 4 studies, as well as strong ties to marketing personnel who are knowledgeable about quality of life needs within marketing groups.

MARKETING PERSPECTIVE

How May Quality of Life Data Be Used in Marketing?

Quality of life studies can provide information to help determine a product marketing strategy and establish the comparative advantage of one product over another.

Information obtained in quality of life studies can help select the niche in which a drug should compete. Data from such studies can help determine which attributes of a product to emphasize in marketing activities. Lastly, the data obtained can address the question of how to approach the different customers that marketing must reach.

Quality of life studies can provide information to enhance the product's efficacy and safety profile. These additional data allow a better comparison of a drug's benefits (efficacy) to risks (adverse reactions) than using efficacy and safety data alone. These studies may demonstrate important advantages of one product over another in terms of benefits viewed by patients. Benefits might include aspects of psychological well-being such as reduced worry or increased happiness, improved physical status such as greater comfort, and increased social interactions. In the area of economic benefits, studies can determine both direct and indirect costs of competing therapies.

Who Wants and Will Use the Data Obtained in Studies?

Among today's customers for the products of the pharmaceutical industry are those who make economic decisions affecting medical care. These groups include national, state, and local governments, managed care systems (including health maintenance organizations, preferred provider organizations), buying groups, and insurance companies. These new groups are utilizing numerous mechanisms to control medical practice through controlling expenditures. The ability to demonstrate improved quality of life, either through an improved product profile or cost savings versus another therapy, increases the probability that these new customers will encourage the product's use.

For decision makers in a health maintenance organization, data from studies conducted in most fee-for-service settings are less meaningful than data from studies conducted in an health maintenance organization setting. Likewise, Medicaid or Medicare studies that focus on their particular patient populations will be accepted more readily by decision makers within those groups than data from studies conducted with other populations. Although it is not possible to situate a single quality of life study to please everybody, study site selection criteria should consider health maintenance organizations and other groups that will eventually review the data obtained.

Hospitals, health maintenance organizations, insurance companies, and government agencies also want information that addresses their economic constraints. For example, hospitals do not need information on the life-time costs of therapy, but they need to know how each therapy affects hospital costs. Health maintenance organizations need information that reflects yearly health care resource consumption and the quality of life of its enrollees. Since premiums and rates are adjusted yearly, longer views of quality of life are possibly of less interest. Government health care agencies have similar interests and constraints. Medicare and Medicaid have strong interest in resource consumption issues. Insurance companies and Blue Cross/Blue Shield provide both inpatient and outpatient coverage, and thus combine information needs of both hospitals and health maintenance organizations. Pharmacy and therapeutics committees at hospitals and health maintenance organizations want data on quality of life and resource consumption. Most physicians and pharmacists desire quality of life information, but have little or no interest in information on resource consumption.

The outlook for quality of life data to be used in reimbursement decision making is less clear. Neither Medicare nor Medicaid requires quality of life information for reimbursement of those (e.g., hospitals, patients) who are using specific drugs. However, quality of life data constitute potentially persuasive information for gaining inclusion on state Medicaid formularies or as support for pricing decisions. The recently enacted catastrophic health bill requires the development of standard operating procedures for the use of medical and surgical procedures, including the use of drugs that will be included in the outpatient drug coverage component of Medicare. Quality of life information will be important in establishing these standard operating procedures.

When Should Quality of Life Data Be Obtained?

When should quality of life information on a new drug be provided to formulary and other groups? Ideally, at the time of product launch. Providing data at the time of a launch creates two major issues about conducting quality of life studies. First, conducting quality of life studies prior to regulatory approval generates data that are not based on real world behavior. The controlled nature of clinical studies, the close supervision of medical practice and patient behavior, and the use of traditional clinical sites produces results that are sometimes difficult to reproduce in physicians' offices, hospitals, or health maintenance organizations after a drug is launched. Benefits demonstrated in controlled settings may diminish or even disappear when physicians are less intensive in their medical treatment. The opposite phenomenon also occurs; some drugs are more effective in practice than in clinical studies.

Clinical studies conducted after marketing approval allow for evaluation of drugs under actual use conditions. Usage on the market may subjectively demonstrate significant quality of life benefits to patients and physicians. These benefits can be most clearly demonstrated in well-controlled, randomized clinical trials. Waiting for regulatory approval before initiating well-designed and controlled studies, however, delays the availability of the information and may reduce the eventual usefulness and profitability of the product.

Which Drugs Should Be Evaluated?

Not all drug products need quality of life studies. The perceived medical advantage of a new product may be so significant that there would be little or no benefit derived from documenting quality of life improvements. Drugs without competition do not generally require these studies. Cost issues of a drug may be so negligible that a study could not add to the drug's commercial value. Other factors may influence the decision for or against conducting a quality of life study. For example, how important is the commercial value of the drug to the company? How important is it to demonstrate quality of life benefits to physicians, patients, and to those who pay for the therapy?

Drugs that are not profitable or not expected to be profitable do not require quality of life studies. Because a product with limited sales potential is less likely to be a candidate for quality of life studies, it is better to place research resources where they will achieve the greatest results. If potential advantages of a drug product have little or no meaning to those who will prescribe, use, or pay for the product, there is little reason to conduct such studies. Though quality of life studies may initially appear to be relevant for all products, a company must be selective in its use of resources for these studies.

The selection of drugs to compare with a company's drug depends on reaching a consensus between medical and marketing interests. Products perceived as competitors from medical's point of view may not be the products that marketing wants to compete against. Marketing may want to reposition a product, to change a product from one market to another, or to find a more suitable niche in the existing market. Medical personnel may feel that marketing's desire for repositioning a product weakens the clinical significance of the product. Joint discussions are often required to resolve differences.

In summary, from a marketing perspective, the specific types of drugs for which quality of life studies should be conducted include (a) drugs in intense competition, (b) "me-too" drugs, and (c) drugs in certain therapeutic areas (e.g., cancer, cardiology) where the data may help speed the drug approval process. In each of these (or other) cases, the costs of quality of life studies must be justified in terms of anticipated commercial benefits.

MEDICAL AND REGULATORY PERSPECTIVES

Medical Perspective on the Conduct of Quality of Life Studies

The most important medical reason for conducting quality of life studies is to establish a comprehensive product profile. Quality of life studies are designed to extend the clinical understanding of a product's effectiveness and the consequences and various costs of its adverse reactions. A quality of life profile provides physicians and other medical care decision makers with additional information to use for arriving at therapeutic decisions. Quality of life data on a drug or other therapy provide medical decision makers with the most meaningful information when these studies are conducted in comparison with standard drugs or nondrug products. When no standard exists, a no-treatment group may be used as control.

Quality of life studies can provide important information on adverse reactions and their impact on patient health. For example, what is the relationship between nonsteroidal anti-inflammatory drugs and the appearance of ulcers? Are all of these drugs the same? Do some have less tendency to cause ulcers? From the patient's point of view, what is the trade-off in terms of pain reduction versus increased risk of an ulcer? If patients take a nonsteroidal anti-inflammatory drug, which ulcer medication should they take if an ulcer occurs. Should they forego the anti-inflammatory until the ulcer is healed? The answers to such questions provide medical benefits to patients and commercial benefits to the company whose drug has demonstrated advantages over the competition.

How May a Quality of Life Plan Be Initiated, Coordinated, and Reviewed?

The responsibility for raising questions about quality of life issues on a new investigational drug belongs with the project team that is involved in its development.

This group has (or should have) both medical and marketing members. If this group is not involved (or is only indirectly involved) in quality of life studies, then appropriate people in marketing or medical groups may contact the project group to raise this issue.

Once quality of life issues are being discussed within a project group, plans will begin to develop as discussed below. This will best be handled by integrating the activities into existing plans within medical and marketing groups, and conducting reviews within the organizational structure that evaluates project activities.

What Elements Should Be Considered in the Development of a Quality of Life Plan?

The development of useful quality of life information for physicians depends primarily on two issues: which product(s) and which attributes are to be compared. Product comparisons should cover five areas: physical status, physical ability, psychological well-being, social interactions, and economic profiles. The clinical efficacy and safety profiles of new drugs are most often compared with standard drugs in phase 3 and 4 clinical trials. Data obtained may influence drug labeling. In addition to basic efficacy and safety data on how drugs compare with others, it is important for physicians to understand differences in how drugs affect quality of life. Improvement in overall quality of life measures is not yet an accepted basis for drug approval, especially if safety and efficacy do not meet the standards of existing therapy.

Several issues about quality of life studies should be addressed before the actual studies are initiated. Is a pilot study required? Should quality of life measures be included as part of other clinical studies (e.g., safety studies, efficacy studies) or should they be conducted on their own? During what phase of development should these studies be conducted? What measurement tools should be used? Before decisions are made about what parameters to evaluate in a quality of life study, it is necessary to determine the goals of the study, plus (a) indications to analyze, (b) patient populations to enroll, and (c) type or nature of sites to use in the study(ies).

If quality of life studies are conducted on their own and not as part of other clinical studies, then factors such as cost, personnel, and timing should be explored. A separate study usually costs more than adding a few questions or tests to an existing study. Determining differences between drugs when measuring them on quality of life issues may require large populations. The larger the study, the larger the commitment of both company personnel and capital. A third factor in the cost equation is the duration of quality of life studies. Often the most important endpoint of a quality of life study is the long-term outcome of drug therapy. Patient enrollment in such studies could range from 1 to several years. The study, from time of protocol development to medical report summarization, could last 1 to 2 years longer than the length of enrollment of any one patient.

Providing necessary resources to conduct a major study of this type may affect other drug development work within the company. However, scarce human resources may be augmented by using outside clinical study vendors. Company culture, capable vendors, importance of rapidly completed studies, and available company resources necessary to manage the contract are the major elements to consider in reaching a decision to use outside contractors.

At What Phase of Clinical Development Should Quality of Life Studies Be Conducted?

Most of the reasons for conducting quality of life studies relate to a drug's marketing. This suggests that at least some quality of life studies should be conducted prior to Food and Drug Administration approval so that the information is available when the drug is initially marketed. Following this reasoning, quality of life considerations could begin as early as phase 2 during the conduct of well-controlled studies. Phase 2 studies could be used to identify which parameters and populations of patients (e.g., severely ill versus mildly ill) should be more completely evaluated in later studies. For example, if a product is thought capable of reducing length of stay in an intensive care unit, then collection of such data in phase 2 could determine if the supposition is warranted, give a sense of how much the stay is reduced, or determine at what levels of drug dosing the best efficacy and stay reduction is achieved. Such information will allow for the design of phase 3 studies that will produce the data necessary to test the hypothesis. Another approach is to use observational methods in uncontrolled treatment-IND (Investigational New Drug) studies to identify parameters.

Three general approaches are described of the most appropriate timing for quality of life studies. The first approach is to conduct studies during phases 2b and 3a if data are likely to enhance the speed of regulatory approval. For chemotherapy products there is a growing acceptance in the industry and regulatory agencies that approval of these drugs could be based, at least in part, on quality of life data. These data should be gathered in studies conducted during phases 2b and 3a (i.e., prior to New Drug Application [NDA] submission). Drugs in a number of other therapeutic areas (e.g., cardiology) may also be candidates for early clinical trials on quality of life.

A second approach to the question of when to conduct quality of life studies is to wait until the NDA has been filed. These studies would be conducted during the period of regulatory review (i.e., phase 3b). This approach does not delay the submission of the NDA and has the possibility of having quality of life information available at the time of product launch. It does require submission of appropriate information to the Food and Drug Administration prior to final drug approval, and this could potentially slow the Food and Drug Administration's review of the drug.

A third approach is to wait until the drug is approved before conducting quality of life studies. Neither the submission nor the regulatory review is delayed. However, the drug is launched without sufficient quality of life information, thereby diminishing and delaying the potential impact of this information. Independent quality of life studies, however, could progress while an NDA was being prepared by a company or was being reviewed by the Food and Drug Administration.

What Methods Should Be Used and What Data Should Be Obtained?

It is much easier to determine which methods should be used than what data should be obtained. The well-controlled, randomized clinical trial is the method that should be used whenever possible. In certain situations observational methods may be used, but it is desirable that findings from such studies are confirmed with more rigorous well-controlled, randomized clinical trial methods.

The next issue is to identify which of the major quality of life domains (i.e., broad categories) to study. These are generally accepted to be physical abilities, social interactions, psychological well-being, and economic factors. Quality of life studies may evaluate one, two, three, or all four of these domains. One may use a single test that evaluates any or all of these domains, or a battery of tests that evaluate one (or more) domains in substantial depth. These considerations illustrate the range of possible choices about the domains and tests used to evaluate them. The specific tests available to evaluate each of the domains are identified and discussed in other chapters of this book.

The specific data to collect depends on its importance to patients and to marketing's customers, plus the ability to collect valid data and to analyze it. If a product is being developed for a disease where the only current therapy is surgery, then the ability to avoid surgery becomes an important economic variable to assess in a quality of life study. If the product under development is going to compete with other drugs, then the economics of concomitant drug usage, length of therapy, and necessity of monitoring drug usage are often important.

In selecting a scale(s) to use in a quality of life study, avoid unvalidated scales whenever possible. A single overall scale, battery of targeted scales, or a single targeted scale (e.g., on psychological well-being) may be used. Confirm that scales to be used have been validated for the population to be studied. Quality of life scales are often validated only for specific populations or for a specific means of administration (self-administered, telephone, mail, physician or other person). Disease-specific scales would superficially appear to be more desirable to use than general scales, but there is a large group of experts that challenge this view. They recommend general scales unless they are inappropriate and validated disease-specific scales exist.

Most scales are developed to measure populations at a single point in time. Such scales are used to compare dissimilar populations (e.g., those capable of walking with those bed-ridden). Few scales have been developed to measure change over a period of time in the quality of life of patients with a specific disease. The ability of existing scales to measure a drug's effect on quality of life of a patient during the course of prolonged treatment is often limited. This is a critical factor in studies of chronic medications.

The issue is complex because a company may demonstrate cost-effectiveness for almost any drug by carefully choosing the treatment to which it is compared or by carefully choosing the specific endpoints used for evaluation. For example, cost-effectiveness may be shown for drug A in terms of lower cost per capsule, for drug B on a per dosage basis, for drug C per course of treatment, for drug D based on the duration of hospital stay, for drug E based on the cost of hospital stay, and for drug F based on days of work gained, and so forth. This implies that endpoints (as well as specific quality of life tests and scales) may be carefully chosen to "prove" a preconceived point. Ethical aspects of this issue are obvious.

How Should Quality of Life Data Be Presented to the Food and Drug Administration

Neither regulation nor law currently requires quality of life information for either Food and Drug Administration approval or government reimbursement. There is no legal requirement for a company to obtain quality of life data to help the Food and Drug Administration make regulatory decisions on a drug's safety and efficacy. Therefore, the decision to provide this information to the agency is based on answers to two questions: What will the Food and Drug Administration do with the information, and how much delay, in the submission of the NDA, will be caused by undertaking quality of life studies prior to NDA submission?

As part of the review process for "life-threatening conditions," the Food and Drug Administration will consider risk-benefit information in its decision making. Although risk-benefit analysis does not have to include quality of life information, it does allow for such data. Quality of life factors could therefore be used by the agency in its current review and approval process. Such information could in theory be requested either prior to approval or in post-marketing studies. This could potentially become the norm for most drugs, and not merely for life saving therapies. It is hoped that the regulatory pendulum does not swing to that extreme position.

CONCLUSION

Although quality of life information is not currently accepted as a major or sole basis for either drug approval or reimbursement, we believe that these steps will occur over the next decade. Pharmaceutical companies should use quality of life scales that have been developed and validated. New scales are almost never relevant to develop. A detailed strategy for quality of life studies should be developed which considers appropriate domains of study, components of each domain to study, endpoints to measure, patient populations to evaluate, and approximate timing. Close working relationships between relevant medical and marketing personnel are required to insure that a company addresses these issues appropriately. A separate group within the medical organization that is heavily influenced by marketing views is one suitable model to achieve these goals.

REFERENCES

1. Croog SH, Levine S, Testa MA, et al. The effects of antihypertensive therapy on the quality of life. *N Engl J Med* 1986;314:1657–1664.

Quality of Life Assessments in Clinical Trials, edited by B. Spilker. Raven Press, Ltd. New York, 1990.

16

A Regulatory Perspective*

†Dale Shoemaker, ‡Gregory Burke, †Andrew Dorr, §Robert Temple, and †Michael A. Friedman

†Cancer Therapy Evaluation Program, Division of Cancer Treatment, National Cancer Institute, National Institutes of Health, Bethesda, Maryland 20892; ‡Division of Oncology and Radiopharmaceutical Drug Products; §Office of Drug Review I; Center for Drug Evaluation and Research, Food and Drug Administration, Rockville, Maryland 20857

Clinical trials to determine the efficacy of new investigational agents in cancer patients have special problems. Placebo-controlled studies are generally impossible. In comparative trials, crossover of patients progressing on investigational agents to salvage therapy confounds survival analysis. There is, therefore, great interest in measures of clinical benefit that can be used, together with evidence of objective tumor response, as a basis for new drug approval. Quality of life assesssments appear to represent a possible method of demonstrating clinical benefit. Indeed, the Oncologic Drugs Advisory Committee of the Food and Drug Administration has recommended survival and quality of life as the key efficacy parameters for consideration in approving new anticancer agents (1). To date most emphasis has been placed on quality of life data in the evaluation of palliative therapies, but these data can also be important for judging curative therapies, especially when such curative approaches employ analogs of approved active agents and aim to reduce toxicity. In this chapter some of the methods of assessing the quality of life and the use of these methods under current Food and Drug Administration regulations will be described, as will some of the problems encountered. The role of quality of life data in the phase 2 setting and new Food and Drug Administration regulations pertaining to drugs intended to treat life-threatening illness will also be briefly presented.

GENERAL METHODS TO ASSESS QUALITY OF LIFE

The following discussion considers four general methods which may be used to measure quality of life and provides examples of anticancer agents recently approved by the Food and Drug Administration based on applications containing data obtained by these methods.

---

*The opinions expressed in this chapter are solely those of the authors and do not necessarily reflect those of any government agency.

Implicit Improvement in Quality of Life

Although there is at present great interest in ways of measuring quality of life, many measures of patient response commonly recorded in the past are in reality also quality of life measurements. Pain, performance status, appetite, and weight are regularly evaluated or measured and reflect a patient's well-being. Certain effects of an agent represent implicit improvements in quality of life, even if no particular measure records this. Implicit improvements in the quality of life of cancer patients have included an increase in disease-free survival and an increased complete response rate. Examples of previously approved anticancer agents which recently were approved for supplemental indications based on this type of measure include tamoxifen and daunorubicin.

Tamoxifen, previously approved for women with metastatic breast cancer, was approved for use as a surgical adjuvant in postmenopausal women with primary breast cancer. The approval of this agent was based on the fact that women with estrogen receptor-positive disease receiving tamoxifen after primary resection had an increased disease-free survival. The evidence from the individual trials supporting a statistically significant impact upon survival was less clear, but the quality of life (knowledge that they were tumor-free) of patients who were disease-free was thought to be better than that of patients with overt metastatic disease. In this case, the relative lack of toxicity of tamoxifen was important in reaching the approval decision despite lack of a formal assessment of quality of life.

Daunorubicin, previously approved for patients with acute myelogenous leukemia, was approved for the treatment of adult patients with acute lymphocytic leukemia based on an improvement in the rate of first complete remission inductions and good duration of the complete response. Daunorubicin added to vincristine and prednisone increased the complete response rate compared to vincristine and prednisone alone, but did not increase overall survival. This apparent lack of survival benefit, however, may have resulted from use of a crossover design in which daunorubicin was given to patients failing vincristine and prednisone inductions.

Improvement in Specific Disease Symptoms

The improvement in specific disease-related symptoms of cancer patients can be demonstrated in many ways, such as fewer infections, fewer transfusions, relief of an obstructed viscus (e.g., esophagus or bronchus), weight (lean body mass) gain in cachectic patients, healing of malignant skin ulcers, or resolution of paraneoplastic endocrine syndromes and relief of pruritus.

Alpha-interferon, which was approved for the treatment of patients with hairy cell leukemia, is an example of this category. This agent was approved on the basis of a showing that patients treated with alpha-interferon had very high objective response rates and required fewer transfusions, suffered fewer infections, and were hospitalized for fewer days compared to their own pretreatment status.

Diminished Acute and/or Chronic Toxicity

A qualitative or quantitative difference in the toxicities between an investigational agent and standard therapy is meaningful only if there is evidence of efficacy (such as improvement in survival or in some disease-related symptom complex or other endpoint). Ordinarily, approval of the new agent would not depend on the demonstration of an improved toxicity profile for the new agent (a new drug need not be superior to available therapy to be approved), but the evidence would be very important for proper labeling and use of the drug. In these studies, the use of concurrent medications (antiemetics, analgesics, stool softeners) and concurrent radiotherapy, blindedness of the observer, and generally accepted toxicity scales should be considered prospectively because they can easily confound comparisons. Specific target populations could be evaluated using these criteria. For example, an analog with potentially less toxicity (such as nephrotoxicity) could be used to treat patients who cannot tolerate the parent agent (a prior nephrotoxic response). In this case the better tolerated analog could be approved by the Food and Drug Administration for use in the subpopulation if efficacy was shown to be preserved on the basis of a much smaller database than would be needed to support treatment for the entire population of patients with the tumor.

A recently developed method for assessing the toxicity profile of a patient on adjuvant therapy is the Time Without Symptoms of disease and subjective toxic effects of Treatment (TWIST) as described by Gelber et al. (2) for the adjuvant treatment of breast cancer. TWIST is calculated by subtracting from overall survival the periods of time during which the patient experienced the toxic effects of the treatment or symptoms of disease recurrence. A similar analysis might be used in advanced disease with an agent demonstrating a decreased time to reach complete response and/or requiring a shortened period of treatment. The time to complete response is applicable only if therapy is not continued after complete response and toxicity is not greater than for the alternative therapy.

Global Measures of Quality of Life

A full discussion of the spectrum of instruments for measuring quality of life in cancer patients is beyond the scope of this chapter but is provided elsewhere in this volume. Although no new anticancer agent has as yet been approved solely on the basis of these quality of life measurements, the instruments developed by Schipper et al. (3) and Spitzer et al. (4), the linear analog self-assessment scales and the performance status measures, warrant discussion as a basis for illustrating important regulatory and scientific issues.

Schipper et al. (3) developed the Functional Living Index–Cancer for determining cancer patients' functional response to their illness and treatment and proposed it as an adjunct to the assessment of response and toxicity in clinical trials. The patient reports his/her own perception of level of function. The Functional Living Index–Cancer instrument is capable of distinguishing patients who are disease-free and off treatment from those receiving adjuvant therapy or those in the midst of treatment for active disease, and from those in the palliative care or preterminal setting. Using this instrument the patient serves as his/her own control to measure the quality of life as a continuous variable over time (5).

Ganz et al. (6) recently utilized the Functional Living Index–Cancer to estimate the quality of life in patients with advanced metastatic non-small cell lung cancer prospectively randomized to supportive care alone versus supportive care in combination with chemotherapy. This was the first published report describing the application of the Functional Living Index–Cancer instrument in measuring quality of life in a clinical trial. Although there was good correlation between the Functional Living Index–Cancer and performance status scores at study entry, the instrument could not be used to assess treatment effect.

Several difficulties were encountered in administering the Functional Living Index–Cancer. Some patients had problems reading the instrument and others refused to complete the form unless it was read to them. Questions were left unanswered and there was variability in how the visual analog scales were completed. In addition, the rate of self-administration declined over time as the performance status decreased and there was variation in the location of administration. Because of inhomogeneity in the data, the two groups could not be statistically compared. The authors concluded that quality control procedures must be developed for collection of quality of life data; these must be used to evaluate the Functional Living Index–Cancer more extensively in clinical trial settings to assess its usefulness. The instrument thus needs validation to demonstrate that it accurately and reproducibly measures the change in quality of life status over time and the response to therapy of patients being treated for cancer.

The Quality of Life Index (QL-Index) developed by Spitzer et al. (4) discriminates between patients in the early (relatively asymptomatic) or middle stages of their disease and patients who are terminally (severely) ill. The authors settled on five items for measurement: activity, daily living, health, support, and outlook on life. The instrument measures the physician's perception of the patient's level of activity. They reported that the index was concise, quantitative, and easy to use (4). This instrument has recently been used by Coates et al. (7) to demonstrate that continuous chemotherapy in patients with advanced breast cancer was associated with significantly better quality of life than intermittent therapy. The authors did not identify any major problems in utilizing this instrument, but a significant dropout rate (24%) from the analysis limits the conclusions.

The application of linear analog self-assessment scales to cancer patients has been described by Priestman and Baum (8). They used the following 10 indices to measure the patient's own view of his or her quality of life: feeling of well-being, mood, level of activity, pain, nausea, appetite, ability to perform housework, social activities, level of anxiety, and whether or not the treatment is helping. The instrument was self-administered to women with recurrent or metastatic breast cancer. Although the technique proved reasonably reliable, the authors indicated that the questionnaire was subject to two major criticisms. First, questions on feelings, performance, and symptoms were mixed indiscriminately and second, all indices were given equal weighting. They felt, however, that a readily comprehensible, convenient, and reliable method for patients to assess their quality of life during and after treatment had been established.

Coates et al. (9) applied a subset of the linear analog self-assessment scales used by Priestman and Baum (8) to determine certain aspects of the quality of life of patients receiving therapy for malignant melanoma, small cell anaplastic bronchogenic carcinoma, and ovarian cancer. They concluded that the linear analog self-assessment scales were a convenient method for assessing the patient's perception of his/her quality of life while receiving cancer therapy. The scales developed to date have measured a limited number of specific factors. New scales developed for specific patient populations and disease states would be a useful addition to the currently available quality of life measures. They would of course need to be validated.

Although Schipper et al. (3) found that performance status scores do not correlate well with measures of psychological well-being, sociability, or even somatic discomfort, they have been proposed as an adjunct to survival data to assess the efficacy of new anticancer agents (10). Orr and Aisner (11) noted that the application of performance status scales has concentrated on four main purposes:

1. As a means to stratify patients at the beginning of a clinical trial (presuming differing prognoses, response to therapy, and/or toxicity).
2. As a means to select patients for entry into clinical trials (in order to achieve greater homogeneity).
3. As a measure of the efficacy of treatment. While a decline in performance status score is interpreted as a deterioration in the health of a patient, the improvement of the score is seen as an improvement of the health status.
4. As a measure of the quality of survival (usually in situations where "cure" is not obtained and partial responses are associated with toxicity).

The Karnofsky Performance Status Scale has been used widely since it measures the ability to perform work and self-care activities as well as symptom status (11). Mor et al. (12) demonstrated the validity of the Karnofsky Performance Status Scale in a research setting and suggested that this scale would be a valuable research tool when employed by trained observers. Recently, Bakker et al. (13) demonstrated that the Karnofsky performance status decreased significantly in both responders and nonresponders being treated with chemotherapy for non-small cell lung cancer. Following discontinuation of the chemotherapy, the performance status approached pretreatment scores in the responders only. However, the changes in performance status in responders and nonresponders did not differ significantly at any time before, during, or after chemotherapy. Previously, Yates et al. (14) observed that the Karnofsky Performance Status Scale had moderately high reliability and validity as a global indicator of the functional status of cancer patients and that deterioration in the scale predicted, to a limited extent, an early death. Hutchinson et al. (15) identified problem areas in using the Karnofsky Performance Status Scale, including interobserver variability and a need for expanded elements to allow for a greater number of patients to be accurately evaluated.

UTILIZATION AND GENERAL PROBLEMS OF QUALITY OF LIFE MEASURES

There have been several obstacles to the incorporation of quality of life endpoints into clinical trials in cancer patients. The multicenter clinical trials groups have had limited experience with systematic evaluation of the patient's quality of life, at least partially because many investigators question whether the effort required to acquire such data is worth the trouble (10). The attempts to date have shown that the collection of quality of life data requires committed staff in both the participating institutions and central data offices. The greatest obstacle may be that currently there is no widely accepted instrument or method for measuring quality of life although the interest in doing so has increased (10). Schipper and Levitt postulated that quality of life instruments have not been used in clinical trials because they are not considered scientific, but rather are an undefinable and unmeasurable gestalt (5). However, quality of life is definable and measurable and can be valuable in assessing clinical trials within the limits of a particular instrument. In addition, as with any clinical trial, patient compliance and protocol compliance (incomplete treatment, unevaluatable patients, etc.) is of great concern. The instrument or method used to measure quality of life must be designed to encourage patient participation over a sometimes prolonged period of time.

General questions which should be considered prior to using quality of life instruments in clinical trials include the following:

1. Is the instrument linear over the range of measurement and is it sensitive to changes occurring in the patient? What is the clinical meaning of a given change in an instrument at each end of the scale? Does each instrument measure the same thing in patients with different cancers and in the same patient at different time points? How do you interpret the instrument when there is significant treatment-related toxicity, especially if the toxicity differs in the treatments being compared? If the scales/scores are to be used to support effectiveness, they must be able to distinguish cancer-related from drug-related effects. Which statistical tests should be used to demonstrate significance?
2. When all the patients entered into a study have good performance status, as is generally required, it will not usually be possible to demonstrate improvement. Instead, time to deterioration, probably using life table methods, must be measured.
3. Should the instrument be used before therapy is initiated, during therapy, and/ or after all treatment is finished?
4. Is it valid and useful to adjust results using baseline scores on the instrument? Is there a correlation between the score and response rate or survival?
5. Should the observer and the patient be blinded as to treatment and whether or not there has been an objective response to treatment?
6. How much training of the patient and observer is necessary? What quality control measures of documentation should be used? Should dropouts be censored?

From this partial list of issues needing consideration, it is obvious that much prospective work remains to be done to develop quality of life measures that will be widely acceptable for routine use in cancer patients. Currently there is no single instrument of convincing value for any particular disease or therapy.

FUTURE REGULATORY ROLES OF QUALITY OF LIFE DATA

The suggestion that quality of life measures become an important effectiveness endpoint for clinical trials with anticancer agents has led to a reconsideration and discussion of how pivotal studies incorporating such measurements might be designed. In 1985 Temple (16) proposed that more attention be paid to resolution of unequivocal cancer symptoms (pain over involved bone, extreme anorexia, decreased pulmonary function) as a potential endpoint that might be attained even when response rates were low. Wittes has proposed that the measurement of decreased toxicity and such symptoms and signs (all certainly elements relevant to quality of life) could be utilized and emphasized in the nonrandomized phase 2 setting along with a measure of the therapeutic activity of the investigational agent (10). The scientific objectives of the phase 2 trial would then include the following:

1. The assessment of the extent of disease and stability of performance status and symptoms during a short period of pretreatment observation. The period would probably be 2 to 3 weeks in most cases and a careful observation during this time frame would serve as a control for the post-treatment comparison.
2. The demonstration of unequivocal tumor diminution.
3. The full characterization of any treatment-related toxic events.
4. The careful description of the disease-related symptoms at the start of therapy and at various intervals through the course of treatment. Although some of the information may be descriptive, the data should be quantitated as often as possible. Much of these data are commonly missing or incomplete in phase 2 studies and are essential in providing evidence of the benefit of the new agent. As discussed above, the improvement of symptoms unequivocally related to the tumor could be interpreted as an improvement in quality of life. Specifically included in this category of significantly improved symptoms are resolution of bone pain at a site of metastasis, a change in appetite accompanied by an increase in lean body weight in a previously cachectic patient, an improvement in pulmonary function in a patient who had an identified pulmonary metastases but no pulmonary infection, and/or significant and sustained decreases in analgesic requirements.
5. The measurement of the longitudinal performance status for each patient entered in the study to determine the effects of therapy (benefits and toxic events) and disease on the function of the patient.
6. Maintenance of a log of all patients considered for entry on the study and documentation of the reasons why those excluded were not entered.

Two or three of these phase 2 studies could be carried out independently following the demonstration of antitumor activity against a specific tumor type in phase 1 or early phase 2 studies (10). Multiple observers would be responsible for making the clinical observations and judging the response, all of which would be subject to external review. Each patient would serve as his/her own control with a determination of pre- and post-treatment status forming the basis of deciding whether the new treatment was effective. The longitudinal estimation of performance status and the extent of symptoms both before and during treatment could be quantitatively assessed using parameters such as body weight, pain, performance status, and exercise tolerance. Even if the data for all patients were not completely quantifiable, it would be possible to develop a good sense of the effect of the various agents tested on the patient's well-being (10). Although the collection of these data would require trained staff and more complex studies, the results could provide convincing evidence of an agent's activity and acceptable toxicity.

In a presentation to the Oncologic Drugs Advisory Committee, Temple (17) discussed the Wittes' proposal outlined above. Temple agreed that more attention to tumor-related symptoms and the refinement of the procedures for assessment are needed. However, he felt the measurement of these symptoms in the context of a comparative trial rather than an uncontrolled phase 2 study would be more persuasive. Controlled clinical trials utilizing all these endpoints would be needed since only a fraction of treated patients usually respond and therefore the impact of the treatment on the entire population must be observed, especially when toxic treatments are used.

PROPOSED REVISIONS TO DRUG APPROVAL REGULATIONS

The Food and Drug Administration recently published new procedures for potentially accelerating the approval of new agents intended to treat patients with life-threatening diseases such as cancer and AIDS (18). The proposed procedures would base the approval of new agents on "phase 2 controlled studies" and eliminate the need for large multicenter phase 3 studies before approval. Early consultation between the sponsor of the agent and the Food and Drug Administration is emphasized and encouraged. Meetings with the agency at both the pre-investigational new drug (IND) stage and at the end of phase 1 studies are necessary to plan the appropriate preclinical and clinical studies to determine as completely and as quickly as possible the safety and efficacy of the agent. These controlled phase 2 studies would probably be larger and more complex than conventional phase 2 trials. Many of the endpoints outlined by Wittes (10) above could certainly be incorporated into these phase 2 studies to measure an effect on toxicity and quality of life in demonstrating an increased benefit versus risk ratio required for approval. The impact of these proposals on the utilization of quality of life data for approving a new agent and for accelerating the approval remains to be determined.

CONCLUSION

Many recent approvals of oncologic drugs have been based on implicit improvement of quality of life (long complete response, increased time to recurrence); improved symptom status has also been a basis for approval. To date, however, quality of life scores and evaluations have not been an important part of applications for approval of new agents. This is likely to change. In particular, early demonstration of improvement in unequivocal tumor-related symptoms in phase 2 studies appears to be an especially promising avenue for further study.

REFERENCES

1. Johnson JR, Temple R. Food and Drug Administration requirements for approval of new anticancer drugs. *Cancer Treat Rep* 1985;69:1155–1157.
2. Gelber RD, Goldhirsch A. A new endpoint for the assessment of adjuvant therapy in postmenopausal women with operable breast cancer. *J Clin Oncol* 1986;4:1772–1779.
3. Schipper H, Clinch J, McMurray A, Levitt M. Measuring the quality of life of cancer patients: The functional living index-cancer: Development and validation. *J Clin Oncol* 1984;2:472–483.
4. Spitzer WO, Dobson AJ, Hall J, et al. Measuring the quality of life of cancer patients. A concise QL-index for use by physicians. *J Chron Dis* 1981;34:585–597.
5. Schipper H, Levitt M. Measuring quality of life: Risks and benefits. *Cancer Treat Rep* 1985;69:1115–1123.
6. Ganz PA, Haskell CM, Figlin RA, et al. Estimating the quality of life in a clinical trial of patients with metastatic lung cancer using the Karnofsky performance status and the functional living index-cancer. *Cancer* 1988;61:849–856.
7. Coates A, Gebski V, Stat M, et al. Improving the quality of life during chemotherapy for advanced breast cancer. *N Engl J Med* 1987;317:1490–1495.
8. Priestman TJ, Baum M. Evaluation of quality of life in patients receiving treatment for advanced breast cancer. *Lancet* 1976;i:899–901.

9. Coates A, Dillenbeck CF, McNeil DR, et al. On the receiving end–II. Linear analogue self-assessment (LASA) in evaluation of aspects of the quality of life of cancer patients receiving therapy. *Eur J Cancer Clin Oncol* 1983;19:1633–1637.

10. Wittes RE. Antineoplastic agents and FDA regulations: Square pegs for round holes? *Cancer Treat Rep* 1987;71:795–806.

11. Orr ST, Aisner J. Performance status assessment among oncology patients: A review. *Cancer Treat Rep* 1986;70:1423–1429.

12. Mor V, Laliberte L, Morris JN, Wiemann M. The Karnofsky performance status scale. An examination of its reliability and validity in a research setting. *Cancer* 1984;53:2002–2007.

13. Bakker W, Van Oosterom AT, Aaronson NK, et al. Vindesine, cisplatin, and bleomycin combination chemotherapy in non-small cell lung cancer: Survival and quality of life. *Eur J Cancer Clin Oncol* 1986;22:963–970.

14. Yates JW, Chalmer B, McKegney FP. Evaluation of patients with advanced cancer using the Karnofsky performance status. *Cancer* 1980;45:2220–2224.

15. Hutchinson TA, Boyd NF, Feinstein AR, et al. Scientific problems in clinical scales, as demonstrated in the Karnofsky index of performance status. *J Chron Dis* 1979;32:661–666.

16. Temple R. Transcript of the Oncologic Drugs Advisory Committee Meeting. June 28, 1985.

17. Temple R. Transcript of the Oncologic Drugs Advisory Committee Meeting. December 8, 1987.

18. 21 CRF 312 *Federal Register* 53, No. 204, 41516–41521, October 21, 1988.

IV

Special Populations and Approaches to Quality of Life

Quality of Life Assessments in Clinical Trials, edited by B. Spilker. Raven Press, Ltd. New York © 1990.

17

Pediatrics:

Assessing Quality of Life

*Peter Rosenbaum, *David Cadman, and †Haresh Kirpalani

Departments of Clinical Epidemiology and Biostatistics, and Pediatrics, McMaster University, Hamilton, Ontario L8N 3Z5 Canada; †Department of Pediatrics, Hospital for Sick Children, Toronto, Ontario M5G 1X8, Canada

Craig was born 10 weeks premature and experienced many complications of prematurity and neonatal intensive care. At 3 years of age he has a mild spastic hemiplegia and mild language delay, but is happy and affectionate. Marissa is 12 years old. At age 11 she developed acute lymphoblastic leukemia, but after a prolonged intensive course of chemotherapy and cranial irradiation, she is now in remission and on maintenance therapy. She has fallen behind in her school work, is an overly anxious child, and her parents have sought counseling because of "stress."

What is the quality of life of these children? What more do we need to know about their functional status to determine quality of life? Who determines what functional domains of childhood define quality of life? From whose perspective and values should quality of life based on function and well-being be judged: parents', professionals', the child's, or the society to which these children and their families belong?

Three important issues central to the challenge of measuring quality of life in childhood are illustrated by the above anecdotes. The first complexity concerns the multiple meanings of the phrase "quality of life," a term which has increasingly entered the common parlance of politicians and commentators as well as health professionals. In the context of health usage, quality of life usually means "health-related" quality of life, and refers to some aspect(s) of functional status. Here there is usually a clear ordering of levels of function in each of several dimensions (such as physical/occupational function, psychological state, social interactions, and somatic discomfort [1]). The various levels of performance are ordinal within each dimension. There is, however, no formally determined value or utility attached to states of function, which are combinations of levels of functioning for each of the dimensions used. The value of the state therefore remains subject to individual interpretation and judgment. The quality of life functional status generally reflects the perceptions and viewpoints of the clinician or health professional who specifies the domains used in the measure, and who may also perform the measurement itself.

Quality of life can also be measured using explicit valued-based judgments about health states. In this form of measurement the "value" of a particular health state is derived by asking respondents to judge (by any of a variety of well-established techniques) the relative importance of different health states. Trade-offs are made until any specific state of health and function has been "placed" relative to "better" and "worse" states experienced by a similar stimulus subject. The purpose is to develop a "utility" value for any particular health state. In this approach the perceptions of the judge (patient or surrogate) are often used both to assess health status and to value that health status. Thus, the quality of life functional status generally refers to evaluation of the quality of life domains by health professionals and utility-based quality of life refers to evaluation of the same domains by patients or surrogates.

A second problem concerns which dimensions of children's function to include in any quality of life evaluation. Measures generally reflect the particular perceptions of the individuals assessing quality of life (especially the quality of life functional status) for a specific purpose, using aspects of function they judge relevant to that purpose and ignoring other dimensions. Such measures therefore rarely reflect a general construct of childhood functional well-being. Furthermore, the dimensions of function applicable to adults, such as economic well-being, are clearly not germane to a child's quality of life functional status, and other dimensions such as psychological well-being or social interactions require reformulation to states of function relevant to children's experience.

Theoretical frameworks for comprehensive but applicable measures of children's health status (quality of life functional status) have been suggested by several authors (2,3). These usually focus on limitations of physical, social, and emotional function, and limitations of normal daily activities (such as play) as experienced by children. Each intends to be more than a catalog of the child's abilities, as shown by the inclusion of more ethereal constructs such as "resilience," in order to encompass aspects of "positive health" (2). These multidimensional conceptual models are intended for use in the general childhood population, and usually have not targeted specific illnesses or outcomes of particular treatments. The literature germane to this discussion reveals a progression from simple functional measures to more global quality of life functional status measures.

The third vexing issue concerns who makes judgments about a child's function. Parents, health professionals, children, and members of the lay public may have very different perspectives on both the dimensions of importance and the values placed on different health states (4). The latter concern lies at the heart of quality of life measures, in which varying states of health or function are quantified systematically. The ultimate goal of a utility-based quality of life measure is to create a databased set of values or utilities associated with specific composite health and functional states. The techniques to measure quality of life are readily available, but the challenge remains to decide *whose* judgments, concerning *what* functions, should be values in the quality of life measure.

According to the World Health Organization, "Health is a state of complete physical, mental and social well-being and not merely the absence of disease and infirmity" (5). Interest in assessing the nonphysical domains of the child health experience reflects an increasing awareness of the impact of chronic health problems in childhood. It is noteworthy that the usual morbidity and mortality markers are inadequate. In fact there is a growing interest in what has been called the "new morbidity" in pediatrics, referring specifically to developmental, behavioral, and learning disorders, as well as to a variety of social dysfunctions of childhood and adolescence. Health-related quality of life tries to describe the impact of the illness and predicament (6) of a biological disorder in order to complement the disease markers measured as incidence, prevalence, physiological dysfunction, or mortality rate.

As we hope to show in this chapter, children's quality of life may be measured for a number of different purposes (see Pantel and Lewis [3] for a useful outline of many of these purposes). Functional health status measures are frequently used in surveys of children's health, usually as some form of quality of life functional status measure. Investigators and clinicians are becoming increasingly involved in assessing disease-specific quality of life functional status, usually with measures created for this purpose. In the future health planners can be expected to show increasing interest in applying utility-based quality of life measures to weigh options for the development or expansion of clinical services, using explicit value-based assessments of clinical outcomes and health status to guide planning. It is therefore incumbent upon clinicians, investigators, planners, administrators, and the public to have a clear understanding of the concepts implicit in the term "childhood quality of life."

FUNCTIONAL MEASURES

A brief review is presented of measures of functional status generally used for specific populations such as developmentally delayed infants, retarded children, or children with learning problems. These measures should be contrasted with the quality of life evaluations (either quality of life functional status or utility-based quality of life) that follow.

Measures of Function for Clinical Use

Currently in clinical practice, most assessments of a child's function rely on subjective judgments. Formal tests are available to distinguish, "What can this child do?" from, "What can this child not do?" and allow functional classification. Validation by reference to a comparative group of normal children allows statements to be made about normal ranges. This approach informs all developmental measurement tools. These measures typically include domains other than the purely physical—for example, personal-social, fine motor adaptive, language, and gross movements—but they remain targeted at a functional assessment of neurological maturation. Examples include the Denver Developmental Screening Test (7), the Bayley Scales Infant Development (8), and the Stanford-Binet Scales (9). Other measures such as the Alpern-Boll Developmental Profile (10), which seeks to assess academic achievement and communication skills as well as physical disability, the Vineland Social Maturity Scales (11), the McCarthy Scales of Children's Abilities (12), and the Adaptive Behavior Scale of the American Association of Mental Deficiency (13), all attempt to tap multiple areas of function. The data for these scales are variously drawn from either parental/caregiver interviews or teacher appraisals and observation of the child. Judgments about quality of life based on the functional performance of the child compared to the "norm" are implicit.

Measures of Health and Function for Use in Populations

Perhaps the best known example of an attempt to operationalize a broad framework of health is the RAND Corporation Measure of Health for Children developed for the United States Health Insurance Study (14,15). This measure is administered to parents. The items were generated by a review of existing measures of health and function in physical, mental, social, and overall general or developmental health domains. The items were aggregated into 14 scales using factor analytic and other scaling techniques (14). The majority of the scales have satisfactory internal-consistency reliability and construct validity (14) for children 0 to 4 and 5 to 14 years of age. Different scales and items are used for these two age groups. The measure results in a profile of scaled scores covering each domain assessed.

The Ontario Child Health Study developed measures to assess the physical, social, and emotional health of children 4 to 16 years of age in a general population survey (16). The scales and measures of this study have generally satisfactory internal-consistency reliability and construct validity. The measures are completed by parents and older children aged 12 to 16 using self-report and interviewer-administered items. Other community child health surveys have used remarkably similar constructs as components of children's well-being. Haggerty et al. (17) and Walker et al. (18) developed general population measures for children employing similar survey items. All of these measures result in multiple scales tapping the different aspects of function included in each, rather than a single summary measure of function. Judgments concerning children's quality of life based on these population measures are made implicitly against population score distributions.

QUALITY OF LIFE MEASURES IN CHILDHOOD

Functional Measures

Many investigators have attempted to measure multidimensional well-being and quality of life functional status as outcomes of medical and surgical care. It is apparent that the measures for general populations may be insensitive to changes in quality of life for children with many specific illness, or undergoing specific treatments. Pantel and Lewis have developed a model of child health-related quality of life to measure the impact of medical care (3). In developing the model the authors were careful to distinguish multidimensional summary meaures and multiple dimension "collections" of scales included in the same interview or assessment.

Few if any studies have been performed using a methodologically sound approach to the construction, validation, and application of instruments (as outlined in Chapter 4). The results have not been validated and remain descriptive measures of uncertain applicability and generalizability. However, some measures are clearly relevant, disease-specific outcomes that describe functional status, capturing outcomes german to children with particular disorders. Two examples from the current literature illustrate the clinical richness of this approach.

In a follow-up study of 120 children treated surgically for high imperforate anus, Ditesheim and Templeton (19) related quality of life (functional status) to the achievement of fecal continence. Their "Quantitative Assessment of Quality of Life" utilized three dimensions of function: school attendance, social problems, and physical (continence) capabilities. Each was operationally defined and a scoring system was devised. Total scores were then categorized into "good," "fair," and "poor" outcomes, which in turn were correlated with several aspects of surgical management, gender, age, and functional fecal continence.

This paper illustrates a rational, focused approach to the measurement of aspects of outcome of a surgical procedure, relating dimensions of fecal continence (the primary surgical goal) to other psychosocial and functional performance. The authors explicitly recognized the confounding influence of age on function. However there is no specified rationale for the selection of items or the scoring system used; no reliability or validity data are presented (although there appears to be some construct validity in the data); and there is no discussion of parental perceptions of the usefulness of this measure or how it might be improved.

In a study of the quality of life after extensive severe burns in children. Herndon et al. (20) state, "the remarkable advances in acute care force us to focus on the quality of life of survivors of these severe burns." They set out to assess a number of aspects of the physical, physiological, social, psychological, and independence functions of a small population of very badly burned survivors. The investigators used a variety of standardized measures (behavior checklists, 12-minute exercise test), unstandardized clinical evaluations (psychoanalysts' mental status assessments), and their own assessments (a 12-item activities of daily living checklist with local norms) with items derived from other measures. The scope of the approach is broad and relevant, based on the authors' judgments of what morbidity indicators they felt from clinical experience were most important.

As with Ditesheim and Templeton (19), there is no discussion of the measurement issues involved in creating this functional profile of burn survivors. Although face validity of the dimensions and items is apparent, the nonstandardized and nonvalidated nature of the measure leaves room for improvement.

What is apparent from both of these efforts to measure nontraditional functional outcomes (quality of life functional status) of specific diseases of childhood is their idiosyncratic nature. In the absence of agreed-on dimensions of functional outcome as judged by parents and/or physicians and/or community citizens, each investigator is likely to report results in an individual manner, consistent with varied perspectives on what elements are important. It will therefore be difficult to compare patterns of quality of life outcomes across studies of the same disorder, let alone across disease categories.

One project currently underway is likely to contribute greatly to our understanding of how to measure function and quality of life functional status in children. It takes a generic approach to the assessment of function in an effort to create a measure applicable to all children and all states of function irrespective of disease or disorder.

For several years a group of investigators at the State University of New York at Buffalo has been developing and using the Functional Independence Measure to quantitate adult functional status across disorders, and after changes in health states as a result of treatment (21,22). Current work is in progress to create and validate a pediatric version of the measure (presently called WeeFIM) to capture many dimensions of function in the childhood age range. The collaborative efforts of a number of experienced child health specialists should enable the investigators to refine the measure to make it relevant to the universe of child health problems, and ultimately suitable as a comparative and evaluative instrument. No formally generated utilities are involved in the scaling of the instrument. Preliminary reliability data are reasonably good, and validity information will be forthcoming as the WeeFIM develops.

Value-Based Measures of Childhood Quality of Life (Utility-Based)

Kaplan and Bush were apparently the first to use social value and preference techniques in generating a scheme of well-being for children (Bush, *personal communication*). They derived this from a measure for adult health status, the Index of Well-Being, which yields a single summary score combining mobility, physical, and social domains (23). The well-being score is derived from preferences placed on the corresponding classification of functional level, as judged by a general adult population sample (23). The resulting measure is less comprehensive than some now available such as the RAND instrument (14) or the Ontario Child Health Study (16). To generate the Index score for children they applied values for adult functional levels. To our knowledge, this Children's Index of Well-Being has never been applied. Presumably this reflects the difficulties of using an essentially adult measure in a pediatric population. Nonetheless this measure was a major step toward the utility approach to measuring health-related quality of life now common in the adult quality of life measurement literature (24).

The major limitation of the available measures of health status, well-being, and utility-based quality of life for the general population of children is that they are all largely based on the conceptualizations of their authors. Recognizing the lack of explicit social value-based scales, Cadman et al. generated an adult *and* child social value, preference, and utility-based definition of quality of life for children (25).

Starting with 16 attributes of health and function measured in the Ontario Child Health Study, these investigators measured the relative importance of each of these attributes to overall children's quality of life as judged by a general population sample of parents and their children in grades 6 through 8 using previously developed preference and utility measurement scaling methods (26). Six attributes met criteria for inclusion in the multi-attribute definition of children's quality of life: sensory and communication ability, happiness, self-care ability, freedom from moderate to severe chronic pain or discomfort, learning and school ability, and physical ability (25).

The researchers went on to develop a weighted utility-based model to create a single summary index value of children's utility-based quality of life applicable to the general population. This work requires replication in other samples in order to validate this multi-attribute construct.

An important illustration of the application of utility-based quality of life data to an assessment of costs and outcomes of neonatal intensive care was provided by Boyle et al. (27). The investigators first defined four dimensions of function, each subdivided into several levels. These included physical function (six levels), role function (five), social and emotional function (four), and health problems (eight) (28).

Applying multi-attribute utility theory, it was possible with category scaling (for single-attribute measurements) and a time trade-off procedure (for multi-attribute measurements) to determine the relative value placed on various potential health states by members of society. Once aggregate preferences (utilities) had been determined, these values were used with actual regional neonatal intensive care outcome data to calculate cost-effectiveness, cost-utility, and cost-benefit estimates for populations of very low-birthweight infants cared for at two time periods (before and after implementation of regional tertiary-care services) in the same community. Using this technique with "standardized" utilities for varying health-and-function outcomes, the authors were able to compare the costs of care required to produce equivalent outcomes at two time periods with considerably different patterns of caregiving for premature infants (27).

A large study currently underway at McMaster University and the Hospital for Sick Children, Toronto is evaluating costs and outcomes of treatment of three forms of childhood cancer (Wilm's tumor, high-risk acute lymphoblastic leukemia, and neuroblastoma) in a multistage process. This study uses and expands on the measurement techniques developed earlier by Torrance et al. (24,28) and applied to costs and outcomes of neonatal intensive care as described above.

A detailed review of the contemporary medical literature has been undertaken to define, as fully as possible, the best quantitative estimates of survival, long-term sequelae, and interim toxicities of the treatments for these conditions. Parallel to this process, the investigators are using a multi-attribute utility function approach (28) to estimate values associated with various levels of health states. The attributes chosen were based on the work of Cadman et al. (25). By employing a multi-attribute measurement technique it is possible, in the course of a 60 to 90 minute interview of randomly selected parents of able-bodied children, to derive information on preferences for a wide range of clinical outcomes, and to impute scores for other health states not included in the interview. By combining the two processes, quantitative estimates of the quality of life outcomes of different childhood cancers will be derived and compared in a standardized manner.

ISSUES IN DEVELOPING QUALITY OF LIFE MEASURES FOR CHILDREN

Children can be distinguished from adults by a number of special characteristics. It is important to recognize these issues since they influence how one tries to evaluate quality of life (whether quality of life functional status or utility-based quality of life) in a pediatric population. In particular, it can be argued that adult quality of life measures are inappropriate for children, and that the development of childhood quality of life instruments requires particular care and special perspectives.

Developmental Change

Developmental change makes it difficult to apply any single measure to all age groups from infancy through adolescence. This problem is most obvious in the preschool years because of the rapid rate of change in normal children.

In a study to determine the attributes comprising well-being or quality of life in young handicapped children, Cadman found that an index applicable to 3-year-old children could not be applied to those 5 years of age (29). In the functional status measurement of the RAND Health Insurance Study, there were separate scales for children aged 0 to 4 and those aged 5 to 13 (14). No attempt was made to assess mental or social health in children under 5 years in that study (14).

Both these examples illustrate that children are a "moving target" for whom levels of function in various dimensions—and even the dimensions themselves—change with age and developmental stage. A unitary concept of childhood quality of life is probably not possible, particularly if it was developed for use with adults.

Furthermore, the cognitive capabilities of children evolve continually throughout childhood and adolescence. Variations in this dimension of children's function can cause practical problems in evaluating responses to abstract ideas. For example

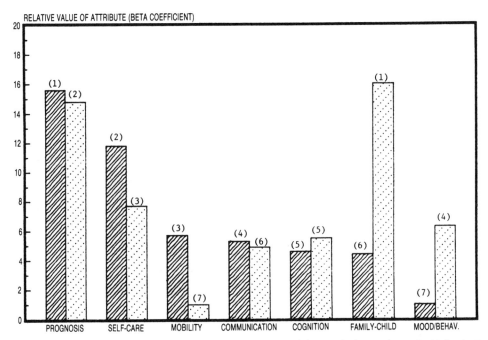

FIG. 1. Care of children with developmental disabilities; relative value of attribute in determining holistic value of multi-attribute description. Parents and community, ▨; Clinicians, ▢; and Ordinal rank in group, (#).

Pantel and Lewis (3) identified a position bias in children's responses, such as a tendency to choose the first answer among response options. They also cautioned about the use of terminology in questions to children (a child may equate the term "diabetes" with "you are about to die"!).

Professional and Parent Perspectives

Parents' perspectives may differ from assessments made from a professional's viewpoint. Cadman et al. found marked differences between health professionals and parents when they explored relative values concerning several dimensions of quality of life for young neurodevelopmentally handicapped children (4). The perspectives of parents, the general adult public, and professionals working with such children and their families were examined. No differences were found between parents and the general population, but professionals differed substantially in their definition of well-being. This is illustrated in Fig. 1, which summarizes the relative importance of each of eight dimensions which are generally accepted treatment goals for such children.

McCormick et al. (30) used a single question from the RAND health profile (14) to judge concordance between maternal assessment of child health and professional judgment of a child's limitations. Parents were asked to assess the child's health over the past year as excellent, very good, good, fair, or poor. Discrepancy between physician and parent perception was found for children with spina bifida and survivors of neonatal intensive care units, but not for patients with rheumatoid arthritis.

Maternal ratings of child health did tend to correlate with a limitation in activities of daily living in patients previously healthy but with a chronic disorder, such as rheumatoid arthritis (30). After making similar observations in another study of children with chronic disability, McCormick et al. (31) concluded, "Despite the children's health problems their parents generally viewed their health positively. Only 15% considered their child to be in fair or poor health."

These observations demonstrate how the values and perceptions of parents may be quite different from those of professionals. Even when impairments produce similar disabilities (as seen by health professionals), judgments about these functional states are influenced by parental perspectives of past health states (loss of previous health versus congenital disability). The parental valuation of their child's health is clearly based on more than present functional status.

Adult and Child Perspectives

It has been shown that a clear developmental progression exists in childhood comprehension of disease causation. The kindergarten-aged "magical" perception evolves gradually to the young adolescent's "complex interactions" model in a developmental progression (32).

When children are presented with health care decisions, they sometimes ask for their parents' assistance. Such was the case when consent for vaccination was sought in the swine influenza vaccine trial, from children between the ages of 6 to 9 years (33). However this occurred within the confines of an experimental therapy for a future health outcome. We are aware of only one study that has used utility and preference measurement techniques to scale quality of life from the perspective of children (25). Children in grades 6 to 8 were able to use reliably Likert-type rating scales of importance, a "feeling thermometer" method, and Time-Trade-Off measures (24).

Children's perspectives on the relative weighting of different aspects of quality of life such as physical ability, learning and school ability, and happiness were only slightly different from those of their gender-matched parent using these methods. Interestingly, the most complicated measurement technique, Time-Trade-Off, was the one most reliably completed by children as well as adults. We believe that with further refinement, these methods of generating children's perspectives on the attributes of quality of life and scaling quality of life measures could be used in children as young as 8 years who have developed abstract reasoning skills. Since children can be asked about health outcomes, what differences do they exhibit compared to parental perceptions? Hospitalization for adults is perceived as a negative health event. It may not be so for children, where some 7 to 10 year olds regard hospitalization as a mark of "courage" that involves feelings of self-esteem (34). This is a dramatic example of a markedly different age-dependent perspective.

Correlations of children's self-reports of functional status and those of parents are good for many aspects of quality of life such as interference of illness with usual activities and impact of illness on independence (3). However, several areas may be poorly correlated (3), demonstrating the need for multiple sources of information in children's quality of life measures. In mental health studies, for example (35), it has been found that checklists of mental and social function may be completed quite differently by parents and children. Whichever perspective is valid or "true," the fact is that these variations in perspective add another complexity to the assessment of quality of life in childhood.

CONCLUSIONS

Several themes emerge from this survey of the literature on quality of life measurement in childhood. First, it should be evident that one cannot directly apply to children measures developed for use with the adult population. The dimensions of function, and the levels therein, are simply too distinct and different to be applicable.

Second, even within the realm of quality of life measurement in childhood, the myriad measures currently in use have different functions. Despite some overlaps at times, these have been developed and applied for varying purposes such as clinical evaluation of function, survey data-gathering, or disease-specific outcome evaluation.

The issue of importance is that the *purpose* of the measure should determine the choice of instrument or the direction of development of a new measure. It should be apparent that the detail required to assess long-term outcome of surgical management of high imperforate anus is simply not present in a survey instrument like the Ontario Child Health Study (16); while conversely the measure developed by Ditesheim and Templeton (19) would obviously be useless as a means of measuring child and adolescent mental health and functional morbidity in the community.

Third, the examples from the literature reported here suggest that good models exist for survey quality of life measurement (14,16), assessment of disease-specific outcomes (19,20), and quality of life evaluations for particular disorders of childhood (28). The best of these instruments have been created systematically with a clear purpose in mind, following principles of measurement development. We recommend that investigators interested in evaluating quality of life in childhood be as clear as possible about the questions they seek to answer, and then find or create measures appropriate to the task. In our judgment these will rarely if ever be measures developed for use in the adult population.

ACKNOWLEDGMENT

The authors wish to acknowledge the support, advice, and insights of Dr. David Feeny whose perspectives were particularly valuable in the development of these ideas.

REFERENCES

1. Schipper H, Levitt M. Measuring quality of life: Risks and benefits. *Cancer Treat Reports* 1985;69:1115–1123.
2. Starfield B. Measurement of outcome: A proposed scheme. *Milbank Mem Fund Q* 1974;52:39–50.
3. Pantel RH, Lewis CC. Measuring the impact of medical care on children. *J Chron Dis* 1987;40(Suppl. 1):99S–108S.
4. Cadman D, Goldsmith C, Bashim P. Values, preferences, and decisions in the care of children with developmental disabilities. *J Dev Behav Ped* 1984;5:60–64.
5. World Health Organization. Constitution of the WHO: Annex 1. WHO, 1958.
6. Taylor DC. The components of sickness: Diseases, illnesses and predicaments. In: Apley J, Ounsted C, eds. *One child*. London: Heinemann, 1982;1–13.

7. Frankenburg WK, Dodds JB, Fandal AW. *Denver developmental screening test reference manual*, rev ed. Denver: Ladoca Publishing Foundation, 1975.

8. Bayley N. *Bayley scales of infant development. Manual*. New York: The Psychological Corporation, 1969.

9. Thorndike RL, Hagen EP, Sattler JM. *The Stanford-Binet intelligence scale, 4th ed*. Chicago: Riverside Publishing Company, 1986.

10. Alpern GD, Boll TJ, Shearer MS. *Developmental Profile II*. Denver: Psychological Development Publications, 1980.

11. Sparrow SS, Balla DA, Cicchetti DV. *Vineland adaptive behavior scales: Interview edition. Survey form manual*. Circle Pines, Minnesota: American Guidance Service, Inc., 1984.

12. McCarthy D. *McCarthy scales of children's abilities*. New York: The Psychological Corporation, 1972.

13. Lambert N, Windmiller M, Cole L, Figueroa R. *AAMD adaptive behavior scale. Public school version*, 1974 revision. Washington: American Association on Mental Deficiency, 1975.

14. Eisen M, Donald C, Ware JE, Brook R. *Conceptualization and measurement of health for children in the Health Insurance Study*. Santa Monica, CA: The Rand Corporation Publication R-2313-HEW, 1980.

15. Eisen M, Ware JE, Donald C. Measuring components of children's health status. *Med Care* 1979;17:902–921.

16. Boyle M, Offord D, Hoffman H, et al. Ontario child health study: Methodology. *Arch Gen Psych* 1987;44:826–831.

17. Haggerty RJ, Roghmann KJ, Pless IB, eds. *Child health in the community*. Toronto: Wiley and Sons, 1975.

18. Walker D, Gortmaker S, Weitzman M. *Chronic illness and psychosocial problems among children in Genessee County*. Boston: School of Public Health, Harvard University, 1981.

19. Ditesheim JA, Templeton JM, Jr. Short term vs. long term quality of life in children following repair of high imperforate anus. *J Ped Surg* 1987;22:581–587.

20. Herndon DN, LeMaster J, Beard S, et al. The quality of life after major thermal injury in children: An analysis of 12 survivors with greater than or equal to 80% total body, 70% third-degree burns. *J Trauma* 1986;26:609–619.

21. Granger CV, Gresham GE. *Functional assessment in rehabilitation medicine*. Baltimore: Williams and Wilkins, 1984.

22. Granger CV. Health accounting—Functional assessment of the long-term patient. In: Kottke FJ, Stillwell GK, Lehmann JF, eds. *Krusen's handbook of physical medicine and rehabilitation*, 3rd ed. Philadelphia: W.B. Saunders Co., 1982;253–274.

23. Kaplan RM, Bush JW, Berry C. Health status: Types of validity and the index of well-being. *Health Serv Res* 1976;11:478–507.

24. Torrance GW. Utility approach to measuring health-related quality of life. *J Chron Dis* 1987;40:593–600.

25. Cadman D, Goldsmith C, Torrance GW. *A methodology for a utility-based health status index for Ontario children*. Final report to the Ontario Ministry of Health. Hamilton, McMaster University, 1986.

26. Torrance GW. Social preferences for health states: An empirical evaluation of three measurement techniques. *Socio-econ Planning Sci* 1976;10:129–136.

27. Boyle MH, Torrance GW, Sinclair JC, Horwood SP. Economic evaluation of neonatal intensive care of very-low-birthweight infants. *N Engl J Med* 1983;308:1330–1337.

28. Torrance GW, Boyle MH, Horwood SP. Application of multi-attribute utility theory to measure social preferences for health states. *Oper Res* 1982;30:1043–1069.

29. Cadman D, Goldsmith C. Construction of social value or utility-based health indices: Usefulness of factorial experimental design plans. *J Chron Dis* 1986;39:643–651.

30. McCormick MC, Atreya BH, Bernbaum JC, Charney EB. Preliminary observations on maternal rating of health of children: Data from three subspecialty clinics. *J Clin Epidemiol* 1988;41:323–329.

31. McCormick MC, Charney EB, Stemmler MM. Assessing the impact of a child with spina bifida on the family. *Dev Med Child Neurol* 1986;28:53–61.

32. Perrin EC, Gerrity PS. There's a demon in your belly: Children's understanding of illness. *Pediatrics* 1981;67:841–849.

33. Lewis C, Lewis M, Ifeckwunigue N. Informed consent by children and participation in an influenza vaccine trial. *Am J Pub Health* 1978;68:1079.

34. Danilowicz DA, Gabriel HP. Post-operative reactions in children: Normal and abnormal responses after cardiac surgery. *Am J Psychiat* 1971;128(2):185–188.

35. Achenbach TM, McConaughy SH, Howell CT. Child/adolescent behavioral and emotional problems: Implications of cross-informant correlations for situational specificity. *Psych Bull* 1987;101:213–232.

Quality of Life Assessments in Clinical Trials, edited by B. Spilker. Raven Press, Ltd. New York, 1990.

18

Geriatrics:

A Perspective on Quality of Life and Care for Older People

T. Franklin Williams

National Institute on Aging, National Institutes of Health, Bethesda, Maryland 20892

The later years of people's lives bring into sharper focus essential features of quality of life and their interrelations with quality of care, which are actually important throughout life. Gerontology and geriatrics have much to contribute to understanding the entire life span. Factors which in earlier years of life at first seem to be optional, become critical in old age for the maintenance of a person's integrity, independence, and autonomy; they become life-or-death matters, figuratively and literally. What are these important elements of quality of life and care, how do they interrelate, and how may we approach more adequate recognition and assessment of them and response to them?

As background for considering these questions, we need an accurate picture of what old age is really like. Fortunately the results of much recent research, as well as increasingly common experiences of all of us with the rapidly increasing numbers of old and very old people, provide much clearer details about old age than were available even as recently as 10 years ago. Table 1 is an attempt to summarize this picture briefly.

It is clear, first, that there are immense individual differences among older people, more than at any earlier age, in virtually all types of characteristics—physical, mental, health, socioeconomic. Thus when we consider what quality of life means to an older person and what features of quality of care may contribute to that quality of life, we *must* arrive at highly individualized conclusions. This principle is of course recommended for all ages, but it may not be so essential in some aspects of earlier life as it is in the lives of older people, as noted below.

Second, we now know that many older persons may continue to be remarkably healthy and functional in all or most ways into very late years. Contrary to pervasive earlier views of inevitable decline in physical and mental functions, changes in personality, and losses of social involvement, much recent research establishes the stability of all of these aspects for many persons into their 80s or beyond—for at least some, even beyond 100 years. Even in organ systems where there are age-related changes, if good lifestyle practices are present and in the absence of overt disease, there is sufficient adaptability and reserve function for most activities (1). This knowledge helps define the challenges for maintenance of quality of life.

TABLE 1.

Older, and especially very old, people:
1. show great individual differences, greater than any other age; and
2. may maintain extraordinarily stable physical, mental, personality, and social characteristics; but
3. are likely to acquire disabilities in any or all of these realms, which may or may not be remediable;
4. may continue to contribute to the life and well-being of themselves, their families, and society;
5. are likely at times to need some or much care by others; and
6. such needs typically occur in clusters of events.

Third, we also know that chronic disabling conditions become progressively more common as persons age, and impinge on reserves and threaten loss of functional independence (1,2). It is also clear that we can do more to restore or compensate for much of this functional loss, through rehabilitative measures (including physical and occupational therapy) and environmental modifications such as specially designed kitchen work spaces, modified controls for driving automobiles, and chairlifts for stairs.

Fourth, contrary to the common view that most older people are burdens on society, we now know that most older persons continue to contribute in personal, informal, and formal ways to their own maintenance and to their families and communities (3). Common examples include daily care of grandchildren while the middle generation is engaged in paid work, and a great variety of volunteer community activities.

Fifth, many older persons at various stages of their later lives do need fluctuating amounts of help from, and care by, others, most of which is provided by family members but also by formal care services. Among persons aged 85 and older—the most rapidly growing portion of our population—40% are disabled to the degree of needing daily help (4). A major challenge here is to focus on respecting the older person's individuality and autonomy.

Sixth, when conditions or events which threaten loss of quality of life such as diseases, injuries, and social losses occur in older people, they typically occur in multiples and against a background of already limited reserves. This is why any single new threat which might appear to be of only limited importance for a younger person is likely to pose a critical problem for an older person. This is also why it is necessary to approach the maintenance of quality of life for older persons with comprehensive consideration of the multiple factors present and the interrelatedness of quality of life and quality of care.

Finally, as background for discussing specific aspects of quality of life and quality of care, an overriding goal and concern of older people for their own quality of life is that *they maintain (or regain) as much personal independence as possible*. This refers to each of the domains of quality of life (i.e., physical, psychological, social, and economic). It is the personal autonomy and the freedom to make choices and to live one's own life according to one's own decisions, both small and large, that means most.

Against such a background, let us first consider characteristics of quality of life which older persons may determine or influence for themselves, and how these may be assessed or measured. Then what is required to provide high quality care to support the desired quality of life will be examined.

QUALITY OF LIFE CHARACTERISTICS DETERMINED OR INFLUENCED BY OLDER PERSONS THEMSELVES

Lifestyle Factors

It is clear from numerous studies that a prudent diet, regular exercise (physical and mental), no smoking, only modest amounts or no alcohol, and adequate sleep are all important for maintaining good health and independence into later years. Regular physical and mental activities, in particular, have been neglected in the past and their benefits have been recently well documented. Regular physical activity has been shown to be as beneficial in older as in younger persons for increasing or maintaining aerobic capacity and muscle mass and strength, minimizing bone loss, and improving blood lipids and glucose tolerance (5–7). Although not specifically studied in older persons, it can be assumed that the beneficial effects on mood produced by physical activity applies in older as well as in younger persons also. Recent studies have also shown that the active use of cognitive functions contributes to their maintenance or improvement in older persons (8,9).

Methods for assessing and measuring these factors exist in epidemiologic and demographic studies such as the Alameda County studies, and studies conducted by the National Center for Health Statistics, the National Institute on Aging, the Bureau of the Census, and others. A bibliographic summary of aging-related statistical studies is available from the National Institute on Aging.

Screening and Early Detection of Potential Problems

Even though there is need for more studies of the benefits of some screening efforts in relation to their costs, reasonable consensus exists on the value of certain procedures which can lead to early detection and effective prevention or treatment of potentially disabling conditions, thus contributing to quality of life maintenance. Professional groups in Canada and the United States have addressed this issue, including its application to older persons (10–12). The Institute of Medicine of the National Academy of Sciences is currently conducting an evaluation of preventive practices "for the second fifty," i.e. ages 50 to 100. A recent review and consensus on recommendations, prepared by an expert committee for the United Seniors Health Cooperative, encompasses these screening procedures at various specified intervals: blood pressure; occult blood in stool; digital rectal examination; breast examination and mammography; pelvic examination with Papanicolaou test; vision; hearing; blood lipids; hematocrit; urinalysis; thyroid function; vaccination for influenza, pneumococcus, and tetanus; specific attention at times of physical examinations to skin, oral health, and feet (13). A diary recording the completion of these tests is recommended for each older person.

PSYCHOLOGICAL, SOCIAL, AND ECONOMIC FACTORS AFFECTING QUALITY OF LIFE

The quality of life of older persons is clearly influenced by psychological, social, and economic factors in the same way that younger persons are influenced, for the most part. At the same time there are features of special importance in the lives of older people which may be highlighted here. In the psychological realm, longitudinal studies establish the remarkable constancy or stability of basic personality characteristics, as seen for example in the studies of McCrae and Costa (14), against which any changes in behaviors or symptoms can appear as signals for further inquiry. Concern about any suspected loss of cognitive function is very frequent among older persons and also deserves explicit attention. The satisfaction of continuing to contribute to others is important to most older persons and should be a part of psychosocial assessment.

In the social realm, contrary to some earlier views, it is clear that most older people maintain as close ties to their families and social networks as they had in earlier life (15). Here again individual variation is important, and longitudinal information is critical in assessing the meaning of current social relationships and activities to the quality of life of a specific older person.

In the economic aspects of their lives, older persons usually have little or no opportunity to add to their fixed retirement income and are concerned first about security and second about unanticipated costs, especially in health care.

All of these realms are important to the quality of life wherever an older person may be, and in whatever state of health or disability: in her/his lifelong home, retirement community, or nursing home, with or without disabilities. They should be part of an assessment of quality of life in any setting.

CHARACTERISTIC NEEDS FOR AND PROVISION OF QUALITY CARE AFFECTING QUALITY OF LIFE IN OLDER PERSONS

Disabling conditions, physical or mental, in older persons are clearly common threats to maintenance of the independence which is a key to their quality of life. Not only is an affected person at risk of losing some control over her/his own life, but also she/he faces the depressing sense of being a "burden" to family members or others, as well as upsetting financial costs. Elsewhere in this volume measures of physical and mental functioning in general, and in certain disease conditions in particular, are addressed. Here the most common disabling conditions for older, and especially very old (age 85 +), persons may be noted: dementia; loss of mobility due to arthritis, stroke, peripheral vascular disease, and hip fractures (usually associated with osteoporosis); loss of vision; loss of hearing; depression; and urinary incontinence. Assessment measures for all of these features exist, but also could use further refinement.

The impact of any of these conditions on the maintenance of independence and quality of life is influenced by the lifestyle factors referred to earlier as well as by the strength and stability of the family and other social and economic resources. It is obvious that all of these factors must be examined simultaneously when assessing their impact on quality of care and quality of life.

What Is High Quality Care?

In the face of threats to independence posed by disabling conditions in older persons as well as the large private and public burdens of care and the associated costs, there is an understandable widespread interest in the types, quantity, and quality of care involved and in its costs. Concerning quality of care, it can be observed that virtually all of the attention has been on documenting and eliminating *poor* or unacceptable care, that is, to aim through assessment and interventions to accomplish *minimum* levels of quality of care. These goals are certainly desirable, but they fall short of seeking or achieving *high* quality care, the care each of us would like for ourselves or our older relatives or friends. Anything less than high quality care will fall short of helping to achieve a high quality of life for those needing care.

High quality care for older persons can be defined as, "care that is desired by the informed patient or client (and family); is based on the sound judgment of the professionals involved, from scientific studies and/or experience; and is agreed upon and carried out in a relationship of mutual trust and respect" (16). Others have given essentially the same definition (17,18). This general definition would apply to care for persons of any age, but let us consider specific features of its application to older persons needing care.

As already emphasized, the older person's highest priority will usually be to regain as much independence as possible; thus the emphasis in the approach to care should be fundamentally *rehabilitative*. A comprehensive rehabilitation philosophy and approach should infuse virtually all care for disabled older persons, in acute as well as in chronic care settings, utilizing the skills of a variety of professionals. Also important is an informed patient and family, so that care plans (which are likely to involve chronic or long-term activities) are mutually understood and agreed upon (19). Fortunately there are good sources of information for the public about most common problems affecting older persons, including help from many support groups such as those concerned with Alzheimer's disease, arthritis, or strokes. Professionals also have a responsibility to provide adequate information.

Second, in carrying out their part in achieving high quality care for disabled older persons, the involved professionals must start with the recognition, emphasized earlier, that multiple complex problems (medical, functional, and psychosocial) are almost always present simultaneously; thus a *comprehensive, multidisciplinary assessment* and development of a comprehensive care plan are essential first steps in achieving high quality care. This necessity has been stressed in the recent Consensus Development Conference on this topic at the National Institutes of Health (20,21). A major focus of the care plan should be on rehabilitative potential and efforts. Sound judgment based on up-to-date knowledge of the scientific literature relevant to the patient's conditions is also an obvious necessity.

The third component of high quality care, namely that the care be conducted in a relationship of mutual respect and agreement (22), is often the weakest link: the fundamental individuality and right to autonomy of the disabled person is not respected. There is much evidence of caregivers—family members as well as professionals—talking *about* the affected person rather than with her or him, and making decisions about and for that person rather than with her or him. This problem is perhaps most obvious in many nursing home settings where the person is "institutionalized," i.e., fitted into the routines of the institution, rather than *individualizing* the care to the preferences as well as the needs of the older person. That truly individualized approaches can be achieved is illustrated in some nursing homes in Scandinavia and elsewhere, as well as a few in this country (23).

Assessing and Accomplishing High Quality Care

There has been little attention paid to developing methods for assessing high quality care in older persons, and perhaps even less to steps taken to achieve it. It appears feasible that measures for documenting the components of high quality care described above can be developed and used. For example, the patient's preferences for daily living routines can be determined and documented, and the performance of caregivers can be assessed against them. The extent of her/his understanding of the disease conditions present and of the options for treatment can be noted, as well as the professionals' responses. Specific efforts in rehabilitative therapy can be noted, as well as response. A consensus panel has identified specific disease conditions for which high quality care can make a real difference in outcome, as well as types of services which may be most important in improving quality of care (24).

To accomplish such care we need to expand the numbers and then take full advantage of the new generation of physicians and other professionals in the health and human services fields who are specially trained in gerontology and geriatrics. Physicians in internal medicine and family medicine are obtaining certification of special competence in geriatrics, and soon special competency certification in geropsychiatry will be available. Similar special competencies are developing in other professions. It should be a matter of policy that all care organizations—hospitals, nursing homes, group practices, retirement communities, etc.—have a team of such specially prepared professionals as part of their staffs, called upon to give leadership in the care of older persons with disabilities or other complex problems.

Further, it is suggested that more responsibility be given to chiefs of services, the directors of caring organizations, for assuring that high quality care, not just meeting minimal standards, is accomplished. This is essentially a personal responsibility for the person in charge to exercise throughout his/her staff and operations. They should be accountable to an informed board including representatives of patients and their families as well as professionals. In essence this is the structure by which we have nominally organized our caring systems; but boards typically have given most attention to capital, financial, and management features, and too little attention to assuring that the key staff leaders are in turn assuring high quality care.

In summary, we should establish ambitious but nevertheless attainable, individualized goals of high quality care for older persons in need of such care, and also establish the expectation that our professionals are going to be prepared for, and supervised in providing, such a level of care that any of us would be pleased to receive it.

REFERENCES

1. Williams TF. Current status of biomedical and behavioral research in aging. In: Andreopoulos S, Hogness JR, eds. *Health care for an aging society*. New York: Churchill Livingstone, 1989;123–137.
2. National Center for Health Statistics, Havlik RJ, Liu BM, Kovar MG, et al. Health statistics on older persons, United States, 1986. *Vital and health statistics*, Series 3, No. 25. DHHS Pub. No. (PHS) 87-1409. Public Health Service. Washington, D.C.: U.S. Government Printing Office, June 1987.
3. Kahn RL. Productive behavior: Assessment, determinants, and effects. *J Am Geriat Soc* 1983;31:750–757.
4. *Americans needing help to function at home*. Public Health Service Advance Data No. 92, DHHS Pub. No. 83-1250, Washington, D.C.: U.S. Department of Health and Human Services, 1983.
5. Seals DR, Hagberg JM, Hurley BF, et al. Endurance training in older men and women. I. Cardiovascular responses to exercise. *J Appl Physiol* 1984;57:1024–1029.

6. Seals DR, Hagberg JM, Hurley BF, et al. Effects of endurance training on glucose tolerance and plasma lipid levels in older men and women. *JAMA* 1984;252:645–649.
7. Dalsky GP, Stocke KS, Ehsani AA, et al. Weight-bearing exercise training and lumbar bone mineral content in postmenopausal women. *Ann Intern Med* 1988;108:824–828.
8. Baltes PB, Lindenberger U. On the range of cognitive plasticity in old age as a function of experience: 15 years of intervention research. *Behav Ther* 1988;19:283–300.
9. Rodin J. Aging and health: Effects of the sense of control. *Science* 1986;233:1271–1276.
10. Canadian Task Force on the Periodic Health Examination. The periodic health examination: 2. 1985 update. *Can Med Assoc J* 1986;134:724–727.
11. Medical Practice Committee, American College of Physicians. Periodic health examination: A guide for designing individualized health care in the asymptomatic patient. *Ann Intern Med* 1981;95:729–732.
12. Council on Scientific Affairs. Medical evaluation of healthy persons. *JAMA* 1983;249:1626–1633.
13. United Seniors Expert Panel. Taking charge of your health. Special Report. United Seniors Health Cooperative, Washington, D.C., 1988.
14. McCrae RR, Costa PT, Jr. *Emerging lives, enduring dispositions: Personality in adulthood.* Boston: Little, Brown, 1984.
15. Shanas E. Social myth as hypothesis: The case for the family relations of older people. *Gerontologist* 1979;19:3–9.
16. Williams TF. Quality of care for older people: Challenges to research and teaching. The Kesten Memorial Lecture. (*Submitted*)
17. Lohr KN, Yordy KD, Thier SO. Current issues in quality of care. *Health Aff* 1988;7(1):5–18.
18. Council on Medical Service. Quality of care. *JAMA* 1986;256:1032–1034.
19. Davies AR, Ware JE, Jr. Involving consumers in quality of care assessment. *Health Aff* 1988;7(1):33–48.
20. National Institutes of Health Consensus Development Conference Statement: Geriatric assessment methods for clinical decision-making. *J Am Geriatr Soc* 1988;36:342–347.
21. Solomon DH. Geriatric assessment: Methods for clinical decision-making. *JAMA* 1988;259:2450–2452.
22. Steffen GE. Quality medical care: A definition. *JAMA* 1988;260:56–61.
23. Williams CC. The experience of long term care in the future. *J Gerontol Social Work* (*in press*).
24. Fink A, Siu A, Brock RH, et al. Assuring the quality of health care for older persons: An expert panel's priorities. *JAMA* 1987;258:1905–1908.

Quality of Life Assessments in Clinical
Trials, edited by B. Spilker. Raven
Press, Ltd. New York © 1990.

19

The Frail Elderly:

Creating Standards of Care

Marsha D. Fretwell

Programs in Geriatric Medicine and Medicine, Brown University, Providence,
Rhode Island 02910

In the preceding chapter, Dr. Williams (1) described some pertinent characteristics
of older persons as background for developing and applying measures of quality to
the experience of older individuals in our acute and long-term care systems. This
chapter focuses on two of these characteristics: (a) the multiplicity of factors (physical, mental, emotional, social, and economic) that interact in a complex fashion at
any point in time in an older person's life; and (b) the resulting enhancement of
interindividual variation among older individuals of a given chronological age. Based
on these attributes, the argument is made that *personal preferences and individualized care plans are intrinsic to the definition of quality of life and care in this
group.* This requirement of individualized clinical therapies and care is then related
to the research methodology used in the creation of standards of care and the evaluation of the effectiveness and efficiency of our medical and social interventions.
The role of an individual's physical, cognitive, and emotional functions as pivotal
outcomes in the evaluation of both quality of life and care is highlighted. The need
for studies using outcome measures that are adequately sensitive and specific is
discussed. The chapter concludes with the description of a systematic approach for
the collection and integration of patient information and the creation of patient care
plans that allow individualization of the therapies within a standard set of domains.

COMPLEXITY AND INDIVIDUAL VARIATION

As humans age, there is a continuous interaction of environmental and genetic
factors that accentuates the uniqueness of each person. Individuals of the same
chronologic age may differ considerably in such physiologic or biologic functions as
vital capacity, cardiac output, creatinine clearance, and visual accommodation (2).
These wide biological differences in individuals of a given chronologic age significantly reduce the usefulness of age as a single criterion for triaging services or
categorizing patients within population-based studies. Additionally, within one individual, age-related changes in one organ system are not necessarily predictive of
similar changes in other organ systems.

In any given individual, the aging process may be better viewed as the ongoing interaction of biological processes, surrounding social forces, idiosyncratic health behaviors, and lifestyle stresses. This complex interactive process is superimposed on the underlying asynchronous physical, cognitive, and emotional development curves (3). Over time, in susceptible individuals, losses in the physical, mental, social, and economic spheres of life become more frequent and require continuous adaptation. How well an individual adapts to change becomes a central factor determining both the length and quality of one's life (4). As one becomes frail and more dependent on the care of others, and particularly if this care is in the setting of an institution, the determinants of the quality of one's life begin to merge with those of the quality of one's care. Eventually, the burden of irreversible changes is so great and the capacity of the individual to respond to environmental stress is so limited that a simple pulmonary pneumonia, even if diagnosed and treated appropriately, may be the patient's final illness.

PERSONAL PREFERENCE AND INDIVIDUALIZED STANDARDS OF CARE

Acute and long-term care of frail older individuals highlights the shift in focus of our health care system. Health care has changed from treating a single disease underlying an illness to managing the individual's entire burden of disease and disability over a sustained period of time (5). The outcome of any illness is usually more dependent on various attributes of the host, positive or negative, than the absolute virulence of the infective organism or the progressive nature of the disease. Assisting each individual to achieve and maintain his or her optimal physical, cognitive, and emotional function for that point in life becomes the overriding goal of care. A critical role for physicians is to provide accurate prognostic information for an individual, i.e., telling patients where they are on their life's course at any given point in time. This enables patients to participate appropriately in decision making about their care.

The inherent complexity of frail older persons offers a significant challenge in diagnosis and prognosis not only for physicians but also for administrators and regulators who are attempting to establish standards of care. A large number of interacting variables influence health outcomes following a single episode of illness in these elderly patients with multiple chronic diseases and functional disabilities. The information base for diagnosis must be large and the treatments multidimensional to achieve an optimal outcome. Generalizations about treatment are unproductive, and may be counterproductive, if one condition greatly influence treatment of another. Additionally, many functional problems of the elderly such as incontinence and immobility have multiple underlying etiologies (6). Failure to identify and treat all underlying etiologies may lead to a persistence of the functional problem despite appropriate treatment of one of the etiologies.

Even if all the information from the multiple domains influencing health outcomes is collected and considered for accuracy of diagnosis and prognosis, the patient's values about the planned treatment could override and determine the actual outcome (1). For instance, the person's attitude about feeding tubes is a major determinant of outcome in instances where malnutrition is the central problem. If a competent frail older person refuses the placement of a feeding tube when it represents the only mechanism for refeeding and survival, he or she has chosen this to be the final illness. If the prognosis for this episode of illness is constructed on the medical illness and functional status of the individual without consideration of personal preference for treatment, the predicted outcome could be very different from the actual outcome. If appropriate application of the standard treatment for medical disease is the only measure of quality, this person has received poor care. If allowing individual autonomy in the decisions that affect him is a measure, then this person has received the highest quality of care.

For frail older persons, the standards established for their health care have a fundamental impact on their quality of life. This concept, taken with the complexity and individual variation among individuals, supports the regular inclusion of personal preference and individualized care plans in our definition of high quality health care.

THE PROBLEM: INDIVIDUAL PATIENTS AND GENERIC STANDARDS

Clinicians have always been challenged by the translation of data obtained from the basic sciences and population-based studies into information that is relevant and useful for decision making with individual patients (7). Clinical investigations and pharmacological studies that exclude very old individuals on multiple medications or those with multiple chronic illnesses have limited application in the care of frail and/or chronically ill older persons. Research utilizing the methodologies of clinical epidemiology may provide data that support the treatment of certain problems. Often, however, the study results summarize the causal factors without identifying the appropriate patients for clinicians to treat (8). Additionally, this approach to study design has focused on asking questions that are amenable to answering with currently available research methodology. These questions may not always be relevant to the clinician caring for individual patients. This tension between a clinician's concern for the individual patient and the use of aggregate data methodology to extend knowledge is a critical feature of our considerations in creating standards of care for frail older persons (9).

"Standard" is one of several words such as criterion, gauge, measure, test, and yardstick that refer to sets of rules or principles by which we evaluate the quality of something. "Standard" itself implies an objective, impartial set of rules that have actually been defined in advance and are usually derived from aggregates of individual information in scientific studies. Once the standard is established, the item that is under scrutiny is usually evaluated in a yes-no comparison with the standard (10). In discussions of the standards used to measure the quality of care, Donabedian's original framework—structure, process, and outcome—is usually applied (11). Currently, much of the attention in the pursuit of quality is focused on assessment of patient outcomes (12). The mechanisms for establishing standards for patient outcomes are most often based on analyses of large aggregates of patient data and use implicit criteria such as "preventable death" and "avoidable hospitalization" (13). These criteria are applied retrospectively to completed episodes of care and therefore may be a source of anxiety to clinicians, rather than a source of learning. Although there is a growing sophistication in the description of an individual's risk factors and outcomes, we are at the very beginning of understanding how patient preference, i.e., the creation of standards that are partial to individual patients, might be included in the evaluation of quality of care.

FUNCTIONAL MEASURES: ISSUES RELATING TO STANDARDS OF CARE

Explicit measures of appropriate care to date have included the benefits, risks, and costs of care. Benefits usually include increased life expectancy, pain relief, reduced anxiety, and improved functional outcomes. Risks include morbidity, decline in functional outcomes, mortality, and psychological distress. *As our population under care ages, the gold standard of care, survival at all costs, is slowly being replaced by relevant measures of physical, cognitive, and emotional function.* Their widespread inclusion in both studies of the quality of life and the quality of care confirms their importance as valid measures of human activity. Function as a focus of care has been elaborated by investigators such as Karnofsky (14), Katz (15), and Lawton (16) in response to the needs of patients undergoing restorative care of chronic arthritis, and treatment of cancer, acute cerebral vascular accidents, and fractures of the hip. Measures of human function range from a cell membrane's pumping sodium to an individual's ability to file her income tax. This chapter focuses on those cognitive and physical functions of frail older persons that are necessary for living independently.

Basic functional measures, such as the Katz Index of Activities of Daily Living have been appropriately applied to (a) predict patient outcomes, (b) measure the effectiveness of restorative interventions, and (c) orient the medical care of frail older individuals toward issues relevant to their independence and dignity (17). Other indexes of functional disability, such as Barthel's Index (18) and the Older Americans Research and Service Instrument (19) also may be helpful for higher levels of function. Additional scales like Spitzer's Quality of Life Scale (20), which includes both the basic and higher levels of human function, may be needed. The choice of a particular scale is determined by an understanding of the norm of activities for a group of individuals at a certain point in the natural history of their life and illness. In the author's study (21), the frailty of the older individual makes the Katz Index the most appropriate test to use. When evaluating the impact of different therapies for a specific illness, quality of life and care scales must focus on the expected change in functional activities in order to be adequately sensitive. For instance, surgeries that affect only the upper body or extremities in otherwise functionally intact individuals, require evaluation instruments that focus on the upper extremities' functions.

The Katz Index was developed in the context of specific neurological and structural impairments, but has been successfully applied to measure change in function in large aggregates of older individuals, regardless of the different etiological factors underlying that change. When used as an outcome measure in acute and long-term care, the activities of daily living score behaves as an integrated summary of multiple physical and cognitive etiological variables and is therefore an accurate and concise source of information for making a statement of prognosis.

If an individual's change in function after treatment is used as an indicator of the quality of care he receives, we need additional baseline information to accurately predict the best possible trajectory of functional change for that person. If our predictors are appropriate, then the comparison of the actual functional outcome following a given treatment with the predicted one offers one measure of the quality of the treatment. Using the change in a functional outcome measure in this manner requires that we not only know the overall degree of functional impairment at baseline, but also have an understanding of: (a) the specific contribution of certain diagnoses, medications, and malnutrition to the functional impairment; (b) the potential for change or reversibility of each of the diagnoses and functional impairments driving the summary Katz score; and (c) the length of time and the change over time of the various functional states.

The best example of this concept is given by examination of the changes in cognitive function that occur in the acute care hospital. In acutely ill older patients, the risk of acute confusional states appears to be about 25% or higher (22), especially for those individuals with chronically impaired cognition. Once a patient becomes delirious, the risk of losing other functions (e.g., continence, mobility) is greater, and, of equal importance, the probability of regaining either continence or mobility is minimal until the confusional state is reversed. Therefore, the prevention or early detention and treatment of delirium is a critical marker for quality in acute hospital care.

If, in examining cognitive function change in a patient during a hospital stay, the only measure used is a summary scale combining the changes of acute (reversible) and chronic (irreversible) confusion, one has a measure of the degree of confusion, but no understanding of its etiology. On the other hand, if a measure is constructed which distinguishes those with acute and reversible changes in cognitive function from those with chronic irreversible impairment, the diagnostic and prognostic accuracy of the measure will be enhanced. Accurate prognosis provides the basis for appropriate expectations and allows evaluation of whether appropriate diagnostic and treatment has occurred for an individual patient.

Once we understand the nature and degree of a patient's dysfunction, there are other issues which affect patient outcomes. These include the availability of treatment, the risk to benefit ratio of treatment, and the patient's personal preference for treatment. These factors must be included in prognosis statements to achieve the most accurate trajectory of functional change. Additionally, as individuals reach the final phase of their lives, small changes in function that may be imperceptible by current measures can have a strong influence on their quality of life (23). For instance, individuals considered completely dependent as assessed by the Katz Index of Activities of Daily Living are no longer able to feed themselves. What are the measures that will help us determine the quality of care and therefore the quality of life for these individuals? For one individual, supporting continued independence in feeding by providing finger foods is the correct approach; for another, hand feeding by a caretaker is better. Unfortunately, in our current approach to care, we are just beginning to be sensitive to the functional decline associated with natural death and to provide resources that allow it to happen in the setting most conducive to meeting individual needs.

CREATING STANDARDS FOR FRAIL OLDER PERSONS

The goal of health care is to assist each individual to maintain and improve her or his ability to function independently in her or his everyday life. As one ages and approaches the last phase of life this goal remains the same, but the level of functioning may be different. Given the degree of variation among persons of the same chronologic age and given the potential complexity of the burden of disease and disability that may occur in the very old or very frail, personal preferences and individualized care plans become central to the definition of high quality care. There appears to be a fundamental conflict involved in our task. Standards, by definition, cannot be individualized; they are impartial rules, based on the average. Yet older persons, physicians, and caring families routinely acknowledge the tremendous need for an individualized approach to care.

How can individualized care plans and the resulting patient outcomes be evaluated? How can a standard of care for frail or very old persons be defined and measured? In this section, we describe one approach for systematic collection and integration of patient information which promotes the creation of care plans that allow individualization of therapies within a standard set of domains.

As a means of organizing the large number of interacting variables that influence health outcomes following a single episode of illness in a frail older patients, Fretwell has developed a patient care process referred to as the Comprehensive Functional Assessment (24). Using a biopsychosocial patient information base and the Katz Index of Activities of Daily Living, each area of function on the Katz Index is examined for its biological (e.g., age, sex, diagnosis, medications, nutrition), psychological (e.g., cognitive function, emotional function, personality, prior coping style), and social (e.g., support system, finances, style of social interactions) determinants. As noted above, function measured by the Katz score is an integrative summary of these multiple etiological determinants or variables and has quantitative characteristics that make it accurate for prediction of outcomes and/or ordering services to compensate for functional deficits.

In this process of systematic collection and integration of patient information, medical diseases change from being considered the central focus of health care to becoming only one of several very significant sources of functional impairment. Other sources of impairment are within the psychological, social, environmental, and economic domains of human reality. For accurate prediction of patient outcomes, these sources of impairment must also be included in the overall evaluation of each patient. The focus of assessment shifts, based on the acuity of the patient's presenting complaint. The interactive nature of these dimensions within the experience of human illness and wellness suggests that a comprehensive knowledge of the patient is essential for safe and effective medical care. Thus, in this method of creating individualized care plans, "comprehensive" refers to the need for a biological, psychological, and social database (see domains, Table 1) and "functional" refers to the focus of care on maintaining and improving the patient's everyday basic function (see functional scales, Table 1).

The writings of George Engel (25) provide support for the biopsychosocial information base and those of Sidney Katz (17) provide support for the focus on functional outcomes. The activities of daily living measure of an individual's function at one point in time offers a mechanism for identifying, within the infinite number of descriptive variables of the biopsychosocial model, those that are pertinent in determining health outcomes.

Based on applying a Comprehensive Functional Assessment in a standardized interdisciplinary team format to 200 patients over the age of 75 years entering a hospital (21), Fretwell derived the following categories within which all of the assessment and recommendation statements could be placed: diagnosis, medications, nutrition, continence/constipation, cognition, emotion, mobility, and social support. These have subsequently become the standard areas of concern for the clinician in the individualized care plan (see Areas of Concern Table 2).

The Individualized Care Plan

For each diagnosis and for each of the seven other areas listed in Table 2, the patient is assessed and all problems are identified. Reversible ones are first identified

TABLE 1. *Biopsychosocial information base*

Biomedical domain	Psychological domain	Social domain
Medical diagnosis	Mental status	Individual social skills
Medications	Emotional function	Marital history
Duration	Depression	Acceptance of help
Adverse drug reaction	Personality type	Presence of
Creatinine clearance	Coping style	confidante
Nutritional status	Specific dysfunction	Support system
Albumin	Hostility	Quantity and quality of
Weight changes	Anxiety	the system
Appetite	Depression	Use of formal support
Communication function	Hallucinations	Financial resources
Hearing	Paranoia	
Speech	Values	
Vision	Concerning medical treatments	

Summary Scales for Function	
Basic activities of daily living	Instrumental activities of daily living
Feeding	Use of transport
Bathing	Shopping
Dressing	Finance
Use of toilet	Telephone
Transfer	Medications
Mobility	Housework
Continence	

(see Table 2, column 1) and recommendations consistent with the standard of medical practice are listed (see Table 2, column 2). Irreversible problems, especially those that influence the overall prognosis, are also noted. In column 3, the patient's preference about the standard recommendations are noted. For instance, if the diagnosis is colon carcinoma, the standard of medical practice is surgery; if the patient is competent and chooses to refuse surgery, this is noted. Column 4 then contains the actual recommendations, i.e., those standard practices modified by the patient preference. Patient preferences are elicited for all recommendations in each of the diagnoses and the seven other areas: medications (patient may refuse chemotherapy or antidepressants), nutrition (patient may refuse a feeding gastrostomy tube), continence/constipation (patient may refuse a Foley catheter), cognition, emotion, mobility (patient may refuse to go to rehabilitation), and social support (patient may refuse to go to day care). The actual recommendations (column 4) include only those treatments and therapies that the patient (or the patient and the family) finds acceptable. Presumably, with this degree of input, the recommendations will be appropriate and compliance will be high.

Based on information about the burden of irreversible problems and the proposed actual recommendations, one sets goals for each of the diagnoses and the other seven domains. For instance, under cognition, the identified problem might be an acute confusional state categorizing the patient as significantly impaired. The provisional and actual recommendations are to "stop" a certain medication and the outcome goal is "improvement" in the domain of cognition. This would be documented as moving from significantly impaired to mildly impaired. Outcome goals for each domain are focused on restoring and/or maintaining each person at an optimal level of physical, cognitive, and emotional function. Despite this adherence to consistent or

TABLE 2.

Area of concern	1. Assessment	2. Standard medical practice	3. Patient preference	4. Actual recommendations	5. Predicted outcomes
Diagnoses Primary Secondary	Reversibility	—	Dialysis Surgery Amputation	—	Improve Maintain Decline
Medications use	Functional impact score	—	Attitude toward drug use; Chemotherapy Antidepressants	—	Improve Maintain Decline
Nutrition	1. Intact 2. Mild impairment 3. Significant impairment	—	Feeding tubes	—	Improve Maintain Decline
Continence	1. Intact 2. Requires assistance 3. Dependent	—	Foley catheters	—	Improve Maintain Decline
Constipation	1. No 2. Yes 3. Impaction	—	—	—	Improve Maintain Decline
Cognition	1. Intact 2, Mild impairment 3. Significant impairment	—	Minimal mental impairment	—	Improve Maintain Decline
Emotion	1. Intact 2. Mild depression 3. Significant depression	—	Pain tolerance	—	Improve Maintain Decline
Mobility	1. Intact 2. Requires assistance 3. Dependent	—	Assistive device Rehabilitation unit	—	Improve Maintain Decline
Social support	1. Intact 2. Stressed 3. Unavailable	—	Return home Temporary nursing home Avoid nursing home	—	Improve Maintain Decline
Placement	1. No change 2. Temporary change 3. Permanent change	—	—	—	

standard domains, within each domain the recommendations can be individualized and made consistent with the personal preference of the patient.

Setting Standards of Care for Frail Older Persons

The above process of developing an individualized care plan can be accomplished by either an independent practitioner or, in the event of high risk or particularly complex patients, an interdisciplinary team. In the setting of a Geriatric Assessment Unit, this approach has demonstrated utility and proven benefits to health care outcomes (26). Among the benefits are better diagnostic accuracy and treatment planning, more appropriate placement decisions with fewer referrals to nursing homes, improved functional and mental status of the patient, prolonged survival of the patient, and lower overall use of costly institutional care services (27).

Assessing Quality of Care at an Institutional Level

This process of creating individualized care plans may be transformed into a system for assessing the quality of care at an institutional level. To do this it is necessary to systematize the assessment within each area of concern. For instance, based on using standard cutoff values in the measurement of serum albumin, an individual is assessed as having intact, mild, or significant nutritional deficiency. For emotion, based on clinical judgment and/or using an existing scale such as the Geriatric Depression Scale (28), an individual is assessed as being either intact, mildly depressed, or significantly depressed. These "current status" assessments and actual recommendations (Table 2, column 4) are used as the information base to predict an outcome in each domain. These "predicted outcomes" must also be categorized systematically, i.e., it is predicted that the individual, after treatment, will improve, maintain, or decline in function in each of the eight domains (see Table 2, column 5). Standard definitions for improvement, such as moving from significantly to mildly depressed, insure consistency.

The optimal period for setting these patient outcome goals or "predicted outcomes" in an acute care hospital is within the first 72 hours after admission. At other points in time (e.g., discharge or set intervals within prolonged hospitalizations), new assessments of each domain are made and compared with these outcomes predicted at admission. Based on this feedback, each individualized care plan is modified and "new" outcomes are established. This process is also repeated at predetermined intervals following discharge.

In any site where health care is provided, this process offers a prospective approach to setting standards and evaluating quality, allows outcome goals to be individualized, and provides timely feedback that may be incorporated into continuing education as well as quality assurance programs. This process does not replace existing quality improvement programs for evaluating the structure and process of medical care. Rather, it extends them by acknowledging the complexity of treating diseases and managing illness in frail older people. If we are to use outcome measures as a means of evaluating the quality of care or life for frail older people, the predicted outcomes against which the actual outcome is compared must be accurate or appropriate for the individual.

By systematizing the patient assessment and cueing the clinician to organize assessment data into a standard patient care plan, this process promotes accurate predictions about patient outcomes. By routinely providing feedback in the form of actual patient outcomes for each of the diagnoses and seven domains discussed above, the complexity of each patient's natural history is clarified and learning is promoted. Including clinicians in the process of setting goals for their patients will improve their ability to make prognosis statements. Including the patient's preferences about treatment and comparing them to a statement of standard treatment not only insure an individualization of care, but may improve compliance. Additionally, the process clarifies issues about patient competency and documents the reasons for variation from standard medical practice.

At the institutional level, the use of standard assessments to establish the current status of the individual in each diagnosis and the other eight domains and standard categories (improve, maintain, decline) for predicted outcomes, allows data from multiple individual patients to be aggregated. Institutional standards for improving or maintaining nutritional status, patient mobility, and cognitive and emotional function may be set. Charts are flagged for review based on a negative differential between the predicted and actual outcomes.

For more complex patients or for patients known to be at high risk for a poor outcome (such as a prolonged length of stay; being placed in a nursing home for the first time or an unaccountable death), a team care and management system can be used. High risk patients are identified at admission, and receive functional assessments from their primary nurse and an interdisciplinary team conference which includes the physician and other traditionally utilized hospital staff, i.e., dietition, pharmacist, physical therapist, and social worker. More recently nontraditional staff from Risk Management and Utilization Review have been included, which allows early and complete integration of the clinical, functional, and financial elements of contemporary hospital care. The interdisciplinary team structure is optimal for providing the necessary subspecialty expertise, professional self-scrutiny, and emotional support for the difficult task of creating appropriate standards for care of those patients who are dying (29) or those for whom no direct knowledge of personal preference is available.

This process of setting and achieving individualized standards of care by evaluating the relationship between predicted and actual outcomes is derived from the theory underlying W. Edward Demming's and other's work on Japanese and American industry over the last 30 years (30). Identified recently in the *New England Journal of Medicine* as "The Theory of Continuous Improvement" (31), it focuses on a prospective and educational approach to quality rather than a retrospective and punitive one. Most importantly, by first addressing the uniqueness and need for personal preference in each older person with a serious illness and then involving the clinician in a self-evaluative approach to the highest quality of care, this process preserves the traditional structure of the patient-clinician relationship.

REFERENCES

1. Williams TF. The future of aging. John Stanley Soulter Lecture. *Arch Phys Med Rehabil* 1987;68:335–338.
2. Gilcrist BA, Rowe JW. The biology of aging. In: Rowe JW, Besdine RW, eds. *Health and disease in old age*, 1st ed. Boston: Little Brown, 1982;15–25.
3. Costa PT, McCrae RR. Concepts of functional or biological age: A critical review. In: Andres R. Bierman EL, Hazzard WR, eds. *Principles of geriatric medicine*. New York: McGraw-Hill, 1985;30–37.
4. Rowe JW, Kahn RI. Human aging: Usual and successful. *Science* (copywrite by AAAS), vol. 237, July 10, 1987;143–149.
5. Fried LP, Bush TL. Morbidity as a focus of preventive health care in the elderly. *Epidemiol Rev* 1988;10:48–64.
6. Judd HL. Prevention of osteoporosis. In: Solomon DH, moderator. New issues in geriatric care. *Ann Intern Med* 1988;108:718–732.
7. Andres R. Normal aging versus disease in the elderly. In: Andres R, Bierman EL, Hazzard WR, eds. *Principles in geriatric medicine*. McGraw-Hill, 1985;30–37.
8. Malenka DJ, Baron JA. Cholesterol and coronary heart disease: The importance of patient-specific attributable risk. *Arch Intern Med* 1988;148:2247–2252.
9. Murphy EA. Commentary: Public and private hypotheses. *J Clin Epidemiol* 1989;(42)1:79–84.
10. Hayakawa SH. Choosing the right word. New York: Perennial Library, Harper & Row, 1968;584.
11. Donabedian A. Evaluating the quality of medical care. *Milbank Q* 1966;44(3):166–203.

12. Knaus WA, Nash DB. Editorial: Predicting and evaluating patient outcomes. *Ann Intern Med* 1988;(109)7:521–522.
13. Dubois RW, Brook RH. Preventable deaths: Who, how often, and why? *Ann Intern Med* 1988;109:582–589.
14. Karnofsky DA, Burcheneal JH. The clinical evaluation of chemotherapeutic agents in cancer. In: Macleod CM, ed. *Evaluation of chemotherapeutic agents.* New York: Columbia University Press, 1949;191–208.
15. Katz S, Vignos PJ, Moskowitz RJ, Thompson HM, Suec KH. Comprehensive outpatient care in rheumatoid arthritis. *JAMA* 1968;206:1249–1254.
16. Lawton MP, Brody EM. Assessment of older people: Self-maintaining and instrumental activities of daily living. *Gerontologist.* 1969;9:179–186.
17. Katz S. Assessing self-maintenance activities of daily living, mobility and instrumental activities of daily living. *JAGS* 1983;37:721–727.
18. Mahoney FI, Barthel DW. Functional evaluation: The Barthel Index. *Maryland S Med J* 1965;14:61–65.
19. Fillenbaum GG. *Multidimensional functional assessment: The Oars Methodology,* 2nd ed. Durham, NC: Duke University, The Center for the Study of Aging and Human Development, 1978.
20. Spitzer WO, Dobson AH, Hall J, et al. Measuring quality of life in cancer patients: A concise QL-index for use by physicians. *J Chron Dis* 1981;34:585–597.
21. Fretwell MD, Raymond PM, McGarvey S, Owens N, Silliman RA, Mor V. The Senior Care Study: A controlled trial of a consultant/unit based geriatric assessment program in acute care. *JAGS (submitted).*
22. Lipowski ZJ. Delirium in the elderly patient. In: Desforges JF, ed. *Medical intelligence, current concepts: Geriatrics. N Engl J Med* 1989;320(9):578–581.
23. Feinstein AR, Josephy BR, Wells CK. Scientific and clinical problems in indexes of functional disability. *Ann Intern Med* 1986;105:413–420.
24. Fretwell MD. Comprehensive functional assessment. In: Hazzard WR, Anders R, Bierman EL, Blass JP, eds. *Principles of geriatric medicine and gerontology.* New York: McGraw-Hill, 1989.
25. Engel GL. The clinical application of the biopsychosocial model. *Am J Psych* 1980;137:535–544.
26. Rubenstein LZ, Josephson KR, Wieland GD, et al. Effectiveness of a geriatric evaluation unit. A randomized clinical trial. *N Engl J Med* 1984;311(26):1664–1670.
27. Epstein AM, Hall JA, Besdine R, et al. The emergence of geriatric assessment units. The "new technology of geriatrics." *Ann Intern Med* 1987;106(2):299–303.
28. Yesavage J, Brink T, Rose T, et al. Development and validation of a geriatric screening scale: A preliminary report. *J Psychiatr Res* 1983;1737–1749.
29. Carlson RW, Devich L, Frank RR. Development of a comprehensive supportive care team for the hopelessly ill on a university hospital medical service. *JAMA* 1988;259(3):378–383.
30. Deming WE. *Quality, productivity, and competitive position.* Cambridge, MA: Massachusetts Institute of Technology, Center for Advanced Engineering Study, 1982.
31. Berwick, DM. Continuous improvement as an ideal in health care. Sounding Board, *N Engl J Med* 1989;320(1):53–56.

Quality of Life Assessments in Clinical Trials, edited by B. Spilker. Raven Press, Ltd. New York © 1990.

20

Substance Abuse:

The Challenge of Assessment

David S. Metzger and Charles P. O'Brien

Center for Studies on Addiction, Department of Psychiatry, Philadelphia Veterans Administration Medical Center and University of Pennsylvania School of Medicine; Philadelphia, Pennsylvania 19104

QUALITY OF LIFE AND DRUG DEPENDENCE

Quality of life assessments attempt to measure the well-being of individuals. Although various definitions of quality of life can be found in the literature, each incorporates a similar set of domains differing primarily in their degree of specificity (1,2). These domains include economic and occupational issues, physical health and somatic concerns, psychological adjustment, familial functioning, and social integration. In many clinical settings these nonmedical, psychological, economic, and social aspects of patient functioning are foreign and are not considered to be an integral part of the disease process. However, in the diagnosis and treatment of individuals dependent on alcohol and other drugs, these quality of life problems define common areas of difficulty and are often central to the prognosis of treatment. Drug-dependent individuals are often first identified as a result of such problems.

Drug dependence is a complex disorder and quality of life assessments among drug dependent individuals present challenges which may not arise in the study of other patient populations. Patient heterogeneity, diagnostic insensitivity, etiological uncertainty, and chronicity are all characteristic of this disorder and each has an impact on the content and process of measurement. This chapter reviews these issues briefly, beginning with a description of the current diagnostic criteria for drug dependence and concluding with the presentation of a set of measures having proven utility in assessing this patient population.

DIAGNOSTIC CRITERIA FOR SUBSTANCE USE DISORDER

In order to gain an overview of the nature of drug dependence, its common symptoms, and its relationship to quality of life, it is appropriate to begin with a review of the criteria used to make a diagnosis of drug dependence. This review also provides a basis for examining the close relationship between drug dependence and functional difficulty in the areas commonly used to define quality of life. Nine criteria for dependence upon a psychoactive substance are presented in the third edition of the

Diagnostic and Statistical Manual of Mental Disorders (DSM-III-R) (3). A diagnosis of dependence is based on the presence of three or more of these criteria. Obviously individuals differ with regard to the severity of their dependence and this is reflected in the number of criteria which are met. In general, the nine symptoms can be seen as grouping into three common areas—loss of control over the timing and amount consumed, interference with the completion of occupational and social obligations, and the development of tolerance.

With regard to the criteria related to an individual's loss of control, a common characteristic of dependence is inability to be successful in attempting to regulate the use of the drug. Substances are consumed more frequently and in larger quantities than intended. A second control-related symptom is the inability to reduce or restrict the use of the drug. This is characterized by frequent attempts and failures to eliminate or reduce consumption. A third related symptom is the increasing amount of time devoted to the acquisition, preparation, administration, and recovery from the effects of the drug.

Dependence is also characterized by its interference with the completion of important obligations. This would include intoxication or withdrawal symptoms being present when important work, school, or family tasks need to be completed. Work might be missed or assignments neglected. The social interference caused by drug use may also appear as a withdrawal or reduction of involvements in important social, familial, or work activities due to the use of drugs or due to the withdrawal from their effects. Dependence is also characterized by the continued use of substances known to have caused or exacerbated chronic or recurrent social, psychological, or physical disorder. Thus, the drug-dependent individual will often present to the clinician with an extensive history of incidents in which drug use resulted in or contributed to social and occupational difficulty. Yet in spite of this history, the patient continues to use the substance. Dependent individuals often have an inability to recognize the extent to which their substance use has interfered with their functioning.

The development of tolerance is also an indicator of dependence. Tolerance is characterized by the need to use increased quantities of the substance in order to achieve intoxication or the desired effect. Withdrawal symptoms often appear when intake of the substance is stopped for several days. The intensity of these withdrawal symptoms varies a great deal among individuals and substances. It is important to note that although in some cases these symptoms can be severe and include delirium, severe depression, tachycardia, nausea, fatigue, and insomnia, for many individuals withdrawal symptoms can be managed safely and effectively on an outpatient basis (4). A final criteria of dependence is the use of the substance in order to ward off the unpleasant feelings of withdrawal. As the physical symptoms of withdrawal appear, the dependent individual becomes increasingly uncomfortable. The uncomfortable feelings of withdrawal serve as cues for the initiation of further drug seeking, thus maintaining the dependence.

These nine symptoms represent the behavioral characteristics that form the basis of a diagnosis of dependence. They are presented here to provide a definitional foundation for understanding drug dependence and its intimate relationship to quality of life concerns. Together the criteria reflect the extent to which drug dependence interacts with the social, psychological, and physical functioning of an individual. Each is linked either directly, as in the case of occupational interference, or indirectly, as with control issues, to the individual's quality of life. In fact, these quality of life problems are so often associated with dependence that they have frequently been viewed as being caused solely by the dependence (5). This widely held belief has resulted in a somewhat narrow interpretation of drug dependence and its treatment.

THE RELATIONSHIP BETWEEN QUALITY OF LIFE AND DEPENDENCE

It is commonly conceived that drug dependence develops in an incremental and progressive manner. As an individual's use of drugs increases, his or her social and productive involvements become less stable and at greater risk of disruption and dissolution. Under this progressive paradigm, the cause of an individual's problems is seen as the direct result of the increasing drug use. Greater amounts of time are devoted to thoughts of the drug, its procurement, and its use. As a consequence of this increased drug use and related behavior, the attention devoted to family and personal relationships, work, and health diminishes, leading to profound problems in an individual's life and the lives of their family and friends.

Given this progressive disease model of dependence and the problems associated with increased use, treatment and measurements have frequently been centered around the quantity and frequency of continued drug use. Specifically, treatment has been focused on abstinence and measurement has focused on quantity and frequency of use. It is reasoned that since the problems of a drug-dependent individual are the result of drug use, these problems will dissipate as the use of the substance diminishes. It is therefore reasonable to expect that improvements in these "collateral" areas of functioning will be observed when the abuse is brought under control. However, several reports (6,7) have provided evidence which calls into question the validity of this model of dependence which causally links a dependent individual's occupational, psychological, and social problems to their drug use. These investigations have found that improvements in these related problem areas do not always occur when drug use ceases. Many patients who stop using drugs continue to experience problems in other areas of functioning. These findings would suggest that an individual may not experience far-reaching changes in their quality of life as a result of the elimination of their drug use.

This issue has important implications in the design of clinical interventions and the measurement of their success. In light of the independence of these problem areas, it is important that the criteria selected for use in clinical trials be tied to the dependence-related problems of the individual. For example, it is appropriate that employment is a goal of treatment and criteria for success for a patient who lost a job due to drug use. However, for an individual who entered treatment with a history of chronic unemployment, the application of employment as a goal of treatment is less valid. Interventions should be directed at the full range of problems experienced by the patient and not merely focused on their substance use. Drug dependence cannot be diagnosed and treated only on the basis of the quantity and frequency of use. This is not meant to minimize the importance of treating and monitoring patients' continued drug use. The elimination of continued drug use may be necessary to produce improvements in a patient's quality of life, but it is not always sufficient.

MEASUREMENT ISSUES IN DRUG ABUSE

In spite of the known relationship between drug dependence and a broad range of functional difficulties, the quality of life of substance abusers has rarely been measured as a distinct construct. This is particularly true of methods which have asked patients to report their perceived quality of life in its various component parts. In fact, the literature contains only one report utilizing subjective assessments of drug-dependent patients' quality of life (8). Not surprisingly, this study found that patients entering treatment reported extremely low ratings of their health, work, housing, and social relationships. Only slight and nonsignificant gains during the 3 and 6 month follow-up periods were observed. Subjective assessments of well-being may be of limited value in isolation of more objective indicators.

As stated earlier, diagnostic and evaluative criteria have typically been centered around assessing quantity and frequency of drug use. Less intensive effort has been focused on the assessment of health and psychological, employment, family, and legal problems. These are the common problem areas of drug-dependent individuals and improvements in these areas of functioning are often expectations of treatment. The measurement of these variables among drug-dependent patients presents some challenges which should be considered in the design of clinical investigations. These include the problems of available data sources, delayed diagnosis, and the timing of assessments.

There is no litmus test for drug dependence. Unlike many other conditions, we have no laboratory tests available which alone can confirm the diagnosis of drug abuse or dependence. Although there are specific diagnostic criteria, much of the information on which these criteria rely is only available from the reports of patients, their families, or others closely involved with the individual. By the time the patient reaches treatment, these individuals may be unavailable or unwilling to provide information. Consequently, patient self-report is the primary and often the only source of information available to make a diagnosis and set treatment goals. Self reports of drug-dependent patients have been shown to be valid and reliable (9,10,11), but investigations must be designed and conducted with an awareness of the limited data sources and a sensitivity to the issues involved in conducting clinical interviews with patients and their family members.

As alluded to earlier, the substance abusing patient is often first identified to the clinician as a result of disruptions or deteriorations in his or her quality of life. Frequently, individuals are identified as drug dependent as a result of incidents which take place on their job or in the community. Patients are sometimes identifed due to accidents, injuries, or illnesses caused by their abuse. Police contact such as an arrest for driving under the influence has become a common first public indicator of abuse. The loss of income or depleted savings is also common among drug-dependent individuals. These are all examples of the types of incidents which motivate individuals to seek treatment after what are often long histories of use. Rarely do patients present themselves to the clinician with a concern that they may be developing symptoms of dependence. As a consequence of this delay in making a diagnosis, serious occupational, social, and physical problems typically predate the diagnosis of substance abuse or dependence. This may be one of the most important features of drug dependence distinguishing it from many other medical conditions— the patient's quality of life is most at risk prior to diagnosis and treatment involvement. This has implications for the measurement process. Any assessment at the point of entry into a treatment episode is likely to define the nadir of a cycle and caution must be used in interpreting such measures as a baseline of pretreatment functioning. Assessments with drug abusers will therefore differ from other patient groups who are struggling to maintain their pretreatment quality of life which is often at greatest risk following diagnosis.

Drug dependence is accurately viewed as a chronic disorder, characterized by periods of abstinence followed by relapse to drug use. This must also be considered in the timing and the frequency of assessments. Patients often respond quickly to interventions, showing rapid improvement over their pretreatment patterns of use. Patients begin to feel better and are more able to control their use. This success often proves to be short lived once the patient is exposed to the environmental and emotional cues that have been intimately linked to their dependence. Frequently, the stress produced by unemployment or family problems is cited as a factor in the return to drug use. The chronic nature of dependence requires that regular follow-up assessments be incorporated into the design of investigations.

QUALITY OF LIFE INSTRUMENTS

Considering the preceding discussion, it should be expected that drug abusing populations will demonstrate difficulties in diverse functional areas and this may be the most important consideration in selecting quality of life instruments. Clinical investigators must be prepared to screen for the presence of these problems, assess their severity, and monitor their status over time. The necessity for such a broad-based approach to assessment limits the range of available instruments. The instruments which will be suggested here are those which have been demonstrated to be useful in measuring quality of life domains and each relies upon self report. The recommended instruments are also able to be administered at follow-up assessment points. Each of these instruments has also been used extensively with drug-dependent patients. Four instruments are presented here: the Addiction Severity Index, the Social Adjustment Scale, the Beck Depression Inventory, and the Symptom Checklist-90. Two of the instruments, the Addiction Severity Index and the Social Adjustment Scale, provide the researcher with coverage on a range of quality of life issues. Given the concordance between the two, both scales need not be used together. The two additional scales, the Beck Depression Inventory and the Symptom Checklist-90, are suggested as instruments able to tap the psychological dimensions of well-being in a direct and valid manner. When used with either the Addiction Severity Index or the Social Adjustment Scale, the investigator is provided with a well-rounded assessment package incorporating subjective and objective indicators of well-being in a complete range of functional areas.

THE ADDICTION SEVERITY INDEX

The Addiction Severity Index is perhaps the most widely used assessment tool in the field of drug abuse treatment and research. The Addiction Severity Index is a structured clinical interview that combines objective and subjective data to produce ratings of problem severity in seven functional areas: medical, employment and support, drug use, alcohol use, legal status, family/social relations, and psychological status. The index was developed to assess "the multiple problems seen in alcohol and drug dependent persons" (12). Its comprehensive coverage of relevant areas of functioning, its incorporation of both objective and subjective information, its widespread use and citation in the published literature and its performance characteristics with regard to validity and reliability make it the most appropriate tool available for quality of life assessments among this patient population.

The Addiction Severity Index is designed to be administered in a personal interview which takes approximately 45 minutes to complete. The administration time will vary somewhat depending on the capacity of the patient to respond clearly and concisely to each item. The interview format alleviates problems caused by poor reading levels of some patients and allows the opportunity to probe responses for clarification and confirmation that the respondent adequately understands the question being asked.

Completion time will also depend on the interviewer's familiarity with the structure and content of the Addiction Severity Index. In this regard it is important that the index be administered by an individual who has an adequate knowledge of the instrument and some practice in its administration. There are a number of items which require awareness of methods and interpretations not clearly obvious from the form itself. A unique strength of the Addiction Severity Index is the training materials available. These include a set of instructional videotapes, a detailed manual, and a scoring guide. The videotapes provide an orientation to the instrument and a sample interview. It is not appropriate to use the index without reviewing these materials.

Two types of quantitative scores are produced by the Addiction Severity Index in each of the seven problem areas: severity ratings and composite scores. Severity ratings are subjective assessments made by the interviewer describing the degree to which the patient is currently experiencing difficulty and consequently their need for additional treatment. Severity scores range from 0, meaning no real problem/additional treatment not necessary, to 9, meaning a life-threatening problem/additional treatment essential. The severity ratings are based on the responses to questions in each particular area and are meant to reflect the amount, duration, and intensity of the symptoms. Specific guidelines are provided to the interviewer to help him or her arrive at a valid and reliable score.

Composite scores are computed from the responses to specific items contained in the Addiction Severity Index. As with severity ratings, the composite scores are produced for each of the seven problem areas. They were developed primarily to provide a numerical basis for determining change and treatment outcome and as such are more appropriate for statistical analyses. The composite scores and severity ratings have been assessed with regard to their validity and reliabilty (12–14). Severity ratings and composite scores have demonstrated high levels of interrater, test re-test, and concurrent reliability.

Aside from the severity ratings and composite scores produced by the Addiction Severity Index, the completion of an interview provides a rich clinical picture of the patient and a sound basis for treatment planning. The questions provide an opportunity to probe and elicit clinically relevant information from the patient. It is this dual clinic/research function which has made the Addiction Severity Index a valuable tool in the field of drug abuse treatment and research.

The Addiction Severity Index has limitations. It has been used most widely with individuals entering substance abuse treatment. There are little performance data available for the index when it is used with non-substance abuse treatment populations. It is difficult to predict the costs to validity and reliability of the instrument when used with other patient populations. Although not necessarily a limitation, the fact that the Addiction Severity Index is administered in a 45-minute personal interview conducted by a trained technician may restrict its application.

THE SOCIAL ADJUSTMENT SCALE

The Social Adjustment Scale is a 42-item assessment which has both an interview (15) and a self-report form (16). The scale measures an individual's performance in six functional areas: (a) work as a worker, housewife, or student; (b) social and leisure activities; (c) relationship with extended family; (d) marital role as a spouse; (e) role as a parent; and (f) member of a family unit. The questions which are asked in each of these areas are directed at determining the subject's success in the performance of the expected tasks, the interpersonal behaviors and conflicts associated with the task, and the feeling and satisfactions associated with the task. The personal interview version of the Social Adjustment Scale takes approximately 45 minutes to complete, and 15 to 20 minutes are required for the self-report form. The two versions have been tested for their agreement with each other and significant correlations were found.

Although the areas of functioning measured by the Social Adjustment Scale overlap with the employment and the family/social functioning scales of the Addiction Severity Index, it is suggested here due to its more restricted focus which is at times advantageous, and because it offers the possibility of using a self-report methodology which might expand its application to projects unable to provide in-depth personal interviews. Concurrent validity was examined in two studies (13,14) which correlated the relevant scores of the Addiction Severity Index with the Social Adjustment Scale, and both found significant levels of agreement.

THE BECK DEPRESSION INVENTORY

Depression is an important construct in the comprehensive assessment of drug abuse and may be considered a good global indicator of perceived quality of life. The Beck Depression Inventory is a 21-item questionnaire that is most frequently self-administered, but can also be completed as part of a clinical interview. If self-administered, a sixth grade reading level is suggested. It is widely used and often cited in the professional literature, and has been shown to validly and reliably assess depression in many patient groups, including drug abusers (17). The form is designed to be self-administered and can be completed by most individuals in 5 to 10 minutes. Individuals are presented with 21 sets of statements about their behaviors and cognitions. Each set contains four statements from which the respondent must choose one that best describes themselves. Each statement within a set is numbered from 0 to 3 indicating increasing severity. The sum of the values of the selected statements forms the individual's depression score. The range of the score is therefore 0 to 63. Since its development (18), the Beck Depression Inventory has appeared in several different versions. A shorter 13-item form is available but is not recommended here due to the possibility that the shorter form may assess only one cognitive dimension of depression (17).

The items included in the scale were selected based on the systematic consolidation of symptoms of depression identified through clinical observation. These items include mood, pessimism, sense of failure, lack of satisfaction, guilt feelings, sense of being punished, self-dislike, self-accusation, suicidal wishes, crying, irritability, social withdrawal, indecisiveness, distortion of body image, work inhibition, sleep disturbance, fatigue, loss of appetite, weight loss, somatic preoccupation, and loss of libido.

THE SYMPTOM CHECKLIST-90-R

The Symptom Checklist-90-R is a self-administered questionnaire that asks patients to rate the degree to which they have been troubled over the preceding week by common symptoms of psychological distress. It is suggested as a useful tool in quality of life studies because of the importance of this symptom domain in understanding the drug abusers' response to treatment. Psychiatric severity has been shown to be the best predictor of response to treatment and the Symptom Checklist-90-R provides a more fine-grained assessment of this symptom dimension than is available using the Addiction Severity Index alone. The scale has been widely used since its introduction and has demonstrated its utility in clinical investigations, its coverage of the content area, and its acceptability to substance abusing populations.

In addition to an overall general symptom score, the 90 items form subscales which yield scores on nine symptom constructs. These constructs include somatization, obsessive-compulsive disorder, interpersonal sensitivity, psychoticism, anxiety, depression, hostility, phobic anxiety, and paranoid ideation.

The Symptom Checklist-90-R has its origins in the 77-item Hopkins Symptom Checklist (19,20) which was developed as an outcome measure for use in psychotherapy research. This early version of the scale formed the basis of the Symptom Checklist-90, which underwent revision to become the Symptom Checklist-90-R. The psychometric properties of the scale have been examined and both internal consistency and test re-test reliability coefficients were quite good for each of the subscales, averaging about .85 (21). The Symptom Checklist-90 has also been shown to correlate highly with the Minnesota Multiphasic Personality Inventory (22), the Hamilton Depression Rating Scale, and the Social Adjustment Scale (23,24).

As stated, the scale is self-administered and takes approximately 15 minutes to complete. The items can be read to individuals who have difficulty reading. The manual states that the scale can be used with individuals as young as 13 with the assistance of a technician. The Symptom Checklist-90-R is appropriate for use with psychiatric and medical patients (with the obvious exception of individuals who are acutely psychotic). It has been widely used with alcoholic and drug abusing populations and is sensitive to the changes produced by psychoactive substances. The scale does not appear to be sensitive to practice effects resulting from repeated administrations and can be used in studies requiring follow-up assessments.

CONCLUSIONS

These four scales provide the clinical researcher with a set of tools having proven utility in the comprehensive assessment of quality of life difficulties among drug-dependent individuals. There is clearly a need for ongoing research and development with regard to both instrumentation and methodologies. Of particular importance is the development of new instruments or the revision of existing tools to be responsive to the changing drugs of abuse and issues associated with their use. For example, all of the scales presented here were developed prior to the widespread use of cocaine and its more virulent form, crack. It is likely that dependent patterns of use develop more rapidly among cocaine users. The measurement implications of these issues have yet to be empirically examined. Similarly, the increasing importance of the role of drug use in the transmission of the HIV virus is not adequately addressed by current instrumentation. The risk of HIV infection is likely to impact not only drug preference, but the method of use and social integration of drug users as well. Continued research is also warranted in the development of valid and reliable scales which can be used in the assessment of adolescents. None of the instruments presented here have been validated with this growing patient poplation. Another important area in need of investigation is the impact on data quality of the method of questioning drug-dependent individuals. There have been no recent assessments of the validity of data collected via personal interview as compared to similar information collected through self-administered questionnaires. Patients may be more accurate in their reports of sensitive information when questioned using the more impersonal questionnaire approach. The degree of disclosure via differing methods may also be a function of demographic and cultural variables. Given the substantial efficiency achieved through the use of this method, it is important that its validity be assessed.

In conclusion, the important role of quality of life issues in the identification and treatment of substance abuse demands that ongoing effort be devoted to the refinement and development of measurement tools and methods. In learning more about the relationship between quality of life problems and substance use, we will expand our understanding of dependence, its causal mechanisms, and its effective treatment.

REFERENCES

1. Flanagan JC. Measurement of quality of life: Current state of the art. *Arch Phys Med Rehabil* 1982;63:56–59.
2. Andrews FM, Withey SB. *Social indicators of well-being: Americans' perceptions of life quality.* New York, London: Plenum Press, 1976.
3. American Psychiatric Association. *Diagnostic and Statistical Manual of Mental Disorders, Third Edition, Revised.* Washington, D.C.: American Psychiatric Association, 1987.
4. Hayashida MD, Alterman AI, McLellan AT, et al. Comparative effectiveness and costs of inpatient and outpatient detoxification of patients with mild to moderate alcohol withdrawal syndrome. *N Engl J Med* 1989;320:358–365.
5. Levine HG. The discovery of addiction. *J Stud Alcohol* 1978;39:41–53.
6. Rounsaville BJ, Kosten TR, Kleber HD. The antecedents and benefits of achieving abstinence in opioid addicts: A 2.5-year follow-up study. *Am J Drug Alcohol Abuse* 1987;13:213–229.
7. McLellan AT, Luborsky L, Woody GE, O'Brien CP, Kron R. Are the "addiction-related" problems of substance abusers really related? *J Nerv Ment Dis* 1981;169:232–239.
8. Irwin PH. Quality of life assessment and drug abuse treatment program evaluation. *Eval Prog Plan* 1981;4:123–130.
9. Amsel Z, Mandell W, Matthais L, et al. Reliability and validity of self-reported illegal activities and drug use collected from narcotic addicts. *Int J Addict* 1976;11:325–336.
10. Bale RN. The validity and reliability of self report data from heroin addicts: Mailed questionnaires compared to face to face interviews. *Int J Addict* 1979;14:993–1000.
11. Pompi KF. The reliability of biographical information obtained from court stipulated clients newly admitted to treatment. *Am J Drug Alcohol Abuse* 1979;6:79–95.
12. McLellan AT, Luborsky L, Woody GE, O'Brien CP. An improved diagnostic evaluation instrument for substance abuse patients: The addiction severity index. *J Nerv Ment Dis* 1980;168:26–33.
13. Kosten TR, Rounsaville BJ, Kleber HD. Concurrent validity of the addiction severity index. *J Nerv Ment Dis* 1983;171:606–610.
14. McLellan AT, Luborsky L, Cacciola J, et al. New data from the addiction severity index: Reliability and validity in three centers. *J Nerv Ment Dis* 1985;173:412–423.
15. Weissman MM, Paykel ES. *The depressed woman: A study of social relationships.* Chicago: University of Chicago Press, 1974.

16. Weissman MM, Bothwell S. Assessment of social adjustment by patient self-report. *Arch Gen Psychiatry* 1976;33:1111–1115.
17. Beck AT, Steer RA, Garbin MG. Psychometric properties of the Beck Depression Inventory: Twenty-five years of evaluation. *Clin Psychology Rev* 1988;8:77–100.
18. Beck AT, Ward CH, Mendelson M, et al. An inventory for measuring depression. *Arch Gen Psychiatry* 1961;4:561–571.
19. Derogatis LR, Lipman RS, Covi L, Rickels K. Factorial invariance of symptom dimensions in anxious and depressed neuroses. *Arch Gen Psychiatry* 1972;27:659–665.
20. Derogatis LR, Lipman RS, Rickels K, Uhlenhuth EH, Covi L. The Hopkins Symptom Checklist (HSCL): A self report symptom inventory. *Behav Sci* 1974;19:1–15.
21. Derogatis LR. *SCL-90 Revised Version Manual-1.* Clinical Psychometrics Research Unit, Johns Hopkins University School of Medicine, Baltimore, 1983.
22. Derogatis LR, Rickels K, Rock AF. The SCL-90 and the MMPI: A step in the validation of a new self report scale. *Br J Psychiatry* 1976;128:280–289.
23. Weissman MM, Sholomskas D, Pottenger M, et al. Assessing depressive symptoms in five psychiatric populations: A validation study. *Am J Epidemiology* 1977;106:203–214.
24. Weissman MM, Pursoff BA, Thompson WD, et al. Social adjustment by self report in a community sample and in psychiatric outpatients. *J Nerv Ment Dis* 1978;166:317–326.

Quality of Life Assessments in Clinical Trials, edited by B. Spilker. Raven Press, Ltd. New York © 1990.

21

Rehabilitation

Ralph R. Turner

Pfizer Central Research, Groton, Connecticut 06340

As rehabilitation has evolved from a narrowly focused compensatory program during the first half of the twentieth century into a broader-based process of reintegrating persons with disabilities into community life, the need for effective assessment methods has been brought into sharp focus (1). Perhaps more than any other health care field, assessment strategies in rehabilitation are influenced by, and reflect fundamental changes in, the models which underlie the conceptual basis for the rehabilitation process. As rehabilitation moves away from acute care toward chronic long-term care, the traditional focus on observable physical pathology and dysfunction and subjective symptoms has proved to be too limiting (2).

Rather, as the goals of rehabilitation have broadened beyond restoration of physical function, the assessment needs have widened to capture the impact of disability across several functional domains and to measure the outcomes of rehabilitation intervention. As Jette points out (3), measures of performance or functional status as health status indicators reflect a psychosocial rather than medically based health concept. The individual rather than the organ becomes the unit of analysis and active pathology is evaluated indirectly through its effect on functioning of the individual. This movement away from the traditional medical model in rehabilitation has accelerated the need for clearer organizational concepts and more effective assessment methods that can be linked to rehabilitation outcomes.

Organizing Concepts and Key Terms

This shift in emphasis has not been smooth and is certainly not complete. However, as chronic conditions—in disease and in the elderly as well as in rehabilitation— overcome acute conditions as the predominant focus in health care, the need for more effective models, concepts, and health assessment tools will continue to strengthen.

The call for better organizing structures has been comprehensively answered by both Nagi (4,5) and Wood (6). Their models, although applying somewhat different emphases, provide a framework for the key rehabilitation concepts: impairment, disability, handicaps, and functional limitations. Recently, Granger (2) presented a synthesis and expansion of the Nagi and Wood schemes which is shown in Fig. 1.

Concepts are organized across three levels: organ, person, and society. Within each, the prevailing condition results, directly or indirectly, in either impairment, disability, or handicap. Anatomical, physiological, or psychological defects deter-

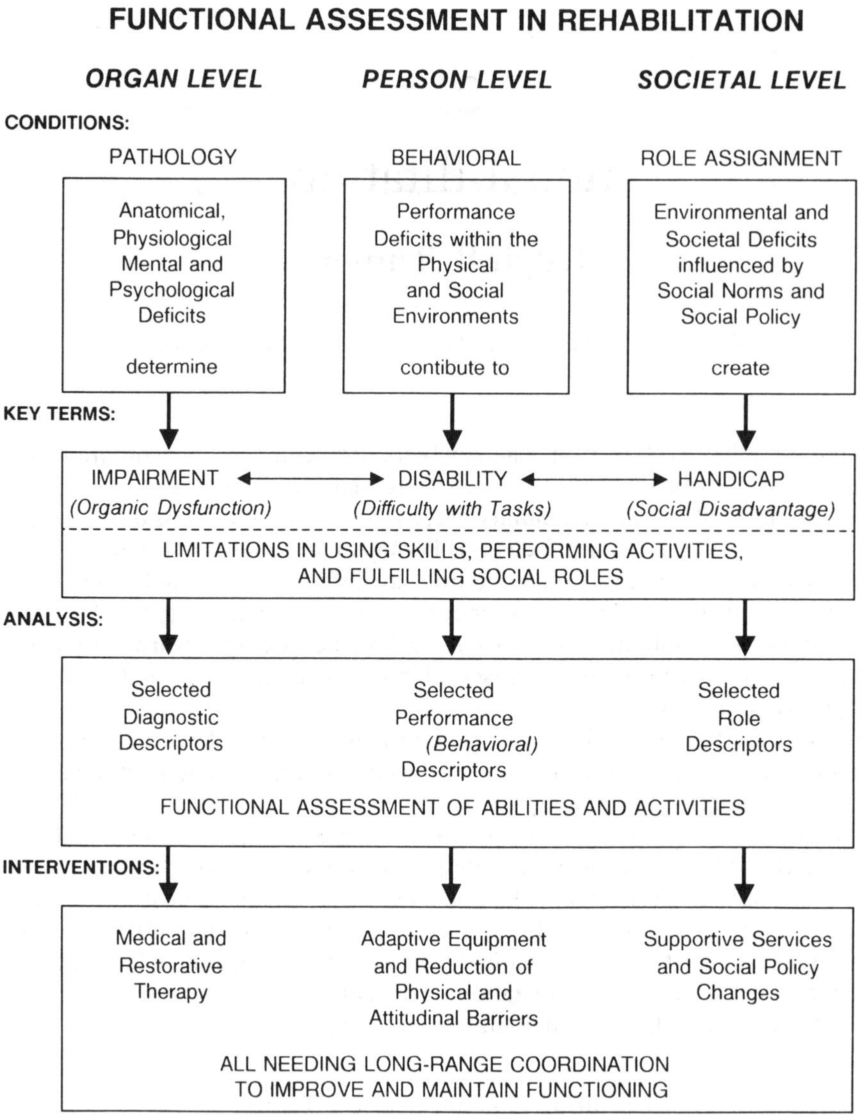

FUNCTIONAL ASSESSMENT IN REHABILITATION

ORGAN LEVEL	PERSON LEVEL	SOCIETAL LEVEL

CONDITIONS:

PATHOLOGY	BEHAVIORAL	ROLE ASSIGNMENT
Anatomical, Physiological Mental and Psychological Deficits	Performance Deficits within the Physical and Social Environments	Environmental and Societal Deficits influenced by Social Norms and Social Policy
determine	contibute to	create

KEY TERMS:

IMPAIRMENT ◄───►	DISABILITY ◄───►	HANDICAP
(Organic Dysfunction)	*(Difficulty with Tasks)*	*(Social Disadvantage)*

LIMITATIONS IN USING SKILLS, PERFORMING ACTIVITIES, AND FULFILLING SOCIAL ROLES

ANALYSIS:

Selected Diagnostic Descriptors	Selected Performance *(Behavioral)* Descriptors	Selected Role Descriptors

FUNCTIONAL ASSESSMENT OF ABILITIES AND ACTIVITIES

INTERVENTIONS:

Medical and Restorative Therapy	Adaptive Equipment and Reduction of Physical and Attitudinal Barriers	Supportive Services and Social Policy Changes

ALL NEEDING LONG-RANGE COORDINATION TO IMPROVE AND MAINTAIN FUNCTIONING

FIG. 1. Integrative model for rehabilitation concepts. In the upper portion, the concepts of impairment, disability, and handicap are related across organ, person, and societal levels. In the lower portion, the role of functional assessment in producing three classes of data are presented leading to rehabilitation intervention. From Granger, ref. 30, with permission.

mine impairment or organic dysfunction. Performance defects within the physical and social environment contribute to disability or difficulty with tasks. And environmental or societal defects influenced by social norms and policy create handicaps or social disadvantage. The unifying concept here is that each of these represents limitations in function, whether in using skills, performing activities, or fulfilling social roles. Although analysis of these functional limitations has a different focus, depending on the level of interest, at the core is the need for outcomes to be conceptualized and defined in measurable terms.

Conceptual Framework for Functional Assessment

As with impairment, disability, and handicap, so too have the terms "functional status," "functional limitations," and "functional assessment" created confusion and confounded attempts to develop and implement effective measures. Early usage of functional limitation stemmed from a predominantly medical focus on impairment which is by itself inadequate to meet rehabilitation's emerging broader goals (1). Jette suggested that functional assessment needs to operate from the perspective of the individual as the unit of analysis and "pathology, as represented by various physical manifestations or symptoms, is evaluated through its effect on functioning of the individual" (3). Jette's subdivision of functioning within rehabilitation includes physical performance, mental performance, emotional performance, and social performance. Brown et al. (7) described an integrated model of functional assessment and rehabilitation outcomes which included as individual level variables demographic, structural, and basic functioning; cognitive and psychological functioning; knowledge; and applied functioning.

These broader views of rehabilitation fit closely with quality of life assessment in the clinical context. Schipper and Levitt (8) has defined quality of life as a pattern of function, measured over time, that incorporates physical ability, psychological well-being, and social interactions. This conceptual framework is consistent with those prepared by Wenger et al. (9) and Patrick and Erickson (10), which incorporate similar domains. In all of these, there is common agreement that measuring performance within these domains through functional assessment provides a comprehensive picture of the interaction between the individual and the environment at the disability and handicap levels. When viewed as an extension of earlier work that focused primarily on physical limitations at the impairment level, a matrix emerges which organizes levels of limitation (i.e., impairment, disability, and handicap) and content domains that can be used to clarify assessment goals.

Functional Assessment Measurement in Rehabilitation

Attempts to apply functional assessment methodology to the rehabilitation setting have been problematic for two reasons. First, the changes in rehabilitation's conceptual models have resulted in changing assessment needs. And second, the quality of measurement technology, especially in early scale development, has been generally weak. As much as two decades ago, the inadequacies of functional assessment in rehabilitation caused concern. Kelman and Willner (11) cited problems in outcome definition, standardization of methods, and technical quality of the measures. Keith (12) and Frey (1), in recent reviews, found that little had changed in the ensuing period.

There are several encouraging trends, however. Genuine progress has been made in addressing the critical issues of conceptual models, terminology, and standardization. As trends in health care measurement arising from chronic disease management, elderly long-term care, and rehabilitation begin to converge, new and different resources are being brought to bear. Measurement is moving from situation and institution-specific scale development to broader-based, coordinated, interdisciplinary work. This cross-fertilization of effort led to a recent call by Ellwood for the development of a national "outcome management" information system with quality of life assessment at its core (13). As well-developed psychometric standards are applied to the selection and development of functional assessment measures within the framework of clearly specified objectives and definitions, the quality of the assessment information will improve, feeding back into the system to further refine the concepts and objectives. This approach, called for by Brown et al. (7) in Bassett (14) and Backer (15), will permit real progress to be made in functional assessment and in rehabilitation.

Users who need effective assessment strategies now, however, do not have the luxury of waiting as the field matures. What they need is a set of practical guidelines to assist in the selection of functional assessment measures that meet their needs. The purpose of this chapter is to provide an introduction to those guidelines, to indicate sources where more comprehensive assistance can be found, and to present a sampling of functional assessment instruments that reflect a proposed conceptual framework for rehabilitation.

CRITERIA FOR FUNCTIONAL ASSESSMENT

The changing nature of rehabilitation models coupled with a problematic assessment history that is rapidly evolving into a conceptually and technically sophisticated future leave the potential user faced with making assessment decisions under difficult circumstances. It is an encouraging sign that the problem has been recognized and sound theoretical and practical advice and guidance have been offered. Especially important contributions have been made by McDowell and Newell (16), and Feinstein (17). Earlier, Brown et al. (7) presented an integrative model that linked functional assessment and outcome measurement. In each of these practical guides there are a series of criteria that serve as tools to be used to select an assessment approach. The approach presented here differs in degree and emphasis rather than in fundamental concepts. All of these recent guides have a great deal in common and the reader is encouraged to pursue them as a means of expanding the scope of this chapter.

Clarification of Purpose

The first step in selecting a functional assessment scale is to ask, "What is the question?" Although seemingly obvious and intuitive, this basic process of identifying and clarifying the measurement objectives is often either inadequately addressed or, more seriously, overlooked altogether. Yet the admittedly difficult process of clarifying, in measurable terms, what the intended outcomes are is often enlightening and greatly facilitates the assessment process.

Matching the user's intentions, once they have been clearly stated, with those of the scale developer is an essential second step. The criteria used in the scale development process may differ substantially from the user's purpose. Scales with evidence that supports one purpose may not serve well when applied to a different task.

Kirshner and Guyatt (18) present a useful taxonomy that classifies assessment scales into discriminative, predictive, and evaluative categories. Each type of scale addresses substantially different objectives. Discriminative scales are designed to separate patients (or clients or subjects) into discrete classes that can be defined according to specifiable diagnostic criteria. Predictive scales serve a similar role. However, here patients are classified into groups against a known criterion, or "gold standard." Evaluative scales differ markedly from the other two since they are intended to reflect clinically important change when it occurs. Each type of scale has a useful role to play in rehabilitation but mismatching the types may result in incorrect assessment information. All too often discriminative scales are used to assess change in function following rehabilitation intervention. Although change may have occurred, the scale may be insensitive to it, resulting in incorrect conclusions.

The criteria for developing each type of scale differ at nearly every step in the test development process. Figure 2 from Kirshner and Guyatt summarizes these differences. Although much of the functional assessment scale development literature does not yet reflect this level of technical sophistication (12), the user should become familiar with the underlying assumptions. Key questions such as, "Do I want to group patients according to their current functional ability?" or "Do I want to classify clients according to prognosis for successful vocational placement?" or "Am I interested in determining how much functional change occurs as a result of my rehabilitation treatment program?" all reflect this basic distinction, help clarify objectives, and set a much clearer course for instrument selection. This distinction in type of measurement adds a third dimension to the conceptual framework which now permits functional assessment to be incorporated into a measurement model that synthesizes the clarification needed in the basic terminology, the domains of interest necessary for a comprehensive assessment of functions and quality of life, and the purposes for which the scale was developed.

A three-dimensional model is presented in Fig. 3 that is based, in part, on the assessment proposal by Frey (1). Along one axis are the areas of assessment—impairment, disability, and handicap. Much of the early functional assessment work focused on the impairment level, but it is now clear that changing models have expanded the scope to disability, with preliminary attention being paid to the handicap level. Along the second axis are the domains of assessment that are generally accepted as relevant for rehabilitation outcomes as well as more broadly based health assessment theories. Along the third axis are the types of measurement classified by Kirshner and Guyatt.

This model can be used to guide the questions the user needs to ask at the onset of the assessment task: What is the appropriate unit of analysis? How many, and which content domains are relevant? What is my assessment goal? Answers to these questions should help identify a preliminary set of instruments which can then be examined more closely for evidence of psychometric quality and practical utility.

Psychometric Properties

Once the central question and purpose are clarified, the user's task is to balance psychometric quality with practical considerations. Both issues have been discussed in recent health assessment and functional assessment publications. Excellent summaries of this theoretical basis for measurement are provided by McDowell and Newell (16) and Feinstein (17), with more technical discussions found in Nunnally (19), Thorndike (20), and Torgerson (21). What follows here is an overview of the key issues and suggested guidelines.

MAJOR ISSUES IN SCALE DEVELOPMENT

	DISCRIMINATIVE CRITERIA	PREDICTIVE CRITERIA	EVALUATIVE CRITERIA
ITEM SELECTION:	– Tap important components of the domain – Universal applicability to respondents – Stability over time	– Statistical association with criterion measure	– Tap areas related to change in health status – Responsiveness to clinically significant change
ITEM SCALING:	– Short response sets which facilitate uniform interpretation	– Response sets which maximize correlations with the criterion measure	– Response sets with sufficient gradations to register change
ITEM REDUCTION:	– Internal scaling or consistency – Comprehensiveness and reduction of random error vs. respondent burden	– Power to predict vs. respondent burden	– Responsiveness vs. respondent burden
RELIABILITY:	– Large and stable intersubject variation: correlation between replicate measures	– Stable inter and intrasubject variation: chance corrected agreement between replicate measures	– Stable intrasubject variation insignificant variation between replicate measures
VALIDITY:	– Cross-sectional construct validity: relationship between index and external measures at a single point in time	– Criterion validity: agreement with criterion measure	– Longitudinal construct validity: relationship between changes in index and external measures over time
RESPONSIVENESS:	– Not relevant	– Not relevant	– Power of the test to detect a clinically important difference

FIG. 2. Summary of issues in functional assessment measurement. From Kirshner and Guyatt, ref. 18, with permission.

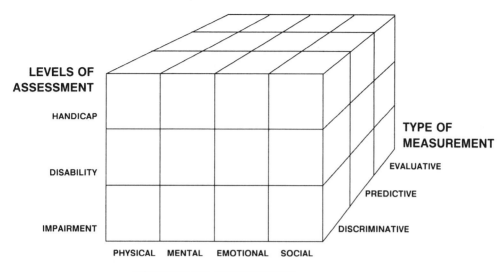

LEVELS OF ASSESSMENT

HANDICAP

DISABILITY

IMPAIRMENT

TYPE OF MEASUREMENT

EVALUATIVE

PREDICTIVE

DISCRIMINATIVE

PHYSICAL   MENTAL   EMOTIONAL   SOCIAL

DOMAINS OF ASSESSMENT

FIG. 3. A three-dimensional model for functional assessment.

Reliability

All measurement involves some degree of error. Although such error cannot be eliminated, the degree to which it is minimized reflects the extent to which the score can be considered stable and reproducible (19). Ware (22) suggested standard where reliability coefficients above 0.90 are required for making comparisons between individuals whereas between-group comparisons require coefficients in the 0.50 to 0.70 range.

Three types of reliability are typically employed in functional assessment scale development, depending on the type and purpose of the measure. Test re-test reliability refers to the stability of a score derived from serial administration of a measure by the same rater. Timing is one of the key factors to consider when judging the evidence for this type of reliability. Enough time has to elapse to minimize the effects of memory, yet too much time may allow the phenomenon under study to change significantly. Professional judgment and experience are required to determine whether the reliability assessment design is adequate. For example, the effects of arthritis fluctuate, creating difficulty for the assessment of reliability, whereas aspects of spinal cord injury are remarkably stable (3).

A second factor is related to the type of scale that is developed. Kirshner and Guyatt (18) suggest that the nature of the reliability data ought to differ across the three types of scales. A useful discriminative index must demonstrate large and stable between-subject variation. So must predictive scales, but with an additional requirement: there should not be any systematic change in subject scores over time. Evaluative indices, however, should evidence small within-subject variation in stable subjects are large change in scores when functional status improves or deteriorates (18). This analysis has rarely been reported in the functional assessment literature, but it is presented here to illustrate the importance of the compatibility between scale construction and use, and to encourage rehabilitation researchers to include such information.

When scores are obtained from measures administered and scored by different raters, interrater or interobserver reliability is assessed. The interrater reliability coefficient is generally determined from correlations between different raters' judgments. The interobserver correlation or Kendall's index of concordance (*W*) are typically used where responses of more than two raters are being compared (10). In rehabilitation settings where staff teams are often used to generate client-level information, good interrater reliability is an essential quality to be considered in scale selection.

Internal consistency assesses the extent to which different items within a particular scale are measuring the same content or characteristic. Several formulas are available for estimating the correlations between all possible pairs of items, e.g., Kuder-Richardson 20 and Cronbach's alpha coefficient (23). Internal consistency is particularly important in judging whether the items being grouped together measure a unified underlying domain. If the coefficient does not meet the proposed 0.80 criterion, the resulting scale score may be too unreliable to accurately detect the presence of the construct (e.g., pain), or to detect change following rehabilitation intervention.

Validity

Reliability is a necessary but insufficient condition for validity. Additional evidence is needed to indicate whether a scale is measuring what it purports to measure. There are several types of validity, and a basic understanding of the role they play in adding evidence of a measure's value is necessary for making informed decisions about test selection. Feinstein (17) offers practical guidance for evaluation validity. A more extensive discussion can be found in Brinberg and Kidder (24).

Most programmatic attempts to establish validity begin with content validity. This refers to how adequately the sampling of questions reflects the aims of the index, as specified in the conceptual definition of its scope (10). Content validity is rarely tested statistically owing, in large part, to the absence of a standard which can be measured. Rather, expert opinion is sought and systematically gathered within a well-specified conceptual framework. The main difficulty does not lie in using a consensus but, rather, with getting a suitable group of authorities (17). In rehabilitation this issue is compounded by substantially different models and world views. Emphasis on impairment or disability creates concern about content validity among users since the distinction directly reflects the differences between the medical and psychosocial models (25). When selecting scales, all of the user groups should be consulted concerning agreement on the models and, subsequently, whether there is sufficient support for content validity within that model.

Criterion validity proceeds when an established measure, or "gold standard" exists against which the new measure can be compared. Both the established and the new measure are administered simultaneously and the results are compared with an appropriate correlation coefficient. Criterion validity appears to be most relevant for functional assessment at the impairment level. For example, several well-established clinical procedures exist for the diagnosis of organ pathology. Functional scales that are intended to be easier and less expensive to administer than these have a useful role to play in the screening process.

For most functional assessment scales, as for most quality of life scales, no gold standard exists. Evidence for construct validity must be gathered but no single procedure provides definitive proof (16). Rather, correlations must be shown to be in the hypothesized direction and of the expected magnitude provided by the authors. Of course, constructs themselves vary in the degree of consensus and supporting evidence they possess. Often, advanced analytical methods such as factor and cluster analysis can be used to provide empirical support for the constructs.

A serious shortcoming for most functional assessment scales is the lack of sound evidence for validity. Validation research is difficult in rehabilitation because of the levels of differences in viewpoint and changes in conceptualization that have been discussed here. Consequently, the user should make an effort to review the case for validity that the developer presents. McDowell and Newell (16) provide assistance. First, it needs to be understood that the magnitude of the validity coefficient is constrained by the reliability of both the proposed and the standard measure (technically, the product of the square root of each reliability coefficient). Reported validities need to approach this upper bound, rather than perfection, as a key criterion. Second, it may be useful to translate correlation coefficients into a more useful concept. The basic assumption is that the functional assessment measure is being used to predict some criterion. The purpose of validity is to estimate how much the accuracy of the prediction is improved based on knowing the score on the measurement. A simple approach is to square the correlation coefficient. If a health measure correlates 0.70 with a criterion, it will provide about a 50% reduction in error compared with guessing. The key point here is that correlation coefficients of 0.50 or lower begin to rapidly lose their predictive utility. More elaborate approaches can be found in Helmstadt (26). More generally, the validation approach taken by scale developers needs to be examined. Validation programs should systematically state and test clear hypotheses, attempt to disprove hypotheses that the scales measure something other than the stated purpose, and employ a variety of validation approaches (16).

Responsiveness

Responsiveness, precision, and sensitivity represent a third consideration for scale selection. Responsiveness refers to the power of a scale to detect clinically important change when it occurs (18) and is similar in concept to precision, which refers to the degree of change in the phenomenon that can be detected. Sensitivity, on the other hand, traditionally refers to positivity in the presence of disease (3).

As shown in Fig. 2, responsiveness is an issue only for evaluative indices. In clinical trials, scales are needed that can detect often small but clinically significant differences. While different across different disease levels, such change may be operationalized as that magnitude which alters prognosis, therapy, or intensity of follow-up (3). In rehabilitation, change is often the key outcome indicator (7), yet many functional assessment scales were not designed to detect meaningful change.

Practical Considerations

The success of systematic functional assessment depends directly on the match between the assessment purpose, the rehabilitation setting, and the characteristics of the scale. These practical issues were discussed by Brown et al. (7) who identified two broad dimensions of functional assessment scales. Brown et al. argued that relevance, i.e., the match between the content and structure of the scale and the user's information needs, is the essential first practical consideration. Obviously if the data are seen as irrelevant to the problem, psychometric quality will not matter; the information will be ignored. Further, the information must be produced feasibly. This analysis of the resource limitations and constraints has been further refined by Ware (22) who presented the useful guide for identifying several areas of consideration summarized below:

Acceptability

> History of use in trials
> Completion rates
> Missing data
> Complaints from study participants
> Respondent burden

Mode of administration required

> Direct observation
> In-person interview
> Telephone interview
> Self-administered questionnaire

Length/administration time

Special training and equipment

With the exception of respondent burden, the issues involved in determining the acceptability of an instrument are rarely reported in the literature or in the users' manuals which accompany the scale. Yet issues such as whether the scale was used successfully in a similar setting and the nature of missing or incomplete data have direct implications for the relevance and feasibility of the information.

Respondent burden is one practical consideration that does receive attention. A key question is how long the scale takes to administer. The majority of patients can complete four standardized items per minute, according to Ware's research (22), with longer time needed for more disabled or disadvantaged respondents. Administrative time is certainly important but it is not the only respondent burden of concern. Attention needs to be directed toward psychologic stress as well. The issues here involve the difficulty or complexity of an interview or questionnaire, and the content. Sensitivity to client needs within the assessment process is an especially important consideration in rehabilitation (27).

Mode of administration is a second component of practical consideration. The modes listed above range from time-consuming and fairly resource intensive direct observation through generally less costly and more easily managed self-administered questionnaires. Each type has advantages and disadvantages that need to be reviewed against the central objectives of the study. Tracking changes in the effectiveness of interpersonal skill training for mildly mentally retarded workers may well require direct observation by trained technicians, for example, whereas pain management and mobility in arthritic patients may be accurately assessed with a self-administered questionnaire.

The final two considerations involve length/administration time and the need for special training or equipment. The time to complete the assessment is important, but so too is the time necessary to prepare for the administration and to deal with the assessment data following the administration. Once completed, one must ask how much "massaging" is needed to transform the responses into usable data. Open-ended questions, for example, yield rich and unique information but are resource-intensive to convert to usable data. Other assessment approaches require special training and equipment. These can represent substantial investment of resources, and trade-offs with data quality need to be considered.

It is not being argued that short, self-administered assessments are the best approach. Rather, users are encouraged to keep the objectives of the assessment in sharp focus and to make informed decisions about the trade-offs associated with producing data necessary to meet those objectives. With this in mind, one final point needs to be made. Time and resources invested in pilot studies often yield tremendous benefit. Good estimates of response burden, issues of administrative complexity, and "bench-testing" of data reduction and analytic procedures are all possible with brief, well-planned pilot studies involving a similar set of respondents.

SUMMARY

Functional assessment in rehabilitation settings can be considered successful if the information produced meets the user's needs with the resources available. The user is required to state the needs in measurable terms, to select from a large collection of scales of decidedly mixed quality those which have the potential to produce the appropriate information, and then refine that set by applying a series of technical and practical guidelines.

This section introduced a measurement model and a set of guidelines which were designed to assist the user in obtaining meaningful functional assessment information. The model makes use of the important distinctions between the key concepts: impairment, disability, and handicap. This distinction can be applied to each of the functional domains that are consistent with those include (physical, mental, emotional, and social) used in other health assessment areas. As users identify the level of interest for their information needs within and across relevant domains, the third dimension of the model comes into play. Scales can be used to categorize respondents according to underlying constructs (discriminative indices), or against some "gold standard" (predictive indices), or according to whether they can detect clinically important change (evaluative indices). The simultaneous application of these dimensions should yield a subset of potentially appropriate scales which can then be examined against the issues of psychometric quality and practicality.

Although guidelines for both reliability and validity are generally well-known and available, many functional assessment scales in rehabilitation, particularly the activities of daily living scales, either do not have adequate evidence or, too often, do not report reliability and validity results at all. Sources of additional help, especially McDowell and Newell, and Feinstein, were identified.

Finally, practical issues (many of which Feinstein included in his "index of sensibility") play a central role in assessment decisions. The scales must conform to the realities of the resources and settings in which they are to be used. Although these issues are settled through judgmental appraisals which may seemingly reduce their importance and worth, Feinstein argued that such appraisals have priority and can be approached with scientific precision and clarity (17).

FUNCTIONAL ASSESSMENT INSTRUMENTS IN REHABILITATION

In the first part of this section the reader is provided with a description of recent comprehensive reviews of functional assessment instruments that will serve as useful resources for scale selection. A listing of functional assessment scales that have been widely used in a variety of rehabilitation settings and for which reasonable validity and reliability date are available is also included. In the second part of this section, a more detailed description is provided for two general rehabilitation scales (one summary and one comprehensive), two scales focused on specific disabilities (physical and psychiatric), and one general health assessment scale relevant to rehabilitation. These reviews are presented as examples of well-established instruments with different purposes and designs which illustrate the diversity of scales within the field of rehabilitation.

Sources of Functional Assessment Information

A comprehensive review of scales can be found in the Tenth Institute on Rehabilitation Issues' *Functional Assessment* (28), published by the West Virginia Rehabilitation Research and Training Center. The document is available from the Center in Dunbar, West Virginia. In addition to a discussion of assessment issues that apply particularly to the vocational rehabilitation setting, this resource comprehensively describes and compares 11 instruments. The comparative analysis is especially useful for making decisions based on practical considerations. The areas covered are breadth of content, measurement and output, information source, time and cost, potential and users, training, and prior utilization.

Each scale is described according to developers, purpose, descriptions, use, administration, scoring, reliability, validity, advantages, limitations, references, and availability. Each description is followed by a useful case summary that provides the reader with an example of the raw data actually produced by the scale. This document is based, in part, on an older review of 40 client assessment instruments published as the monograph *Client Assessment Measures in Rehabilitation* (29), which is now available from the National Rehabilitation Information Center (NARIC) at the Catholic University of America.

A third important resource has been cited previously in this chapter. McDowell and Newell's *Measuring Health: A Guide to Rating Scales and Questionnaires* (16) takes a broader view of health assessment than just rehabilitation. However, this book proceeds from the World Health Organization definition of impairment, disability, and handicap and the authors use that framework to review functional disability and handicap measures, along with others that are relevant to rehabilitation. Scales are compared in a particularly useful summary chart that includes numerical characteristics, number of items, applications, administrative mode, an assessment of current usage, and assessment of both the thoroughness and results of reliability and validity testing. Further, each scale is summarized according to a standard format that describes the purpose, conceptual basis, description, exhibits, reliability and

FUNCTIONAL ASSESSMENT SCALES IN REHABILITATION

SCALE NAME	PRINCIPAL AUTHORS
Barthel Index	*Mahoney & Barthel*
Disability and Impairment Interview Schedule	*Bennett & Garrad*
Functional Activities Questionnaire	*Pfeffer*
Functional Assessment Inventory	*Crewe & Athelstan*
Functional Assessment Profile Commission	*Massachusetts Rehabilitation*
Functional Status Index	*Jette*
Functional Status Rating System	*Forer*
Independent Living Behavior Checklist	*Walls, Zane, & Thvedt*
Index of Independence in Activities of Daily Living	*Katz*
Kenny Self-Care Evaluation	*Schoening*
Lambeth Disability Screening Questionnaire	*Patrick*
Level of Rehabilitation Scale	*Carey*
Longitudinal Functional Assessment System	*Alexander*
OECD Long-Term Disability Questionnaire	– – – –
Patient Evaluation Conference System	*Harvey & Jelinek*
Physical Self-Maintenance Scale	*Lawton & Brody*
Preliminary Diagnostic Questionnaire	*Moriarity*
PULSES Profile	*Moskowitz & McCann*
Rapid Disability Rating Scale-2	*Linn*
Rehabilitation Indicators	*Brown, Diller, & Fordyce*

FIG. 4. Functional assessment instruments for rehabilitation settings.

validity, alternative forms, reference standards, commentary, availability, and references.

Beyond these comprehensive scale reviews are a series of articles and relevant volumes that together form a solid foundation of conceptual and technical issues for critically examining functional assessment in rehabilitation:

Brown, Gordon, and Diller. ''Functional assessment and outcome measurement: An integrative review'' (7).
Granger and Gresham. *Functional assessment in rehabilitation medicine* (30).
Halpern and Fuhrer (eds). *Functional assessment in rehabilitation* (31).
Indices, Inc. *Functional limitation: A state of the art review* (32).
Wallace. ''Functional assessment in rehabilitation'' (33).
Gresham and Labi. ''Functional assessment instruments currently available for documenting outcomes in rehabilitation medicine'' (34).

Listed alphabetically in Fig. 4 are functional assessment scales frequently cited in the literature and reviewed by measurement specialists. Where relevant, the principal author or developer has been listed to assist the reader in literature searching.

Although not comprehensive (many more activities of daily living scales exist, as do disability-specific scales), this is a useful preliminary set of the user to examine.

Examples of Functional Assessment Scales

In this section five scales that reflect different components of the three-dimensional functional assessment model are summarized. All have well-documented psychometric quality and together they have been used in a variety of studies with large numbers of rehabilitation patients and clients. These scales were selected as examples, in part, because of their diversity. The intent is to demonstrate that careful consideration of the assessment objectives and guidelines discussed previously can (and should) result in functional assessment scales demonstrating variety in content and format. It is not the intent of this section to recommend these as priority scales that should be given first consideration. Since each of these examples has well-documented reliability and validity evidence, those aspects of the guidelines are not presented here.

General Rehabilitation—Summary

User objective: To obtain a low burden and comprehensive overview of the client's functional limitations and strengths that are relevant for vocational rehabilitation.

Scale example: Functional Assessment Inventory (FAI) (Crewe and Athelstan, 35–37).

Functional assessment model: Levels: disability, handicap
Areas: physical, mental, emotional, social
Type: discriminative (possibly evaluative)

Purpose: To provide a summary of a rehabilitation client's functional limitations and strengths based on existing case file, interview, and counselor knowledge and information.

Description: The Functional Assessment Inventory is a rating scale containing 30 four-point limitation ratings and a 10-item strength checklist. The rating items are operationally defined in behavioral terms with levels of limitation corresponding to none, mild, moderate, or severe. The inventory is completed by the rehabilitation counselor using information from medical and other relevant records, interviews, and observations.

Practical issues: The Functional Assessment Inventory is relatively short, requiring 5 to 10 minutes to complete by a knowledgeable counselor. Training is not required but is preferred to insure interobserver and test re-test reliability.

Scoring and use: The Functional Assessment Inventory produces an overview of functional limitations that are relevant for vocational rehabilitation outcomes based on existing information. No new diagnostic information is produced by this inventory. Both a total numerical score and seven subscale scores are produced from ordinal ratings. The subscales result from factor analysis and evidence for responsiveness (i.e., change in response to services) has been reported. The user is cautioned about interpreting change scores (see Section II).

The Functional Assessment Inventory can provide information for problem identification, eligibility determinations, information organizations, goal setting, and service planning within the vocational rehabilitation setting.

General Rehabilitation—Comprehensive

User objective: To obtain a broad-based and comprehensive description of patient
functioning in a variety of rehabilitation settings.

Scale example: Rehabilitation Indicator (RI) (Brown, Diller, Fordyce, and Jacobs,
37).

Functional assessment model: Levels: disability, handicap
                                       Areas: physical, mental, emotional, social
                                       Type: discriminative, evaluative

Purpose: To describe comprehensively and in behavioral terms the diverse aspects
of client functioning that are relevant for rehabilitation outcome.

Description: The Rehabilitation Indicator is a system of assessment instruments,
rather than a single scale, that can be used independently or in combination. Three
instruments provide information from different perspectives and approaches to data
gathering about the patient's functioning.
    Status Indicators consist of 51 descriptions in six areas of functioning: vocation,
income, education, self-care, transportation, and family role. Status indicators
are recorded by interviewing the client or significant other, by examining existing records, or through self-report.
    Activity Pattern Indicators describe an individual's pattern of daily activity,
including types of activity, location, use of assistance, and level of social contact
through direct observation.
    Skill Indicators contain a catalog of several hundred skills which represent be-
haviors necessary for functioning in vocational, educational, recreational, family
role, self-care, and other settings. The skills are organized into groupings, or
"packets," which are preselected by the user according to relevance to the
objectives.

Practical issues: The Rehabilitation Indicator is a comprehensive system and actual
respondent/user burden depends on which, and how much of, the component instruments are used. The Status Indicators require from 5 to 15 minutes, depending
on format; Activity Pattern Indicators vary from 10 to 60 minutes, depending on
detail required; and Skill Indicators require from 10 minutes to several hours, depending on the number of skills selected and the data gathering approach. Training
in the Rehabilitation Indicator system is required and can be accomplished by self
study or directed instructions.

Scoring and use: Rehabilitation Indicators provide a comprehensive behavioral description of the client's functioning. None of the three components produce a numerical score. Skill Indicators provide a composite score and both Activity Pattern
Indicators and Skill Indicators provide item-by-item analysis. Change is assessed
through changes in frequencies in behaviors or acquisitions/demonstrations of skills,
and through change in status.

Specific Rehabilitation—Physical Disability

User objective: To describe the functional limitation in activities of daily living of patients with primarily physical disabilities.

Scale example: Rapid Disability Rating Scale (RDRS) (Linn and Linn, 38).

Functional assessment model: Levels: Impairment, disability
Areas: physical (one-item overview of mental and emotional)
Type: discriminative

Purpose: The Rapid Disability Rating Scale was designed to summarize the physical capacity of elderly chronic hospitalized and community-based patients.

Description: The Rapid Disability Rating Scale is an 18-item, 4-point rating scale designed to be completed by an expert who is knowledgeable of the patient. The rating scales for each question range from None (completely independent or normal behavior) to Total (person cannot, will not, or may not [because of medical restriction] perform the behavior). The scale is composed of three parts. One describes assistance with activities of daily living (e.g., eating, bathing, grooming), the second describes the degree of disability (e.g., communication, diet, incontinence), and the third consists of three general questions about confusion, uncooperativeness, and depression.

Practical issues: The Rapid Disability Rating Scale can be completed in less than 5 minutes when rated by an expert knowledgeable of the patient. No special training is required.

Scoring and use: The items are weighted equally in calculating an overall score which ranges from 18 to 72. The items may be combined according to the parts of the scale. The ratings have been used successfully to classify patients according to level of disability. Community dwelling individuals average about 21, hospitalized patients average about 32, and nursing home patients average about 36.

Specific Rehabilitation—Psychiatric Disability

User objectives: To assess the functional adjustment of chronically mentally ill to community living.

Scale example: Social Adjustment Scale (SAS) (Weissman and Gothwell, 39).

Functional assessment model: Levels: disability
Areas: emotional, social
Type: discriminative, evaluative

Purpose: To assess patient functioning, generally and interpersonally, and patient satisfaction in six instrumental role areas.

Description: There are two versions of the Social Adjustment Scale, an interview form and a self-report version, both of which contain 42 items. Each covers functioning in work, social-leisure activities, relationship with extended family, and marital roles as spouse, parent, and member of family unit.

Scoring and use: Two scoring methods are used: a mean score for each section and an overall score. The focus on social adjustment provides a framework for designing a rehabilitation treatment program.

Health Assessment Applied to Rehabilitation

User objective: To obtain comprehensive functional information that can be used for program planning, health surveys, and patient progress.

Scale example: Sickness Impact Profile (SIP) (Bergner et al., 40).

Functional assessment model: Levels: disability
                                    Areas: physical, emotional, social
                                    Type: discriminative

Purpose: To provide a behaviorally based measurement of perceived health status that reflects "universal patterns" of limitations that may be affected by sickness or disease, regardless of specific conditions, treatments, individual characteristics, or prognosis.

Description: The Sickness Impact Profile consists of 136 statements in 12 categories. Each item describes a change in behavior and specifies the extent of limitation (e.g., I stay away from home only for brief periods of time). Respondents check (self-report) or indicate (interview) only the items that describe them on a given day.

Practical issues: As a self-administered scale, the Sickness Impact Profile requires 20 to 30 minutes. The interview version may take longer and is recommended for more impaired respondents.

Scoring and use: The Sickness Impact Profile is one of the few interval scales available in health assessment. Scores are calculated using items weights that indicate relative severity of each statement. The weights are derived from equal-appearing scaling procedures and permit the production of a total score and scale score with interval properties.

Because the Sickness Impact Profile has undergone extensive validation and normative testing, it permits direct comparison across a variety of groups within rehabilitation settings, and between clients and other disabled or nondisabled groups.

Summary

The purpose of this section was to identify important resources that provide comprehensive reviews of functional assessment instruments used in rehabilitation settings and health assessment scales that are appropriate for rehabilitation specialists. Scales with sound scale development properties were listed in Table 2 and specific examples of the diversity of scales were provided in more detail. Because the field is changing rapidly, the user is advised to keep current with respect to reported validity and applications research reported for the scales under consideration.

APPLICATION OF FUNCTIONAL ASSESSMENT INFORMATION

Functional Assessment in Rehabilitation Settings

There are three main activities in rehabilitation for which functional assessment information can be gainfully used: client management, program evaluation, and research. In client management settings, functional information can provide useful information at each of the critical decision points. In medical rehabilitation settings, the focus is on the individual patient and the information is used to assess initial status, design treatment plans, monitor programs, evaluate the patient's status at the end of treatment to determine whether treatment goals have been achieved, and communicate results (25,41).

In vocational rehabilitation, client management issues are similar and functional assessment has an important role to play. At screening, functional assessment information can be used to assess current levels of functioning and predict probability of a successful rehabilitation, although current rehabilitation outcome measures need further refinement (see Backer [15]). A second important application is at the diagnostic level. Often, batteries of time-consuming (and costly) tests are ordered regardless of the particular needs of the client or counselor. Functional information can be used to organize existing information and target specific areas where additional in-depth information is needed using, for example, the Functional Assessment Inventory. Or, functional assessment information can provide an initial diagnosis based on new information as is the case with the Preliminary Diagnostic Questionnaire (42). Or, further, the situation may require an in-depth and fine-grained analysis of the patient's capabilities and limitations of the sort provided by the Rehabilitation Indicator system.

Once specific client problems have been identified and described functionally, specific services targeted toward those functional limitations can be planned and implemented. During the course of service delivery, progress toward intermediate goals can be tracked as change in functional status and, at case closure, rehabilitation outcomes can be recorded as change in functional problem area as well as enhancements (e.g., cognitive skills) as a result of service delivery.

The second major purpose of functional information is in program evaluation (41). Evaluation activities can be grouped into four classes: program planning and development, program monitoring, impact assessment, and cost-outcome comparison (43). For each of these, functional assessment information can be applied for specific evaluation tasks such as identifying appropriate target populations (the severely disabled, for example), determining if service delivery has produced an improvement, or if there has been a change in status which can be attributed to the intervention, and determining whether those outcomes were delivered economically. This latter point has received a great deal of attention in rehabilitation settings and the role of functional information is becoming more prominent (44).

The third application of functional assessment information is in *research*. A prime example is the use of functional data as descriptors in epidemiological and clinical research. The addition of functional status descriptors to the traditionally collected mortality and clinically diagnosed morbidity data provides an integrative component not only for rehabilitation, but for health care in general (13,45). Further, it is through research that the models and concepts discussed in Section I have become increasingly clarified. Through the process of identifying terms, research methodologists have been obligated to define more precisely what variables should be included in functional assessment (45).

Technical Considerations

When using functional assessment scales, there are a number of technical considerations that influence the analysis and interpretation of functional information across each of the rehabilitation applications.

Scaling

Scaling methods are used to translate the descriptive items in the measure into numerical estimates of functional level (19–21). The most adequate numerical scale possible is the most desirable, but constructing such scales is complex and respondent burden often increases (16,21).

A brief review of the four types of scaling methods is useful in placing functional assessment scales along the continuum of mathematical adequacy. At the low end are nominal (or classification) methods which simply label categories using numbers. No inferences can be drawn since the coding is arbitrary. The most frequently used method in functional assessment occurs at the next level where ordinal scales use numbers as labels for increasing levels of functional limitation (e.g., mild, moderate, severe). The actual value of the numbers, and the numbering distances between them, do not have intrinsic value (16). Virtually all activities of daily living scales and most of the general health scales used in rehabilitation are ordinally scaled. Assessing change using these scales is the topic of methodologic debate (16,21) and the user is advised to seek technical input. Whereas the purists argue that the scale properties violate the necessary mathematical assumptions, the pragmatists point out that the resulting errors are small and there is a substantial trade-off in scale development effort (19).

Interval scales do permit some advanced mathematical assumptions because distances between scale values are constant and unit change is constant change across the range of possible scale scores. Although rare in functional assessment scales developed for rehabilitation settings, the Sickness Impact Profile (40) represents one example of an interval scale.

The most mathematically sophisticated scaling methods produce a ratio scale that has constant unit change properties and a zero point which permit conclusions such as a score of 10 measuring twice the limitation as a score of 5 (16).

In most cases, the instrument requires the combination of scale items into composite measures or scales. A number of key assumptions underlie this procedure and the user should try to ascertain the degree to which they are met in the scales being considered (46):

1. Each item contributes to the pool of information about the construct.
2. The method of combination is consistent with the relationships among the items.
3. All items are scored in the same direction.
4. All items measure the construct in approximately the same units (or they have been standardized and weighted).
5. The resulting measure (or construct) has a meaningful interpretation.

Three approaches to weighting the components have been used but most of the functional assessment work to date has relied simply on investigator-defined scores. The scale developer assigns higher scores to items that reflect, in the developer's opinion, a higher level of functioning. Problems arise with the assumption of social consensus and when respondents rate combinations of attributes (10). Some advanced methods are available, but they are rarely used in functional assessment scales in rehabilitation. A variety of category scaling methods, for example, the equal-appearing index, can be used to produce interval scales, although criticism has been leveled at the use of fixed categories. Magnitude estimation techniques are used for producing ratio scales that are rare in health assessment in general and functional assessment in particular (16).

CONCLUSIONS

Functional assessment in rehabilitation is tied closely to the process of rehabilitation itself. As a result, approaches to assessment reflect the conceptual models that define the rehabilitation process. As these change from acute treatment of impairment to chronic management of disability and handicap, the assessment needs and approaches change as well.

Most functional assessment scale development has not benefited from either long-standing psychometric methods or new advances in health assessment conceptualizations. As users become more knowledgeable and interdisciplinary cross-fertilization becomes more prevalent in rehabilitation settings, greater demand will be made for improved assessment tools.

To be effective, these need to be developed from a conceptual framework that accurately reflects the distinction among impaired, disability, and handicap, and recognizes the array of functional areas that reflect the psychosocial model. Such methods require the application of the best technology and highest standards available to health assessment scaling.

The conditions for these changes are in place. Both disabled and nondisabled persons are living longer and require more long-term care. Also, acute diseases are giving way to chronic conditions in developed countries. Health care resource planning in general is beginning to reflect the convergence of these factors. In rehabilitation, effective management of client services, program evaluation, and research all require accurate and useful information. Functional assessment, produced from conceptually and technically sound measures, is a valuable source of much of that information.

REFERENCES

1. Frey WD. Functional assessment in the '80's: A conceptual enigma, a technical challenge. In: Halpern AS, Fuhrer MJ, eds. *Functional assessment in rehabilitation*. Baltimore: Paul H. Brookes, 1984.
2. Granger CV. A conceptual model for functional assessment. In: Granger CV, Gresham GE, eds. *Functional assessment in rehabilitation medicine*. Baltimore: Williams and Wilkins, 1984.
3. Jette AM. Concepts of health and methodological issues in functional assessment. In: Granger CV, Gresham GE, eds. *Functional assessment in rehabilitation medicine*. Baltimore: Williams and Wilkins, 1984.
4. Nagi SZ. *Disability and Rehabilitation*. Columbus, OH: Ohio State University Press, 1969.
5. Nagi SZ. Some conceptual issues in disability and rehabilitation. In: Sussmann MB, ed. *Sociology and rehabilitation*. Columbus, OH: Ohio State University Press, 1965.
6. Wood PHN. Classification of impairment and handicap. Document WHO/ICDP/REV-CONF/75.15. Geneva: World Health Organization, 1975.
7. Brown M, Gordon W, Diller L. Functional assessment and outcome measurement: An integrated review. In: Pan EL, Backer TE, Vash CL, eds. *Annual review of rehabilitation*, vol. 3. New York: Springer, 1983.
8. Schipper H, Levitt M. Measuring quality of life: Risks and benefits. *Cancer treatment reports* 1985;69:1115–1122.
9. Wenger NK, Mattson ME, Furberg CD, Elinson J. *Assessment of quality of life in clinical trials of cardiovascular therapies*. New York: LeJacq, 1984.
10. Patrick DC, Erickson PE. Assessing health-related quality of life for clinical decision making. Walker SR, Rosen RM, eds. *Quality of life: Assessment and application*. Lancaster: MTP Press, 1988.
11. Kelman HR, Willner A. Problems in measurement and evaluation of rehabilitation. *Arch Phys Med Rehabil* 1962;43:172–181.

12. Keith RA. Functional assessment measures in medical rehabilitation: Current status. *Arch Phys Med Rehabil* 1984;65:74–78.
13. Ellwood PM. Outcome management: A technology of patient experience. *N Engl J Med* 1988;318:1551–1556.
14. Bassett TE. *Measurement of outcomes: A report from the study group on measurement of outcomes.* First Institute on Rehabilitation Issues; Denver, CO; April 15-17, 1974. Institute of West Virginia: Research and Training Center, 1974.
15. Backer TE. New directions in rehabilitation outcome measurement. In: Pan EL, Backer TE, Vash CL, eds. *Annual review of rehabilitation*, vol. 1. New York: Springer, 1980.
16. McDowell I, Newell C. *Measuring health: A guide to rating scales and questionnaires.* New York: Oxford University Press, 1987.
17. Feinstein AR. *Clinimetrics.* New Haven: Yale University Press, 1987.
18. Kirshner B, Guyatt G. A methodological framework for assessing health indices. *J Chron Dis* 1985;38:27–36.
19. Nunnally JC. *Psychometric theory*, 2nd ed. New York: McGraw-Hill, 1978.
20. Thorndike RL. *Applied psychometrics.* Boston: Houghton-Mifflin Co., 1982.
21. Torgeson GS. *Theory and methods of scaling.* New York: Wiley, 1978.
22. Ware JE. Methodological considerations in selection of health status assessment procedures. In: Wenger NK, Mattson ME, Furberg CD, et al., eds. *Assessment of quality of life in clinical trials of cardiovascular therapies.* New York: LeJacq, 1984.
23. Gilford JP. *Psychometric methods*, 2nd ed. New York: McGraw-Hill, 1954.
24. Brinberg D, Kidder LH. *Forms of validity in research.* San Francisco: Jossey-Bass, 1982.
25. Alexander J, Fuhrer M. Functional assessment of physical impairment. In: Halpern AS, Fuhrer MS, eds. *Functional assessment in rehabilitation.* Baltimore: Paul H. Brookes, 1984.
26. Helmstadt GC. *Principles of psychological measurement.* London: Methus, 1966.
27. Vash CL. Evaluation from the client's point of view. In: Halpern AS, Fuhrer MJ, eds. *Functional assessment in rehabilitation.* Baltimore: Paul H. Brookes, 1984.
28. Tenth Institute on Rehabilitation Issues. *Functional assessment.* Dunbar, WV: Rehabilitation Research and Training Center, 1983.
29. Michigan Studies in Rehabilitation. *Client assessment measures in rehabilitation.* Utilization Series 5. Ann Arbor: University of Michigan Press, 1981.
30. Granger CV, Gresham GE. *Functional assessment in rehabilitation medicine.* Baltimore: Williams and Wilkins, 1984.
31. Halpern AS, Fuhrer MJ. *Functional assessment in rehabilitation.* Baltimore: Paul H. Brookes, 1984.
32. Indices, Inc. Functional limitations: A state of the art review. Monograph of Dept. of Health, Education, and Welfare, Rehabilitation Services Administration. Doct. No. 13-p-559220/3-01, 1978.
33. Wallace CJ. Functional assessment in rehabilitation. *Schizophr Bull* 1986;12:604–624.
34. Gersham GL, Labi ML. Functional assessment instruments currently available for documenting outcomes in rehabilitation medicine. In: Granger CV, Gresham GE, eds. *Functional assessment in rehabilitation medicine.* Baltimore: Williams and Wilkins, 1984.
35. Crewe NM, Athelstan GT. Functional assessment in vocational rehabilitation: A systematic approach to diagnosis and goal setting. *Arch Phys and Rehabil* 1981;62:299–305.
36. Turner RR. Functional assessment in vocational rehabilitation: Validation, extension, and applications. Final Report. National Institute of Handicapped Research. Grant G008300163. October, 1987.
37. Brown M, Diller L, Fordyce W, Jacobs D, Gordon W. Rehabilitation indicators: Their nature and uses for assessment. In: Bolton B, Cook D, eds. *Rehabilitation client assessment.* Baltimore: University Park Press, 1980.
38. Linn MW, Linn DS. The Rapid Disability Rating Scale-2. *J Am Geriatr Soc* 1982;30:378–382.
39. Weissman MM, Gothwell S. Assessment of social adjustment by patient self-report. *Arch Gen Psychiatry* 1976;33:1111–1115.
40. Bergner M, Bobbitt RA, Carter WB, Gilson BS. The Sickness Impact Profile: Development and final revision of a health status measure. *Med Care* 1981;19:787–805.
41. Keith RA. Functional assessment in program evaluation for rehabilitation medicine. In: Granger CV, Gresham GL, eds. *Functional assessment in rehabilitation medicine.* Baltimore: Williams and Wilkins, 1984.
42. Moriarity JB. Preliminary Diagnostic Questionnaire: PDQ. Dunbar: West Virginia Rehabilitation Research and Training Center, 1981.
43. Rossi PH, Freeman HC, Wright SR. *Evaluation: A systematic approach.* Beverly Hills, CA: Sage, 1979.
44. Berkowitz M. Benefit-cost analysis in rehabilitation. In: Granger CV, Gresham GE, eds. *Functional assessment in rehabilitation medicine.* Baltimore: Williams and Wilkins, 1984.
45. Labi ML, Gresham GE. Some research applications of functional assessment instruments used in rehabilitation medicine. In: Granger CV, Gresham GE, eds. *Functional assessment in rehabilitation medicine.* Baltimore: Williams and Wilkins, 1984.
46. Ware JE, Brook RH, Davis-Avery A, Williams KN, Stewart AL. *Conceptualization and measurement of health for adults in the health insurance study: Vol. I, Model of health and methodology.* Santa Monica, CA: Rand Corporation, 1980 (R-1987-HEW).

Quality of Life Assessments in Clinical
Trials, edited by B. Spilker. Raven
Press, Ltd. New York © 1990.

22

Chronic Pain Management

Victor C. Lee and John C. Rowlingson

*Pain Management Center, University of Virginia Health Sciences Center,
Charlottesville, Virginia 22908*

Pain, one of the most fundamental human experiences, defies simple characterization or definition, being a phenomenon that bridges multiple levels of understanding and appreciation. The English word *pain* has its roots in the Latin *poena* and the Greek *poine,* both of which signify penalty, or punishment. In a biological sense, pain is a form of penalty for failing to avoid such actions or environmental elements which threaten injury or destruction of an organism. Pain therefore functions to protect the organism from injury. The definition of pain proposed by the International Association for the Study of Pain also reflects this element of injury: "an unpleasant sensory and emotional experience associated with actual or potential tissue damage, or described in terms of such damage" (1). Pain is clearly essential for existence. Evidence for this is provided by accounts of children born with congenital insensitivity to pain and adults suffering from sensory impairment brought on by infectious, toxic, metabolic, or traumatic neuropathies. Such patients repeatedly injure themselves because of failure to avoid tissue-damaging stimuli and eventually succumb to the complications arising from multiple self-injuries.

The impact of pain on the human experience goes beyond sensation and tissue damage. Emotional pain, the anguish of bereavement, and the torment of desperation are psychological experiences not involving tissue damage, and yet produce suffering within the individual. Suffering is the affective counterpart to the sensorineural experience of pain, and the degree of emotional distress may not necessarily correlate with the intensity of the actual pain sensation. The affective component of pain is very fundamental to the experience of pain, in many cases spawning anxiety and depression which must be managed accordingly before a favorable outcome can be realized.

In addition to the sensory and affective components of the pain experience, there are also distinct behavioral alterations that accompany pain. The individual suffering from pain may display hypervigilance, dependency, anger, distrust, avoidance, and guarding. Pain as a "cry for help" may direct the behavior of other individuals as well, in the form of pity, caring, and nurturing; pain can become a powerful manipulative tool. Doctor shopping, disability seeking, and emergency room visits for narcotic medication take their toll on our health care system. The behavioral alterations that accompany chronic pain can in many cases far overshadow the actual medical problems.

A multilayered representation of pain as it is experienced within sensory, affective,

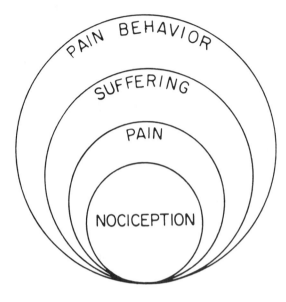

FIG. 1. Loeser's chronic pain model. From Fordyce, ref. 2, with permission.

and behavioral spheres is proposed by Loeser (2) (Fig. 1). Such a scheme provides a useful means of understanding the pain patient and forms a conceptual basis for directing pain management interventions. Effective pain management may necessitate intervention at each of these levels, hence the rationale for a "multidisciplinary" approach to the management of pain (a concept to be discussed in greater detail later in this chapter).

A further distinction must be made with regard to the clinical context of the patient who is experiencing pain, since this defines the role of the physician in managing the pain problem. Three clinical categories are defined: acute pain, chronic pain of malignant disease, and chronic pain of nonmalignant origin. Patients in each of these three categories experience their pain within the sensory, affective, and behavioral constructs described above. The approach to each category of patient, however, is distinctly different, and the options available to the physician, whether they be primarily pharmacological, psychological, or physical therapy-oriented, must be tailored to each patient in the most appropriate fashion.

The following discussion will touch on the different categories of pain patients encountered in clinical practice and the issues surrounding the management of their respective pain problems. Current approaches to managing these categories of pain patients as well as means of quantifying pain and assessing efficacy of pain relief will be addressed. Considerations in the functional organization of the pain management practice and the manner in which multidisciplinary pain management is applied to individual patients will illustrate the means by which intervention in chronic pain has an impact on quality of life of such patients.

IMPACT ON LIFESTYLE AND QUALITY OF LIFE

The chronic pain patient may experience dramatic changes in lifestyle as a result of the persistent pain he suffers; this will quite likely result in a deterioration in what the patient perceives as quality of life. Both chronic malignant and chronic nonmalignant pain produce alterations in daily functioning and perceptions of well-being and satisfaction which determine the quality of a patient's existence. Issues such as restricted physical activity, chronic depression, and preoccupation with pain may be shared by both groups of patients; however, the limited life span of the patient with cancer changes the context of life quality and the modalities which may be appropriately used for management of pain.

The patient with terminal cancer has a number of issues with which to deal. His struggle with malignant disease has likely involved a number of major therapeutic interventions such as surgery, chemotherapy, and radiation treatments. His battle to overcome his cancer has led him through a multitude of emotional ups and downs involving anger, depression, hope, desperation, denial, and acceptance of approaching death. His sense of life purpose and fulfillment have changed drastically and previous long-term goals have turned into short-term ones. His pain has escalated with his progressing disease and may be far more difficult to deal with compared to other problems such as loss of mobility, impaired urinary and bowel function, even the acceptance of death itself.

Zweibel, in a recent editorial addressing the quality of life issue with the terminally ill (3), suggested a number of factors of particular relevance to this group of patients, including the following: amount of pain, level of independent functioning (ambulation, capacity for self-care), level of cognitive functioning (ability to relate in a meaningful way with family, etc.), and burden of terminal care on the family. Listed first is pain, and not surprisingly so. Given our present limitations in cancer therapy, it is quite important not to stop working with the patient after conventional cancer treatments have been completed and/or have failed. It certainly does not end here for the patient, and adequate pain medication may be one of the few meaningful things that a physician can provide for the patient who is losing the cancer battle.

The patient suffering from chronic nonmalignant pain is likewise beset with a deteriorating lifestyle and dissatisfaction with quality of life. In spite of multiple visits to physicians, he is informed that either there is no satisfactory diagnosis or there is simply nothing that can be done for the painful condition. The situation is frustrating for both patient and doctor alike: the patient is faced with unrelieved suffering and the physician with a medical puzzle he is unable to solve; the patient is angered with the "quack" who has subjected him to multiple examinations, laboratory studies, X-rays, exorbitant fees, and has failed to produce a cure; the physician is angered with the "crock" who is obviously either imagining his pain or faking illness in order to obtain medications and/or a financial settlement, and who has plagued him with phone calls from lawyers, has challenged his professional acumen, and has wasted his time. The patient grows increasingly distrustful of physicians as he doctor-shops and visits emergency rooms in the middle of the night for doses of narcotic analgesics which enigmatically "don't take the pain away" but yet are "the only thing that helps the pain," while the physician grows less sympathetic toward chronic pain patients and less willing to seek or acknowledge complaints of pain, especially when he feels that he has "done all he can."

In addition to unsatisfying doctor-patient relationships, litigation, and inappropriate use of medication, chronic pain patients are likely to experience depression, have disarrayed family life, and be disabled. Multiple doctor's office visits are encouraged by attorneys. Work is discouraged, since this detracts from the overall appearance of impairment and perhaps lessens the amount of the final disability settlement. The physician may feel differently, believing the patient's complaints to be out of proportion to his physical findings; he may encourage a period of light duty for the patient. On the other hand, the employer, frequently strapped by insurance companies and labor unions, refuses to grant light duty to the injured patient, maintaining that either the patient receive a full work release or agree to a settlement. The physician refuses to issue a full work release for fear of being later sued if the patient reinjures himself. The prospects for finding alternative employment are poor, with the patient often lacking training for jobs involving less physical activity. The history of prior injury is certainly unattractive on any new job application. The disability check is frequently the patient's only source of income. The result of all of this is a patient whose "path of least resistance is . . . to strive to maintain his disabled status" (4). Not only does the prolonged period of unemployment and physical inactivity result in deconditioning of the patient (i.e., the "disuse syndrome" [5] of musculoskeletal atrophy and decreased strength, range of motion, and work capacity), but the likelihood of ever returning to gainful employment becomes increasingly remote as well.

The above profile is quite typical of the patient suffering from chronic nonmalignant pain and disability, e.g., the "low back loser" (6) or the "whiplash" patient. A recognizable pattern of clinical features emerges, resulting in descriptions such as Strang's "chronic disability syndrome" (7), or the "chronic pain syndrome" (8) of Crook and Tunks, from which the following list of features is adopted:

1. Compared to other patients, the chronic pain patient is less likely to have objective findings and less likely to have a satisfactory diagnosis.
2. Pain is likely to be attributed to a specific event, such as a work-related injury or motor-vehicle accident, and litigation is quite common.
3. These patients are likely to report a greater level of pain compared to other patients, and have a greater likelihood of experiencing psychological disturbances such as depression, social withdrawal, substance abuse, and diminished appetite, energy, and libido.
4. These patients are more likely to fail conservative treatment and are poor surgical candidates as well.
5. These patients consume a disproportionate share of medical and compensation costs and are frequent and inappropriate users of the health care system.
6. These patients are less likely to return to work, particularly if the period of unemployment has exceeded 6 months.

QUANTIFYING PAIN: MEASURING PAIN AND ITS COSTS

Pain, in spite of being such a universally appreciated experience, remains a largely elusive entity due in part to its highly subjective nature. Pain defies simple characterization or quantification. As presented in the introduction to this chapter, pain bridges multiple levels of human experience and expression (sensory, affective, behavioral). Measuring pain therefore depends largely on the particular aspect of pain to be examined. Each aspect of pain which is measured becomes a dimension of pain.

Examples of the sensory dimension of pain are the intensity of pain sensation, temporal aspects of pain (frequency of occurrence, duration), spatial (geographical or topographical) representation of pain, and the comparison of relative pain intensity to previous pain experiences. Emotional, or affective, aspects of pain, often assessed by interview and psychometric testing, strive to characterize the impact of pain on the patient's sense of well-being and the degree of distress or suffering experienced by the patient within the psychosocial context of the pain experience. Behavioral aspects of pain, often the most objective and measurable phenomena of the pain experience, include functional measures (i.e., activity and work history), as well as various other observable events associated with pain such as vocalization, guarding, withdrawal, avoidance, dependence on significant others, medication use, and so on.

Although these dimensions of pain are interdependent, they may at times appear incongruous; e.g., verbal denial of pain intensity in the presence of expression of severe pain through body language and guarding behavior, or verbally reporting severe pain but demonstrating inappropriate responses on physical examination or functional evaluation. To further complicate matters, the circumstances under which the patient reports pain may largely dictate the nature of that pain report; e.g., the child who, following an injury, is stoic in the midst of his peers, but cries in distress before his parents. The subjective aspects of the pain experience, i.e., the sensory and affective dimensions of pain, can be evaluated only if adequate communication exists between the patient and the evaluator. Language ability and other cognitive skills largely determine the extent to which the patient adequately conveys his pain experience to the evaluator. The cultural background of a patient may have an impact on other aspects of pain expression such as willingness or reluctance to vocalize pain, preconceptions and expectations of pain intensity, or the social roles assumed by the patient as reflected in the need to display either stoicism or distress.

The above considerations underscore the complex nature of pain evaluation and our imperfect ability to measure the pain experience. Certain types of pain measurements do, however, appear frequently in pain studies and have proven to be useful. Each study may have its own particular yardstick by which pain is measured, and attention to this, as well as the setting in which the measurement is made, will permit a better understanding of the significance of that study's findings.

SENSORY ASPECTS OF PAIN

The sensory aspect of pain is probably the first to be examined by the physician, providing one of the foremost clues of pathophysiology in diagnostic medicine. The medical student is directed to the mnemonic "PQRST"—Pain, Quality, Region, Strength, and Time—a summary of those qualifying descriptors of pain sensation which aid in diagnosing acute illness. Such sensory characteristics become important in describing chronic pain as well, although the identification of pathophysiology may or may not be relevant in this circumstance.

Pain intensity is most directly evaluated by patient reporting. Although electrophysiologic techniques for sensory evaluation exist, including nerve conduction studies, electroencephalography, somatosensory evoked potential monitoring, and microneurography (Bromm [9]), each has its own technical difficulties, limitations, and uncertainties in interpretation which have limited the widespread use of these electrophysiologic techniques as evalutive tools for quantification and characterization of clinical pain. These techniques do, however, continue to provide fascinating information in the setting of experimentally induced pain. It should be noted here that important differences exist in the evaluation of experimentally induced pain (evoked

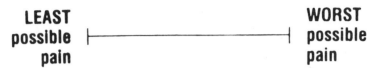

FIG. 2. The 10 cm visual analog scale.

by stimuli such as electrical stimulation, thermal stimulation, mechanical pressure, tourniquet ischemia, or injection of chemical irritants) as opposed to acute and chronic clinical pain. Experimentally induced pain is often employed in the evaluation of the efficacy of analgesic agents and provides a substrate for evaluating neurophysiological parameters of pain sensation and responses to pain. The differences between experimental and clinical pain have been reviewed by Wolskee (13), and involve affective and cognitive factors which distinguish the experimental subject from the patient experiencing clinical pain. Experimental pain focuses almost exclusively on the sensory aspect of pain, removing the affective and sociobehavioral variables which are a necessary accompaniment of clinical pain.

The sensory dimension of pain is most often quantified in a linear fashion, although some attention has been given to nonlinear measures of pain (9). Linear scales can be discontinuous "ordinal" scales (9) which contain descriptive words (no, little, mild, moderate, severe pain), or continuous graphic representations, such as the widely used "visual analog scale," a 10 cm line representing a linear spectrum of pain intensity, the opposite ends of which are labelled with descriptions such as "no pain" and "worst possible pain" (Fig. 2). The patient is asked to make a mark at a point along the line which represents the intensity of his pain on this scale. Visual analog scales require cognitive understanding of linear representation of pain intensity and presuppose an intellectual capacity appropriate for such an exercise. There are other limitations of the visual analog scale having to do with reproducibility (14), although on the whole these scales continue to be widely used in clinical pain studies.

Pain intensity is often measured in an indirect fashion by analysis of analgesic requirements, particularly in settings such as postoperative pain. Such an analysis equates narcotic "requirement" with intensity of pain and assumes that patients will demand and receive pain medication until a certain level of pain relief is experienced, that the amount of medication demanded and administered correlates with pain intensity, that a certain consistently reproducible lowering of pain is achieved in all patients receiving similar doses of medication, and that some common endpoint of satisfaction is reached by all patients. Such assumptions, needless to say, may prove dangerously false when subjected to more careful scrutiny. More properly, medication usage is a behavioral phenomenon which may only remotely reflect actual pain intensity. Nevertheless, it remains an interesting and quantifiable phenomenon in studies of pain if the study is designed with care and excessive liberties are not taken in drawing conclusions from such a study.

The temporal (onset, duration, frequency) and spatial elements of clinical pain properly belong to the sensory universe of pain and are important characteristics

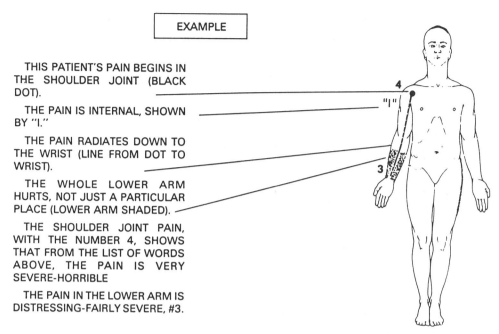

THIS PATIENT'S PAIN BEGINS IN THE SHOULDER JOINT (BLACK DOT).

THE PAIN IS INTERNAL, SHOWN BY "I."

THE PAIN RADIATES DOWN TO THE WRIST (LINE FROM DOT TO WRIST).

THE WHOLE LOWER ARM HURTS, NOT JUST A PARTICULAR PLACE (LOWER ARM SHADED).

THE SHOULDER JOINT PAIN, WITH THE NUMBER 4, SHOWS THAT FROM THE LIST OF WORDS ABOVE, THE PAIN IS VERY SEVERE-HORRIBLE

THE PAIN IN THE LOWER ARM IS DISTRESSING-FAIRLY SEVERE, #3.

FIG. 3. The pain drawing, from the UVA Pain Management Center, *Pain Assessment Inventory and Narrative.*

and qualifiers of pain sensation. As a means of assessing the latter, "pain drawings"—diagrammatic representations of the human body—are often included in pain questionnaires such as the University of Virginia Department of Anesthesiology Pain Assessment Inventory and Narrative (Fig. 3). The patient is asked to shade in the portion of the diagram corresponding to the distribution of his somatic pain. Quality of pain is frequently assessed by asking the patient to select from a list of descriptive adjectives those which best characterize the pain. An example of qualifying descriptors of pain appears in the McGill Pain Questionnaire (Fig. 4), which is discussed in the following section.

AFFECTIVE AND BEHAVIORAL ASPECTS OF PAIN: PSYCHOMETRIC TESTING

In recognition of the multidimensional nature of the experience of pain, Melzack created the McGill Pain Questionnaire (15), which was compiled from a list of adjectives that characterize pain with regard to its sensory, affective, and evaluative attributes (Fig. 5). The sensory properties of pain are discussed above. The affective properties of pain are those qualities which elicit an emotional response from the patient, e.g., tension, fear, and suffering (as from punishment). The evaluative aspect of pain correlates with pain intensity, but additionally reflects the patient's level of tolerance of the pain experience. The McGill Pain Questionnaire is a prototypical psychometric tool engineered specifically for the measurement of the pain experience.

A number of other psychometric tests have been utilized in the study of the af-

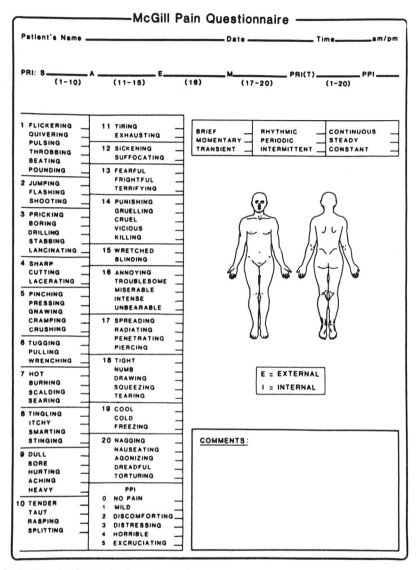

FIG. 4. The McGill Pain Questionnaire. From Melzack, ref. 15, with permission.

fective and behavioral aspects of pain. Notably, the Minnesota Multiphasic Personality Inventory, a widely used tool for psychological assessment, has been examined for its ability to characterize pain states. Sternbach et al. reported statistically significant findings after administering the inventory to patients suffering from chronic pain; affective and behavioral differences were apparent in chronic pain versus acute pain patients, and the presence of litigation correlated with a potentiation of psychoneurotic features compared with patients not involved in such litigation (6). Furthermore, they concluded that the Minnesota Multiphasic Personality Inventory did not differ in patients with "positive" physical findings as compared to patients with "negative" physical findings. The inventory has proven not to be a means of discriminating organic from psychogenic pain (6,16). As a prognosticator of favorable

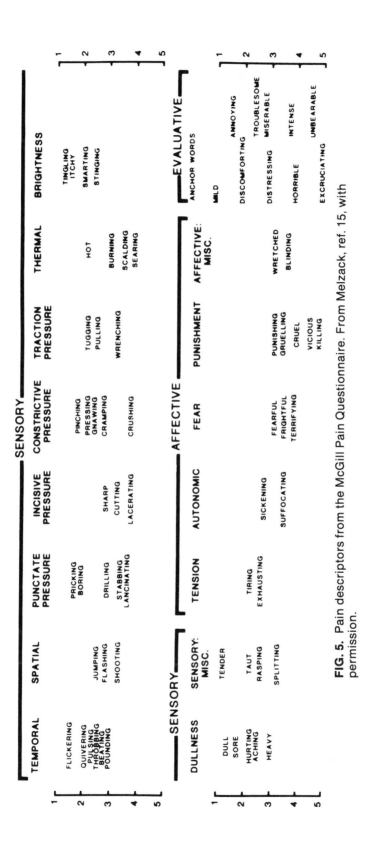

FIG. 5. Pain descriptors from the McGill Pain Questionnaire. From Melzack, ref. 15, with permission.

or unfavorable response of chronic pain patients to treatment, some of the surgical literature supports the use of the Minnesota Multiphasic Personality Inventory for predicting response to surgical interventions such as lumbar disc surgery (17) and chemonucleolysis (18), although response to multidisciplinary pain management (19,20) is not well predicted by the inventory scores. The difference may lie in the way that "favorable" outcome is measured. Return to work does appear to correlate with scores, and the need for vocational rehabilitation may also be predicted (21).

The concept that groups of patients may be separated on the basis of "positive" and "negative" physical findings has focused attention on the qualitative interpretation of the patient physical examination with regard to anatomic versus nonanatomic findings or organic versus nonorganic findings (10). In fact, the outward signs of pain and dysfunction elicited in a patient during the physical examination may indeed reflect complex behavioral phenomenology relating to the patient's psychosocial background and conditioning and may be an index of overall psychobehavioral distress (11). It may offer parameters by which to follow the patient's progress during the course of treatment (12). The use of such findings in predicting treatment outcome should be viewed cautiously.

The use of psychobehavioral indicators as a test of the patient's sincerity or whether or not he is faking his pain, is to be discouraged. On the whole, presumption of a dichotomy between organic and functional pain is viewed by many as being counterproductive to the goal of an effective doctor-patient relationship and effective pain management. True psychogenic pain, or conversion hysteria, is quite rare in the chronic pain patient population (6). An appreciation of pain as a complex interaction between somatogenic pain and overlying psychosocial and behavioral factors permits more effective intervention in the pain problem. Psychometric or psychobehavioral testing therefore should not be used as a screen for accepting or rejecting the validity of patient complaints, nor as a litmus test for discriminating real from imagined pain. On the other hand, a patient may be steered away from certain therapeutic approaches based on psychobehavioral factors. For example, nonorganic physical findings may predict a poor response to surgery and therefore a poor surgical candidate.

MEASURING THE COST OF PAIN

Data from workers' compensation boards are frequently presented in discussions of costs of injuries. For example, the Workers' Compensation Board of New York State paid over a half billion dollars in 1982 for 121,082 claims that had been closed that year, with more than $40 million of that sum being paid for 1,595 back injury claims (medical and hospitalization costs are not included in these figures) (22). Similarly, the Quebec Workers' Compensation Board paid $21 million in medical costs and $129 million in salary compensation for 45,858 claims relating to spinal disorders (23). Extrapolations of such figures leads to staggering estimates of the national costs for chronic pain and injury. Bonica's estimate of 1980 costs for low back pain alone in the United States is $23.2 billion, a composite estimate of direct medical costs, diability costs, lost earnings and services, and mortality (24).

When other chronically painful conditions, such as cancer pain, headache pain, cardiovascular pain, orofacial pain, visceral pain, and neuralgic pain are included in the picture, as Bonica estimates, more than 50 million Americans experience varying periods of disability due to chronic pain, resulting in over 700 million lost work days. The impact on our health care and socioeconomic system is obvious. More efficient utilization of our health care resources must be an obvious goal of effective pain management; i.e., the chronic pain patient must be steered away from costly and often ineffective treatments and particularly those invasive therapies that are administered for questionable indications, and which may result in costly iatrogenic complications. Other necessary improvements include more effective measures aimed at rehabilitation of the injured worker and his reintegration into the workplace, avoidance of communication breakdown with the patient, minimization of doctor-patient game-playing, doctor shopping, and the indiscriminant use of addictive medication. A medical and socioeconomic system as complex as ours certainly is not easily changed, but the recognition of chronic pain as a problem that extends well beyond the patient to include families, employers, insurance companies, and the health care system, is necessary before change can even be contemplated.

MEASURING OUTCOME OF PAIN MANAGEMENT INTERVENTION

Of the many measurements that are made in the assessment of the chronic pain patient, one of the most important is certainly the measurement of outcome. The situation is similar to that of measuring pain with regard to the multiple levels touched on by the pain experience: just as pain is a sensory, affective, and behavioral phenomenon, any measurement of improvement of clinical status must reflect the changes at each of these respective levels. As discussed in a later section, improvement at any one of these levels does not necessarily generalize to improvement at all of these levels.

Given the abundance of chronic pain syndromes and the contribution of many specialties in the management of pain, each specializing in certain pain syndromes or a specific repertoire of modalities for treating pain (e.g., massotherapy, acupuncture, nerve blocks, surgery, stimulation analgesia, etc.), the manner in which success is measured may vary from specialist to specialist. Measuring a response to nerve block therapy may rely heavily on a subjective rating of pain sensation over a very specific window of time (25,26), and other phenomena such as temperature changes and swelling as in the situation of causalgia, or pain thresholds in response to pressure applied to soft tissue trigger points as in the situation of myofascial pain. Using the patient's subjective report of symptomatic improvement and the duration of that improvement makes possible a rating system for assessment of outcome of symptom-directed therapies such as nerve blocks (26). The use of psychometric evaluations such as the Minnesota Multiphasic Personality Inventory (27), and other psychometric testing such as the Community Epidemiological Scale-Depression, and the Personal Adjustment and Role Skills Test, as discussed by Heinrich et al. (28), forms the basis for quantifying psychological and behavioral improvement with therapeutic intervention in chronic pain. Physical rehabilitation programs rely heavily on strength, range of motion, and work capacity assessments in documenting improvement with physical rehabilitation (12,29).

Multidisciplinary pain management centers employ combinations of the types of measures cited above in assessing outcomes of their patients, and include other factors such as return to work, medication use, participation in recreational activities, and utilization of medical care resources (30–33). Often, verbal reports of pain may persist but patients report an improved ability to cope and decrease their utilization of medical resources (34), a decidedly favorable outcome but one that would not be appreciated if only an assessment of pain sensation were made. When one adds to this the recovery of income and services following return to work, and the diminished costs of compensation and of medical care utilization, a cost-benefit analysis is possible, such as that presented by Stieg et al. in which a cost-benefit of greater than $200,000 per patient following completion of a multidisciplinary pain program was reported (35).

ORGANIZATIONAL APPROACHES TO PAIN MANAGEMENT

The patient with chronic pain carries the burden not only of the unpleasant sensations related to his pain, but also the so-called psychosocial consequences thereof—disrupted family life, activity restriction, work interruption, intimidating legal involvement, uncertain income, reinforced pain behaviors, and growing frustration with the failure of the medical system to solve the problems (36–38). This contrasts the patient's previous experience with acute pain in which he has been accustomed to rapid resolution of aches and pains based on the natural history of most such ordinary experiences. Now, he is trapped by symptoms that concurrently result in suffering and disability for which no apparent cause is found (36,39,40). The expense to the patient, let alone to society, who continues to seek to be cured can be enormous (39,40). As the symptoms persist and treatments fail, more doctors are seen, more therapy is provided, and iatrogenic side effects are added to the total symptom complex. The end result can be a patient who overwhelms and frustrates his doctors with demands for office visits, diagnostic tests, alternate therapy, and testimonies to document disability.

Such patients frequently can benefit from an evaluation done by someone outside of the patient's usual cadre of doctors. Although Bonica highlighted the differences between acute and chronic pain in the late 1940s (39), it has not been until the past 20 years that practitioners around the world who were interested in pain management have begun to devote significant time to pain management and to organize themselves into affiliated groups with the intent of more efficiently evaluating and treating patients with chronic pain from many etiologies (40–42). No matter how extensive the group of specialists (from a single practitioner to a university medical center-based pain management center), factors common to all dolorologists are a genuine *interest* in (even fascination with) patients with chronic pain, a practice set up to guarantee sufficient *time* for necessarily thorough evaluation and subsequent treatment planning, and the realistic *attitude* that no one specialist will have all the answers for a given patient. These characteristics rest on a foundation of information that acknowledges the significant differences between acute and chronic pain, and appreciates the need to keep current in neurophysiology, neuropharmacology, the mechanisms of pain, behavioral assessment, etc. These practitioners are likely to keep abreast of the advances in pain management by devoting time to the literature and attending meetings. Frequently, the largest organization of pain specialists exists in academic/university centers where there can be ready collaboration with colleagues of multiple specialties, flexibility in clinical scheduling to allow for attendance at scientific meetings, and collaboration of basic science and clinical research to advance the whole of pain management.

The primary purpose of evaluating any patient is to establish an accurate diagnosis. Only after this can treatment that is appropriate and logical be prescribed. In the patient with a complex chronic pain problem, the accurate diagnosis must include not only the physical generators of the pain but also the consequences of the pain *on* the patient's emotional framework and *in* the patient's life. Thus, the goal of the evaluation that assesses the patient's medical, psychological, occupational, social, and treatment history is to rule in or rule out serious or progressive physical or psychological disease, identify adverse sick role behaviors, discover what "pain" means to the patient, appraise functional impairment, and determine the patient's true motivation to re-achieve "wellness" through compliance with therapy (37,39,43).

Because contemporary pain management may involve an incredible amount of time for treatment initiation and follow-up, it is important that the evaluation scheme used by the practitioner allocates the patients into one of the following groups:

1. Those likely to have enough flexibility left so they can make changes in attitudes, behavior, and lifestyle that will define successful therapy.
2. Those with such extensive psychological investment in the "pain" that this issue must be dealt with before other therapy can be expected to work.
3. Those with binding legal contingencies related to the pain such that interference with therapeutic effects is likely.
4. Those who truly are or should be declared disabled, given the extent of their physical and/or nonphysical "pain" problems.
5. Those who are seeking disability but who do not have any reasonable likelihood of qualifying.
6. Those who are primarily dissatisfied with their entire medical care and will never be pleased no matter what is done.

Therapy planning is not denied to any patient and the patient's classification may change with time and/or treatment. However, frank discussions about all the factors acting on the patient and the realistic expectations of treatment must be provided to the patients in each category.

The philosophical approach to patients with complex problems with chronic pain is maintained by those specialists involved in a referral practice and is fundamental to patient assessment and management. It endorses that not all pain (i.e., acute versus chronic versus cancer pain) can be evaluated and treated with the same protocol because when pain is understood to be an unpleasant sensory and emotional experience (1), the nonsensory aspects of the pain *must* always be concurrently evaluated. There is an understanding that negative laboratory test results do *not* indicate that there is no pain. There is an awareness that challenging the authenticity of the patient's pain is *not* likely to be as productive an approach as is encouraging the patient to become more functional in spite of their residual pain. There is an appreciation that just taking away the physical pain does *not* solve all the consequences of the "pain" in the patient's life. The patient must be active in his own care and expect a decrease in the pain from a number of contributing treatment modalities rather than a singular, magic cure (44,45).

Forms of Organization

Given the complexity of the patient with chronic pain, it is logical that no one physician should try to provide all aspects of the patient's care. Anesthesiologists became involved years ago because of their ability to provide at least prompt, temporary relief of pain by the use of local anesthetics and regional anesthetic procedures. It was apparent, however, that these specialists, as well as many others, did not always have the breadth and depth of knowledge to manage all pain syndromes and that a collaborative interaction among specialists would be of greater benefit to the patient (41). A variety of practice styles have emerged (40,42,43,46).

There are a number of dedicated individuals who have devoted a large percentage of their practice to algology or who have made this a full-time commitment. They apply their specialty training in the evaluation and treatment sequence, and refer patients out of the practice for all consultations. They may choose to evaluate only one particular type of pain patient, working in a so-called syndrome-specific practice (i.e., a neurologist dealing with patients with headaches), or provide only one major therapeutic intervention, thereby embodying the modality-specific practice (i.e., an anesthesiologist doing nerve blocks). The cooperation among specialists is casual and communication is largely by letters of introduction and reply. So, there are headache, low back pain, and orofacial pain specialists and acupuncture, biofeedback, physical therapy, and nerve block services.

The next level of practice is the pain clinic. This may be a free-standing facility, as in a nonhospital doctor's office, or an outpatient hospital clinic. The pain clinic provides patient evaluation and treatment on a daily, outpatient basis and represents a slightly more intimate coordination of services. Because more than one individual and more than one specialty is involved, no one practitioner must make a full-time commitment. Rather, with a few individuals working in a conjoint effort and with each one offering his expertise, the evaluation protocols can be broadened and the treatments offered more numerous than from a single physician. Fundamental treatment programs that involve a number of components being applied in a coordinated fashion can be provided. Programs that provide for patient education and teaching about chronic pain are available in this setting.

The ultimate standards of contemporary pain management are defined by the multidisciplinary or comprehensive pain management center. The very name connotes the interaction of many full-time specialists in a designated locale. Indeed, such organizations have a full-time director and ancillary/support staff; dedicated physical space for patient interviews and examinations, diagnostic testing, plus medical, psychological, and exercise therapy, small group discussions, and storage; ample equipment for diagnosis and therapy; at least a daily outpatient program, if not an inpatient program; and, specific protocols for patient screening, selection, evaluation, and treatment. Patients with all types of pain problems will be seen. Teaching programs for health care professionals, including residents and fellows of diverse specialties, are common as are weekly academic conferences, on-site library facilities, and ongoing research. Although the development of such a comprehensive service requires time and a commitment to improved patient care, the entire team, as proposed by Bonica in the late 1940s, might include neurologists, neurosurgeons, orthopedists, anesthesiologists, psychologists, psychiatrists, social workers, specialized RNs, physiatrists, physical and occupational therapists, and vocational rehabilitation specialists (41).

The advantages of such an enormous association of specialists are many (41,43). The broad-based resource of knowledge and the variety of expertise provide for the necessarily thorough and systematic evaluation of patients. This can be conducted in a time-efficient manner since the necessary personnel are located in one center.

The specialist applies the most reputable therapeutic options, and ongoing research feeds the vitality and creativity of the entire staff. They become experts in pain management, not in the sense of "knowing it all," but rather because of the concentrated experience gained, the integration of many specialty inputs, and sharing perspectives while involved in patient management on a daily basis.

The primary disadvantage of such a system is its expense. Reimbursement is usually not commensurate with the costs of providing such intensive care. There may be a lack of support by administrative personnel who do not appreciate the many benefits of such an endeavor because of preoccupation with economic return. Research and teaching are expensive, yet these vital components must be expected of the pain management center. A second disadvantage is the risk that the patient's care can become fragmented unless a patient manager is appointed so that coordinated care is provided (40,41,43). Many such centers work diligently to educate the referring doctors to be the qualified patient manager with open lines of communication back to the pain center.

FUNCTIONAL ASPECTS OF THE PAIN MANAGEMENT CENTER

The referred patient enters a systematic procedural network that aims to be efficient and thorough, and to satisfy the patient that all issues have been examined to his satisfaction. The primary doctor has likely been stymied by the patient's ongoing symptoms and lack of response to therapy. The patient may be losing confidence in that doctor. The doctor-patient relationship is strained and both parties worry that a frank discussion will so alienate the other that the relationship will be destroyed. A neutral third party, eager to help both reach a new level of understanding, is needed. Unfortunately many referrals come late, after much treatment has failed, when learned behaviors have become entrenched and iatrogenic disease is present.

The pain management center collects pertinent records dealing with the patient's pain problem. Added to these are the center's evaluation instruments. These pencil and paper tests collect the multitude of information needed to establish the pain, drug and treatment, general medical, occupational, and psychosocial history of the patient and also provide attitude assessment and a screening for major psychological dysfunction. Because standard protocols are followed to yield information for the database in a consistent manner which is familiar to the pain center staff, the process is highly productive.

Because there is no single test that can quantitate "pain," identify every organic generator, or discriminate the percentage of physical from psychological pain, the three traditional tools of patient assessment—history-taking, physical examination, and laboratory tests—will be relied on. It is crucial that the doctor acknowledge that the lack of physical findings does *not* automatically indicate the presence of major psychopathology as an explanation for the ongoing pain. Also, he must realize that negative laboratory results do not by default indicate the absence of "real," i.e., physical pain. Often, challenging the authenticity of the patient's pain only provokes more obnoxious pain behavior which leads to further deterioration of the doctor-patient relationship.

The history-taking component is vital because the patient's story told the patient's way must be heard by someone. The pain specialist, with his interest and the attitude that everything may be important, can win the patient's confidence just by being a good listener. Having reviewed the patient's records will allow for a directed interview, but not one so rigid that the patient feels suffocated. This same freedom of discussion will be equally crucial at the end of the evaluation process because the patient *must* be given the opportunity to reveal what his understanding of the pain is—what does he think it's due to, what does he think should be done?

As the sophistication of the pain practice grows, the greater will be the interest shown in the details of the patient's workup, the capability for extensive physical and psychosocial assessment, and the availability of contemporary laboratory evaluation tests. In essence, the medically oriented pain specialist gathers information from the record review and history, physical examination, and laboratory studies, whereas the psychology specialists have a parallel evaluation scheme in which the psychological interview replaces physical examination and psychometric/neuropsychological tests replace laboratory investigation.

The purpose of the evaluation process is to arrive at a diagnosis of the patient's entire pain condition from which a logical treatment program can be devised. Reality dictates that the correct diagnosis is not made every time, nor is every patient "cured." Because the treatment program must address the many needs important to the patient, the patient's choices for treatment options based on a thorough explanation of the likely contribution of each to his condition will be paramount. The patient must live with the consequences of his choices and realistic expectations of the treatment must be discussed frankly and openly with him and his significant others.

Monitoring the Patients

The realistic goals of treatment, as they must be explained to the patient, are to decrease the frequency and intensity of the pain as much as possible (N.B.—elimination of the pain is not the first and foremost goal), enhance the patient's ability to cope with (live with) residual pain by providing insight into the physical and nonphysical contributions to the pain and striving for a degree of environmental control, and encourage the patient to achieve and maintain the highest functional level possible. A combination of pain management techniques will be necessary.

Pain can be reduced by the judicious use of medications, nerve blocks, surgery, and nervous system stimulation techniques. As pain reduction begins to occur, the patient must be encouraged to gradually increase his participation in productive activity. Then, as the pain is decreased and activity is restored, the patient with chronic pain is likely to be confronted with the reality that, as his doctors have been telling him, some portion of the "pain" will be slower to disappear and may in fact not change at all. This patient will require supportive therapy that may range along a continuum from a strong, understanding family system to formal psychotherapy. Ultimately as pain is decreased and physical and psychosocial restoration are manifest, the patient may qualify for rehabilitation to part-time or full-time work at or away from home.

The fundamental idea is that just as no one practitioner is likely to have all the answers for the chronic patient, neither is it likely that any option available when applied in singular fashion will be totally therapeutic. Rather, each component chosen in the treatment program contributes a percentage of decrease in the pain, symptoms, and suffering, such that the end result is a better quality of life for the patient.

Analgesic medications that are generically prescribed for pain and used long past the expected period of safety or reasonable effectiveness can add drug-related side effects to the patient's symptom profile. When pain persists as well, logically the medications must be changed. Safer combinations of nonaddictive medications are to be recommended (47–49). The lesser potency of these drugs does not trivialize the pain complaints, but rather acknowledges that medications are but one component of a treatment program.

Invasive treatments such as surgery or nerve blocks are used in patients for specific reasons. The patient must make decisions about such therapy based on a presentation of his diagnosis, and the expected result of and rationale for the application of the proposed procedures. Given the invasive nature of these therapies, scar tissue, a failed procedure, and even adverse consequences might result which make the "pain" worse. Sites of neural injury can become foci for pain generation (50). Synaptic areas in the pain transmission system within the central nervous system can be so chronically stimulated that reflex activity there is established which spontaneously triggers pain even in the absence of afferent input from peripheral somatic sites (50).

The physical consequences of pain can be devastating (7,36,51). Activity reduction may result in decreased tone, bulk, and strength of muscles; decreased range of motion of major joints; weight gain; postural limitations; decreased energy and intolerance of physical activity; and unproductive emotions such as anger, frustration, and desperation. As pain treatment results in lessened discomfort, and when the workup fails to reveal that the patient's ongoing pain represents ongoing tissue damage, the patient must cooperate with physical restoration programs. The purpose of graduated, guided therapy is to reverse the detrimental physical consequences of prolonged inactivity. For short periods of time (2 to 6 weeks), formal physical therapy may be necessary to teach the patient the proper techniques for exercise, to demonstrate and encourage compliance, and to provide follow-up such that exercise of a progressive nature can be recommended (52). Numerous authors have found no correlation between a patient's complaint of pain and the performance of prescribed exercises and physical activity (53–55).

The provocation of the patient to increased activity in spite of pain is, again, an acknowledgment that chronic pain does not have a direct, biological, signal-of-harm function as does acute pain, and that chronic pain alone is not necessarily a reason to curtail activity. The prescription of exercise is not a denial of the severity of the pain, however, but rather a pain-reduction and coping technique with the expected result of increased function without a major increase in pain. The patient improves his fitness, finds great satisfaction in the addition of activity to his daily routine, and gains a sense of mastery over some of the pain. The initial goal of formal physical therapy should be to increase range of motion and restore strength and endurance for common activities of daily living and then approximate the more aggressive, work-related activities. The patient's cooperation with physical therapy may be an early indication of his true motivation to improve through his adopting self-help attitudes (44,45,54,56).

The patient must deal with the reality that some of the chronic "pain" will not disappear. Even though the physical generators are diminished, there still may be interpersonal, vocational, socioeconomic, and legal consequences of the patient's pain. Thus, the patient has many emotions to deal with and management of anxiety-depression and stress are frequently recommended concurrent with other aspects of the treatment program (43). The basic idea is to help the patient cope with his residual pain, i.e., to improve the quality of his life by providing techniques far beyond the practitioner's hollow recommendation to "go home and learn to live with it." Thus, the patient's social support network must be evaluated, starting with the patient's individual strengths and proceeding through those of his spouse and family and beyond into the local community and his doctors (37,38). Formal psychotherapy on an individual or group basis may be necessary (43).

The most desired consequence of pain management is physical and psychosocial rehabilitation to such a point that the patient can return to employment (56,57). What must happen before this can logically occur is the restoration of home-based activity and social reintegration. Then, a return to work serves as the ultimate manifestation of the patient's increasing his function and coping with his pain. Unfortunately, return to work is held out as the gold standard but is truly a lesser index of successful overall therapy because of the innumerable barriers in the legal and compensation system that may complicate achieving this enviable goal (40,58). Deyo et al. suggest that there is a window of time during which many factors must come together so that a return to work is manifest (59). Taking the pain away does not necessarily solve all of the consequences of chronic pain in the patient's life or predict a successful return to work status (7,33,37). Catchlove et al. showed that the best results are obtained when plans for returning a patient to work are included early in the treatment goals statement and a target date is set (60).

There is substantial evidence that multidisciplinary pain centers make a useful and important contribution in the management of complex pain syndromes (33,46,61–64). The follow-up of patients treated for chronic pain generally shows that the shorter the period of follow-up, the better the results. There are clearly those patients who benefit from the syndrome-specific approach and from modality-specific therapy offered by single practitioners. As the complexity of the patient's problems with pain increases or as the structure of a pain facility becomes more comprehensive, the success rate of treatment may fall off. However, improving a percentage of the patients referred, remembering that they are selected for referral because of the difficulty of their overall pain problem, is a significant achievement. The schedule for follow-up may be at regular intervals or progressive as the patient accepts more and more responsibility for the treatment program. Published studies indicate that most problems encountered by patients seen in a pain management center are behavioral and socioeconomic rather than physical (36,37,40,65). An organization of specialists confronts and overcomes many of the obstacles of the thorough evaluation and treatment planning for patients with chronic pain. With the emphasis on improving the patient's quality of life and a mutual understanding of what is possible, a modicum of success can be achieved for the majority of patients.

PAIN MANAGEMENT AND OPTIMIZATION OF LIFE QUALITY

Pain is the most widely shared of human afflictions (40). Bonica et al. wrote that beyond disabling disease and nutritional problems, chronic pain is one of the most important and pressing issues of modern health care (41). Chronic pain is a frequent cause of suffering and disability and seriously impairs the quality of life of millions of people throughout the world (36,39,41,65,66). Furthermore, not just the patient is affected. The family and society share indirectly in the severe physical, emotional, social, and economic stresses of the chronic pain (7). The pain disrupts the family's lifestyle, financial resources, and routines. Fitness and activity are replaced with a progressive deterioration of physical conditioning that is characterized by fatigue, inability to do work, and inactivity. Sleep becomes restless and fitful. Time and money are spent in medical evaluation and treatment. Interpersonal relationships suffer from strain, excessive worry, and innuendo such that the patient becomes isolated. Suspicion arises, given the vague diagnoses and nonprovable subjective complaints. The patient grows desperate and may resort to excessive medication or substance use; dangerous, unproven surgery; neurolytic nerve blocks; quackery; or suicide.

There are risks that patients with chronic pain that is poorly understood or managed will suffer iatrogenic consequences of therapy. The prolonged application in chronic pain treatment of the many therapeutic modalities that are so beneficial and familiar in acute pain management can eventually add to the patient's problems. Patients can develop signs of drug interaction, toxicity, or withdrawal, as analgesics and sedatives are continuously used or rearranged. Multiple operative procedures can result in scar tissue formation that only becomes another site of pain generation. Recommendations to rest-and-it-will-get-better from the time of the acute injury, when followed for too long, result in physical deconditioning, unnecessary bedrest, imposed activity restriction, and the entrenchment of learned behaviors that adversely influence the patient's attitude and lifestyle.

The patient's pain customarily will be primarily reduced with some combination of appropriate medications, judicious choices about appropriate surgery, the use of therapeutic nerve blocks in selected cases, and counterstimulation techniques such as acupuncture, transcutaneous electrical nerve stimulation, massage, and ultrasound. A key concept is that each component of therapy chosen is expected to contribute a percentage of decrease in the total pain. Any option used alone would likely result in an insignificant degree of pain reduction, but when two or three or four are used concurrently, the additive result is pain reduction that is rated by the patient as worthwhile enough to justify all the energy involved in applying the treatment. Once the pain's intensity and frequency decline, the patient is encouraged to resume or increase his physically oriented activity. This allows physical rehabilitation, relieves the emotional stress of isolation and the disruption of daily routines, and puts the patient in an advantageous position to confront the sociovocational rehabilitation system. In summary, the patient with chronic pain requires a coordinated program of management consisting of choices from the reputable, available treatment options that are appropriate for his diagnosis.

Rehabilitation is defined as a process of restoring one to a former capacity or to a condition of health or useful and constructive activity. Just taking the physical pain away does not instantly or permanently solve all of the patient's consequential problems with "the pain." If this were so, there would be no need in treatment for more than the above-suggested sequence of medications-surgery-nerve blocks-stimulation techniques. Clearly then, the patient with chronic pain who suffers a significant alteration in lifestyle, a failure to show progressive improvement, and the inability to make realistic plans for his future, needs to be involved in a rehabilitation process.

The need for a psychosocial assessment of the patient was explained previously.

Basically, one is looking at the patient with an intent to more than rule out the presence of psychiatric illness. One is trying to assess the nonphysical factors that are operative in the patient's pain; analyze the positive and negative consequences of the pain; compare his behavioral response and level of function now to other periods of disruption or change in his life; and clarify his beliefs about, understandings of, and expectations for the pain. With this information at hand, a logical treatment/management program that involves the numerous psychotherapeutic interventions available can be offered to the patient (40,41,43). It is crucial that the patient understands his diagnosis and the reasons why the recommended treatment is logical before he can be expected to make informed decisions about therapy. Common options of treatment within this realm include individual, group, or family counseling; biofeedback; relaxation training; hypnosis; and formal psychotherapy (43). By these means, the social reintegration of the patient becomes an achievable goal of therapy (37).

The system of vocational rehabilitation is complex. So enormous is the task of rehabilitating patients to return to work status that hardly any method does it well. Sophisticated agencies will do elaborate assessments of the patient to determine their physical and mental aptitudes for work but can do little to match the patient with available openings in that field, especially if it means relocating the family to another community, more years of school work, or a marked reduction in pay (21). Compensation for pain may or may not be an influential factor in a patient's response to treatment, but the receipt of money for up to 500 weeks for pain complaints is easily perceived as a deterrent to motivating the patient to be aggressive in reestablishing his employment (7,56,58,67). The occasional legal hassles that workers and employers engage in over culpability for injury and the payment of medical bills and compensation clearly affect the patient's quality of life in an adverse way.

Prolonged inactivity over weeks to months results in physical deconditioning (7,51). The physical consequences of pain can only fuel the patient's desperation and frustration that have developed because the pain continues in spite of repeated medical evaluation, diagnostic tests, and treatment regimens. A crucial endpoint of the patient's thorough workup must be the determination that the ongoing pain is *not* related to ongoing tissue damage, because, if this is true, the chronic pain should no longer be interpreted to mean that the patient must stop activity. Furthermore, many patients have tried restricting their activity for weeks to months prior to pain clinic evaluation with no major change in the pain or at least no improvement.

Thus, one thrust of the treatment must be to reverse the state of deconditioning. This will generally require weeks to months of progressive physical exercise. So that no further time will be wasted, the patient should be enrolled in a formal physical therapy program for 3 to 4 weeks (this is an arbitrary amount of time!). This is recommended so that the patient can have a thorough physical assessment after which an exercise program that addresses the patient's unique physical needs can be explained and demonstrated. This participation under guidance will insure the proper performance of exercise right from the start. The patient will benefit from the therapist's feedback about his progress. Obviously, the patient must be motivated to cooperate with this mode of therapy (33,44,52,62). This is most likely to be manifest if the patient had a pain assessment and then an explanation with which he is satisfied. He must be so motivated that he performs exercise on a daily basis at home and in spite of the lack of all the conducive trappings of the physical therapist's office.

The practitioner should be prepared to defend his recommendation that the patient with chronic pain be more active. This recommendation is not a denial of the reality nor the severity of the pain. Rather, it is an admission that although little may be done about the complaints of chronic pain, the patient's *reaction*—both physical and emotional—to that pain need not be inactivity and frustration. Studies by numerous researchers have failed to show a positive correlation between a patient's activity level or performance of exercise with complaints of pain intensity (53–55). The ultimate goal is to gain a marked increase in activity, not just for activity's sake, but in a manner that the patient finds productive and satisfying.

A modern response to the combined needs of organized physical rehabilitation and realistic return to work assessment is embodied in work hardening programs (29). An assessment of the referred patient's medical and psychological status as well as the physical and mental demands of the patient's usual job is done. While the patient receives 2 to 4 weeks of progressive physical therapy and group counseling, he is also involved in workplace simulation activity. The end result of such goal-specific treatment is the dual achievement of the restoration of physical capabilities of the patient, as well as his confidence about performing his job. With this approach, uncertainty about his work performance is allayed before his return to work, as compared to the more typical scenario where 100% performance from a worker is demanded on day number one back to work when he has been away from the job for a lengthy period of time. There is no realistic way that the physical demands of an 8-hour workday can be approximated at home where the patient "putters around the house."

The referring physician performs a crucial function in realizing that another specialist or group of specialists may be more appropriate to manage a given patient's pain. He may have done all that is necessary in referring the patient to a pain management facility. Since most pain centers send the patients back through the referring physician to the patient's local community, the referring doctor should remain in the patient's network of health care workers. He may no longer be directly involved in the patient's care but will be a valuable resource. The referring physician should be sent a complete letter of consultation so that he will understand the patient's diagnosis and the rationale for the treatment options chosen.

The patient's primary physician is instrumental in the total management of the patient. This crucial team member must thoroughly understand the patient's diagnosis, the physical and nonphysical factors involved, the rationale for the treatments chosen, and the predicted contribution of each option in the control of the patient's pain. This trusted physician may be the one who ultimately helps the patient truly see what is being offered and why it is the most reasonable approach to the management of the pain. This doctor will provide the serial evaluation of the patient and should be the most discriminating as to progression of a chronic disease or the presence of new pathology, physical or not, that may require re-referral. He should be able to manage flare-ups of pain above the patient's baseline with appropriate therapy, but know the patient and his life situation so well that "pain" due to changes in the patient's vocational or social status will be reacted to sensitively and in a pattern consistent with the recommendations from the consultants.

There will be patients who are declared disabled and for whom this status is reasonable given their age, physical or psychological condition, or realistic chances of rehabilitation. This patient's quality of life can be severely affected when he is hassled repeatedly in waiting for a declaration of disability or when maintaining as productive a lifestyle as possible after this status is clarified. Those patients who are inappropriately seeking disability must have the reality of their status quickly made plain to them and be encouraged to cooperate with pain management protocols and rehabilitation. Difficult decisions have to be made about the allocation of resources for patients with chronic pain. Some advocate closed-ended compensation which gives the patient a finite period of time during which benefits will be received, but also helps them maintain a goal-oriented approach toward the application of rehabilitative therapy. In essence, the patient must understand and agree with the diagnosis of his total condition and take an active posture in the compliance with all therapeutic recommendations.

SUMMARY

The experience of pain is universal, serving in large part a protective role by promoting withdrawal and avoidance responses to environmental elements which threaten potential tissue damage and destruction of that organism which perceives the pain. This protective role is most clear in the setting of acute pain, wherein tissue damage, acute pathophysiology, and pain are intimately linked. In the setting of chronic pain, however, this protective role is no longer relevant since ongoing tissue damage and acute pathophysiology are not necessary conditions to the pain experience. It is in this context that pain has an adverse effect on quality of life by disrupting work, leisure time, sleep, and social relationships.

Pain is a sensory phenomenon, but vastly transcends the sensory experience by producing alterations in affect and behavior as well. Any effort to analyze pain and its repercussions must take into account this multidimensional nature of pain. Measurement, or quantification, of the pain experience, must likewise reflect at least these three dimensions of the pain experience. Pain sensation may be measured with regard to intensity and quality, by the use of a number of pain scales, and by selection from lists of descriptive words which characterize the nature of pain. Affective and behavioral factors may be examined by use of psychometric inventories, with which the impact of pain management interventions may be assessed. The use of such psychometric testing is of little value as a discriminator between "real" pain and "psychogenic" pain, since true conversion hysteria is rare in the chronic pain population and most chronic pain situations involve a complex interplay of somatogenic as well as psychosocial factors. The assessment of clinical improvement following pain management intervention involves quantification of the above variables as well as assessment of functional (return to work) as well as economic (compensation, utilization of the medical system) factors.

The goal of pain management is to improve quality of life by intervening in such a way as to improve subjective and objective measures of the pain experience. There are pain clinics which may specialize in certain pain syndromes or specific treatment modalities, and employ those measurements of treatment response which best reflect the benefit of that specific treatment modality. However, a more global view of the impact of pain on life quality mandates a multidisciplinary approach to the pain problem, with treatment modalities directed at symptom management (directed at the sensory aspect of chronic pain), psychobehavioral intervention (directed at affective and behavioral factors), and physical and vocational therapy (directed at the functional and work aspects of chronic pain). Such a multidisciplinary approach requires specialists in each of the respective areas noted. Correct and timely exchange of information is crucial to the working of such a multidisciplinary team of specialists and requires a coordinator, or manager, of the pain intervention effort, who in many cases can and should be the patient's referring physician, or primary medical doctor. With the participation of many specialists coordinated by a team manager, the efforts directed at management of the patient's pain problem are far more likely to have an impact on the patient's quality of life than the efforts of a single physician or specialist. This concept lies at the heart of multidisciplinary management of chronic pain.

REFERENCES

1. IASP subcommittee on taxonomy. Classification of chronic pain. *Pain* 1986 (Suppl. 3):S217.
2. Fordyce WE. Environmental factors in the genesis of back pain. In: Bonica JJ, Liebeskind JC, Albe-Fessard DG. *Advances in pain research and therapy,* vol 3. New York: Raven Press, 1979:659–666.
3. Zweibel NR. Measuring quality of life near the end of life. *JAMA* 1988;260:839–840.
4. Carron H, DeGood DE, Tait R. A comparison of low back pain patients in the United States and New Zealand: Psychosocial and economic factors affecting severity of disability. *Pain* 1985;21:77–89.
5. Bortz WM. The disuse syndrome. *West J Med* 1984;141:691–694.
6. Sternbach RA, Wolf SR, Murphy RW, Akeson WH. Traits of pain patients: The low-back "loser." *Psychosomatics* 1973;14:226–229.
7. Strang JP. The chronic disability syndrome. In: Aronoff GM, ed. *Evaluation and treatment of chronic pain.* Baltimore: Urban and Schwarzenberg, 1985;603–623.
8. Crook J, Tunks E. Defining the "chronic pain syndrome": An epidemiological method. In: Fields HL, Dubner R, Cervero F. *Advances in pain research and therapy,* vol. 9. New York: Raven Press, 1985;871–877.
9. Bromm B. *Pain measurement in man.* New York: Elsevier Science Publishers, 1984;3–13.
10. Waddell G, McCulloch JA, ZKummel E, Venner RM. Nonorganic physical signs in low-back pain. *Spine* 1980;5:117–125.
11. Korbon GA, DeGood DE, Schroeder ME, Schwartz DP, Shutty MS. The development of a somatic amplification rating scale for low-back pain. *Spine* 1987;12:787–791.
12. Khalil TM, Goldberg ML, Asfour SS, Moty EA, Rosomoff RS, Rosomoff HL. Acceptable maximum effort (AME): A psychophysical measure of strength in back pain patients. Spine 1987;12:372–376.
13. Wolskee P. Clinical and experimental pain assessment. In: Wu WH, Smith LG, eds. *Pain management: Assessment and treatment of chronic and acute syndromes.* New York: Human Sciences Press 1987;83–101.
14. Huskisson EC. Visual analog scales. In: Melzack R, ed. *Pain management and assessment.* New York: Raven Press, 1983;33–37.
15. Melzack R. *Pain measurement and assessment.* New York: Raven Press, 1983;41–61.
16. Rook JC, Pesch RN, Keeler EC. Chronic pain and the questionable use of the Minnesota Multiphasic Personality Inventory. *Arch Phys Med Rehabil* 1981;62:373–376.
17. Pondaag W, Oostdam EMM. Predicting the outcome of lumbar disc surgery by means of preoperative psychological testing. In: Bonica JJ, Liebeskind JC, Albe-Fessard DG, eds, *Advances in pain research and therapy,* vol. 3. New York: Raven Press, 1979;713–717.
18. Wiltse LL, Rocchio PD. Preoperative psychological tests as predictors of success of chemonucleolysis in the treatment of the low-back syndrome. *J Bone Joint Surg* 1975;57-A:478–483.
19. Moore JE, Armentrout DP, Parker JC, Kivlahan DR. Empirically derived pain-patient MMPI subgroups: Prediction of treatment outcome. *J Behav Med* 1986;9:51–63.
20. Cummings C, Evanski PM, Debendetti MJ, Anderson EE, Waugh TR. Use of the MMPI to predict outcome of treatment for chronic pain. In: Bonica JJ, Liebeskind JC, Albe-Fessard DG. *Advances in pain research and therapy.* New York: Raven Press, 1979;667–670.
21. Hammonds W, Brena SF. Pain classification and vocational evaluation in chronic pain states. In: Melzack R, ed. *Pain management and assessment.* New York: Raven Press, 1983;197–203.
22. Haddad GH. Analysis of 2932 worker's compensation back injury cases, the impact on cost to the system. *Spine* 1987;12:765–769.
23. Spitzer WO, Leblanc FE, Dupuis M. Scientific approach to the assessment and management of activity-related spinal disorders. *Spine* 1987 (Suppl. 1);12:S9–S59.
24. Bonica JJ. The nature of the problem. In: Carron H, McLaughlin RE, eds. *Management of low back pain.* Boston: J Wright, PSG Inc. 1982;1–15.

25. Abram SE, Anderson RA, Maitra-d'Cruze AM. Factors predicting short-term outcome of nerve blocks in the management of chronic pain. *Pain* 1981;10:323–330.
26. Evans PJD. Simple rating system for assessing treatment outcome in chronic pain patients. In: Fields HL, Dubner R, Cervero F, eds. *Advances in pain research and therapy,* vol. 9. New York: Raven Press, 1985;377–385.
27. Roberts AH, Reinhardt L. The behavioral management of chronic pain: Long-term followup with comparison groups. *Pain* 1980;8:151–162.
28. Heinrich RL, Cohen MJ, Naliboff BD, Collins GA, Bonebakker AD. Comparing physical and behavior therapy for chronic low back pain on physical abilities, psychological distress, and patient's perceptions. *J Behav Med* 1985;8:61–78.
29. May VR. Work capacity evaluation and work hardening: Process and application in private sector rehabilitation. In: Deutsch PM, Sawyer HW, eds. *A guide to rehabilitation.* New York: Matthew Bender, 1987;6A1–6A46.
30. Seres JL, Newman RI. Results of treatment of chronic low-back pain at the Portland Center. *J Neurosurg* 1976;45:32–36.
31. Swanson DW, Swenson WM, Maruta T, McPhee MC. Program for managing chronic pain. I. Program description and characteristics of patients. *Mayo Clin Proceedings* 1976;51:401–411.
32. Malec J, Cayner JJ, Harvey RF, Timming RC. Pain management: Long-term followup of an inpatient program. *Arch Phys Med Rehabil* 1981;62:369–372.
33. Sturgis ET, Schaefer CA, Sikora TL. Pain center followup-study of treated and untreated patients. *Arch Phys Med Rehabil* 1984;65:301–303.
34. Newman RI, Seres JL, Yospe LP, Garlington B. Multidisciplinary treatment of chronic pain: Long-term followup of low-back patients. *Pain* 1978;4:283–292.
35. Stieg RL, Williams RC, Timmermans-Williams G, Tafuro F, Gallagher LA. Cost benefits of inter-disciplinary chronic pain treatment. *Clin J Pain* 1986;1:189–193.
36. Crook J. Rideout E, Browne G. The prevalence of pain complaints in a general population. *Pain* 1984;18:299–314.
37. Roy R. Pain clinics: Reassessment of objectives and outcomes. *Arch Phys Med Rehabil* 1984;65:448–451.
38. Rowat KM, Knafl KA. Living with chronic pain: The spouse's perspective. *Pain* 1985;23:259–271.
39. Bonica JJ. Introduction. *Evaluation and treatment of chronic pain.* Aronoff GM, ed. Baltimore: Urban & Schwarzenberg, 1985;xxxi–xliv.
40. Ng LKY (ed.). New approaches to treatment of chronic pain: A review of multidisciplinary pain clinics and pain centers. NIDA Research Monograph 36, May 1981.
41. Bonica JJ, Benedetti C, Murphy TM. Functions of pain clinics and pain centers. In: Swerdlow M, ed. *Relief of intractable pain.* Oxford: Elsevier Science publishers B.V., 1983;65–84.
42. Kroening RJ. Pain clinics structure and function. *Sem Anesth* 1985;4(3):231–236.
43. Rowlingson JC, Toomey TC. Multidisciplinary approaches to the management of chronic pain. In: Ghia JN, ed. *The multidisciplinary pain center.* Boston: Kluwer Academic Publishers, 1988;45–74.
44. Aronoff GM. The role of the pain center in the treatment for intractable suffering and disability resulting from chronic pain. In; Aronoff GM, ed. *Evaluation and treatment of chronic pain.* Baltimore: Urban & Schwarzenberg, 1985;503–510.
45. Williams RC, Stieg RL. Validity and therapeutic efficacy of individual patient goal attainment procedures in a chronic pain treatment center. *Clin J Pain* 1987;2:219–228.
46. Hallett EC, Pilowsky I. The response to treatment in a multidisciplinary pain clinic. *Pain* 1982;12:365–374.
47. Khoury GF. Therapeutic use of pain relieving drugs in chronic pain patients. *Sem Anesth* 1985;4(4):300–304.
48. Monks R, Merskey H. Psychotherapeutic drugs. In: Wall PD, Melzack R, ed. *Textbook of pain.* New York: Churchill-Livingstone, 1985;526–537.
49. Aronoff GM, Evans WO. Pharmacological management of chronic pain. In: Aronoff GM, ed. *Evaluation and treatment of chronic pain.* Baltimore: Urban & Schwarzenberg, 1985;435–449.
50. Abram SE. Pain pathways and mechanisms. *Sem Anesth* 1985;4(4):264–274.
51. Wilensky J. Physiatric approach to chronic pain. In: Aronoff GM, ed. *Evaluation and treatment of chronic pain.* Baltimore: Urban & Schwarzenberg, 1985;199–230.
52. Dolce JJ, Crocker MF, Moletteire C, Doleys DM. Exercise quotas, anticipatory concern and self-efficacy expectancies in chronic pain: A preliminary report. *Pain* 1986;24:365–372.
53. Fordyce W, McMahon R, Rainwater G, et al. Pain complaints—Exercise performance relationship in chronic pain. *Pain* 1981;10:311–321.
54. Fordyce WE, Lansky D, Calsyn DA, et al. Pain measurement and pain behavior. *Pain* 1984;18:53–69.
55. Skevington S. Activities as indices of illness behaviour in chronic pain. *Pain* 1983;15:295–307.
56. Dworkin RH, Handlin DS, Richlin DM, et al. Unraveling the effects of compensation, litigation, and employment on treatment response in chronic pain. *Pain* 1985;23:49–59.

57. Mayer TG, Gatchel RJ, Kishino N, et al. Objective assessment of spine function following industrial injury: A prospective study with comparison group and one-year follow-up. *Spine* 1985;10:482–493.
58. Carron H. Compensation aspects of low back claims. In: Carron H, McLaughlin RE, eds. *Management of low back pain*. Littleton, MA: John Wright–PSG Inc., 1982;17–26.
59. Deyo RA, Tsui-Wu Y. Descriptive epidemiology of low-back pain and its related medical care in the United States. *Spine* 1987;12:264–268.
60. Catchlove R, Cohen K. Effects of a directive return to work approach in the treatment of workman's compensation patients with chronic pain. *Pain* 1982;14:181–191.
61. McArthur DL, Cohen MJ, Gottlieb HJ, et al. Treatment chronic low back pain. II. Long-term follow-up. *Pain* 1987;29:23–38.
62. Lutz RW, Silbret M. Olshan N. Treatment outcome and compliance with therapeutic regimens: Long-term follow-up of a multidisciplinary pain program. *Pain* 1983;17:301–308.
63. Aronoff GM, Evans WO, Enders PL. A review of follow-up studies of multidisciplinary pain units. *Pain* 1983;16:1–11.
64. Guck TP, Skultety M, Meilman PW, Dowd ET. Multidisciplinary pain center follow-up study: Evaluation with a no-treatment control group. *Pain* 1985;21:295–306.
65. Margolis RB, Zimny GH, Miller D, Taylor JM. Internists and the chronic pain patient. *Pain* 1984;20:151–156.
66. Oosterhuis WW. Early screening of pain to prevent it from becoming intractable. *Pain* 1984;20:193–200.
67. Mendelson G. Compensation, pain complaints, and psychological disturbance. *Pain* 1984;20:169–177.

Quality of Life Assessments in Clinical Trials, edited by B. Spilker. Raven Press, Ltd. New York © 1990.

23

Cardiovascular Surgery Patients

James M. Raczynski and Albert Oberman

Division of General and Preventive Medicine, Department of Medicine, University of Alabama at Birmingham, Birmingham, Alabama 35294

Quality of life is being examined in patients receiving a variety of cardiovascular procedures, including: cardiac transplants (1,2), valvular surgeries (3,4), angioplasty (5), and other types of open heart procedures (6). Out of the estimated 2.46 million cardiovascular operations and procedures conducted in 1985, the 230,000 coronary artery bypass graft operations were by far the most frequent (7), and this number is estimated to be increasing each year. Prolonged life with coronary artery bypass graft surgery was demonstrated first for those patients who have left main coronary artery disease (8–10) and later for those who have triple-vessel disease and left ventricular dysfunction (11). Yet the enhanced survival for other patient groups remains controversial, and the financial cost of coronary artery bypass graft is high (12). In addition, almost 9% of 743 coronary artery bypass graft patients were found to require reoperation within 15 years, substantially adding to overall surgery costs (13). Some patients require reoperation for a third time or more (14). Since the number of coronary artery bypass graft procedures performed annually is increasing, the cost of these procedures is escalating, and, for most patients, the procedure does not prolong life, a strong argument exists for emphasizing changes in quality of life after coronary artery bypass graft surgery.

With the rapid changes in technical aspects of the procedures and advances in medical treatment, we have confined our review to coronary artery bypass graft studies published since 1980. We have restricted tabulations to those studies representing data on at least 100 coronary artery bypass graft patients and have excluded analyses not explicitly dealing with quality of life issues.

RECOMMENDED ASSESSMENT METHODS FOR QUALITY OF LIFE AMONG CARDIOVASCULAR SURGERY PATIENTS

As discussed by others (15,16), no specific measures have been developed for assessing the quality of life of cardiovascular surgery patients. However, a variety of standardized instruments are already available for assessing quality of life in general, and these may be used in the assessment of cardiovascular surgery patients. Assessment approaches should include those domains which are expected to be relevant for the particular types of patients being examined. For cardiovascular surgery patients, the major domains include psychological and neuropsychological functioning, social interactions, functional capacity, and economic measures.

For psychological and neuropsychological functioning, individual measures include: global satisfaction and mood; specific measures of anxiety, depression, and focus on symptoms; and neurological and cognitive changes. Psychological measures to quantify global changes in well-being and emotional changes are available, including the Psychological General Well-Being Index (17). This index also provides specific measures of anxiety, depression, perceptions or focus on health, and three other subscales. The State-Trait Anxiety Inventory (18) and the Center for Epidemiologic Studies-Depression scale (19) are also recommended as measures of anxiety and depression. Neurologic variables as well as standardized neuropsychological testing should be evaluated. Comprehensive neuropsychological assessment batteries are available to fully assess subtle changes in cognitive abilities, including the Halstead-Reitan Battery and Allied Procedures (20,21) and the Luria-Nebraska Neuropsychological Battery (22). However, the time requirements of these comprehensive test batteries make them unfeasible as measures of quality of life. Nonetheless, quality of life batteries should include at least a few standardized neuropsychological tests, such as the Reitan Trail Making Test (23), a measure of attention and concentration, and the Wechsler Memory Scale (24,25), a measure of attention and immediate, short-term, long-term, and distant memory.

Changes in familial and nonfamilial social interactions should be assessed. Social interaction may be measured by standardized self-report instruments such as the Social Participation Index (26) and the Social Support Questionnaire (27). In assessing social interactions, measures should span not only the degree to which patients are engaging in social activities but also their level of satisfaction with activities. For family social interactions, the degree of protectiveness shown by family members toward patients also appears to be a relevant variable which some investigators (28) have assessed through specific self-report questionnaires.

Evaluation of functional capacity should include changes in global functional capacity as well as capacity to perform and satisfaction in specific functional areas such as work, avocational activities, and sexual performance. Objective measures of functional capacity should be assessed through procedures such as graded exercise testing, general fitness testing, or a 6-minute walk test (29). Standardized measures of functional status are also available, such as the New York Heart Association (NYHA) functional classification (30), the Canadian Cardiovascular Society classification (31), or the Specific Activity Scale (32). Functional status in particular areas may also be assessed with standardized measures, such as with work performance and satisfaction (33).

Measures of economic factors should include: global cost-effectiveness variables; change in standard of living; and the vocational impact of the surgery, involving not only work status but also expectations about work since patients may voluntarily stop working if they have sufficient economic resources. Methods are certainly available for examining the cost-effectiveness of cardiovascular surgery (34,35). Since most of the costs are borne by third-party payers, these analyses generally reveal the cost-effectiveness of the surgery from a societal perspective. Work status can be objectively determined with relative ease, and changes in standard of living may be determined through self-report questions administered to patients.

To evaluate the influence of the coronary artery bypass graft, measures should be taken preoperatively and then periodically after surgery. The baseline preoperative measures should be collected before perioperative emotional responses confound measures such as well-being, emotional responses, and even performance on cognitive tests. Although historical objective baseline data such as work status and absenteeism may be useful, such data raise concerns about validity. Since data suggest a decline in postoperative quality of life improvements after 10 years, at least in comparison to medically treated patients (36,37), long-term follow-up of patients is desirable. With relatively little known about quality of life changes over long periods of follow-up among nonpatient populations, the inclusion of nonpatient comparison groups may be important. Finally, the examination of age, severity of disease, and sex subgroups of patients may be important. Older patients may be more subject to neuropsychological impairment, have a higher rate of surgical complications, and have a higher average cost for surgery (38). Since enhanced survival for particular groups of patients is controversial, it may be important to examine separately the quality of life of groups according to severity and type of their disease. Rates of surgical mortality, incomplete revascularization, early and late graft occlusion, and recurrent angina have also been found to be more common among women than men (39).

PSYCHOLOGICAL FACTORS

The emotional and neuropsychological dimensions of psychological well-being among patients after cardiovascular surgery have been examined in the literature. These studies are summarized in Table 1. Studies examining cognitive and emotional sequelae of neurological effects are summarized in the table, but studies of neurological changes alone, without consideration of functional status, are not included.

Emotional Measures

Among the studies which have examined emotional aspects of quality of life, the measures utilized range from global measures of satisfaction with surgery to specific emotional changes with surgery.

Global Indices of Satisfaction and Psychological Functioning

Generally, nonrandomized and uncontrolled studies which have examined global measures of satisfaction with either the surgery or with the patients' quality of life have reported favorable findings with surgery. Kornfeld et al. (53) sampled 100 consecutive coronary artery bypass graft patients 3½ years postsurgery; 77% of the patients reported an improvement in their general pleasure in life. Jenkins et al. (3,28) found general satisfaction with the surgery but noted that the percentage of patients who reported that they would undergo surgery again declined from those indicating an unqualified yes of 71% at 6 months to 56% at 12 months. However, 91% of the respondents at 12 months indicated that they were better off after surgery than before. The authors interpret this change in findings not as a general decline in satisfaction with the surgery, but as a loss of enthusiasm and a trend toward weighing alternatives rather than late dissatisfaction with the surgery. This interpretation appears difficult to justify without specific data.

Alternatively, these findings might be interpreted by suggesting that patients' expectations are not being realized. In fact, some data suggest that patient expectations

TABLE 1. *Psychological aspects of quality of life*

Study	Population	Measures	Duration of follow-up	Results
Kornfeld et al. (40)	100 CABG patients	Interview; standardized questionnaires[a]	4½ years	At 3½ years, 60% extremely pleased and only 4% displeased; 77% reported improved pleasure in life
Jenkins et al. (3)	318 CABG patients	Standardized cognitive tests[b]	9 days and 6 months	At 6 months, anxiety, depression, and fatigue decreased and positive well-being, helplessness, and vigor increased
Roberts et al. (38)	291 CABG patients	CNS deficit; psychosis[c]	120 days	Postoperative psychosis more common among older group
Shaw et al. (41,42)	312 CABG patients	Neurologic measures; cognitive tests; psychosis[kd]	7 days	1% with postoperative psychosis; 17% showed serious functional disability during hospital stay; 79% showed some cognitive impairment
Folks et al. (43)	96 CABG patients	Standardized questionnaire[e]	6 months	Greater health concerns found after surgery; greater age associated with less psychologic distress
Jenkins et al. (28)	366 CABG patients	Psychological symptom self-report[b]	6 and 12 months	Anxiety, depression, fatigue, and life change decreased postsurgery; well-being and vigor increased after surgery; hostility did not change

[a] Modified version of Psychiatric Evaluation Form (44), Cattell 16 Personality Factor (PF) Questionnaire (45), Type A/B Structured Interview.
[b] Trailmaking Test (23), Visual Reproduction (Form II) and Logical Memory (Form I) from the Wechsler Memory Scale (46), Profile of Mood States (POMS) (47), State-Trait Anxiety Inventory (18), scales for well-being (48), self-esteem (49), hope (50), dependency, locus of control, willingness to accept help, and other psychological constructs.
[c] Clinical judgment.
[d] Clinical judgment and Halstead-Reitan Trail Making Test (Part B) (23), Wechsler Memory Scale (24), Wechsler Adult Intelligence Scale (51).
[e] Psychological Adjustment to Illness Scale (52).
CABG, coronary artery bypass graft.

prior to surgery may be inappropriately positive, setting patients up to be disappointed with the realistic gains in their functioning (43,54). While Mayou and Bryant (54) report that only 10% of their sample of 79 patients anticipated any problems with surgery, considerable dissatisfaction occurred across the sample when postsurgical difficulties were encountered.

Also, global measures of psychological functioning have generally shown improvement from the preoperative to the postoperative period (3,4,28). Although these findings certainly look favorable for coronary artery bypass graft surgery, these findings were uncontrolled, and Raft et al. (5) have already reported in a small sample that percutaneous transluminal coronary angioplasty patients reported more improved functioning than coronary artery bypass graft patients. Percutaneous transluminal coronary angioplasty patients rated their overall functioning better at work, their sexual performance more improved, and their family relationships more positive than coronary artery bypass graft patients at 6 months, with continued better functioning at work through 15 months. Larger randomized studies need to compare global measures of satisfaction for percutaneous transluminal coronary angioplasty and coronary artery bypass graft patients.

Specific Emotional Measures

Studies which have examined depression and anxiety, the two most commonly examined specific emotional measures, have generally indicated favorable outcome with surgery, at least in the long term. Raymond et al. (55) initially found an increase in depression 1 to 2 weeks postoperatively among 31 coronary artery bypass graft patients, but depression decreased 4 to 6 weeks later to a level comparable to that seen after surgery. Anxiety ratings persisted for 1 to 2 weeks postoperatively but decreased significantly by 6 to 8 weeks later. Jenkins et al. (3) note that their preoperative measure of anxiety was only slightly higher than reference norms for general medical and surgical patients. However, they found substantial decreases large enough to be of real clinical importance in both anxiety and depression from the few days prior to coronary artery bypass graft surgery to 6 months later. These findings were replicated at 1 year among a slightly larger group of coronary artery bypass graft patients (28). Magni et al. (4) similarly report significant decreases in anxiety and depression from pre- to post-surgery at 1 year among a mixed group of coronary artery bypass graft and valvular surgery patients. Again, however, it must be cautioned that these findings are uncontrolled and nonrandomized.

Other psychological measures have yielded mixed results. Jenkins et al. (3) found that measures of hostility, hopelessness, self-esteem, sense-of-mastery, and willingness to depend on others showed no significant changes. Significant improvement in obsessiveness and compulsiveness from prior to surgery to 1 year later was reported for a mixed group of 99 coronary artery bypass graft and valvular patients (4).

The degree to which patients focus on their symptoms after surgery has been a conceptually relevant dimension which few studies have examined. Magni et al. (4) reported a decrease in somatization, a measure of focus on physical symptoms, from just prior to surgery to 1 year after the surgery among combined vascular and coronary artery bypass graft patients. Although these results appear consistent with a general picture of improved psychological functioning of patients from immediately prior to surgery to long-term follow-up, Folks et al. (43) noted greater health concerns 6 months after surgery than they had prior to the surgery. As mentioned earlier, Folks and colleagues suggest that this discrepancy in their findings may be a function of the unrealistic expectation that their patients had about outcome prior to surgery. Other findings indicate that patients' expectations are not always realized by their outcomes (54,56). To enhance psychological adjustment to surgery, patients might benefit from an evaluation of their expectations and an educational or psychological program focused on what to expect after surgery.

Neuropsychological Measures

Neurological changes with coronary artery bypass graft surgery have been examined less often than with other types of cardiac surgery involving more extensive bypass techniques and patients who are often more ill (57). With other types of cardiac surgery, some neurological impairment was found in approximately 35% of the patients (58). With coronary artery bypass graft surgery, major neurological complications have been described in approximately 2% of the patients (57). These neurological complications can be categorized as follows (57): delirium following a lucid interval, attributed to metabolic disturbances, medications, or sleep disturbances; hypoxic-ischemic syndrome; focal neurologic problems; seizures; or peripheral nervous system injuries. A similar incidence of 1% with major neurological sequelae was found for 3,206 patients who were examined after surgery and while still in the intensive care unit (59). Suspected causative factors among the unresponsive patients and those who developed immediate postoperative focal neurological signs were atheromatous embolism, perioperative hypotension, carotid artery occlusive disease, and air embolism. In a prospective study, Breuer et al. (60) found encephalopathy in 11.6%, signs of stroke in 5.2%, and major signs of stroke indicated by functional disability in 2% of the 421 consecutive patients whom they examined presurgically and one to four times beginning on the fourth day after surgery. These rates of stroke compare closely to the 5% rate of stroke reported by others (41).

Peripheral nervous system problems have received little attention. In one of the few uncontrolled studies in the area, Lederman et al. (61) reported a range of peripheral problems among 13% of 421 patients. The most common of these problems was brachial plexus injuries with other injuries including: mononeuropathies, persistent singultus, unilateral vocal cord paralysis, isolated partial Horner syndrome, and facial neuropathy. Males were more likely to develop these problems than females, and hypothermia during surgery was associated with increased risk for these peripheral problems. This number compares closely to the 12% of patients with brachial plexus problems noted by Shaw et al. (41). These problems are most probably due to nerve compression from surgery or postoperative care (57), and though not considered to be a major consideration for quality of life, these problems may have considerable impact on patients who engage in activities requiring fine motor activity. Nonetheless, most of the peripheral nerve problems have been noted to be transient with only rare lasting disability (61).

Postoperative psychosis, a transient phenomenon, probably should not be considered to be a major quality of life variable, at least over the long term, since there is no evidence that it recurs. These phenomena have been found to be infrequent in coronary artery bypass graft patients 60 years of age or less (8% of 77 patients) but significantly more frequent among those 65 years or older (44% of 66 patients) (38). Others have reported rates as low as 1% of postoperative psychosis among 312 coronary artery bypass graft patients (41).

Of greater relevance for quality of life are neuropsychological changes that affect cognitive and psychological functioning, resulting in functional impairment. In a mixed group of coronary artery bypass graft and valvular surgery patients, Savageau et al. (62,63) reported that 28% of their 227 patients sampled 9 days after surgery were definitely impaired on at least one of three neuropsychologic measures. Six months later, only 5% of the patients had decreased performance relative to preoperative measures, suggesting that the earlier transient effects were related to medication, mood change, or fatigue. Decrements of function at 6 months were associated with total estimated blood loss greater than 3,000 ml, propranolol administration during surgery, and higher levels of postoperative fatigue, depression, and worries. These data thus suggest that both physiologic and psychologic factors contribute to the decreased test performance and associations which may warrant examination among coronary artery bypass graft patients.

In a controlled comparison of 31 coronary artery bypass graft patients and 16 general surgery patients, similar declines in performance measures of cognitive functioning relative to the general surgery patients have been reported at 1 to 2 weeks postsurgery (55), but these differences disappeared 6 to 8 weeks after surgery. Uncontrolled observations on a more extensive cognitive battery, administered prior to surgery and again 1 week after surgery, indicated that 61% of 312 patients showed new clinical abnormalities after surgery (42).

As noted by Mayou (57), neuropsychological test performance change both transiently and over the long term may be accounted for by psychological reaction. In fact, Jenkins et al. (3) suggest that their findings among 318 post-coronary artery bypass graft patients of improvements in test performance of speed and concentration from presurgery levels may be due to decreased anxiety and depression and reduced medication usage among their patients.

Summary of Psychological Factors

Although most reports in this area are uncontrolled and no investigations could be found which address these variables using a randomized design, data on emotional and neuropsychological aspects of quality of life suggest that coronary artery bypass graft patients are globally satisfied with their surgical outcome. However, there appears to be some long-term lessening of enthusiasm for surgery, a finding possibly related to inappropriately optimistic presurgical expectations. Assessing patient expectations and educating patients about postsurgical complications and results might be a fruitful area for exploration. Although there may be short periods after surgery in which at least depression may worsen, coronary artery bypass graft patients' anxiety and depression appear to improve from measures taken immediately prior to surgery, but a measure of mood taken so close to surgery may be an inappropriate baseline. The anticipation of surgery alone would be expected to increase anxiety and depression and not yield a true baseline level for these variables. Overall, coronary artery bypass graft patients appear to suffer few long-term emotional consequences from their surgery.

Transient neuropsychological deficits lasting up to several weeks do occur from medication or emotional changes. Additional data are needed to investigate subtle neuropsychological sequelae of surgery. A propensity for transient changes among the elderly suggest that research should focus on or differentiate between both the short- and the long-term neuropsychological sequelae of coronary artery bypass graft surgery in these patients. Some patients endure long-term neurological deficits, but generally short-term effects of surgery appear to diminish over time. Some predictors of neuropsychological changes have been identified, but future research should attempt to identify those at risk of such complications.

SOCIAL INTERACTION FACTORS

Social interaction with family and others has been examined to determine the effects of cardiovascular surgery on quality of life. Social support also appears to be an important predictor of outcome with some patients. The Beta-Blocker Heart Attack Trial found that social isolation in combination with a high level of stress increased the risk of death fourfold (64). The effects of surgery on social interactions

TABLE 2. *Social interaction aspects of quality of life*

Study	Population	Measures	Duration of follow-up	Results
Kornfeld et al. (40)	100 CABG patients	Self-report	Up to 3½ years	Improved family satisfaction with only 4% reporting worsening family relations
Jenkins et al. (3)	318 CABG patients	Self-report	6 months	Friends and social support stayed same; participation in social activities increased; 81% reported receiving as much affection as desired; 36% reported overprotection
Folks et al. (43)	96 CABG patients	Standardized questionnaire[a]	6 months	Significant strengthening of relations with nuclear family and in social activities
Jenkins et al. (28)	366 CABG patients	Self-report	6 and 12 months	Decline from 6 to 12 months in calling on others for assistance; no change in visits from friends and relatives; increase in going out to social activities; decrease in worrying by family; high level of marital satisfaction

[a] Psychological Adjustment to Illness Scale (52).
CABG, coronary artery bypass graft.

thus have importance beyond being a measure of quality of life. Studies which have examined social interaction aspects of quality of life among coronary artery bypass graft patients are summarized in Table 2.

Familial Interaction

Quality of life studies which have examined family relationships in coronary artery bypass graft patients suggest that family interactions do not worsen and often improve after surgery. Raft et al. (5) reported that bypass patients continue to report significant improvement in functioning with their families 6 months after surgery, although the sample was small and this effect did not persist at 15 months. Over a longer period of follow-up, Kornfeld et al (40) found 3½ years after surgery that the majority of 57 patients examined reported an improvement in their family relations.

In a more comprehensive evaluation, Jenkins et al. (3) reported that 81% of their 318 post-coronary artery bypass graft patients reported receiving as much affection as they wanted from those with whom they lived, and 74% of the sample reported that they felt that people closest to them understood how they felt most or all of the time. Half of the patients reported feeling that their surgery brought their families closer together, whereas only 3% reported adverse effects on their families. During recovery from surgery, 36% of the patients felt that they were overprotected compared to only 5% who felt that others expected too much of them during recovery. Half of the patients felt that their families worried more about their health after surgery, and only 14% reported a decline in their families' worries about them. At 1 year of follow-up, the trend in family worry about the patients was reversed (28). This latter finding may represent a decline in family concern about the patient or alternatively may reflect an increase in the patient's expectations of family concern or protection. Patients generally maintained high levels of involvement with their families. For both sexes, 88% of those living with their spouse reported that they were happy or very happy with their marital relationship.

Nonfamilial Social Interactions

In social interactions outside of the family, coronary artery bypass graft patients also report improved social activities. Jenkins et al. (3) reported that the number of friends with whom patients reported that they could discuss problems remained about the same after surgery; when changes did occur, they tended to be increases in social interactions. Patients reported that numbers of visits from friends and relatives from pre- to postsurgery remained the same for 48%, decreased for 24%, and increased for 28%. However, 42% of the patients reported an increase in social interactions, suggesting that they engaged in more self-initiated social activities after surgery. After a year of follow-up assessment, patients reported maintained levels of high social activity outside of the household (28).

Summary of Social Interaction Factors

Again, investigations examining social interaction measures have been uncontrolled and have not utilized randomized designs. From the uncontrolled studies, bypass patients appear to show high levels of social interaction with both family and friends. They may initially feel that family are overprotective, but this phenomenon appears to ameliorate and even perhaps to shift in the opposite direction in the longer term. It is not yet clear, though, whether this changed perception of overprotectiveness is actually a reduction in overprotectiveness by family or a shift in patient's perceptions of how much they should be protected by family.

FUNCTIONAL CAPACITY FACTORS

Functional capacity has been examined from both a general perspective and a more specific focus on functional ability to engage in particular types of activities. Studies which have examined functional capacity measures as part of quality of life among coronary artery bypass graft patients after surgery are summarized in Table 3. Studies which have only examined changes in functional capacity through changes in self-report or medical testing are not included.

General Functional Capacity

Many controlled and randomized studies have indicated improved myocardial perfusion after surgery (70). Self-reported improvement in function has also been consistent. Among the clinical trials which have examined the effects of coronary artery bypass graft surgery, all have demonstrated improvement in reports of angina (9,66, 71). Most centers report at least significant improvement in angina in 90% of their patients (72). The finding that these subjective improvements correlate with graft patency (71) suggests that this effect is not attributable merely to nonspecific effects.

TABLE 3. *Functional capacity aspects of quality of life*

Study	Population	Measures	Duration of follow-up	Results
Kornfeld et al. (40)	100 CABG patients	Self-report; functional capacity[a]	Up to 3½ years	Mean NYHA functional class of 3.2; sexual frequency decline postoperatively which was related to preoperative cardiac impairment, return to work, and Type A behavior
Barboriak et al. (65)	350 CABG patients	Self-report	1 year	Significant increase in light and sports activities after surgery; no change in frequency of sexual activity
CASS Principal Investigators (66)	390 medical and 390 CABG patients	Functional status measures; self-report	6, 18, and 60 months	CABG patients reported less activity limitation than medical patients; no difference in recreational status
Jenkins et al. (3)	318 CABG patients	Physical functioning self-report; dyspnea rating[b]	6 months	69–85% of patients with angina reported complete angina relief at 6 months; 54% of patients reported complete relief from dyspnea at 6 months; usual daily physical activity increased; few changes in sexual functioning
Misra et al. (67)	120 English CABG patients	Self-report	6–23 months	50% of employed reported normal work capability
Haze et al. (68)	272 Japanese CABG patients	Self-report of activity and health status	Average of 29 months	73% reported no activity limitation; most frequent cause of activity limitation was angina
Folks et al. (43)	96 CABG patients	Standardized questionnaire[c]	6 months	Sexual dysfunction and frequency of sexual contact showed improvement at 6 months
Jenkins et al. (28)	366 CABG patients	Functioning self-report; dyspnea rating[b]	6 and 12 months	Few changes from 6 to 12 months; 62% free of dyspnea at 12 months

[a] New York Heart Association (NYHA) functional classification (30).
[b] London School of Hygiene Dyspnoea Questionnaire and London School of Hygiene Cardiovascular Questionnaire (69).
[c] Psychological Adjustment to Illness Scale (52).
CABG, coronary artery bypass graft.

Further, improvements in exercise tolerance and decreased use of antianginal drugs have been noted (9,66).

Specific Functional Capacity

Vocational, avocational, and sexual functioning measures have tended to rely on self-report recall rather than potentially more valid measures of behavior such as self-monitoring, reports by others, or more objective indices of functional capacity in specific settings.

Vocational Measures of Functional Capacity

With the general improvements in functional capacity (9,66) and the observation that most jobs do not have heavy exertional requirements (73), work capacity should also be improved after recovery from surgery. However, data examining the relation between work status and functional status relations are contradictory. Some studies have found no relation between employment and physical activity (74) and even between employment and physical findings (75). Other investigations have found return to work much greater among patients who had a greater degree of revascularization (76), higher exercise tolerance (77), and better relief of angina (78). Activities at work are further complicated by legal considerations involving insurance and workmen's compensation. These data suggest that work activities appear to be complex phenomenon of physiologic, psychologic, economic, and societal interactions rather than a simple measure of functional capacity.

Avocational Measures of Functional Capacity

Avocational functioning at worst appears to change little with surgery. Although Barboriak et al. (65) reported an increase in both light activities and sports, other studies have reported little change in avocational activity. More than half of 318 coronary artery bypass graft patients reported no change in their work around the home and outside tasks after surgery (3). Of the remaining patients, an almost equal split of those who report increases and decreases in general activities was seen. Consistent with this finding, the randomized, controlled findings of the Coronary Artery Surgery Study suggest no change in recreational status (66).

Sexual Measures of Functional Capacity

Although sexual functioning may be taken as a measure of functional capacity, a number of other variables enter into determining sexual activity. Aside from functional capacity, sexual activity is related to emotional and psychological variables. Additionally, patients' spouses contribute to determining sexual frequency, and some spouses may avoid sexual activity out of concern over stressing their husband or wife. Among the investigations that have addressed sexual functioning of patients, the results have been mixed.

Kornfeld et al. (40) report a sample of 100 coronary artery bypass graft patients where those patients who were sexually active at least once a week declined from 67% preoperatively to 38% 9 months after surgery. Sexually functioning remained worsened for approximately one-fourth of their sample 3½ years postsurgery. Jenkins et al. (3), on the other hand, found that half of the 318 post-coronary artery bypass graft patients reported no change in their satisfaction with sexual activities, with the remainder about equally divided between improvement and worsening of sexual satisfaction. At one year of follow-up, Jenkins et al. (28) report essentially no changes in sexual satisfaction measures among both sexes. Folks et al. (43), on the other hand, reported an improvement in sexual functioning 6 months after surgery. Among females, Althof et al. (79) reported an initial decline in intercourse frequency postsurgery in a small sample of female coronary artery bypass graft patients. At one year postsurgery, intercourse frequency increased to presurgery levels for the females but remained lower than frequencies reported prior to the onset of symptoms.

Summary of Functional Capacity Factors

In contrast to the other quality of life areas, some randomized, controlled findings of functional capacity effects with surgery are available. Objective data of coronary artery bypass graft patients' functional capacity strongly suggest an increase from preoperative levels in their exercise tolerance, a decrease in angina symptom report, and a decrease in use of medication. Subjectively, patients generally report an increase in vigor and a decrease in fatigue. When specific behaviors are addressed, work status does not appear to be a good measure of functional capacity but appears to be related to a number of variables, many of which are unrelated to outcome. Patients report no overall change in avocational activities. Although sexual functioning is also a dimension which is influenced by many variables other than merely capacity for the activity, uncontrolled self-reports of sexual functioning changes after surgery appear mixed, with some studies suggesting increases and others declines in sexual activity. Overall, it appears that there is little change in sexual activity.

ECONOMIC FACTORS

Economic factors have generally been viewed from two perspectives—return to work and cost-effectiveness. Return to work has often been a focus of quality of life assessment among coronary artery bypass graft patients, not only because this measure is easy to collect and is an indicator of economic factors, but also because it is an indirect measure of functional capacity. Due to the magnitude of economic implications for society, cost-effectiveness analyses have been undertaken. Studies which have addressed economic factors in the quality of life of post-coronary artery bypass graft patients are summarized in Table 4.

Return to Work

The percentage of patients returning to work varies across samples, although there appears to be fair consistency in findings among studies conducted in the United States. Recent reviews suggest that there is little net change in the number working before surgery and the next few years after surgery (87,94–96). There is also the suggestion of about a 10% reduction in employment among patients who survive for more than 2 years after surgery (94).

One major exception to the return to work rates among coronary artery bypass graft patients after surgery in the United States is the report by Liddle et al. (82). Among the 352 patients, 85% of the total sample and 97% of those working preoperatively were found to be working 6 months after surgery. As Mayou (57) noted, this difference in postoperative employment rates may be at least partially attributable to a strong work focus among Mormons living in Utah. Alternatively, this high rate may be due to psychological preparation and support of the patients as Liddle et al. suggest (82).

Greater variability in return to work is evident in studies conducted outside of the

TABLE 4. *Economic aspects of quality of life*

Study	Population	Measures	Duration of follow-up	Results
Anderson et al. (80)	564 CABG patients	Work status	1 and four years	Age, postsurgical angina, previous MI, physical requirements of job related to 4-year employment.
Niles et al. (81)	105 CABG patients	Work status	12–31 months	60% of total sample returned to work; increase by 10% in those working after surgery
Liddle et al. (82)	565 CABG patients	Work status; surgical costs and income	6 months	85% of those <65 returned to work; education and preoperative employment status related to return to work; postoperative income of employed 4.5 times medical and disability costs of entire sample
Boulay et al. (83)	1,602 CABG patients	Work status	From 1 to over 3 years	69–72% returned to work; length of preoperative unemployment most predictive of work status; preoperative occupation, noncardiovascular illness, education, anginal class, and symptom duration also predictive of employment.
Gutmann et al. (84)	358 CABG patients	Work status	4–22 months	58% working at follow-up; presurgical employment best predictor of work status; income, job classification, ejection fraction, subjective improvement also related; age, symptoms, disability compensation negatively related
Guvendik et al. (85)	100 CABG patients	Work status	Over 5 years	90% employment at 1 year; decreased to 73% at 5 years
Johnson et al. (86)	2,354 surviving CABG patients	Work status	Up to 10 years	Increase of 20% in those working after operation; main reason for not working was physical disability
Kornfeld et al. (40)	100 CABG patients	Work status	Up to 3½ years	Patients who returned to work were significantly younger, showed more angina improvement, and were more likely to be Type A pre- and postoperatively
Haze et al. (68)	272 Japanese CABG patients	Work status	Average of 29 months	84% of patients desiring to return to work were working at follow-up; main reasons for not working included angina, shortness of breath, general fatigue, leg pain, anxiety, lack of confidence, and doctor's advice

TABLE 4. *Continued.*

Study	Population	Measures	Duration of follow-up	Results
Maddern et al. (92)	4,001 Australian CABG patients	Work status; procedure cost; visits to physician	Mean of 3.1 years	Overall unemployment increase of 163% postoperatively; female homemakers reported improved work; 44% seeing physician less frequently and only 20% seeing physician more frequently; mean cost of CABG = $3,476
Sergeant et al. (93)	250 Belgium CABG patients	Work status	2 years	Months of preoperative unemployment, type of employment, and number of preoperative MIs predicted return to work
Jenkins et al. (28)	366 CABG patients	Economic changes; work status	6 and 12 months	73% reported no major change; 21% reported reduction in standard of living; few changes from 6 to 12 months in work status
Rogers et al. (37)	390 medical and 390 CABG patients	Work status	10 years	Similar work status between two groups
Hemenway et al. (12)	478 patients; some medical, some surgical	Economic data; work status	Up to 3 years	Average costs for 6-month treatment = $5,705 for medical patients and $27,862 for CABG patients; follow-up costs over 3 years higher for CABG than medical patients; treatment unrelated to work status
Misra et al. (67)	120 English CABG patients	Work status	6–23 months	72% employed before operation returned to work
Roberts et al. (38)	143 CABG patients	Hospital costs	120 days	Older group had greater hospital cost than younger group
Rodis et al. (76)	109 consecutive CABG patients	Working status	11–19 months	94% of age-eligibles (<65 yrs.) returned to work; preoperative work status most predictive of return to work; educational level, postoperative symptom relief, and degree of revascularization also related to work status
Rogers (91)	390 CABG and 390 medical patients	Number working	6 and 18 months, and 5 years	Slightly more CABG patients working at baseline; no differences between groups during postsurgical period
Folks et al. (43)	96 CABG patients	Work status	6 months	Vocational status showed marked improvement; patients reported less interference of illness with job activities and less absenteeism with better physical performance

TABLE 4. *Continued.*

Study	Population	Measures	Duration of follow-up	Results
Oberman et al. (87)	416 medical and 444 CABG patients	Work status	3 years	Higher percentage working among CABG patients after 1 year, but after 3 years little difference; patients in professional or managerial occupations or manorial industries more likely to work
Smith et al. (74)	579 medical and 769 surgical patients	Work status	2 years	Little difference between groups; preoperative work status, postoperative angina, type of work, and age predictive of work status
Almedia et al. (88)	1,602 CABG patients	Work status	10–56 months	66% returned to work postoperatively; 12% reported lowered job satisfaction; return to work influenced by absence of chest pain, preoperative working status, younger age, fewer jobs before surgery, higher education, male sex, completeness of revascularization, not taking propranolol, normal myocardial contractility, and no or fewer preoperative myocardial infarctions
CASS Principal Investigators (66)	390 medical and 390 CABG patients	Work status	6, 18, and 60 month	Work decrease in both groups during follow-up; no difference in work status between groups at 1, 3, and 5 years of follow-up
Jenkins et al. (3)	318 CABG patients	Economic changes; work status	6 months	Family income remained about same for 77%; income of others mostly declined; among preoperative employed, 75% remained working at 6 months
Rosenfeldt et al. (89)	702 Australian CABG patients	Work status	2–9 years	Of 591 patients ≤55 years, 68% were working after surgery; young age, short time off work before operation, and absence of postoperation angina associated with return to work
Holmes et al. (90)	2,250 PTCA patients; 25.3% with CABG	Work status	Mean of 1.5 years	Employment reduced in all groups; no difference between groups; PTCA patients returned to work sooner than those with both PTCA and CABG

CABG, coronary artery bypass graft; MI, myocardial infarction; PTCA, percutaneous transluminal coronary angioplasty

United States. In Japan, of 190 patients judged as needing to return to work, 160 or 84% returned to work on at least a part-time basis (68), a rate considerably higher than most return to work rates found after surgery in the United States. On the other hand, Misra et al. (67) report that a quarter of a British sample had retired from work even before the onset of angina. In Australia, Maddern et al. studied 4,001 patients following coronary artery bypass graft surgery (92) and found decreased employment among the male patients that was similar to the decline in employment for the general male population. For females, an increase in those able to maintain full-time work duties was noted after surgery. In Israel, 100 consecutive coronary artery bypass graft patients were followed over an average of 14 months postsurgery (76), with a 6% increase in working after surgery. A number of hypotheses account for these differences in return to work rates, including: the influence of cultural and ethnic factors which affect patients' support from their physicians, family, and employers, as well as the patients' own attitudes toward work; different economic factors influencing economic pressures to return to work; differences in other patient characteristics of those who receive elective coronary artery bypass graft surgery; and differences in employment exertional requirements.

More rigorous, randomized studies comparing return to work of medical treatment versus coronary artery bypass graft surgery demonstrated little differences in return to work related to treatment type. A sample of patients from the Coronary Artery Surgery Study (66) found reductions in work over 5 years of follow-up to be similar between the medical and surgical groups. In the Minnesota Coronary Artery Surgery Study sample (74), similar declines among the patients working in both treatment groups were also found. At 10 years after surgery, there continue to be no differences between the medical and surgery groups in the number working (37). Declines in work status appear to be attributable to treatment for coronary artery disease rather than to specific treatment type.

This interpretation is strengthened by the observation that the percentage of patients who return to work after percutaneous transluminal coronary angioplasty (PTCA) appears to be the same as for those who undergo coronary artery bypass graft surgery. Holmes et al. (90) examined the data from the National Heart, Lung, and Blood Institute's Percutaneous Transluminal Coronary Angioplasty Registry. They analyzed data from 2,250 patients who had undergone PTCA, classified into groups according to those who successfully underwent PTCA without myocardial infarction and without coronary artery bypass graft surgery, those who had coronary artery bypass graft surgery after unsuccessful PTCA, and those who had other forms of medical management following unsuccessful PTCA. At 1.5 years postprocedure, there was a small decline in employment in all groups. Among the 1,150 patients who were working before their procedure and were 60 years of age or younger, 81% to 86% remained working after an average of 1.4 years postprocedure regardless of PTCA outcome. Although PTCA did not improve return to work any more than coronary artery bypass graft surgery, PTCA did reduce the time interval for the patients returning to work.

A number of investigations have examined predictors of return to work for coronary artery bypass graft patients after surgery (53,74,82,90). In an elaborate approach, Boulay et al. (83) examined return to work predictors over successive years. They subjected their data to a stepwise discriminant analysis of a variety of variables on work status postoperatively for 1,217 patients. No major differences were noted in the variables over 1-, 2-, 3-, and 4-year periods. Nine independent variables correlated significantly with postoperative working status, including: age, anginal class, duration of symptoms, associated vascular disease, noncardiovascular illness, length of preoperative unemployment, education, types of physical activity in preoperative occupation, and total annual income. The most strongly associated variable was preoperative employment status. Oberman and Finklea (97) summarized the predictive data by suggesting that these factors include work status at baseline, nonwork income, occupation, postoperative symptoms, age, perception of health, severity of disease, and education. The factors which appeared most strongly related to work status are full-time work at baseline, occupation, and type of industry (87). Patients in professional or manorial industries, i.e., those which encouraged loyalty and internal promotion, were more likely to return to work.

Among cross-cultural samples, the rates of return to work have differed from United States samples, but predictors of return to work have been surprisingly similar to those in the United States. Sergeant et al. (93), in a sample of 443 male Belgium coronary artery bypass graft patients, found that preoperative working status, type of employment, and number of preoperative infarctions were the best independent predictors of return to work. In Israel, preoperative work status was found to have the strongest relation to postoperative working, with educational level, postoperative symptom relief, and degree of revascularization also relating to postoperative work status (76).

Patients' satisfaction with work has also been addressed by several studies. Folks et al. (43) found that their sample of patients reported significantly less interference by their illness in their jobs and less absenteeism after surgery. However, there appears to be a subsample of patients who return to work but report adverse effects of the surgery. Mayou and Bryant (54) note that 20% of those who returned to work postoperatively in their sample were very dissatisifed at work. Their reasons for dissatisfaction were largely due to switching to less interesting, and often less well paid, positions, often with fewer promotion possibilities and with less of a pension. A further 13% of their sample reported feeling anxious and insecure and had lost enjoyment in their jobs. Some patients may also equate their work with the development of their disease, which influences their attitude toward work (97). Thus, return to work cannot be equated simply with positive quality of life. Type of occupation, socioeconomic factors, and psychological adjustment impact greatly on decisions to return to work and likely satisfaction.

Return to work has usually been classified as a dichotomous variable of patients either returning or not returning to work. However, examining delay in return to work may reveal process information which will enable us to better understand and to promote earlier return to work and perhaps improve overall return to work rates. Dupuis et al. (98) report that of the variables examined 2 months prior to coronary artery bypass graft surgery among 66 patients, length of preoperative unemployment, anxiety, and depression significantly predicted return to work delay. These data suggest that it is not just the postoperative psychological adjustment of patients which influences return to work, but also the preoperative psychological functioning of patients may be related to work parameters.

Cost-Effectiveness Analyses

Cost-effectiveness analyses suggest that coronary artery bypass graft surgery compares favorably with most interventions for chronic problems. Liddle et al. (82) even note that the total postoperative earnings of their sample of 565 single-surgery patients at the time of their report were 4.5 times the cost of these patients' surgeries. The costs and effectiveness of treatment approaches may differ somewhat depending on whether the approach is viewed from the societal perspective or from individual patients' perspectives.

From society's perspective, a considerable amount of effort has been made to conduct cost-effectiveness analyses for coronary artery bypass graft surgery. Weinstein and Stason (34) reviewed the cost-effectiveness data available at the time, including analysis of data from the European trial (99), the Veterans Administration Cooperative Study (100–102), and other published reports. This analysis took into account the quality of patients' lives in using symptom reports to calculate measures of quality-adjusted life-years as the measure of health effectiveness. They found that the estimated net cost per quality-adjusted life-year gained from coronary artery bypass graft surgery ranged from $3,800 in left main disease to $30,000 in one-vessel disease. These data were reported to compare favorably with those for other accepted medical therapies such as treatment for moderate diastolic hypertension. Costs of surgery itself ranged from $15,000 to $20,000 with a mean of $17,500 and included: the differences in costs of medical management with and without the surgery, savings attributable to the prevention of sequel events, and the difference between surgically and medically treated patients in costs of repeated or subsequent operations. This analysis revealed that the estimated net resource cost of surgical treatment is $14,000 (range, $10,500–$17,500) for patients with severa angina, and $15,500 (range, $12,000–$19,000) for patients with mild angina. The authors concluded that coronary artery bypass graft with symptomatic patients with coronary artery disease appears to be reasonably cost-effective.

In a similar analysis, Pliskin et al. (35) suggest that a simplified cost-effectiveness analysis for patients in whom surgery was the optimal treatment reveals a range of costs from $1,500 to $250,000 per year of life gained and from $1,500 to $32,000 per quality-adjusted life-year gained. As Pliskin et al. note, however, major factors in this analysis are patient characteristics, including patient preferences for physical activity. Patients with preferences for more active lifestyles, of course, will enjoy lower costs per quality-adjusted life-year gained.

As Rogers (91) has noted, there are a number of hidden, sometimes ignored, costs such as the cost of the medical management of coronary artery disease among patients who do not undergo coronary artery bypass graft surgery. However, Hemenway et al. (12) reported that the higher costs of medical therapy over a 3-year period offset only about 11% of the higher initial costs of surgery. For patients who are able to be maintained on medical therapy alone, medical management appears to be the more cost-effective approach. In the Coronary Artery Surgery Study, 38% of the patients with three-vessel disease and about 75% of all patients in the randomly assigned medical group crossed over to receive coronary artery bypass graft surgery during the 5 years of follow-up (91). These patients who were initially treated without surgery endured the highest costs of all of the patients, having incurred both the medical management and surgical costs (103). If these trends continue, it may be financially advantageous for most patients to endure the initial higher costs of surgery and save the costs of medical management and higher medication usage (37). On the other hand, the frequency of repeat coronary artery bypass graft surgeries over 8 to 10 years (13) suggests that total costs may be contained best by delaying the initial surgery for as long as possible.

While the costs of coronary artery bypass graft surgery are high, these costs may be lessened somewhat by cost-containment procedures (104). Procedures such as outpatient testing may prove effective in containing costs (105). Further, surgical costs vary widely between countries, averaging only $3,476 in Australia during 1981 to 1982 (98), suggesting different cost-effectiveness outcomes in different countries. Costs are probably also lower in hospitals where procedures are conducted frequently. Age of the patient is an important variable determining cost. The average cost of hospital stay for the elderly (aged 65 and over), largely influenced by an increased number of complications and longer hospital stays by the elderly, has been estimated to be $28,000 in the United States, but only $18,000 for those age 60 and younger (38).

Issues that are significant from an individual patient's standpoint are also important when discussing costs and effectiveness. Examination from this perspective suggests that substantial individual differences may exist between patients in both their benefits from treatment and the impact of the costs of surgery upon their standard of living. As suggested by the Pliskin et al. (35) analysis, patient preferences for physical activity may influence the benefits of surgery from the individual's viewpoint. Jenkins et al. (3) reported no major change in family income or living standard after surgery in 77% of their 318 coronary artery bypass graft patients. Not surprisingly, a change in the primary breadwinner was usually accompanied by a major drop in family income. However, 21% of their sample reported reduced living standards, depleted savings, or incurred debt, whereas only 6% of the sample reported financial gains. In one year, 15% of the patients reported outstanding large unpaid doctor and hospital bills. Considerable financial burden is experienced by at least a modest number of coronary artery bypass graft patients and differential benefits of the surgery may be seen between patients.

Summary of Economic Factors

Work status, extensively examined including during controlled, randomized investigations of coronary artery bypass graft patients, appears to be one easy approach to evaluating quality of life. Work histories also provide an adequate baseline comparison as opposed to other quality of life variables in which only perioperative baseline measures may be available. However, nonwork dimensions of quality of life may be more important for patients.

In the United States, the general consensus suggests no net change in return to work among patients after surgery. Among studies outside of the United States, a wide variation in the rate of return to work after coronary artery bypass graft surgery has been noted. These differences may relate to differences in population variables (including both demographic, economic, and psychological dimensions), differences in societal variables and social support, and different periods of follow-up. Measures of return to work are complex, involving not only measures of capacity to return to work but also aspects of satisfaction with job, opportunities and resources for retirement, and psychologic and social factors. Russell et al. (103) suggested other possibilities for not seeing greater return to work: the lengthy postsurgical recovery time may result in patients' becoming accustomed to not working; the pain, fear, and anxiety of surgery may enable postsurgical patients to qualify for disability more easily; and the collective expectations of employers, families, and friends about working after major surgery may discourage patients from returning to work. Oakley (106) has recently pointed more directly to the influence of a chronic period of disability which some patients endure before and/or after surgery. From a social learning perspective (107), patients who go through a long period of disability and unemployment may be learning a disabled role which may require more than mere symptom relief to overcome.

In examining predictors of return to work, a general consensus appears to emerge (108). Patients more likely to return to work appear to be those who were working preoperatively, who expect that they will return to work and perceive that their health is adequate, and who have jobs where less strenuous physical activity is involved. A number of other factors also seem related to work return to a lesser degree, including age, educational level, sex, symptoms after surgery, anxiety and depression, and economic resources.

Data suggest that the cost-effectiveness of coronary artery bypass graft surgery is similar to treatment for other chronic medical problems. Although most patients do not suffer major financial problems after their surgery, at least some patients do experience a decline in their standard of living. Despite the patient's financial status, even medically treated patients will be likely to eventually undergo surgery according to current medical opinion. Delaying surgery for those who will eventually require coronary artery bypass graft surgery burdens the patient with both medical and surgical expenses. The high frequency of repeat surgeries after 8 to 10 years adds additional controversy to the medical as well as the financial analysis. These issues need to be addressed by future long-term cost-effectiveness analyses.

SUMMARY OF QUALITY OF LIFE AMONG BYPASS SURGERY PATIENTS

Overall, the quality of life of coronary artery bypass graft patients after surgery appears much improved in perioperative and some preoperative measures of quality of life. These studies generally remain poorly controlled for type of treatment and, with the exception of return to work and functional capacity areas, are observational rather than randomized studies. Quality of life through the first few weeks postoperatively may be low, but is likely to show an improvement over the succeeding several months (3,43). Improvements in quality of life among coronary artery bypass graft patients compared to medically treated patients suggest that differences between the groups appear to diminish at 10 years, probably resulting from the return of symptoms in surgical patients but also the number of coronary artery bypass graft surgeries conducted in the previously treated medical patients (36,37).

METHODS OF IMPROVING QUALITY OF LIFE AMONG CARDIOVASCULAR SURGERY PATIENTS

Although the quality of life of cardiovascular surgery patients is in need of further examination, attention should also be focused on methods to improve quality of life. A preliminary study has already suggested beneficial effects of a combined rehabilitation, psychologic, and social support intervention to further improve the quality of life among coronary artery bypass graft patients after surgery (83). Other researchers have suggested that interventions targeted at rehabilitation, behavioral, social support, and/or education areas may improve the quality of life of post-coronary artery bypass graft patients.

Rehabilitation Programs

Observational studies indicate that a supervised exercise rehabilitation program for coronary artery bypass graft patients improves work capacity (109,110). Further, one nonrandomized but controlled investigation supports the beneficial effects of exercise not only on functional capacity but also on work status, anginal complaints, and overall ratings of well-being and quality of life (111). The one randomized, controlled study (112) reported that patients in a rehabilitation program improved their functional capacity by 15% to 20% more than those receiving usual care. Low-level exercise also appears to stimulate positive psychosocial changes among participants (73). Exercise testing alone may provide objective evidence to patients to assist in their overcoming perceptions of disability (113). Beyond the testing, exercise offers a positive and constructive approach by helping to encourage participation in new activities and dispelling fears associated with physical exertion (114–116). Such changes allow patients to view themselves in the context of health, strengthening feelings of well-being, self-esteem, and self-confidence (73).

Despite the variety of potential mechanisms through which rehabilitation programs may have beneficial effects on quality of life, only 10% of a sample of patients were found to have attended a cardiac rehabilitation program and fewer than half of those who attended a program remained in the program for 12 or more weeks (28). These data suggest that further exploration of rehabilitation programs as they impact on quality of life of cardiovascular surgery patients may be an important avenue of future research.

Behavioral Programs

Data from several recent studies of post-myocardial infarction patients indicate that behavioral intervention alone or in combination with other interventions favorably impacts on prognosis (117–120). Although the effects of behavioral interventions on prognosis of coronary artery bypass graft patients has not been examined, behavioral or psychological programs both prior to and after surgery may be effective in improving quality of life. Several studies have suggested that presurgical expectations may influence patients' later assessment of their quality of life (43,54), and patients report far-reaching unrealistic expectations that are not being adequately addressed (121). Additionally, Radley and Green (122) report that styles of coping or adjusting to coronary artery bypass graft surgery relate to recovery from the surgery, and anxiety and depression 2 months prior to surgery have even been found to be related to return to work delay (98). Limited data similarly suggest that behavioral characteristics and social interactions may actually influence postoperative mortality (4). Determining whether these presurgical expectations and styles of adjustment may be modified to affect long-term quality of life is an important empirical question for future research. Certainly, the elective nature of coronary artery bypass graft surgery allows ample time for educational and behavioral interventions prior to surgery (113).

After surgery, behavioral and psychological interventions may also prove beneficial in improving quality of life. Studying patients after myocardial infarction, Ott and Bergner (116) have examined the randomized control effects of an early exercise rehabilitation program versus a rehabilitation program plus a teaching and counseling program. It is impossible to differentiate the effects of education from counseling, but significantly greater improvements in psychosocial quality of life variables were obtained with the combined educational and counseling component. In coronary artery bypass graft patients, Mayou and Bryant (54) found that functioning in early convalescence was a good indicator of return to work, mental state postsurgery, and overall outcome. This may suggest that patients at high risk for poor quality of life outcome may be identified early and targeted for intervention. In multivariate analysis, when other factors are held constant, patients who perceive themselves as healthier after either medical or surgical treatment are more likely to return to work (103). These data suggest that interventions aimed at cognitive restructuring of patients' perceptions of health status after surgery may be effective in improving quality of life measures.

Social Support Programs

Social support programs designed from the perspective of physicians, families, employers, and other sources may also be important in improving quality of life measures. Psychological preparation of patients and their families as well as the attitudes toward rehabilitation expressed by attending physicians and employers enhance the likelihood of successful convalescence (73,82). This strongly suggests the importance of medical practitioners' working with patients' families and employers to improve return to work measures (97).

Coronary clubs and similar community organizations where patients receive support and rehabilitation would be expected to have beneficial effects on the quality of life of surgery patients and their families. Although most coronary artery bypass graft patients already appear to be highly involved in social activities, service clubs, community projects, and service organizations should not be overlooked as means to involve patients. Employers and other employees should also be encouraged to assist in the socialization of patients at work. The more that coronary artery bypass graft patients are involved with coworkers at work and during social activities, the more they are likely to function effectively on the job.

Educational Programs

As noted by Walter and Amsel (95), physician advice has commonly been given as the main reason for patients' not returning to work postoperatively. These data must be interpreted cautiously, since they were based on patients' interpretation of what their physicians said rather than a direct assessment of physicians' advice. Nonetheless, this common finding suggests that physicians need to deal directly with return to work issues. Data further suggest that cardiac surgery patients perceive that they are well educated and prepared about issues concerning activities, but are not well educated about emotional reactions and changes in social interactions (121). Unrealistic expectations of patients may have to be dealt with as a psychological issue; however, adequate patient education is an important first step in promoting realistic expectations. Since few patients may spontaneously express all of their fears

TABLE 5. *Subjective estimates of CABG surgery on quality of life dimensions*[a]

Dimension	Effect of surgery
Psychological	+
Anxiety	+
Depression	+
Neuropsychological	−
Social interactions	+ +
Family	+
Nonfamilial	+ +
Functional capacity	+ + +
General	+ + +
Vocational	0
Avocational	+
Sexual	0
Economic	0
Return to work	0
Cost-effectiveness	+
Individual economic impact	0

[a] Number of pluses on scale indicates degree of beneficial effect; number of minuses indicates degree of negative effect of surgery; and 0 indicates no effect from surgery.
CABG, coronary artery bypass graft.

and the range of their concerns to their physicians and these concerns may not even be addressed by patient education (121), encouraging patients to ask questions may be important, potentially reducing their anxiety and depression and improving quality of life (73,123).

CONCLUSION

Coronary artery bypass grafting increases the survival rate of patients with left main coronary artery disease and of patients with three-vessel disease and left ventricular dysfunction (8–11,100). Even among patients for whom there is a prolongation of life but especially among those for whom there is questionable prolongation of life, issues of quality of life are paramount. The effects of surgery on specific dimensions of quality of life have been subjectively summarized in Table 5. Pluses indicate a positive change in a particular quality of life dimension, whereas minuses suggest negative effects of surgery on the variable. Most patients benefit from coronary artery bypass graft for at least 5 years, with beneficial effects appearing to diminish prior to 10 years after operation.

Overall, it is difficult to determine the net gain in quality of life for several reasons. Foremost is the lack of controlled, randomized investigations examining quality of life changes. In addition, the few controlled studies are particularly difficult to interpret due to the large number of patients who have crossed over from medical to surgical treatment, the lack of a comprehensive quality of life assessment battery, and grouping all of the patients together rather than considering age, severity of disease, and sex subgroups. With PTCA becoming a more common procedure, more quality of life comparison studies between PTCA and coronary artery bypass graft surgery need to be undertaken.

One basic issue that influences quality of life after surgery is the preoperative adjustment of the patient. Preoperative adjustment is affected by the course of the disease and the time at which coronary artery bypass graft surgery is undertaken. The return to work literature clearly demonstrates the adverse effects of sustained periods of disability upon this dimension of quality of life; patients who undergo longer periods of disability are less likely to return to work. Although return to work is influenced by many factors, social learning theory (107) suggests that at least part of what mediates length of disability effects on employment and other measures of quality of life is learning the disability role, an effect which surgery and relief from symptoms alone would not be expected to overcome. Quality of life after coronary artery bypass graft surgery might be improved by endeavoring to minimize periods of disability. Current data indicate that most medically treated patients will eventually cross over to surgical treatment. Earlier coronary artery bypass graft surgery may have implications for improved quality of life unless otherwise indicated. However, patients who require repeat vascularization obviously endure some of the highest financial costs and potentially the greatest adverse effects on quality of life. The answer to this dilemma appears to lie in determining the optimal time for surgical intervention both medically and in terms of quality of life.

Other research needs also exist. Analysis of quality of life among patient subgroups based on age and severity of disease needs to be undertaken. More comprehensive approaches to understanding predictors of quality of life changes for patients need to be undertaken so that more effective surgical decision rules are determined.

Despite the paucity of randomized, controlled studies, coronary artery bypass graft surgery does appear to improve the functional capacity and overall quality of life of patients with coronary artery disease. The issue with quality of life of coronary artery bypass graft patients is not whether improvement is seen, but rather uncovering ways of maximizing and maintaining improvement, shifting the focus from longitudinal to treatment-outcome research. Rehabilitation and psychologic, social support, and patient education programs appear promising for improving many dimensions of quality of life, but have not been adequately evaluated.

REFERENCES

1. Wallwork J, Caine N. A comparison of the quality of life of cardiac transplant patients and coronary artery bypass graft patients before and after surgery. *Quality Life Cardivasc Care* 1985;1:317–331.
2. Baldwin JC, Stinson EB. Quality of life after cardiac transplantation. *Quality Life Cardivasc Care* 1985;1:332–335.
3. Jenkins CD, Stanton BA, Savageau JA, et al. Coronary artery bypass surgery: Physical, psychological, social, and economic outcomes six months later. *JAMA* 1983;250:782–788.
4. Magni G, Unger HP, Valfre C, et al. Psychosocial outcome one year after heart surgery: A prospective study. *Arch Intern Med* 1987;147:473–477.
5. Raft D, McKee DC, Popio KA, et al. Life adaptation after percutaneous transluminal coronary angioplasty and coronary artery bypass grafting. *Am J Cardiol* 1985;56:395–398.
6. Neil CA. Quality of life issues in the adult with congenital heart disease. *Quality Life Cardivasc Care* 1987;3:5–14.
7. American Heart Association. *1988 heart facts*. Dallas: American Heart Association, 1988.
8. The Veterans Administration Coronary Artery Bypass Surgery Cooperative Study Group. Eleven-year survival in the Veterans Administration randomized trial of coronary bypass surgery for stable angina. *N Engl J Med* 1984;311:1333–1339.
9. European Coronary Artery Surgery Study Group. Long-term results of prospective randomized study of coronary artery bypass surgery in stable angina pectoris. *Lancet* 1982;2:1173–1180.
10. Passamani E, Davis KB, Gillespie MJ, et al. A randomized trial of coronary artery bypass surgery: Survival of patients with a low ejection function. *N Engl J Med* 1985;312:1665–1671.
11. Scott SM, Luchi RJ, Deupree RH, et al. Veterans Administration Cooperative Study for treatment of patients with unstable angina. *Circulation* 1988;78(Suppl. 1):I-113–I-121.

12. Hemenway D, Sherman H, Mudge GH, et al. Comparative costs versus symptomatic and employment benefits of medical and surgical treatment of stable angina pectoris. *Med Care* 1985;23:133–141.

13. Cameron A, Kemp HG, Green GE. Reoperation for coronary artery disease: 10 years of clinical follow-up. *Circulation* 1988;78(Suppl. 1):I–158–I–162.

14. Brenowitz JB, Johnson WD, Kayser KL, et al. Coronary artery bypass grafting for the third time or more: Results of 150 consecutive cases. *Circulation* 1988;78(Suppl. 1):I–166–I–170.

15. Oberman A, Mattson ME, Alderman E, et al. Report of the working group: Coronary artery bypass graft surgery. In: Wenger NK, Mattson ME, Furberg CD, Elinson J, eds. *Assessment of quality of life in clinical trials of cardiovascular therapies.* New York: Le Jacq. 1984;311–314.

16. Wenger NK, Mattson ME, Furberg CD, et al. Assessment of quality of life in clinical trials of cardiovascular therapies. *Am J Cardiol* 1984;54:908–913.

17. Dupuy HJ. The psychological general well-being (PGWB) index. In: Wenger NK, Mattson ME, Furberg CD, Elinson J, eds. *Assessment of quality of life in clinical trials of cardiovascular therapies.* New York: Le Jacq. 1984;170–183.

18. Speilberger CD, Gorsuch RL, Lushene RE. *Manual for the State-Trait Anxiety Inventory (Self-Evaluation Questionnaire).* Palo Alto: Consulting Psychologists Press, 1970.

19. Radloff LS. The CES-D scale: A self-report depression scale for research in the general population. *App Psycholog Measurement* 1977;1:385–401.

20. Reitan RM. An investigation of the validity of Halstead's measure of biological intelligence. *Arch Neurol Psychiatr* 1955;73:28–35.

21. Reitan RM. *Manual for administration of neuropsychological test batteries for adults and children.* Indianapolis: R.M. Reitan, 1969.

22. Golden CJ, Hammeke T, Purisch A. *The Luria-Nebraska Neuropsychological Battery: Manual (revised).* Los Angeles: Western Psychological Services, 1980.

23. Reitan RM. *Trail making manual for administration, scoring, and interpretation.* Indianapolis: Department of Neurology, Section of Neuropsychology, Indiana University Medical Center, 1958.

24. Wechsler D, Stone CP. *Instruction manual for the Wechsler Memory Scale.* New York: The Psychological Corporation, 1973.

25. Russell EW. A multiple scoring method for assessment of complex memory functions. *J Consult Clin Psych* 1975;43:800–809.

26. Croog SH, Levine S. *Life after a heart attack: Social and psychological factors eight years later.* New York: Human Sciences Press, 1982.

27. Sarason IG, Levine HM, Basham RB, et al. Assessing social support: The Social Support Questionnaire. *J Pers Soc Psychol* 1983;44:127–139.

28. Jenkins CD, Stanton BA, Berger RL, et al. The quality of life 12 months after coronary artery bypass surgery. *Qual Life Cardiovasc Care* 1988;4:29–36.

29. Burtland RJA, Pang J, Gross ER, et al. Two-, six-, and twelve-minute walking test in respiratory disease. *Br J Med* 1982;284:1007–1008.

30. Harvey RM, Doyle EF, Ellis K, et al. Major changes made by the Criteria Committee of the New York Heart Association. *Circulation* 1974;49:390.

31. Campeau L. Grading of angina pectoris. *Circulation* 1976;54:522.

32. Goldman L, Hashimoto B, Cook EFL, et al. Comparative reproducibility and validity of systems for assessing cardiovascular functional class: Advantages of a new specific activity scale. *Circulation* 1981;64:1227–1234.

33. Croog SH, Levine S, Testa MA, et al. The effects of antihypertensive therapy on the quality of life. *N Engl J Med* 1986;314:1657–1664.

34. Weinstein MC, Stason WB. Cost-effectiveness of coronary artery bypass surgery. *Circulation* 66(Suppl. III):III–56–66.

35. Pliskin JS, Stason WB, Weinstein MC, et al. Coronary artery bypass graft surgery: Clinical decision making and cost-effectiveness analysis. *Med Decision Making* 1981;1:10–28.

36. Peduzzi P, Hultgren H, Thomsen J, et al. Ten-year effect of medical and surgical therapy on quality of life: Veterans Administration Cooperative Study of coronary artery surgery. *Am J Cardiol* 1987;59:1017–1023.

37. Rogers WJ, Coggin CJ, Gersh BJ, et al. Ten-year followup of quality of life in patients randomized to medicine vs CABG: Coronary Artery Surgery Study (CASS). *Circulation* 1988;78(Suppl. II):II–258.

38. Roberts A, Woodhall DD, Conti CR, et al. Mortality, morbidity, and cost-accounting related to coronary artery bypass graft surgery in the elderly. *Ann Thoracic Surg* 1985;39:426–432.

39. Becker RC, Corrao JM, Alpert JS. Coronary artery bypass surgery in women. *Clin Cardiol* 1988;11:443–448.

40. Kornfeld DS, Heller SS, Frank KA, et al. Psychological and behavioral responses after coronary artery bypass surgery. *Circulation* 1982;66(Suppl. 3):III–24–28.

41. Shaw PJ, Bates D, Cartlidge NEF, et al. Early neurological complications of coronary artery bypass surgery. *Br Med J* 1985;291:1384–1387.

42. Shaw PJ, Batres D, Cartlidge NEF, et al. Early intellectual dysfunction following coronary bypass surgery. *Q J Med* 1986;225:59–68.
43. Folks DG, Blake DJ, Fleece L, et al. Quality of life six months after coronary artery bypass surgery: A preliminary report. *South Med J* 1986;79:397–399.
44. Spitzer R, Endicott J. *Progress Report Biometric Research.* New York: New York State Department of Mental Hygiene, Research Division, Washington Heights Community Service, New York State Psychiatric Institute, Department of Psychiatry, 1966.
45. Cattell RB, Eber HW. *Handbook for the 16PF Questionnaire.* Urbana, IL: Institute for Personality and Ability Testing, 1962.
46. Wechsler D. A standardized memory scale for clinical uses. *J Psychol* 1945;19:87–95.
47. McNair DM, Lorr M, Droppleman LF. *Profile of mood-states: Manual.* San Diego: Educational and Industrial Testing Service, 1971.
48. Bradburn NM. *The structure of psychological well-being: NORC monograph in social research.* Chicago: Aldine, 1969.
49. Robinson JP, Shaver PR. *Measures of social psychological attitudes.* Ann Arbor: University of Michigan Institute for Social Research, 1969.
50. Beck AT, Weissman A, Lester D, et al. The measurement of pessimism: The hopelessness scale. *J Consult Clin Psychol* 1974;42:861–865.
51. Wechsler D. *Wechsler adult intelligence scale manual.* New York: The Psychological Corporation, 1955.
52. Derogatis LR. *The Psychosocial Adjustment to Illness Scale (PAIS and PAIS-SR) scoring, procedures and administration manual—I.* Baltimore: Clinical Psychometric Research, 1983.
53. Kornfeld DS, Heller SS, Frank KA, et al. Psychologic and behavioral responses after coronary artery bypass graft surgery. In: Wenger NK, Mattson ME, Furberg CD, Elinson J, eds. *Assessment of quality of life in clinical trials of cardiovascular therapies.* New York: Le Jacq, 1984;233–238.
54. Mayou R, Bryant B. Quality of life after coronary artery surgery. *Q J Med* 1987;62:239–248.
55. Raymond M, Conklin C, Schaeffer J, et al. Coping with transient intellectual dysfunction after coronary bypass surgery. *Heart Lung* 1984;13:531–539.
56. Stanton BA, Jenkins CD, Savageau JA, et al. Perceived adequacy of patient education and fears and adjustments after cardiac surgery. *Heart Lung* 1984;13:525–531.
57. Mayou R. The psychiatric and social consequences of coronary artery surgery. *J Psychosom Res* 1986;30:255–271.
58. Pedley RA, Emerson RG. Neurological complications of cardiac surgery. In: Matthews WB, Blaser GH, eds. *Recent advances in clinical neurology,* vol. 4. Edinburgh: Churchill Livingstone, 1984.
59. Bojar RM, Najafi H, Delaria GA, et al. Neurological complications of coronary revascularization. *Ann Thorac Surg* 1983;36:427–432.
60. Breuer AC, Furlan AJ, Hanson MR, et al. Central nervous system complications of coronary artery bypass graft surgery: Prospective analysis of 421 patients. *Stroke* 1983;14:682–687.
61. Lederman RJ, Breuer AC, Hanson MR, et al. Peripheral nervous system complications of coronary artery bypass graft surgery. *Ann Neurol* 1982;12:297–301.
62. Savageau JA, Stanton BA, Jenkins CD, et al. Neuropsychological dysfunction following elective cardiac operation: I. Early assessment. *J Thorac Cardiovasc Surg* 1982;84:585–594.
63. Savageau JA, Stanton BA, Jenkins CD, et al. Neuropsychological dysfunction following elective cardiac operation: II. A six-month reassessment. *J Thorac Cardiovasc Surg* 1982;84:595–600.
64. Ruberman W, Weinblatt E, Goldberg JD, et al. Psychosocial influences on mortality after myocardial infarction. *N Engl J Med* 1984;311:552.
65. Barboriak JJ, Anderson AJ, Rimm AA. Changes in avocational activities following coronary artery bypass surgery. *J Card Rehab* 1983;3:214–216.
66. CASS Principal Investigators and Their Associates. Coronary Artery Surgery Study (CASS): A randomized trial of coronary artery bypass surgery: Quality of life in patients randomly assigned to treatment groups. *Circulation* 1983;68:951–960.
67. Misra KK, Kazanchi BN, Davies GJ, et al. Determinants of work capability and employment after coronary artery surgery. *Eur Heart J* 1985;6:176–180.
68. Haze K, Hiramori K, Sumiyoshi T, et al. Current status and problems in long-term management of patients undergoing coronary artery bypass surgery in Japan. *Jpn Circ J* 1986;50:895–902.
69. Rose GA, Blackburn H. *Cardiovascular survey methods.* Geneva: World Health Organization, 1968.
70. Hurst JW, King SB, Briesinger GC, et al. Atherosclerotic coronary heart disease: Recognition, prognosis, and treatment. In: Hurst JW, Logue RB, Rackley CE, et al., eds. *The heart,* 6th ed. New York: McGraw-Hill, 1985;882–1008.
71. Peduzzi P, Hultgren HN. Effect of medical vs. surgical treatment on symptoms in stable angina pectoris: The Veterans Administration Cooperative Study of Surgery for Coronary Arterial Occlusive Disease. *Circulation* 1979;60:888.
72. King SB, Hurst JW. The relief of angina pectoris by coronary artery bypass surgery. In: Hurst JW, ed. *Update II: The heart.* New York: McGraw-Hill, 1980;71.

73. Oberman A. Rehabilitation of patients with coronary artery disease. In: Braunwald E, ed. *Heart Disease: A textbook of cardiovascular medicine*, 3rd ed. Philadelphia: W.B. Saunders, 1987;1395.

74. Smith HC, LaVon NH, Gupta S, et al. Employment status after coronary artery bypass surgery. *Circulation* 1982;65(Suppl. 2):II-120-125.

75. Gray RJ, Matloff JM, Conklin CM, et al. Perioperative myocardial infarction: Late clinical course after coronary artery bypass surgery. *Circulation* 1982;66:1185-1189.

76. Rodis E, Shapira I, Miller HI, et al. Work status after coronary artery bypass operation. *J Cardiovasc Surg* 1985;26:228-230.

77. Skupin M, Reifart N, Satter P. Incidence of return to work in relation to invasive, noninvasive, and social parameters. In: Walter PJ, ed. *Return to work after coronary artery bypass surgery: Psychosocial and economic aspects.* New York: Springer-Verlag, 1985;93-101.

78. Anderson AJ, Barboriak JJ, Hoffmann RG, et al. Age- and sex-specific incidence and main factors. In: Walter PJ, ed. *Return to work after coronary artery bypass surgery: Psychosocial and economic aspects.* New York: Springer-Verlag, 1985;3-12.

79. Althof SE, Coffman CB, Levine SB. The effects of coronary bypass surgery on female sexual, psychological, and vocational adaptation. *J Sex Marital Therapy* 1984;10:176-184.

80. Anderson AJ, Barboriak JJ, Hoffman RG, et al. Retention or resumption of employment after aortocoronary bypass operations. *JAMA* 1980;243:543-545.

81. Niles NW, Salm TJV, Cutler BS. Return to work after coronary artery bypass operation. *J Thorac Cardiovasc Surg* 1980;79:916-921.

82. Liddle HV, Jensen R, Clayton PD. The rehabilitation of coronary surgical patients. *Ann Thoracic Surg* 1982;34:374-382.

83. Boulay FM, David PP, Bourassa MG. Strategies for improving the work status of patients after coronary artery bypass surgery. *Circulation* 1982;66(Suppl. III):III-43-49.

84. Gutmann MC, Knapp DN, Pollock ML, et al. Coronary artery bypass surgery. *Circulation* 1982;66(Suppl. 3):III-33-III-42.

85. Guvendik L, Rahan M, Yacoub M. Symptomatic status and pattern of employment during a five-year period following myocardial revascularization for angina. *Ann Thorac Surg* 1982;34:383-387.

86. Johnson WD, Kayser KL, Pedraza PM, et al. Employment patterns in males before and after myocardial revascularization surgery. *Circulation* 1982;65:1086-1093.

87. Oberman A, Wayne JB, Kouchoukos NT, et al. Employment status after coronary artery bypass surgery. *Circulation* 1982;65(Suppl. II):II-115-II-119.

88. Almedia D, Bradford JM, Wenger NK, et al. Return to work after coronary bypass surgery. *Circulation* 1983;68(Suppl. 2):II-205-II-213.

89. Rosenfeldt FL, Lambert R, Burrows K, et al. Hospital costs and return to work after coronary bypass surgery. *Med J Aust* 1983;1:260-263.

90. Holmes DR, Van Raden MJ, Reeder GS, et al. Return to work after coronary angioplasty: A report from the National Heart, Lung, and Blood Institute Percutaneous Transluminal Coronary Angioplasty Registry. *Am J Cardiol* 1984;53:48C-51C.

91. Rogers WJ. Medical vs. surgical management of ischemic heart disease: Implications of the Coronary Artery Surgery Study. *Ala J Med Sci* 1985;22:416-422.

92. Maddern GJ, Craddock DR, Leppard PI, et al. The costs of coronary artery surgery to the community. *J Cardiovasc Surg* 1986;27:469-476.

93. Sergeant P, Lesaffre E, Flameng W, et al. How predictable is the postoperative work resumption after aortocoronary bypass surgery? *Acta Cardiol* 1986;41:41-52.

94. Oberman A, Wayne J, Charles E. Socioeconomic costs of coronary artery bypass grafting. In: Hammermeister KE, ed. *Coronary bypass surgery: The late results.* New York: Praeger Publishers, 1983;389-412.

95. Walter PJ, Amsel BJ. Return to work after coronary artery bypass graft surgery: The role of the primary care physician. *Quality Life Cardivasc Care* 1987;3:31-35.

96. Kinchla J, Weiss T. Psychologic and social outcome following coronary artery bypass surgery. *J Cardiopulm Rehab* 1985;5:274.

97. Oberman A, Finklea JF. Return to work after coronary artery bypass grafting. *Ann Thorac Surg* 1982;34:353-355.

98. Dupuis G, Perrault J, Kennedy E, et al. Delay in return to work after coronary artery bypass surgery: A biobehavioral analysis. *Circulation* 1988;78(4)(Suppl. II):II-227.

99. European Coronary Surgery Study Group. Coronary artery bypass surgery in stable angina pectoris: Survival at two years. *Lancet* 1979;2:889.

100. Takaro R, Hultgren HN, Lipton MJ, et al. The VA cooperative randomized study of surgery for coronary occlusive disease. II. Subgroup with significant left main lesions. *Circulation* 1976;54(Suppl. III);III-107-III-117.

101. Murphy ML, Hultgren HN, Detre K, et al. Treatment of chronic stable angina. A preliminary report of survival data of the randomized Veterans Administration Cooperative Study. *N Engl J Med* 1977;297:621.

102. Takaro R, Hultgren HN, Detre K, et al. The Veterans Administration Cooperative Study of Stable Angina: Current status. *Circulation* 1982;65(Suppl. II):II-60.
103. Russell RO, Wayne JB, Oberman A, et al. Return to work after treatment for coronary artery disease: Role of the physician. *Prim Cardiol* 1981;7(5):12-23.
104. Konttinen M, Frick MH, Harjola PT, et al. Hospital cost development in coronary bypass surgery. *Ann Chir Gynaecol* 1986;75:250-253.
105. Loop FD, Christiansen EK, Lester JL, et al. A strategy for cost containment in coronary surgery. *JAMA* 1983;250:63-66.
106. Oakley CM. Is there life after coronary artery surgery? *Q J Med* 1987;62:181-182.
107. Bandura A. *Social learning theory*. Englewood Cliffs, New Jersey: Prentice-Hall, Inc., 1977.
108. Oberman A. Summary of the discussion. In: Walter PJ, ed. *Return to work after coronary artery bypass surgery: Psychosocial and economic factors*. New York: Springer-Verlag, 1985;58-59.
109. Hartung GH, Rangel R. Exercise training in post-myocardial infarction patients: Comparison of results with high risk coronary and post-bypass patients. *Arch Phys Med Rehabil* 1981;62:147-150.
110. Waites TF, Watt EW, Fletcher GF. Comparative functional and physiologic status of active and dropout coronary bypass patients from a rehabilitation program. *Am J Cardiol* 1983;51:1087-1090.
111. Ben-Ari E, Kellerman JJ, Fisman E, et al. Benefits of long-term physical training in patients after coronary artery bypass grafting—A 58-month follow-up and comparison with a nontrained group. *J Cardiopul Rehab* 1986;6:165.
112. Stevens R, Hanson P. Comparison of supervised and unsupervised exercise training after coronary bypass surgery. *Am J Cardiol* 1984;53:1524-1528.
113. Wenger NK. The coronary patient: Psychological, societal, and vocational aspects of recovery. *Quality Life Cardivasc Care* 1988;4:86-94.
114. Prosser G, Carson P, Phillips R. Exercise after myocardial infarction: Long-term rehabilitation effects. *J Psychosom Res* 1985;29:535.
115. Fontana AF, Kerns RD, Rosenberg RL, et al. Exercise training for cardiac patients: Adherence, fitness, and benefits. *J Cardiopul Rehabil* 1986;6:4.
116. Ott C, Bergner M. The effect of rehabilitation after myocardial infarction on quality of life. *Quality Life Cardiovasc Care* 1985;1:176.
117. Oldenberg B, Perkins RJ, Andrews G. Controlled trial of psychological intervention in myocardial infarction. *J Consult Clin Psychol* 1985;53:852.
118. Ornish D, Scherwitz LW, Doody RS, et al. Effects of stress management training and dietary changes in treating ischemic heart disease. *JAMA* 1983;249:54.
119. Friedman M, Thoresen CE, Gill JJ, et al. Alteration of type A behavior and reduction in cardiac recurrences in postmyocardial infarction patients. *Am Heart J* 1984;108:237.
120. Thoresen CE, Friedman M, Powell LH, et al. Altering type A behavior pattern in postmyocardial infarction patients. *J Cardiopul Rehab* 1985;5:258.
121. Stanton BA, Jenkins CD, Savageau JA, et al. Perceived adequacy of patient education and fears and adjustments after cardiac surgery. *Heart Lung* 1984;13:525-531.
122. Radley A, Green R. Styles of adjustment to coronary graft surgery. *Soc Sci Med* 1985;20:461-472.
123. Tesar GE, Hackett TP. Psychologic management of the hospitalized cardiac patient. *J Cardiopul Rehab* 1985;5:219.

Quality of Life Assessments in Clinical Trials, edited by B. Spilker. Raven Press, Ltd. New York © 1990.

24

Gastrointestinal Surgery

Robin S. McLeod

University of Toronto, Toronto General Hospital, Toronto, Ontario M5G 2C4, Canada

Traditionally, the major outcome measures for the assessment of surgical procedures have been morbidity and mortality. Length of hospital stay may also be reported as an indirect assessment of morbidity. In procedures such as appendectomy, where patients are cured of the illness for which they underwent surgery and do not experience side effects related to the operation, such measures are appropriate. It would be an unusual circumstance in which a patient who had an appendectomy experienced long-term reduction in his quality of life. Thus, measuring quality of life would appear to be trivial.

Morbidity and mortality may be appropriate for assessing some procedures, but they are inadequate for others. For example, although there are objective methods such as manometry, barium studies, and esophagoscopy for documenting reflux esophagitis, ultimately the indication for surgery is the persistence of intractable symptoms. Similarly, in determining the success of an operation, the patient's symptoms and overall satisfaction with the operation are the important outcome measures. Operative complications and mortality rate, although important, incompletely assess the procedure. Follow-up must be long-term, and both the side effects of surgery as well as the effect of surgery in alleviating the patient's initial complaints must be considered.

Postoperative quality of life has been considered sporadically in the surgical literature since the turn of the century. However, it tended to be of secondary importance to the greater emphasis placed on the mortality rate and operative complications. Recent interest in quality of life probably reflects the changing patterns of surgical diseases and the evolution of surgical procedures. At the turn of the century, operative morbidity and mortality for most abdominal procedures tended to be high. As a result, surgery was often reserved for conditions where medical therapy had failed and there was little else to offer the patient. Thus, survival was the important variable in assessing the success of the operation. With improvements in anesthetic techniques, the discovery of antibiotics, and advances in nutrition and other supportive measures, both mortality and morbidity have been significantly reduced. As a result, surgery tends to be performed earlier and not only in lifesaving situations. Mortality following surgical therapy tends to be low and not significantly different from that observed with medical treatment. Consequently, the success of an operation must be evaluated by other parameters. These have tended to be measures of functional results such as stool frequency for operations on the bowel and the presence or absence of dumping symptoms for gastric surgery. "Softer" measures in the domain of quality of life (such as the ability to work and participate in sports) have also been considered in comparing preoperative and postoperative health.

It is likely that the need to assess operations in terms of their effect on overall health will become more and more important. Newer operations are being developed for the express purpose of improving quality of life without any improvement in survival rates or decrease in morbidity. The developments in the field of reconstructive surgery for ulcerative colitis are a good example. Recognizing the difficulty some patients had in adjusting to a conventional Brooke ileostomy, the Kock continent ileostomy and later the ileal reservoir and ileoanal anastomosis were developed. Since the complication rate following both of these procedures tends to be higher than following total proctocolectomy and ileostomy, it is imperative that the patient's quality of life is indeed improved. Thus, tools to quantitatively evaluate and compare the three operations are required. Highly selective vagotomy and stricturoplasty in Crohn's disease are other examples of newer operations which must be evaluated against the standard operations to determine their role and relative value.

As indications for surgery expand, changes in the assessment of surgical results are required. Failure of medical therapy is not an uncommon indication for surgery in gastrointestinal disease. In these patients, objective assessments such as radiological, endoscopic, or pathological findings are of secondary importance in evaluating the success of the procedure. Instead, the success of the operation is determined by whether the patient is cured of his symptoms and hence his quality of life is improved. Surgery is also being performed more frequently for prophylaxis (e.g., colectomy in patients with a long history of ulcerative colitis) or palliatively (e.g., debulking procedures in patients with cancer) and quality of life is as important as quantity of life in both of these situations.

As knowledge of and interest in medicine by lay people increases, patients are participating more, not only in decision making about when to operate, but also about which operation to have. In order to provide them with information upon which to base their decisions, it may be necessary to evaluate quality of life. Patients are naturally reluctant to undergo surgery if the negative impact of surgery is greater than the effects of the disease and side effects of medical therapy. In evaluating surgical procedures in order to make a decision, long-term outcome may be as or more important to the patient than the complication rate. This was borne out in a survey of patients with continent ileostomies, in which we found that 94% of patients stated they would rather have revisionary surgery, should complications occur, than have a conventional ileostomy re-established (1). This included one patient who had already had six operations because of complications associated with the continent ileostomy.

Despite the recognized need for measuring quality of life, validated instruments to measure it are lacking in most areas of gastrointestinal surgery. Most studies assessing quality of life have been qualitative in nature. Often questionnaires containing a variety of items covering physical and possibly social and psychological function have been administered to patients. The obvious limitation of this technique is that a quantitative assessment which considers all aspects of health is not obtained. Thus, one cannot compare different procedures nor the preoperative with the postoperative status of patients. Statistical testing cannot be performed.

TABLE 1. *Conditions where quality of life measures are appropriate*

1. Gastrointestinal diseases in which the major indication for surgery is persistent symptoms:
   a) Reflux esophagitis
   b) Peptic ulcer disease
   c) Crohn's disease
   d) Ulcerative colitis
   e) Portal hypertension
   f) Chronic pancreatitis
2. Cancer surgery:
   a) Palliative cancer surgery
   b) "Mutilating" surgery
3. Transplantation surgery

Because of this lack, this chapter will not be devoted to a discussion of the various instruments available for measuring quality of life as in the other chapters. Instead, it will summarize work that has been done to measure quality of life following gastrointestinal surgery and discuss areas where future efforts might be directed.

AREAS WHERE QUALITY OF LIFE ASSESSMENTS ARE APPROPRIATE

Table 1 lists some conditions which are appropriately evaluated with quality of life measures. These conditions have been divided into three general categories. The first category includes gastrointestinal diseases for which the major indication for surgery is failure of medical management or intractable symptoms. It could be argued that portal hypertension does not fit into this category since the major indication for surgery is bleeding. However, because hepatic encephalopathy is commonly present preoperatively and is a major concern when performing surgery, quality of life is a very important issue in assessing surgery for this condition. The second category is cancer surgery. Although survival remains the most important outcome measure for assessing surgery for primary cancers, quality of life is an important consideration in operating on patients for palliation. It is also of major concern if the surgery is mutilating (e.g., pelvic exenteration). Finally, the third category is transplantation surgery. Quality of life has aroused considerable interest because of the economic impact of transplantation surgery.

In the following sections, the status of quality of life measurements as they pertain to these areas will be discussed. Once again it must be emphasized that quality of life assessment is, for the most part, in its infancy within this field so there are relatively few instruments for measuring quality of life in any of these areas.

Gastric Surgery

Gastric surgery was one of the first areas of surgery in which postoperative quality of life came under scrutiny. Although bleeding and perforation are sometimes indications for surgery in peptic ulcer disease, most often the indication is the persistence of intractable symptoms. Side effects such as dumping symptoms are not uncommon postoperatively. Thus, surgery can be a trade-off of intractable ulcer symptoms for other symptoms of varying severity related to the operation. At one time gastric surgery was one of the most common procedures performed by the

TABLE 2. *Modified Visick Scale for assessing peptic ulcer surgery*

Category	Definition
i. Excellent	Absolutely no symptoms. Perfect result.
II. Very good	Patient considers result perfect, but interrogation elicits mild occasional symptoms easily controlled by minor adjustment to diet.
III. Satisfactory	Mild or moderate symptoms not controlled by care, causing some discomfort, but patient and surgeon satisfied with result. Symptoms do not interfere seriously with life or work.
IV. Unsatisfactory	Moderate or severe symptoms or complications which interfere considerably with work or enjoyment of life; patient or doctor dissatisfied with result. Includes all cases with proven recurrent ulcer and those submitted to further operation even though the latter may have been followed by considerably symptomatic improvement.

abdominal surgeon, so it is not surprising that there was considerable interest in the assessment of postoperative results.

Approximately 40 years ago, the Visick Scale was devised to evaluate postoperative results following gastrectomy (2). Using this scale, an overall rating on a scale of 1 to 4 is assigned to each patient (Table 2). It is not "operation-specific" so it can be used to compare the various surgical procedures performed for peptic ulcer disease. Indeed, it has been used as one of the major outcome measures in several clinical trials evaluating peptic ulcer surgery (3–7).

There are several limitations to this scale. First, it is an extremely subjective assessment of the result. Second, although patients are interviewed to elicit symptoms and their satisfaction with the procedure, ultimately the interviewer rates the result. The interviewer's assessment may not correlate with the patient's, especially if the surgeon who performed the operation is also the person interviewing the patient. Hall et al. found this to be true when both the surgeon and patient were asked to grade the result (8). When interobserver reliability was tested, agreement on the overall Visick gradings was low although there was high agreement on whether symptoms were present and the severity of them. Test re-test reliability and validity have not been formally tested. Despite these limitations, the Visick Scale continues to be used in the assessment of peptic ulcer surgery, probably because it has been used for many years and surgeons are familiar with it. However, a new instrument is needed to undertake future trials evaluating peptic ulcer surgery.

Troidl et al. have developed an instrument to measure outcome following gastrectomy for gastric carcinoma (9). This instrument contains disease-specific variables as well as those relating to overall physical and social function. The total score assigned to the patient can range from 0 to 14. This instrument has been tested against a modification of the Visick Scale and the Spitzer Index of Quality of Life and was found to be better at discriminating patients than either of the other two. The literature does not clearly state whether the instrument has been tested for reliability.

Crohn's Disease

In 1970, the National Cooperative Crohn's Disease Study group was formed to plan controlled trials to determine the effectiveness of several treatments of Crohn's disease (10). This group recognized that Crohn's disease is a chronic illness characterized by spontaneous exacerbations and remissions. Changes in symptoms and signs may not be accompanied by changes in objective measures such as radiological or endoscopic findings. Thus, they developed the Crohn's Disease Activity Index in order to measure disease activity. Subsequently other instruments have been developed, many of them modeled after or modifications of the Crohn's Disease Activity Index (11–14). A major component of all of them is the assessment of bowel function. Other symptoms and physical signs as well as certain laboratory measures are incorporated into them. General well-being also is considered in some; otherwise, all items refer only to physical function. Reliability and validity have been variably assessed. Although they have been used to measure outcome in clinical trials, there is considerable debate as to their validity and sensitivity in measuring changes in disease activity (12).

Despite being used to assess medical therapy, these instruments have not been used in the evaluation of surgical treatment. The major limitation of using them for this purpose is that the important attributes for measuring health status may differ postoperatively. For instance, preoperative bowel function tends to correlate with disease activity and is therefore responsive to a change in the patient's status. This is not necessarily true in the postoperative patient. Patients may experience excessive stool frequency due to their resection, without any impairment of their physical health or quality of life. Furthermore, items related to bowel function would be totally irrelevant in assessing the patient in whom an ileostomy was constructed. On the other hand, this patient might have psychological problems related to the stoma which would not be considered in these disease activity indices. Thus, in designing an instrument to measure outcome following surgery, it would need to be responsive to change and in addition, contain items which were relevant both preoperatively and postoperatively. One situation where these instruments might be of value is in the evaluation of stricturoplasty. Provided a resection was not performed, the confounding effects of a resection would not be present and the diseased segments would still be present. Items related to pain, bowel function, nutritional status, and general well-being should be responsive to change, although it is unlikely that items related to extraintestinal manifestations or perianal complications would be affected.

Recently, Guyatt et al. have developed an instrument for measuring the subjective health status of patients with inflammatory bowel disease (15). Unlike the other instruments, this instrument includes items related to patients' subjective evaluation of their functional status. It contains attributes pertaining to four aspects of their lives: symptoms directly related to primary bowel disturbance, systemic symptoms, emotional status, and social function. No physical signs or laboratory values are included. It was developed for measuring outcome in clinical trials of patients with either ulcerative colitis or Crohn's disease.

This instrument attempts to measure quality of life based on items relevant to the patient's functional status. This is noteworthy because, ultimately, the most important judge of quality of life is the patient himself. Items such as the presence of a mass or fever, which are contained in the other activity indices, may correlate well with a feeling of well-being but one cannot presume that this is the case. This instrument may prove to have several shortcomings, however. It was tested in only 61 subjects, most of whom were outpatient volunteers. Only a small number were inpatients and it seems that none of these subsequently underwent surgery. Thus, it appears that all patients probably had mild disease and whether this instrument will be of value in discriminating between patients with a wide spectrum of disease activity is yet to be determined. It has also been developed for use in patients with ulcerative colitis or Crohn's disease. However, at least some of the symptoms and problems encountered differ depending on the disease. Thus, some of the items, especially those that are disease-specific, may not be responsive with one or the other diseases. For example, urgency and the need to find a toilet are common complaints of patients with ulcerative colitis but rarely do patients with Crohn's disease experience this. Like the other instruments, this instrument has not been used in evaluating postsurgical results. It too may be of limited value in this setting since it contains attributes that may not pertain to the postoperative patient.

Other than these instruments, there are no instruments available which have been developed specifically for measuring quality of life of Crohn's disease patients post-operatively. To date, quality of life has only been assessed with patient surveys (16,17).

Ulcerative Colitis

There has been great interest in quality of life in this area since the development of the Kock continent ileostomy and the ileal reservoir and ileoanal anastomosis procedure. These procedures were developed to improve quality of life. It is recognized, however, that both are technically more difficult to perform than a proctocolectomy and conventional ileostomy so the complication rates tend to be higher.

There are multiple articles in the literature assessing the quality of life of patients with conventional ileostomies, ileorectal anastomosis, Kock continent ileostomies, and ileal reservoirs (1,18–26). In all of these, results of patient surveys were reported. Various items covering physical function, psychological well-being, and social function were assessed, as were subjective global perceptions.

The major limitation of all of these studies is that quality of life was not measured quantitatively. Thus, the usefulness of this information is limited in that it is virtually impossible to compare the quality of life achieved by patients with a conventional ileostomy to that of patients with a continent ileostomy or ileal reservoir. Additionally, the preoperative status cannot be compared to the postoperative status. There are, however, no instruments available which have been developed specifically to measure quality of life of ileostomates. There is an interest in this area but it is difficult to develop a multiple-item instrument. Choosing items which are relevant and important to all patients is virtually impossible. For instance, in assessing quality of life in patients with an ileal reservoir, the number of bowel movements per day might be an important item. However, it would be totally irrelevant to a patient with any type of ileostomy for whom fear of leakage or odor might be an important item.

We have used two different techniques which provide a global assessment of the patient's health status: the time trade-off technique and direct questioning of objectives (27,28). The time trade-off technique was developed by Torrance for utility estimation where the utility of a health state is its perceived worth (27). To do this, the patient is presented with a choice between two hypothetical situations. The first is to continue in his present health state for a lifetime (t) which has been determined from actuarial data. The alternative choice is a shorter time (x) in a state of full health. The interviewer then adjusts x until a point of equivalence is reached (i.e., where the patient cannot decide between full health for x time versus present health for *t* time). The value x/t is the utility of the health state for the individual. A utility of 0 indicates death, and 1 indicates full health.

The second technique is the direct questioning of objectives which was developed by Detsky et al. for assessing quality of life in patients on home parenteral nutrition (28). There are three steps. First, a list of objectives or goals which are important to the patient is elicited from each patient. A category scaling is used to derive importance weights, on a scale of 0 to 10, for each of the patient's objectives. Then a category scaling is used to measure, on a scale of 0 to 1.0, the patient's ability to achieve each objective in the present health state. Quality of life is estimated as a weighted average of the patient's ability to achieve his or her objectives with the weights determined by the importance values.

These techniques were used in two situations: the quality of life of patients with a conventional ileostomy, Kock continent ileostomy, or ileal reservoir were compared by studying approximately 100 patients who had had one of these procedures at least 1 year previously. In addition, 25 patients were studied preoperatively to assess their quality of life with ulcerative colitis and compare it with their quality of life 12 months postoperatively. Several standard psychological tests were administered and assessments by the patient, surgeon, and family member were ascertained to test the construct validity of the instruments in this patient population. Reliability was not tested since this had been tested previously (28). Our results indicated that the postoperative patients, irrespective of the surgical procedure, had a high quality of life with mean utilities of over 0.90 in each of the three groups (29). Quality of life was significantly improved over the preoperative status in the group studied before and after surgery.

In assessing the usefulness of these instruments in this patient population, there are several points to consider. Both instruments were highly acceptable to patients and easy to use by the interviewer after only a short training period. The average time to administer both the time trade-off technique and the direct questioning of objectives was less than 15 minutes. Quantitative assessments considering all aspects of health were obtained. Results were amenable to statistical testing. Both instruments were able to detect changes between the preoperative and postoperative states of patients. However, no significant differences were detected among the three postoperative groups of patients. This may be due to the fact that patients do, indeed, achieve equally high quality of life. Patients choose the procedure they want to have. It seems that postoperatively, most patients adjust well to having an ileostomy. On the other hand, it is possible that these instruments are not sensitive enough to detect small differences in quality of life. A final point is that although these instruments are useful for assigning mean utilities for groups of patients, they appear to be imprecise in measuring attitudes of individuals (28).

Currently, we are developing an instrument to measure quality of life of patients with ileal reservoirs. This will be a multiple-item instrument for use in clinical trials assessing this procedure. Items have been chosen which are most important to the patient and best discriminate between results. Our preliminary results have shown that the items measuring social function (e.g., ability to work, perform activities of daily living, and do hobbies) are most important to these patients. Items which pertain to physical function such as stool frequency, urgency, and continence are of lesser importance (*unpublished data*). Most of the surgical literature tends to concentrate on items pertaining to bowel function in assessing the results. This may be of concern to the surgeon but it appears to be of lesser importance to most patients. It emphasizes the discrepancy that may exist between assessments made by the surgeon and the patient.

Cancer Surgery

Quality of life measurements are as important in the evaluation of surgery in cancer patients as they are in evaluating medical therapy. Although there are no instruments which have been developed especially for use in surgical oncology, instruments such as the Spitzer Quality of Life Index, Karnofsky Scale, and Eastern Co-Operative Oncology Group Performance Scale have been used frequently (30–32). These instruments will not be discussed further as they are discussed in other chapters.

Liver Transplantation

The University of Pittsburgh group has performed more liver transplants than any other group in the world, and have also studied quality of life of patients post-transplant most extensively (33,34). Various neuropsychological tests have been used as well as the Sickness Impact Profile. No instrument specifically designed to assess outcome in this patient population has been used.

CONCLUSIONS

It is well recognized that quality of life is an important consideration in performing surgery for gastrointestinal diseases. However, to date, most attempts at measuring it have been relatively unsophisticated and much work is needed to measure quality of life quantitatively. In this chapter, an attempt was made to outline areas where quality of life assessments are needed and to review the literature on work performed to date.

Future efforts should be directed toward developing instruments which measure quality of life in patients undergoing gastrointestinal surgery. Surgeons have been criticized for not evaluating surgical procedures critically in controlled clinical trials. To a large extent, this criticism is valid. However, in order to perform clinical trials, appropriate outcome measures must be chosen. Thus, the need for instruments to measure quality of life is apparent. Disease-specific or operation-specific instruments appear to be required (35). Measures of general health, for the most part, tend to be insensitive to measuring changes in postoperative health or in comparing different procedures. Prior to developing an instrument, its purpose should be explicitly stated because the items included will vary accordingly. As has been mentioned repeatedly in this chapter, for instruments used to compare the preoperative and the postoperative status, items must be chosen which are important and relevant to the patient before and after surgery. In some situations this may not be possible, so instruments which measure the global health status of patients may be more appropriate.

REFERENCES

1. McLeod RS, Fazio VW. Quality of life with the continent ileostomy. *World J Surg* 1984;8:90–95.
2. Visick AH. A study of the failures after gastrectomy. *Ann R Coll Surg Engl* 1948;3:266–284.

3. Goligher JC, de Dombal FT, Duthie HL, Latchmore AJC, Smiddy FG. Five- to eight-year results of Leeds/York controlled trial of elective surgery for duodenal ulcer. *Br Med J* 1968;1:781–787.

4. Jordan PH. A prospective study of parietal cell vagotomy and selective vagotomy-antrectomy for treatment of duodenal ulcer. *Ann Surg* 1976;183:619–627.

5. Stoddard CJ, Vassilakis JS, Duthie HL. Highly selective vagotomy or truncal vagotomy and pyloroplasty for chronic duodenal ulceration: A randomized, prospective clinical study. *Br J Surg* 1978;65:793–796.

6. Dorricott NJ, McNeish AR, Alexander-Williams J, et al. Prospective randomized multicentre trial of proximal gastric vagotomy or truncal vagotomy and antrectomy for chronic duodenal ulcer: Interim results. *Br J Surg* 1978;65:152–154.

7. Christiansen J, Jensen HE, Poul EP, Bardram L, Henriksen FW. Prospective controlled vagotomy trial for duodenal ulcer. Primary results, sequelae, acid secretion, and recurrence rates two to five years after operation. *Ann Surg* 1981;193:49–56.

8. Hall R, Horrocks JC, Clamp SE, de Dombal FT. Observer variation in results of surgery for peptic ulceration. *Br Med J* 1976;1:814–816.

9. Troidl H, Kusche J, Vestweber KH, Eypasch E, Koeppen L, Bouillon B. Quality of life: An important endpoint both in surgical practice and research. *J Chron Dis* 1987;40:523–528.

10. Best WR, Becktel JM, Singleton JW, Kern F Jr. Development of a Crohn's disease activity index. National Cooperative Crohn's Disease Study. *Gastroenterology* 1976;70:439–444.

11. Myren J, Bouchier IAD, Watkinson G, Softley A, Clamp SE, de Dombal FT. The O.M.G.E. Multinational Inflammatory Bowel Disease Survey 1976–1982. A further report on 2,657 cases. *Scand J Gastroenterol* 1982;19(Suppl. 95):1–27.

12. de Dombal FT, Softley A. IOIBD Report No. 1: Observer variation in calculating indices of severity and activity in Crohn's disease. *Gut* 1987;28:474–481.

13. Harvey RF, Bradshaw JM. A simple index of Crohn's disease activity. *Lancet* 1980;1:514.

14. Van Hees PAM, Van Elteren PH, Van Lier HJJ, Van Tongeren JHM. An index of inflammatory activity in patients with Crohn's disease. *Gut* 1980;21:279–286.

15. Guyatt GI, Mitchell A, Irvine EJ, Singer J, Williams N, Goodacre R, Tompkins C. A new measure of health status for clinical trials in inflammatory bowel disease. *Gastroenterology* 1989;96:804–810.

16. Meyers S, Walfish JS, Sachar DB, Greenstein AJ, Hill AG, Janowitz HD. Quality of life after surgery for Crohn's disease: A psychological survey. *Gastroenterology* 1980;78:1–6.

17. Lindhagen T, Ekelund G, Leandoer L, Hildell J, Lindstrom C, Wenckert A. Pre- and post-operative complications in Crohn's disease with special reference to duration of preoperative disease history. *Scand J Gastroenterol* 1984;19:194–203.

18. Jagelman DG, Lewis CB, Rowe-Jones DC. Ileorectal anastomosis: Appreciation by patients. *Br Med J* 1969;1:756–757.

19. Oakley JR, Jagelman DG, Fazio VW, Lavery IC, Weakley FL, Easley K, Farmer RG. Complications and quality of life after ileorectal anastomosis for ulcerative colitis. *Am J Surg* 1985;149:23–30.

20. Roy PH, Sauer WG, Beahrs OH, Farrow GM. Experience with ileostomies. Evaluation of long-term rehabilitation in 497 patients. *Am J Surg* 1970;119:77–86.

21. Morowitz DA, Kirsner JB. Ileostomy in ulcerative colitis. A questionnaire study of 1,803 patients. *Am J Surg* 1981;141:370–375.

22. McLeod RS, Lavery IC, Leatherman JR, Maryland PA, Fazio VW, Jagelman DG, Weakley FW. Factors affecting quality of life with a conventional ileostomy. *World J Surg* 1986;10:474–480.

23. McLeod RS, Lavery IC, Leatherman JR, Maryland PA, Fazio VW, Jagelman DG, Weakley FW. Patient evaluation of the conventional ileostomy. *Dis Colon Rectum* 1985;28:152–154.

24. Kock NG, Darle N, Kewenter J, Myrvold H, Philipson B. The quality of life after proctocolectomy and ileostomy. A study of patients with conventional ileostomies converted to continent ileostomies. *Dis Colon Rectum* 1974;17:287–292.

25. Nilsson LO, Kock NG, Kylberg F, Myrvold HE, Palselius I. Sexual adjustment in ileostomy patients before and after conversion to continent ileostomy. *Dis Colon Rectum* 1981;24:287–290.

26. Pezim ME, Nicholls RJ. Quality of life after restorative proctocolectomy with pelvic ileal reservoir. *Br J Surg* 1985;72:31–33.

27. Torrance GW, Thomas WH, Sackett DL. A utility maximization model for evaluation of health care programs. *Health Services Res* 1972;7:118–133.

28. Detsky AS, McLaughlin JR, Abrams HB, L'Abbe KA, Whitwell J, Bombardier C, Jeejeebhoy KN. Quality of life of patients on long-term total parenteral nutrition at home. *J Gen Int Med* 1986;1:26–33.

29. McLeod RS, Cohen Z, Churchill DN, Lock AM, Isbister S. Measurement of quality of life of patients with ulcerative colitis undergoing surgery (*submitted*).

30. Spitzer WO, Dobson AJ, Hall J, et al. Measuring the quality of life of cancer patients. A concise QL-index for use by physicians. *J Chron Dis* 1981;34:585–597.

31. Karnofsky DA, Burchenal JH. The clinical evaluation of chemotherapeutic agents in cancer. In: Macleod CM, ed. Evaluation of chemotherapeutic agents. New York: Columbia University Press, 1949;191–205.

32. Kalser MH, Barkin J, MacIntyer JM. Pancreatic cancer—Assessment of prognosis by clinical presentation. *Cancer* 1985;56:397–402.
33. Tarter RE, Van Thiel DH, Hegedus AM, Schade RR, Gavaler JS, Starzl TE. Neuropsychiatric status after liver transplantation. *J Lab Clin Med* 1984;103:776–782.
34. Tarter RE, Erb S, Biller PA, Switala J, Van Thiel DH. The quality of life following liver transplantation: A preliminary report. *Gastroenterol Clin North Am* 1988;17:207–217.
35. Goligher JC. Judging the quality of life after surgical operations. *J Chron Dis* 1987;40:631–633.

V

Specific Problems and Diseases

Quality of Life Assessments in Clinical Trials, edited by B. Spilker. Raven Press, Ltd. New York © 1990.

25

Cardiovascular Disorders

*Nanette K. Wenger and †Curt D. Furberg

*Emory University School of Medicine, Grady Memorial Hospital, Atlanta, Georgia 30303; †Center for Prevention Research and Biometry, The Bowman Gray School of Medicine, Winston-Salem, North Carolina 27103

RATIONALE FOR QUALITY OF LIFE STUDIES IN CARDIOVASCULAR DISORDERS

The contemporary practice of cardiology deals predominantly with the care of patients with chronic illness. The goal of therapy of a chronic illness is generally not to cure the disease, but rather to alleviate its symptoms, improve the patient's functional capabilities, and retard the progression of the underlying disease. Thus an evaluative component that addresses the way in which a patient's life is affected by the illness and its care, in addition to the traditional measures of morbidity and mortality, appears warranted. Spitzer has termed this the assessment of "clinically relevant human attributes" (1).

The rationale for quality of life studies differs with different subsets of patients with cardiovascular disease. For example, in patients with advanced congestive cardiac failure, morbidity and mortality are perhaps insensitive measures for comparing outcomes because this is a highly symptomatic disorder with a generally poor prognosis. The goals of therapy, the relief of symptoms with resultant comfort of the patient for the remaining duration of life and the maintenance of a limited functional capacity, are more likely to be influenced by therapy and can be ascertained by assessment of quality of life attributes.

Very different considerations apply when preventive therapies are instituted for cardiovascular disorders, typically in asymptomatic individuals; examples include persons with mild systemic arterial hypertension, asymptomatic hypercholesterolemia, and asymptomatic ventricular dysfunction. These disorders are characterized by an excellent prognosis and very low incidence of complications, at least in the short term, and often a relatively low rate of individual complications even over months to years; here, morbidity and mortality data are typically not helpful for characterizing treatment outcome. However, since most therapies for these conditions may cause symptoms in an otherwise symptomless individual, it is important to address those features that may adversely alter the subject's functional status and sense of well-being.

Considerations differ further when an intervention for a serious and often life-threatening illness may entail manifestations of drug toxicity and resultant morbidity.

335

An example is the use of most anti-arrhythmic drugs designed to control potentially life-threatening arrhythmias. To determine the appropriate role of these interventions, one must compare the patient's quality of life with standard care of the arrhythmias and the potential for urgent intermittent hospitalizations for these life-threatening problems, versus the possibly reduced mortality and likely toxicity associated with an otherwise effective control of the arrhythmia.

A final category of problems involves acute life-threatening illnesses, the prototype being myocardial infarction, for which invasive and high-risk interventions, acute thrombolysis and acute angioplasty to name a few, have the dual goals of improving short-term survival and limiting morbidity, despite the potential discomforts and high risk of complications in the short term.

BACKGROUND INFORMATION

Advantages and Problems of General Quality of Life Measures

Global or generic quality of life measures address a variety of domains or dimensions of life quality, most prominent of which are physical function, social and emotional function, intellectual function, symptoms and their consequences, occupational activities and job satisfaction, leisure activities, sexual adjustment, perceived health status, life satisfaction, and interpersonal relationships. Examples of such measures include the Nottingham Health Profile (2), the Quality of Well-Being Scale (3), and the Sickness Impact Profile (4). It is obvious that one can overestimate the benefits of a therapy if adverse or unwanted effects are not considered. Examination of a variety of dimensions of a patient's life are of value in identifying both unanticipated benefits and side effects of therapy; moreover, these bidirectional effects can sometimes be integrated. General health profiles that encompass the major areas of quality of life can identify those aspects that are affected by the disease and its management.

However, general measures may fail to examine adequately detailed aspects of treatment for specific symptoms or functions related to a disease.

Advantages and Problems of Disease-Specific Measures

Disease-specific measures are designed to address selected changes that are unique to an identified population or illness. As such, the New York Heart Association functional classification can be used to assess limitations of ability to perform physical activity in a variety of cardiovascular diseases (5). The Specific Activity Scale (SAS), also a measure of the ability to perform physical activity, is thought by some to be more precise (6) and correlates well with measured maximal oxygen uptake at graded exercise testing (7). Chest pain in patients with coronary heart disease can be classified by the Rose chest pain questionnaire (8) or the Canadian Cardiovascular Society (CCS) measure of severity (9); several indices are available for the measurement of dyspnea, and are particularly useful in patients with heart failure (10,11).

A problem with disease-specific measures is that many domains of interest, even in a specific illness, vary with the stage or severity of that illness, the setting of the disease, the age of the patient, and the comorbidity. For example, quality of life attributes of concern to coronary patients differ when the patient is in an intensive care unit setting, during the remainder of the hospital stay, and during long-term ambulatory care. Different attributes may also be of interest to the coronary patient with stable angina pectoris as compared with one who has acute myocardial infarction or who is undergoing coronary angioplasty or coronary bypass surgery.

Another major problem of disease-specific measures is that they do not enable comparison of quality of life features or outcomes between populations with different diseases, which is a feasible comparison when global or generic quality of life measures are employed. The difficulty with disease-specific measures further reflects the complex relationships among the quality of life dimensions. For example, increasing severity of physical symptoms and resultant decrease in physical capacities may cause depression or other emotional dysfunction. On the other hand, depression or emotional dysfunction may lead to limitations of physical function. Although some specific aspects are addressed with more detail when disease-specific measures are used, the total scope of quality of life attributes should also be surveyed: general well-being, functional capacity, cognitive function, emotional function, social participation, economic status, and the like.

Perceptions, Expectations, and Patient-Family Interrelationships

It is often advisable to address the impact of the disease on the family and significant others, in addition to the patient; the effects of illness, disability, and their therapies often extend beyond the target individuals.

The perceptions of the patients and their families reflect their personal value systems and judgments regarding general health status, well-being, and life satisfaction. The perceptions of family members as to the effect of the disease and the therapy on the patient are important, and may be different from that of the patient. Often there is lack of congruence between perceived health status and actual health; in a number of studies, it was the rating of perceived health status that correlated significantly with the risk of mortality (12–14). Perceived health status has also been described as correlating better with work performance than objective measures of functional capacity.

Expectations (both the patient's and the family's) constitute important determinants of satisfaction with the outcome of therapy. In many chronic and progressive illnesses, with time, as symptoms become increasingly severe and activities become more stringently restricted, patient expectations are likely to lessen as to the degree of improvement that can be obtained. As new therapies improve the outlook for both morbidity and mortality, excessively limited patient expectations may curtail the scope of benefit that may be ascertained from an intervention.

There is particular concern about the impact of patient expectations when the querying for quality of life variables is done in the capability mode, i.e., "Can you do . . . without difficulty?" versus the performance mode, i.e., "Did you do . . . without difficulty?" Obviously, lessened expectations can alter the former to a greater extent.

Return to Work as a Component of Quality of Life

Many recent studies have been characterized by an inordinate and probably disproportionate focus on return to work as a measure of quality of life, so much so that in a number of reports, work appears to have been used almost as a surrogate for quality of life. Whereas return to work may be an important component of life quality for many patients, and indeed for many populations under study, return to work measures only one aspect of life quality and does not, even for that aspect, address job satisfaction, job performance, the opportunity for advancement, adequacy of income, and the like.

In many populations, particularly the severely impaired and the elderly, return to remunerative work is not a reasonable goal of most interventions, and therefore can be an inappropriate aspect of quality of life to use as an outcome measure. Further, there is abundant evidence that many other nonmedical (nonintervention-related) aspects predominantly influence return to work, including the pre-illness employment history, patient and family preferences, the job category and skill level, the level of unemployment in the community, financial status, and the employer's and the patient's perceptions of limitations. Indeed, in a number of studies, the patient's pre-intervention expectation of the ability to return to work was the most important determinant of employment outcome. In many return to work studies, perception of health status, rather than actual health status, and perception of ability to work, rather than objective measures of functional capability, often proved the overwhelming determinant.

Other Uses of Quality of Life Data

Increasingly, quality of life data will be considered in determining the cost-effectiveness of care, i.e., the resources required relative to the health benefits obtained. Life quality issues are among the attributes of effectiveness; easily determined attributes include independent function and productivity, which encompass return to remunerative work, but life satisfaction is a more difficult area to define precisely. Life satisfaction derives from the sense of well-being, physical status, emotional state, and intellectual functioning, as well as work performance.

SYSTEMIC ARTERIAL HYPERTENSION

The management of patients with asymptomatic or minimally symptomatic mild to moderate systemic arterial hypertension is used as a prototype of an asymptomatic cardiovascular illness that requires long-term therapy, whether alteration of lifestyle or pharmacotherapy; therapies are designed not for immediate benefit, but for the life-long prevention of late complications. These are predominantly preventive interventions. Comparable concerns will be encountered in the management of patients with asymptomatic hypercholesterolemia (15) and in the treatment of asymptomatic ventricular dysfunction (as discussed below in association with congestive heart failure).

These are far different considerations than for the therapy of severe uncontrolled accelerated hypertension, wherein the short-term, life-threatening consequences of cerebrovascular accident, heart failure, myocardial infarction, and renal failure, among others, far outweigh any short-term impact on quality of life.

Both nonpharmacologic and pharmacologic therapies for patients with mild asymptomatic hypertension have provided the greatest longitudinal experience in assessing aspects of quality of life as outcome measures. As stated previously, the prognosis for these patients, based on the traditional biomedical measures of morbidity and mortality, is so favorable (at least in the short term, such as 4 or 5 years), that these measures typically will not discriminate among therapies, nor will they commonly identify the positive and negative impacts on quality of life exerted by each.

Because these patients are essentially asymptomatic, a prominent feature of both nonpharmacologic and pharmacologic therapeutic assessments must involve an extensive spectrum of quality of life attributes. Important among these are the patients' perceptions since long-term adherence to the recommended interventions, if effective, will undoubtedly influence outcome. There is abundant evidence that patients' perceptions of the seriousness of the problem and the importance and value of the therapy influence adherence.

An additional problem, thus far well-documented only in the setting of hypertension, relates to the "labeling effect": an alteration in the sense of well-being, general activity level, and work attendance related solely to the information that hypertension is present, even prior to the initiation of therapy. These adverse responses occurred whether or not hypertension was subsequently determined to be present (16–19). The "labeling effect" must be included in the weighting of positive and negative effects of any antihypertensive treatment. On the other hand, even randomization to the placebo group of a clinical trial has been described as enhancing the patients' perceived symptomatic status (20,21).

Nonpharmacologic interventions, such as substantial changes in lifestyle including dietary modification to effect weight reduction and decrease sodium intake, increased activity level (exercise), smoking cessation, moderation in alcohol use, and the like may significantly alter the patient's perceived life quality (17).

Further, since there are now available a number of categories of antihypertensive medications that can effect a comparable reduction in blood pressure, presumably with comparable long-term benefit, their impact on diverse categories of quality of life must be examined because adherence to medication will be substantially influenced by perceived interference with the desired lifestyle. Among the issues examined in a number of clinical trials comparing categories of antihypertensive drugs are their effect on depression, alertness, intellectual function, sleep dysfunction, activity limitation, and sexual dysfunction, but these features must be combined with consideration of medication-taking problems (particularly the dose frequency), the cost, the requirements for tests for surveillance of therapy, and for office visits for surveillance of care (22,23). Because these patients are asymptomatic, therapy does not have the potential to improve their functional status and sense of well-being, but can only cause new symptoms, decrease the ability to function, and ultimately result in poorer adherence to therapy if the unwanted effects are substantial.

These considerations were highlighted in the 1988 report of the U.S. Joint National Committee on the Detection, Evaluation, and Treatment of High Blood Pressure (24), which included their recommendation to individualize or "profile" patients for treatment of their hypertension. Items addressed were the resultant quality of life of the patient, and the costs of care. Quality of life outcomes have also been cited as concerns in the management of hypertension in the deliberations of the British Cardiac Society and European Atherosclerosis Society and in their recommendations for preventive therapy (25,26).

A number of intellectual and emotional problems are among the unwanted responses to the treatment of patients with hypertension. These include depression; impaired alertness, memory, and intellectual function; sleep dysfunction including nightmares; mood alterations; irritability; lack of initiative; impaired complex cognitive functioning (27), and more. A number of these features have been compared in clinical trials, and the perceptions of the patients, their physicians, and their close relatives have been compared as well (22,23,28–31). In a number of these studies, a combination of the labeling effect and pharmacotherapy resulted in impaired memory and learning, depression, irritability, and lack of initiative, to name a few.

CONGESTIVE HEART FAILURE

Patients with congestive heart failure represent the other extreme of the spectrum of cardiovascular illness. These patients are characteristically chronically and progressively ill, severely symptomatic, often elderly, are usually receiving multiple drugs, and have concomitant restrictions of dietary intake and of activity. Most important, however, is that even with recent improvements in therapy and in short-term survival, their overall prognosis remains poor. Therefore, the major goal of therapy for patients with this problem is the limitation of symptoms with resultant comfort for the remaining duration of life, as well as the maintenance of the current level of physical functioning. Because the physical capacity of these individuals is borderline, the maintenance of independence is often precarious and may be adversely impacted by any unwanted effect of therapy. It is this outcome—maintenance of autonomy and independent living, rather than return to work (as will be discussed below for the coronary patient)—that should be addressed as an outcome variable.

Because virtually all components of life quality may be influenced by an intervention for heart failure, a broadly based assessment instrument using multivariant measures is recommended (32). Among the features to be considered are the effect of the therapy on the ability to ambulate and to perform self-care; to continue home management; to get adequate sleep and rest; to engage in pleasurable activities such as hobbies, recreational activities, and sexual activity; to perform social roles with family and friends; to retain a sense of control and self-reliance; to retain intellectual and cognitive function; to require and use health resources; to continue the coping behaviors and appropriate denial; and to exhibit other features of emotional stability that involve expectations, mood, life satisfaction, and reasonable optimism about the future.

Most important are the expectations of the patients regarding the outcome of their illness and particularly the outcome of therapy. With the demonstration in recent years that newer pharmacotherapies can improve survival as well as improve symptoms and functional capacity, it will be important to determine if patients' expectations of subjective improvement are met (33–35).

As previously noted, the New York Heart Association functional classification, often used to define whether "usual" activities can be performed without resultant symptoms, may be misleading in that "usual" activities at the time of intervention may be significantly less than those typically undertaken months or years previously (36). The Specific Activity Scale (6), although perhaps overcoming some of these problems, appears able only to detect sizable improvements in functional capacity. The New York Heart Association functional classification is similarly insensitive to change. Other indices are available for the clinical assessment of dyspnea, defining the magnitude of effort needed for its precipitation (10,11).

Because cerebral blood flow may change with alterations in cardiac output and peripheral vascular resistance, it appears prudent to assess the finer and more detailed aspects of cognitive function, including attention, concentration, memory, learning ability, and recall, among others, as has been done in some studies of antihypertensive medications (37). Preliminary data from patients with dilated cardiomyopathy referred for cardiac transplantation showed a high incidence of moderate to severe verbal cognitive deficits and deficits of higher cortical function at baseline evaluation (38). The ongoing National Heart, Lung, and Blood Institute Study of Left Ventricular Dysfunction (SOLVD) should provide some information about this aspect via a brief quality of life questionnaire that is included in the composite data collection for all patients. A more detailed substudy on quality of life that addresses personal, social, and role functioning; emotional functioning; cognitive functioning; economic status; and stress, coping measures, and social resources and support will be used to validate the short inventory.

Among the newer data derived from clinical studies of heart failure is the information that exercise capacity correlates poorly with left ventricular ejection fraction. Despite the fact that left ventricular ejection fraction is a good predictor of survival, many patients with a very poor ejection fraction have a reasonable exercise capacity (39,40). Exercise capacity, however, does not reliably predict survival. In other patients, it is the pace at which an activity is performed that is a significant determinant of exercise tolerance (41). Similarly, the symptomatic status of patients with heart failure correlates poorly with indices of ventricular function (39,40), but little is known about the relationship between the objectively determined physical work capacity and features of quality of life. This lack of consistency among exercise capacity, hemodynamic changes, symptoms, prognosis, and quality of life attributes may pose problems in the assessment of outcomes of therapeutic interventions for heart failure. Improvement in physiologic parameters, without comparable improvement in functional status and in the quality of life characteristics deemed important by the patient, probably should not be termed a favorable outcome (39).

In the National Heart, Lung, and Blood Institute's SOLVD trial, the other end of the spectrum of heart failure is also addressed, i.e., asymptomatic left ventricular dysfunction. As noted above, this aspect is more akin to asymptomatic systemic arterial hypertension than it is to severe and symptomatic congestive cardiac failure. Because of the generally unfavorable prognosis once heart failure becomes clinically manifest, the question has appropriately been raised as to the potential benefit of pharmacotherapy in the asymptomatic stage of ventricular dysfunction.

This is one reason why a disease-specific or a problem-specific measure cannot be reasonably considered for "heart failure" as a general problem. In the asymptomatic stage of ventricular dysfunction a therapy has only the potential, at least in the short term, to produce symptoms and adversely affect the perception of health status and well-being. Therefore, the considerations that must be addressed should span most of the life quality variables, and a generic or global measure seems most appropriate. Certainly physical and emotional symptoms should be considered, as should interpersonal relationships, sexual adjustment, leisure activity, and work function. In this asymptomatic population, indices of physical work capacity or dyspnea will not differentiate among outcomes. However, in this population, it is important to ascertain whether a "labeling effect," as described above, will occur in the placebo group even before the initiation of therapy. Although most patients are aware of their heart disease, their predisposition to "heart failure" probably has not been previously addressed.

A recent review of quality of life ascertainment in treatment trials of heart failure (42) emphasized the inability of currently available validated test instruments to capture the range of features that require evaluation and to be responsive to the magnitude of changes that are anticipated. Thus several quality of life measures are often included in clinical trial designs for evaluating heart failure (as well as other cardiovascular) therapies (21).

CORONARY ATHEROSCLEROTIC HEART DISEASE—ANGINA PECTORIS AND MYOCARDIAL INFARCTION

Very different quality of life attributes are appropriate for stable ambulatory patients with angina pectoris than for patients with an acute and unexpected serious illness such as acute myocardial infarction. Still other features are applicable for the same coronary patients undergoing coronary angioplasty or coronary bypass surgery (see Chapter 23).

For the patient with stable angina pectoris, the major concerns relate to functional status, including the effects on the patient's emotional, occupational, and social status, with attention to the requirements for follow-up medical care. Because this is a prominently symptomatic illness, the degree to which the intervention ameliorates function-limiting symptoms is often an important outcome measure. In this regard, disease-specific measures may be of value, particularly those that address the major symptom of coronary heart disease, chest pain. The Rose Questionnaire (8) and the Canadian Cardiovascular Society (CCS) classification (9) are frequently used measures. The impact on function can frequently be measured by the New York Heart Association (NYHA) classification, although the features of "usual" activity as a precipitant of symptoms present the problems previously cited (6); this probably accounts for the less than satisfactory correlation of the New York Heart Association classification with exercise capacity. The Specific Activity Scale (SAS) is purported to overcome some of these problems, but cannot measure small degrees of change; it does, however, correlate well with measured maximal oxygen uptake at exercise testing (7). In the Veterans Administration Cooperative Study of Coronary Artery Bypass Surgery for stable angina pectoris, an angina scoring system combined the severity of angina and a medication score (43). A more recently developed instrument (44) is described as combining features of both the New York Heart Association classification and survival data.

The management of chronic, stable angina pectoris is an area where several categories of comparably effective therapeutic options are available for reduction of myocardial ischemia and the attendant relief of chest pain. Therefore, the choice among the therapies—nitrate drugs, calcium blocking drugs, and beta blocking drugs—is often dependent on their impact on quality of life attributes, as well as on the patient's comorbid conditions.

The setting of acute myocardial infarction poses far different quality of life issues, and these differ both in the intensive care setting and during the remainder of the hospital stay. Previously in the traditional intensive care setting, the degree of discomfort; the ability to achieve sleep and rest; and the impact on responsiveness, alertness, emotional state, orientation, and the like were important. Although these remain important, the acute invasive interventions such as acute coronary thrombolysis and acute coronary angioplasty must be examined for their impact on all aspects of life quality, in addition to the traditional measures of morbidity and mortality. There should be particular emphasis on physical, emotional, and cognitive functioning. Particularly with this acute, unanticipated, yet life-threatening illness, the need for the patient to make immediate decisions and choices among potentially equal but often high-risk therapies must be addressed.

Following transfer from the intensive care setting and during the remainder of the hospital stay, the primary quality of life areas of concern for measurement include the effects of the intervention on mobility, emotional status, cognitive and intellectual function, self-reliance, attentiveness, interactions with family and friends, and the like.

In recent years it has been determined that there are a number of clinical settings and arteriographic characteristics where both coronary angioplasty and coronary bypass surgery are reasonable therapeutic options. At least two clinical trials currently in progress under the sponsorship of the National Heart, Lung, and Blood Institute are comparing the morbidity and mortality aspects of patients randomized to either of the two interventions. However, if survival benefit appears comparable and if morbidity benefits, albeit different, are also comparable, then quality of life issues will assume extreme importance. The comparison will be between the early intensive perioperative morbidity related to surgery and the potential late angioplasty failure with the attendant fear, anxiety, and subsequent acute symptoms. An area of intensive investigation is the impact on subtle features of neuropsychological functioning by the cardiopulmonary bypass procedure needed for coronary bypass surgery. Comparing coronary angioplasty with coronary bypass surgery is an ideal setting in which to examine, by a variety of tests of neuropsychological functioning, whether there is an impact on neurologic deficits (45), memory, motor coordination, recognition, and reasoning, among others from cardiopulmonary bypass.

ARRHYTHMIAS

Primarily in association with coronary atherosclerotic heart disease, but also in the setting of cardiomyopathy of a variety of causes, there has been major concern with life-threatening ventricular arrhythmias. A number of drugs have been studied, initially in the Cardiac Arrhythmia Pilot Study and subsequently in the Cardiac Arrhythmia Suppression Trial of the National Heart, Lung, and Blood Institute, to determine the morbidity and mortality impact of a variety of newer anti-arrhythmic compounds. Also to be considered, should there be comparable benefit from any of the therapies tested, is their impact on a wide variety of quality of life attributes. The setting is that of a life-threatening cardiac problem, but one where the anti-arrhythmic therapies entail considerable risk of morbidity and mortality, in addition to their impact on various aspects of life quality.

In this instance, although the drugs are typically administered on an ambulatory basis, there is need for frequent tests and office visits for surveillance. The impact on quality of life of this aspect of care must be considered, in addition to the actual issues of medication-taking and life quality changes.

SUMMARY

In a number of surveys, the satisfaction of patients with the outcomes of their medical care reflected preponderantly quality of life issues, essentially those attributes valued by patients. Prominent among these were their resultant comfort or sense of well-being; the extent to which they were able to maintain reasonable physical, emotional, and intellectual function; and the degree to which they retained their ability to participate in valued activities within the family, in the workplace, and in the community.

In order to ascertain the full impact of an intervention on patients with specific cardiovascular problems, these attributes, as well as the traditional measures of morbidity and mortality, must be examined. Further, this information must be subsequently reformatted so that the pivotal items can be assessed readily during a brief clinical encounter, as at an office visit. The data gathered in the research setting should enable the clinician to track the areas of quality of life that have clinical relevance for each problem category, in order to tailor treatment to an individual patient's preferences and values. Comparing a brief quality of life measure which is part of routine data collection on all patients involved in a randomized trial of a drug, with a more detailed life quality evaluation of a subsegment of the population, can provide needed validation. If successful, the prototype of this approach in several National Heart, Lung, and Blood Institute trials may serve as an excellent model.

REFERENCES

1. Spitzer WO. Keynote address: State of science 1986: Quality of life and functional status as target variables for research. *J Chron Dis* 1987;40:465–471.
2. Hunt SM, McKenna SP, McEwen J. A quantitative approach to perceived health. *J Epidemiol Community Health* 1985;34:281–295.
3. Bush JW. General health policy model/quality of well-being (QWB) scale. In: Wenger NK, Mattson ME, Furberg CE, et al., eds. *Quality of life in clinical trials of cardiovascular therapies*. New York: LeJacq, 1984;189–199.
4. Bergner M, Bobbitt RA, Carter WB, et al. The Sickness Impact Profile: Development and final revision of a health status measure. *Med Care* 1981;19:787–805.
5. Harvey RM, Doyle EF, Ellis K, et al. Major changes made by the Criteria Committee of the New York Heart Association. *Circulation* 1974;49:390.
6. Goldman L, Hashimoto B, Cook EF, et al. Comparative reproducibility and validity of systems for assessing cardiovascular functional class: Advantages of a new Specific Activity Scale. *Circulation* 1981;64:1227–1234.
7. Lee TH, Shammash JB, Ribeiro JP, et al. Estimation of maximum oxygen uptake from clinical data: Performance of the Specific Activity Scale. *Am Heart J* 1988;115:203–204.
8. Rose GA, Blackburn H. *Cardiovascular survey methods*. Geneva: World Health Organization 1986;56:1–188.
9. CASS Principal Investigators and their Associates. Coronary artery surgery study (CASS). A randomized trial of coronary artery bypass surgery. Quality of life in patients randomly assigned to treatment groups. *Circulation* 1983;68:951–960.
10. Foxman B, Lohr KN, Brook RH, et al. *Conceptualization and measurement of physiological health in adults, v. congestive heart failure*. Santa Monica, CA: Rand Corporation, September 1982.
11. Mahler DA, Weinberg DM, Wells CK, et al. The measurement of dyspnoea. Content, interobserver agreement and physiologic correlates of two new clinical indexes. *Chest* 1984;85:751–758.
12. LaRue A, Bank L, Jarvik L, et al. Health in old age: How do physicians' rating and self-ratings compare? *J Gerontol* 1979;34:687–691.
13. Kaplan GA, Camacho TC. Perceived health and mortality: A nine year follow-up of the human population laboratory cohort. *Am J Epidemiol* 1983;117:292–295.
14. Mossey JM, Shapiro E. Self-rated health: A predictor of mortality among the elderly. *Am J Public Health* 1982;72:800–808.

15. Lefebvre RC, Hursey KG, Carleton RA. Labeling of participants in high blood pressure screening programs. Implications for blood cholesterol screenings. *Arch Intern Med* 1988;148:1993–1997.
16. Johnston ME, Gibson ES, Terry CW, et al. Effects of labeling on income, work, and social function among hypertensive employees. *J Chronic Dis* 1984;37:417–423.
17. MacDonald LA, Sackett DL, Haynes RB, et al. Hypertension: The effects of labeling on behavior. *Qual Life Cardiovasc Care* 1985;1:129–139.
18. Polk BF, Harlan LC, Cooper SP, et al. Disability days associated with detection and treatment in a hypertension control program. *Am J Epidemiol* 1984;119:44–53.
19. Haynes RB, Sackett DL, Taylor DW, et al. Increased absenteeism from work after detection and labeling of hypertensive patients. *N Engl J Med* 1977;296:732–739.
20. Mann AH. Hypertension: Psychological aspects and diagnostic impact in a clinical trial. *Psychol Med* 1984: Monograph Suppl. 5.
21. Fletcher A, McLoone P, Bulpitt C. Quality of life on angina therapy: A randomized controlled trial of transdermal glyceryl trinitrate against placebo. *Lancet* 1988;2:4–8.
22. Croog SH, Levine S, Testa M, et al. The effects of antihypertensive therapy on the quality of life. *N Engl J Med* 1986;314:1657–1664.
23. Jachuck SJ, Brierley H, Jachuck S, et al. The effect of hypotensive drugs on quality of life. *J R Coll Gen Pract* 1982;32:103–105.
24. 1988 Joint National Committee: The 1988 Report of the Joint National Committee on Detection, Evaluation, and Treatment of High Blood Pressure. *Arch Intern Med* 1988;148:1023–1038.
25. Shultz NR, Dineen JT, Elias MR, et al. W.A.I.S. performance for different age groups of hypertensive and control subjects during administration of a diuretic. *J Gerontol* 1979;34:246–253.
26. Bulpitt CJ, Fletcher AE. Quality of life in hypertensive patients on different anti-hypertensive treatments: Rationale for methods employed in a multicentre randomized controlled trial. *J Cardiovasc Pharmacol* 1985;7:S137–S145.
27. Streufert S, DePadova A, McGlynn T, et al. Impact of β-blockade on complex cognitive functioning. *Am Heart J* 1988;116:311–315.
28. Solomon S, Hotchkiss E, Saravay SM, et al. Impariment of memory function by antihypertensive medication. *Arch Gen Psych* 1983;40:1109–1112.
29. Lichter I, Richardson PJ, Wyke MA. Differential effects of atenolol and enalapril on tests of memory during treatment for essential hypertension. *J Hypertension* 1984;2:560.
30. Franchesci M, Tancredi A, Smirne S, et al. Cognitive processes in hypertension. *Hypertension* 1982;31:226–229.
31. Avorn J, Everitt DE, Weiss S. Increased antidepressant use in patients prescribed beta blockers. *JAMA* 1986;255:357–360.
32. Jessup M, Brozena S. Assessment of quality of life in patients with chronic congestive heart failure. *Qual Life Cardiovasc Care* 1988;4:53–57.
33. Cohn JN, Archibald DG, Ziesche S, et al. Effect of vasodilator therapy on mortality in chronic congestive heart failure. Results of a Veterans Administration Cooperative Study. *N Engl J Med* 1986;314:1547–1552.
34. The CONSENSUS Trial Study Group: Effects of enalapril on mortality in severe congestive heart failure. Results of the Cooperative North Scandinavian Enalapril Survival Study (CONSENSUS). *N Engl J Med* 1987;316:1429–1435.
35. Packer M. Prolonging life in patients with congestive heart failure: The next frontier. *Circulation* 1987;75(Suppl. IV):1–3.
36. Goldman L, Cook EF, Mitchell N, et al. Pitfalls in the serial assessment of cardiac functional status. How a reduction in "ordinary" activity may reduce the apparent degree of cardiac compromise and give a misleading impression of improvement. *J Chron Dis* 1982;35:763–771.
37. Rajagopalan B, Raine AEG, Cooper R, et al. Changes in cerebral blood flow in patients with severe congestive cardiac failure before and after captopril treatment. *Am J Med* 1984;76(Suppl. 5B):86–90.
38. Petrucci RJ, Jessup M, Cavarocchi J, et al. Cognitive function in patients with symptomatic dilated cardiomyopathy before and after cardiac transplantation (abstract). *Transplant Proc* 1988;20:810.
39. Guyatt GH. Methodologic problems in clinical trials in heart failure. *J Chron Dis* 1985;38:353–363.
40. Franciosa JA. Epidemiologic patterns, clinical evaluation, and long-term prognosis in chronic congestive heart failure. *Am J Med* 1986;80(Suppl. 2B):14–21.
41. Feinstein AR, Joseph BR, Wells CK. Scientific and clinical problems in indexes of functional disability. *Ann Intern Med* 1986;81:641–664.
42. Bulpitt CJ, Fletcher AE. Measurement of the quality of life in congestive heart failure—influence of drug therapy. *Cardiovasc Drug Ther* 1988;2:419–424.
43. Peduzzi P, Hultgren H. Angina scoring method in the Veterans Administration Randomized Study of Bypass Surgery. *Am J Epidemiol* 1985;122:477–484.
44. Olsson G, Lubsen J, van Es GA, et al. Quality of life after myocardial infarction: Effect of long-term metoprolol on mortality and morbidity. *Br Med J* 1986;292:1491–1493.
45. Shaw PJ, Bates D, Cartlidge NEF, et al. Neurologic and neuropsychological morbidity following major surgery: Comparison of coronary artery bypass and peripheral vascular surgery. *Stroke* 1987;18:700–707.

Quality of Life Assessments in Clinical Trials, edited by B. Spilker. Raven Press, Ltd. New York © 1990.

26

Neurologic Illness

*Robert S. Wilson and †Christopher G. Goetz

Rush Alzheimer's Disease Center; †Department of Neurological Sciences, Rush University; Rush-Presbyterian St. Luke's Medical Center, Chicago, Illinois 60612

Quality of life studies have particular relevance in neurology. The brain, spinal cord, and peripheral nerves control neurologic function for the entire body, and damage to these organs can have highly specific or widespread consequences. Neurologic measures must accommodate implicitly the gamut of possible anatomic involvements, sensory and motor dysfunction, and cognitive impairment of both mild and severe intensity. For example, some neurologic conditions will cause highly focal abnormalities like a weak hand, involuntary eye closure, or isolated facial pain. Other degenerative conditions affect function throughout the body and may involve all neurologic spheres. On the other hand, diffuse encephalopathies may cause few motor or sensory problems, but cause cognitive and emotional abnormalities that devastate quality of life. Pharmacologic treatment of some disorders may succeed in alleviating signs and symptoms of neurologic illness, but at the cost of side effects that adversely affect quality of life. In short, the diverse manifestations of neurological disorders and the agents used to treat these disorders underscore the importance of quality of life to any consideration of neurologic disorders or their treatment.

The heterogenous manifestations of neurological illness have made it difficult to apply a simple or single set of quality of life measures to all disorders. Age and level of cognitive dysfunction, in particular, are critical considerations in the selection, adaptation, or construction of various scales. However, in some domains of quality of life, such as physical function, the behaviors of interest are relatively finite so that use of more general and psychometrically established scales may be feasible. The present chapter is organized into two sections. In the first section, four dimensions of quality of life are discussed: physical, financial, social, and psychological. Within each of these domains, available measures and pertinent considerations are addressed. In the second section, specific neurological applications of these measures are considered.

QUALITY OF LIFE MEASURES

Physical Function

The impact of illness on the ability to perform activities of daily living has long been recognized as an important and practical matter in the management of neurologic patients. As a result, a range of scales has been developed. Two problems in this proliferating area exist, however. First, some scales do not exclusively focus on physical disability, so social and cognitive dysfunction contaminate activities of daily living scores. Such scales lack construct validity and can create dilemmas for the neurologic rater when different functions deteriorate at different rates. For example, the Schwab and England Scale (1) currently used in Parkinson's disease and the Shoulson-Fahn Scale (2) used in Huntington's disease require the examiner to consider simultaneously multiple sources of physical and nonphysical disability in order to arrive at a single measure of functional capacity. Such unidimensional ratings of multidimensional behavior are inherently limited, and although convenient, they lack the capacity to determine changes in discrete areas of neurologic dysfunction. Second, the scales are often restricted to only one disease or disease type, precluding comparisons across the broad spectrum of neurologic illnesses. Historically, some of the more widely used scales were constructed with a single disease in mind or have evolved into a relatively exclusive applicability to one type of disease. For example, the Northwestern University Disability Scale has been used repeatedly to measure the activities of daily living function in Parkinson's disease and has not been widely applied to other disorders (3). Nevertheless, since it rates six functional domains (walking, dressing, feeding, hygiene, speech, and eating), which are reasonably representative of the activities of daily living domain, the scale is potentially applicable to a far wider range of neurologic disorders.

In fact, the number of physical activities of daily living is finite and the range of neurologic competence in such activities can be specified. Within the domain of physical function, therefore, use of the same scale in different disorders may be entirely feasible. Perhaps the most widely used measures of activities of daily living in neurology are those developed by Lawton and Brody (4), Katz et al. (5), and Mahoney and Barthel (6). Lawton and Brody's Physical Self-Maintenance Scale (PSMS), for example, identifies six areas of rudimentary physical activity: eating, dressing, bathing, toileting, walking, and hygiene. Each function is scored on a 5-point behaviorally anchored interval scale. The scale was originally developed to evaluate disability among the elderly and hence is particularly appropriate for such varied neurologic disorders as cerebrovascular accident, Alzheimer's disease, and Parkinson's disease. The Physical Self-Maintenance Scale is often used in conjunction with the Instrumental Activities of Daily Living Scale of Lawton and Brody which assesses more cognitively mediated activities critical to independent living. Items address activities such as shopping, use of transportation and telephone, and handling finances. Used in conjunction, the Physical Self-Maintenance Scale and Instrumental Activities of Daily Living Scale are unique and provide comprehensive, psychometrically sound measurements of two specific subdomains of activities of daily living.

The scale developed by Katz et al. (5) is an ordinal measure of six activities of daily living functions that are presumed lost and regained sequentially. The Barthel Index (6) is perhaps the most widely used activities of daily living scale. There are 11 items, and scoring is on an interval system which is helpful for statistical analyses. The items are rationally weighted such that mobility and continence contribute disproportionately to the total score.

Psychological Function

Psychological function is critical to any concept of quality of life, particularly in patients with neurological disease. Both cognitive and affective functioning have been assessed in a wide variety of measures. Arguably, the most disabling aspect of neurological illness is cognitive dysfunction. Damage to the cerebral cortex, basal ganglia, thalamus, limbic system, or adjacent structures can dramatically compromise diverse intellectual functions. These effects can be seen with focal pathology resulting in various forms of amnesia, aphasia, and cognitive disorganization. Alternatively, diffuse encephalopathies seen with degenerative disorders like Alzheimer's disease or Huntington's disease may produce global cognitive deterioration usually referred to as dementia.

Review of measures of specific cognitive functions is beyond the scope of this chapter. The interested reader may refer to Lezak (7) and Heilman and Valenstein (8). A number of psychometrically adequate dementia screening measures are available (9–11). In selecting any psychological performance measure, however, it is critical that the difficulty level of the scale be appropriate for the population of interest.

As an alternative or supplement to direct measurement of cognitive functioning, the investigator may select rating scales. Scales have been developed that make use of the patient, a significant other, a trained clinician, or some combination of these raters. For example, the Brief Cognitive Rating Scale (BCRS) (12) and the Global Deterioration Scale (GDS) (13) require the clinician to rate either a single (GDS) or multiple (BCRS) dimensions of cognition. The Katz Adjustment Scale (14) and the Sickness Impact Profile (15) allow for rating by either the patient or significant other. In assessing cognitive decline, ratings by a significant other and/or clinician are preferable to the patient's rating.

In the authors' opinion, some direct performance measure should also be included in a cognitive assessment of quality of life. Although subjective evaluations of cognitive functioning have a place in quality of life assessment, such evaluations can be influenced by extraneous factors (e.g., depression). Use of objective measures provides a means of evaluating the validity of the subjective ratings.

Affective changes are the second area of psychological investigation. Such changes are common in neurological disease and are potentially disabling, particularly if they remain unrecognized. Such affective alterations may be the direct result of the neurological lesion; when damage to the frontal lobes or limbic system occurs, a range of disordered emotional behavior, including disinhibition, depression or hypomanic episodes, or hallucinations may result and affect quality of life. In such instances, patients may show few or no cognitive changes. In other instances, when affective changes do not occur as part of the neurologic lesion, emotional reactions to neurological disability still can dramatically alter quality of life. Depressive reactions frequently develop as a secondary result of new disability or chronic illness. In some conditions, like Parkinson's disease, it may be especially difficult to separate the direct emotional effects of the disease from the reactive components. Regardless of the source, however, depression of at least a mild degree is common with diffuse encephalopathies like Parkinson's disease, Huntington's disease, and Alzheimer's disease (16).

Measurement of affect within the context of quality of life has not always focused on clinical dimensions of emotional behavior like depression or anxiety. Rather, constructs such as life satisfaction and psychological well-being are commonly employed. A range of instruments are available for measurement of these or similar constructs (17–22). To a certain extent, the proliferation of such measures is an index of the elusiveness of concepts such as life satisfaction. In fact, no "gold standards" exist in this domain, and it may not be reasonable to expect a single measure to be equally applicable in all situations. Since the sources of life satisfaction change as patients age (23), selection of such measures requires adaptation of tools to the target population.

Economic Function

The financial impact of neurological disease has received significant attention in public health studies, but much less in clinical neurologic assessments. A number of measures have been developed and issues of concern have been raised. Among the latter is the issue of how economic function should be measured: objectively versus subjectively, and directly versus indirectly. Objective measures of the economic impact of disease might include days of work missed, hospital days or outpatient visits to health care professionals, medication, etc. These direct costs can be supplemented by indirect costs like residential alterations necessitated by the disease and days of work missed by family members providing care to the patient. Alternatively, the evaluations may focus on the perceived economic impact of the illness. Thus, on the OARS (18), ratings of directly relevant medical costs supplement the subjective impact on finances of the illness. On the Sickness Impact Profile (15), a multidimensional and psychometrically sound measure of quality of life, the Work and Home Management scales measure the extent to which the patient is able to perform occupational and household duties, respectively. Disability in these domains has clear financial implications although no direct estimate of this cost is provided in the scale. The choice of measurement approaches in the economic domain is complex and depends on the purposes to be accomplished. In a cost-benefit analysis of a specific neurologic treatment, for example, direct estimates of cost are preferable. From a broader perspective in which economics is one of several domains being evaluated, measures of perceived financial burden may suffice.

The economic impact of a given disease will of course largely relate to the patient's economic status before the disease began. Two patients may have similar cerebrovascular accidents and require the same nursing care at home. The wealthy patient will engage a daily nurse with little economic impact, whereas the same care for the poorer patient may have far-reaching economic consequences. Premorbid financial status is not typically considered in objective measurement of economic impact but may implicitly influence ratings of perceived financial burden.

Social Function

Evaluation of the quality and quantity of an individual's social interaction is the fourth area of quality of life measurement. In practice, most measures have tended to focus on social networks, access to community services, and recreational activities. The impact of neurologic disease on the patient's social network has not been well studied, since in many cases the social changes are a mere consequence of the three other domains already discussed. However, many scales are available (e.g., 15,18,24) and could reasonably be incorporated into neurologic evaluations.

The usual approach to assessing social networks begins with the patient or an informant identifying a set of key individuals in the patient's life. Each is rated along several dimensions. Thus, in the Philadelphia Geriatric Scale (24), the extent to which each individual provides emotional support, encouragement, companionship, and advice is rated. In other inventories, the focus is on more objective variables, such as the proximity of these key individuals and their frequency of contact with the patient. In either case, the intent is to determine if the patient's social world has contracted as a result of illness.

On the Social Interaction subscale of the Sickness Impact Profile, the same construct is assessed less tediously through a series of questions requiring only a yes/no response. It is noteworthy that on the Sickness Impact Profile, the Social Interaction scale is part of the psychosocial factor; the other scales that define this factor (e.g., Communication, Emotional Behavior) are clearly psychological rather than social in nature. In fact, the lack of attention to social interaction in neurologic disease may reflect the fact that such effects are indirect. That is, the social impact of neurological diseases may be mediated by the physical and psychological sequelae. In this regard, it is noteworthy that adverse effects on social networks have been studied more in persons responsible for the care of neurologic patients, those with Alzheimer's disease in particular, than in patients themselves (25,26).

Scales for assessing utilization of community services and participation in recreational or leisure time activities are available as well (15,18,24,27). The application of such scales to patients with neurological disorders has been limited, however. Once again, such higher order social activities, though quite relevant to quality of life, may be only secondary reflections of the more fundamental physical and psychological sequelae of neurologic illness.

SPECIFIC EXAMPLES OF QUALITY OF LIFE APPLICATIONS IN NEUROLOGIC STUDIES

In this section, two examples in which quality of life outcome measures were used to address specific issues in neurological disorders in our research center are presented. The first example involves a comparison of two forms of dementia where quality of life measures were used to assess comparative type and severity of clinical dysfunction. In the second example, quality of life measures were used to help evaluate outcome of a new surgical treatment for Parkinson's disease.

Disability Assessment in Dementia

Alzheimer's disease and vascular disease are the leading causes of dementia among the elderly. Vascular disease, alone or in combination with Alzheimer's disease, accounts for 20% to 30% of such cases (28). Subcortical arteriosclerotic encephalopathy (Binswanger's disease) is one of the more common forms of vascular dementia. Clinically, these patients exhibit progressive dementia, often accompanied by focal motor signs, incontinence, and gait disturbance (29). Differential diagnosis of Alzheimer's disease and subcortical arteriosclerotic encephalopathy is often difficult but important since subcortical arteriosclerotic encephalopathy may be a treatable disorder. Although the dementias of Alzheimer's disease and subcortical arteriosclerotic encephalopathy are similar in some ways, clinical reports have suggested more physical disability in subcortical arteriosclerotic encephalopathy, perhaps reflecting the concentration of pathology in periventricular white and gray matter. To address this issue of differential physical disability in the two dementias, we evaluated patients with clinical diagnoses of Alzheimer's disease ($N = 23$) and subcortical arteriosclerotic encephalopathy (N = 26) using Lawton and Brody's (4) Physical Self-Maintenance Scale and Instrumental Activities of Daily Living Scale. Used in conjunction, these scales provide specific measures of rudimentary physical and cognitively mediated, instrumental activities of daily living. Separation of these two facets of activities of daily living is critical when evaluating patients with dementia.

All patients had a standard diagnostic evaluation including a neurological examination, neuropsychological testing, and magnetic resonance imaging (MRI). The clinical diagnosis of probable Alzheimer's disease was based on inclusion and exclusion criteria of the National Institute of Neurological and Communicative Diseases and Stroke/Alzheimer's Disease and Related Disorders Association (NINCDS/ADRDA) study group (30). The diagnosis of subcortical arteriosclerotic encephalopathy required that NINCDS/ADRDA criteria for dementia be met, a modified ischemia scale (31) score of 3 or more, and two or more areas of increased signal intensity on MRI T_2 weighted images in a periventricular distribution. The groups were selected to be equivalent in dementia severity, as measured by the Mini-Mental State (MMS) examination (9).

As hypothesized, these two groups differed on the Physical Self-Maintenance Scale (F [1,46] = 11.1, p < .01) with the subcortical arteriosclerotic encephalopathy patients showing more disability than the Alzheimer's disease patients. In contrast, the groups were equivalent on the Instrumental Activities of Daily Living Scale. In subcortical arteriosclerotic encephalopathy, but not Alzheimer's disease, total Physical Self-Maintenance Scale score (R = .53, p < .01) and each item (all p < .05) correlated with lateral ventriculomegaly, as measured by the width of the lateral ventricles at the most lateral boundaries of the frontal horns. These findings confirm clinical impressions that subcortical arteriosclerotic encephalopathy entails more physical disability than does Alzheimer's disease at comparable levels of cognitive dysfunction. The increased physical disability may be expected to result in management problems and to hasten institutionalization (32). The dissociation between the Physical Self-Maintenance Scale and Instrumental Activities of Daily Living Scale underscores the importance of specificity in scaling physical functioning. Finally, the correlations between function and anatomy support the hypothesis that tissue loss in the periventricular region is the primary source of disability in subcortical arteriosclerotic encephalopathy.

Treatment Evaluation in Parkinson's Disease

Although pharmacological treatment of Parkinson's disease has proven to be effective, disease progression and chronic medication side effects limit therapeutic efforts. Recently, adrenal medullary autografts to caudate nucleus have been used in severely impaired Parkinson's disease patients who no longer respond adequately to dopaminergic replacement therapy. Madrazo et al. (33) reported dramatic improvement in several patients who underwent the procedure, although other investigators have had more modest results (34). The procedure involves a caudate nucleus biopsy and placement of the patient's adrenal medullary cells onto the biopsy site in contact with the ventricular cerebrospinal fluid. Proposed mechanisms for the amelioration of Parkinson's disease by this graft have included enhanced dopamine production by the adrenal medulla cells and possibly the transfer or synthesis of trophic growth factors in the brain.

We have evaluated seven severely impaired Parkinson's disease patients who have undergone the adrenal medulla transplant surgery. Each patient was seen preoperatively and at regular intervals through 6 months postoperatively. Prior to surgery, all patients had severe Parkinson's disease and had serious balance problems or could not stand alone (37) during part of the day. All suffered severe fluctuations in their motor response, spending a mean 39.3% of the waking day "off" and 60.7% "on." "Off" time referred to the hours each day when the patient functioned poorly because of resistance to medication effects, and "on" time referred to the hours each day when the patients functioned well with good medication response. No patient had prior psychiatric impairment and none was demented.

Five men and two women were studied. Their mean age at surgery was 50.3 years, mean age of Parkinson's disease onset was 38.7 years, mean Parkinson's disease duration was 11.6 years, and mean duration of levodopa treatment was 11.0 years.

The scales chosen to study motor efficacy in this protocol were the Unified Parkinson's Disease Rating Scale (UPDRS), the Hoehn and Yahr (HY) stage, and the Schwab and England (SE) Scale (1). The Unified Parkinson's Disease Rating Scale was selected because it provided objective measurements of Parkinsonian motor problems and had subscales that assessed subjective complaints by the patient and activities of daily living. The Hoehn and Yahr stage summarized the major category of global dysfunction and the Schwab and England Scale provided a global measure of independence. In addition, we administered cognitive and neuropsychological tests to assess changes in mental and affective function. Finally, the Sickness Impact Profile (15) was selected to address quality of life. The Sickness Impact Profile is among the most comprehensive and psychometrically sound measures of quality of life. There are 12 internally consistent subscales which yield two summary factor scores. The items are readily observable behaviors and are scored on the basis of an interview with either the patient or a collateral source. The latter option is particularly important in evaluating neurological patients who may not be capable of rating their own behavior.

After surgery, there was a significant decrease in "off" time and improvement in the severity of "off" dysfunction as measured by the Schwab and England Scale and the Unified Parkinson's Disease Rating Scale, (using motor and activities of daily living subscales). There were no changes in psychometric measures of cognitive or affective function. On the Sickness Impact Profile, significant changes were found (Fig. 1) in sleep and rest, emotional behavior, social isolation, ambulation, communication, and overall psychological functioning (all $p < .05$, one tailed). No significant changes were found for body care maintenance, home maintenance, mobility, alerting behavior, work, recreations and pastimes, eating, physical functioning, or overall functioning.

The Sickness Impact Profile proved especially useful in this study for two reasons. First, most of the improvements documented on the Sickness Impact Profile were not detectable by the other measures used. The changes in psychological function and social integration were particularly impressive clinical changes, but would have remained undocumented without a quality of life assessment tool. Second, the Sickness Impact Profile data suggested clues to understanding certain seeming discrepancies in the data from the other measures. Whereas the "off" time improved in duration and severity so that patients ambulated better, patients reported that they

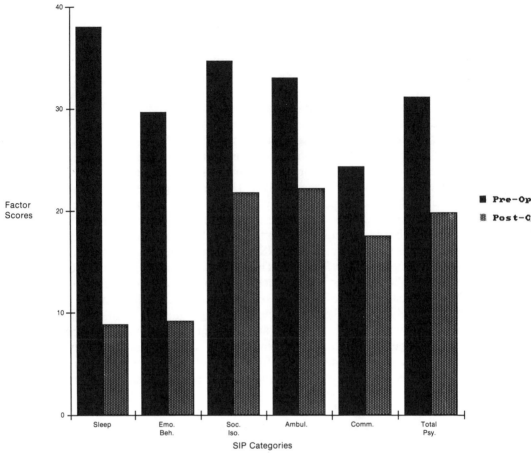

FIG. 1. Significant changes in Sickness Impact Profile scores. Pre-op, ■ and Post-op,
▩.

were not actually doing more independent activities than before. Their assessment
of unchanged physical and overall function on quality of life measures reflected their
attitude about postoperative motor changes. We have found these differences in
objective and perceived improvement particularly important in dealing with rehabilitative efforts in patients with chronic illness.

FUTURE PERSPECTIVES

The incorporation of quality of life measures in neurologic evaluations of disease
or treatments is an increasing practice. Scales are now available that can provide
assessment of specific facets of quality of life relevant to patients with neurologic
disease. Although disease-specific scales are sometimes a necessity, they tend to be
less psychometrically established and do not permit comparisons across disease
categories. In the final analysis, however, the choice of scales for a given study will
depend on the research objectives. Wider extension of quality of life studies to

caregivers and families may reveal a more complete assessment of the impact of neurologic disease and putative therapies.

In the coming decade, one major focus of pharmacologic research in neurology will be the improvement in drug delivery systems. Documenting objective improvement from one formulation to another can be difficult, however, since the drug is the same in both instances. Quality of life measures may prove particularly applicable in measuring the impact of these new formulations. As an example, levodopa was developed in the 1960s as a treatment for Parkinson's disease. It still remains the mainstay of therapy, although its delivery has been altered by more modern pharmacologic manipulations. The addition of carbidopa to levodopa permits more efficient delivery to the central nervous system. More recently, a long-acting protein-bound formulation has been developed to decrease the frequent dosing schedule that is so often necessary with this drug.

In spite of these innovations, the drug itself remains levodopa and objective measures of improvement from one formulation to another are difficult to establish. Nevertheless, incorporation of quality of life measures into the assessments would likely document the impact of fewer side effects with the levodopa/carbidopa combination and the enhanced independence that patients feel when they switch from the short-acting to the long-acting form. These assessments may offer an improved means of monitoring new or more subtle therapies in the future.

REFERENCES

1. Schwab RS, England AC. Projection technique for evaluating surgery in Parkinson's disease. In: Gillingham FJ, Donaldson MC, eds. *Third symposium on Parkinson's disease*. Edinburgh: Livingston, 1969;152–157.
2. Shoulson I, Fahn S. Huntington's disease: Clinical care and evaluation. *Neurology* 1979;29:1–3.
3. Koller WC. *Handbook of Parkinson's disease*. New York: Decker, 1987;482–488.
4. Lawton MP, Brody EM. Assessment of older people: Self-maintaining and instrumental activities of daily living. *Gerontologist* 1969;9:179–186.
5. Katz S, Ford AB, Moskowitz RW. Studies of illness in the aged: The index of ADL, a standardized measure of biological and psychosocial function. *JAMA* 1963;185:914–919.
6. Mahoney FJ, Barthel DW. Functional evaluation: The Barthel Index. *Md Med J* 1965;61–65.
7. Lezak M. Neuropsychological assessment. New York: Oxford University Press, 1983.
8. Heilman KM, Valenstein E. *Clinical neuropsychology*. New York: Oxford University Press, 1979.
9. Folstein MF, Folstein SE, McHugh PR. Mini Mental State. A practical guide for grading the cognitive state of patients for the clinician. *J Psychiat Res* 1975;12:189–198.
10. Mattis S. Mental status examination for organic mental syndrome in the elderly patient. In: Bellak L, Karasu T, eds. *Geriatric psychiatry*. New York: Grune & Stratton, 1976.
11. Mohs RC, Rosen WG, Greenwald BS, Davis KL. Neuropathologically validated scales for Alzheimer's disease. In: Crook T, Ferris S, Bartus R, eds. *Assessment in geriatric psychiatry*. New Canaan, CT: Mark Powley Associates, 1983.
12. Reisberg B, Schneck MK, Ferris SH, Schwartz GE, de Leon MJ. The Brief Cognitive Rating Scale (BCRS): Findings in primary degenerative dementia (PDD). *Psychopharm Bull* 1983:47–50.
13. Reisberg B, Ferris SH, de Leon MJ, Crook T. The Global Deterioration Scale (GDS): An instrument for the assessment of primary degenerative dementia (PDD). *Am J Psychiat* 1982;139:1136–1139.
14. Katz MM, Lyerly SB. Methods for measuring adjustment and social behavior in the community: 1. Rationale, description, discriminative validity and scale development. *Psychol Reports* (Monograph Suppl. 4-V13) 1963;13:503–535.
15. Bergner M, Bobbitt RA, Carter WB, Gilson BS. The Sickness Impact Profile: Development and final revision of a health status measure. *Med Care* 1981;19:787–805.
16. Cummings JL, Benson DF. *Dementia: A clinical approach*. Boston: Butterworths, 1983.
17. Anderson JP, Bush JW, Berry CC. Classifying function for health outcome and quality-of-life evaluation. *Med Care* 1986;454–470.
18. Duke University Center for the Study of Aging. *Multidimensional functional assessment. The OARS methodology*, 2nd ed. Durham, NC: Duke University Press, 1978.

19. George LK, Bearon LB. *Quality of life in older persons*. New York: Human Sciences Press, 1980.
20. Lawton MP. The varieties of well-being. *Exp. Aging Res* 1983;7:65–72.
22. Neugarten BL, Havighurst RJ, Tobin S. The measurement of life satisfaction. *J Gerontol* 1961;16:134–143.
23. Neugarten BL. Personality and aging. In: Birren JE, Schaie KW, eds. *Handbook of the psychology of aging*. New York: Van Nostrand Reinhold, 1977.
24. Lawton MP, Moss M, Fulcomer M, Kleban MH. A research and service oriented multilevel assessment instrument. *J Gerontol* 1982;37:91–99.
25. Cantor MA. Strain among caregivers: A study of the experience in the United States. *Gerontologist* 1983;23:597–604.
26. Rabins RV, Mace NL, Lucas MJ. The impact of dementia in the family. *JAMA* 1982;248:333–335.
27. Phillips L. *Human adaptation and its failures*. New York: Academic Press, 1968.
28. Katzman R. Alzheimer's disease. *New Eng J Med* 1986;314:964–973.
29. Olszewski J. Subcortical arteriosclerotic encephalopathy. *World Neurology* 1962;3:359–374.
30. McKahnn G, Drachman D, Folstein M, Katzman R, Price D, Stadlan E. Clinical diagnosis of Alzheimer's disease: Report of the NINCDS-ADRDA Work Group under the auspices of Department of Health and Human Services Task force on Alzheimer's disease. *Neurology* 1984;34:939–944.
31. Rosen WG, Terry RD, Fuld PA, Katzman R, Peck A. Pathological verification of ischemic score in differentiation of dementias. *Ann Neurol* 1980;7:486–488.
32. Linn MW, Linn BS. Assessing activities of daily living in institutional settings. In: Crook T, Ferris S, Bartus R, eds. *Assessment in geriatric psychopharmacology*. New Canaan, CT: Mark Powley Associates, 1983.
33. Madrazo I, Drucker-Colin R, Diaz V, et al. Open microsurgical autograft of adrenal medulla to right caudate nucleus in 2 patients with intractable Parkinson's disease. *N Engl J Med* 1987;316:831–834.
34. Goetz CG, Olanow CW, Koller WC. Adrenal medullary transplant to the striatum of patients with advanced Parkinson's disease: Multicenter study. *N Engl J Med* 1989;320:337–340.

Quality of Life Assessments in Clinical
Trials, edited by B. Spilker. Raven
Press, Ltd. New York © 1990.

27

Severe Mental Illness in the Community

*Anthony F. Lehman and †Barbara J. Burns

*Department of Psychiatry, University of Maryland Medical Center,
Baltimore, Maryland 21201; †Department of Psychiatry, Duke University
Medical Center, Durham, North Carolina 27706

DISEASE PROTOTYPES

Within the field of psychiatric research the principal focus of quality of life assessment has been on the severely mentally ill: persons suffering from long-term and disabling illnesses such as schizophrenia, chronic depression, manic-depressive illness, severe personality disorders, and the like. The reason for this focus lies in the pervasive effects that these psychiatric disorders can have on individuals' lives, limiting their range of life experiences, and perhaps rendering general population measures of quality of life insensitive to the issues faced by this disabled population. Conversely, for persons with nondisabling mental health problems, such as short-term depression and anxiety reactions, instruments available to assess quality of life in the general population are probably adequate. These will not be addressed in this chapter; instead, measures available to assess the quality of life of persons with severe mental illnesses are summarized.

Further explanation of the predominant disease model for these disorders will clarify why quality of life assessments may be of particular relevance in this population. Although the pathophysiologies of these various disorders are not yet well understood and undoubtedly differ from each other, all are currently conceptualized in terms of a "stress-vulnerability" model (1). That is, persons so afflicted have a biological vulnerability to developing characteristic symptoms of the disease (for example, hallucinations and delusions in schizophrenia; anhedonia, suicidal ideation, and dysphoria in depression; hyperactivity, flight of ideas, and hypersexuality in mania), and stress tends to activate this vulnerability to produce symptoms. This conceptualization has led researchers to take an interest in the patients' psychological and social contexts as sources of stress. Quality of life indicators such as social well-being (functioning and environmental resources) and psychological well-being (life satisfaction, self-esteem, morale) may therefore capture important aspects of a person's life that relate to stress and in turn to illness course and outcome.

AVAILABLE TESTS

Characteristics of seven measures available for assessing quality of life in the severely mentally ill are summarized here. For each instrument the following in-

formation is provided: name of instrument, key reference(s), original purpose, patients studied, type of instrument, number of items, length of administration, summary content, psychometric properties, method of data analysis, and availability of
comparative data.

Satisfaction with Life Domains Scale

Key reference: Baker and Intagliata, 1981 (2).

Purpose: To evaluate the impact of the community support program in New York
State on the quality of life of chronically mentally ill patients.

Patients studied: Chronically mentally ill outpatients, age 18 to 86, in two community
support programs, $N = 118$.

Type of instrument: Self-report scale administered by interview.

Number of items: 15.

Length of administration: "Brief," probably less than 10 minutes.

Summary of content:
a. Physical functioning: None.
b. Social functioning: None.
c. Economic functioning: None.
d. Psychological functioning, individual items: Satisfaction with housing, neighbor-
   hood, food to eat, clothing, health, people lived with, friends, family, relations
   with other people, work/day programming, spare time, fun, services and facilities
   in area, economic situation, place lived in now compared to state hospital, total
   life satisfaction score.

Psychometric properties: Total score correlates 0.64 with Bradburn Affect Balance
Scale (3); total score correlates 0.29 with Global Assessment Scale (4).

Data analysis: Data are reported as item score frequencies and means (7 level;
interval scale).

Comparative data: The frequencies and means on these items can be compared with
item scores in a national quality of life survey of the general population (5).

Oregon Quality of Life Questionnaire

Key reference: Bigelow et al., 1982 (6).

Purpose: To assess quality of life outcomes for evaluating community mental health
service delivery.

Patients studied:
a. Sample of patients at intake to community mental health programs in Oregon, N
   $= 874$ (includes chronically mentally ill, drug abusers, alcoholics, and general
   psychiatric patients).
b. Sample of community mental health program patients at follow-up (later in treatment), $N = 380$.

c. Nonpatient community sample, $N = 100$.

Type of instrument: Structured interview administered by a trained (not necessarily clinical) interviewer.

Number of items: 246.

Length of administration: 45 to 90 minutes.

Summary of content:
a. Physical functioning: Meaningful use of leisure time.
b. Economic functioning: Work at home, employability, work on the job, school.
c. Social functioning: Independence, friend role, close friend role, spouse role, parent role, social support.
d. Psychological functioning: Psychological distress, well-being, tolerance of stress.
e. Other: Negative consequences—alcohol; negative consequences—drugs.

Psychometric properties:
Internal consistency reliabilities: .17 to .89 (median reliability $= .65$).
Discriminant validity: differences detected as predicted across the three samples studied.
Test re-test reliabilities (interval not specified): .37 to .64 (median reliability $= .50$).
Sensitivity: Detected treatment effects of service system changes across time and sites.

Data analysis: Analyses of variance comparing three cohorts.

Comparative data: Available on the three cohorts studied.

Standardized Social Schedule

Key reference: Clare and Cairns, 1978 (7).

Purpose: To assess the nature and extent of social maladjustment and dysfunction in chronic neurotic patients seeing their family doctors.

Patients studied:
a. Nonpsychiatric patients with "adverse" social circumstances, $N = 48$.
b. Chronic neurotic outpatients, $N = 221$.
c. Women with premenstrual complaints, $N = 104$.

Type of interview: Semistructured interview with patient (and key informant, if available) by trained interviewer; ratings by interviewer and subject.

Number of items: Varies from 17 to 48, depending on version.

Length of administration: Not given.

Summary of content: Scales include Material Conditions, Social Management, Satisfaction and Housing, Occupation/Social Role, Economics, Leisure/Social Activities, Family and Domestic Relations, Marital.
a. Physical functioning: Extent of leisure activities.
b. Economic functioning: Housing conditions, occupational stability, family income.
c. Social functioning: Household care; housekeeping; quality of relations with work-

mates, neighbors, and family; marital relationship quality; extent of social activities.

d. Psychological functioning: Satisfaction with housing, work, income, leisure, social relationships, family relationships, parental role, marriage.

e. Other: Residential stability, opportunities for leisure and social activities, interaction with neighbors, interactions with relatives.

Psychometric properties: Interrater K_w on items range from .55 to .94 (median κ = .76). Factor structure *not* stable across populations. Differentiated as predicted across populations studied.

Data analysis: Data presented mainly as frequencies of persons scoring in the maladaptive range on various items across populations.

Comparative data: Compared three populations studied according to percent of each group functioning in the maladaptive range.

Comment: Emphasizes "maladaptation."

Quality of Life Scale

Key reference: Heinrichs et al., 1984 (8).

Purpose: To assess deficit syndrome in patients with schizophrenia.

Patients studied: Outpatients with schizophrenia, N = 111 (described as not applicable to inpatients).

Type of instrument: Semistructured interview by trained clinician.

Number of items: 21.

Length of administration: 45 minutes.

Summary of content: Scale scoring: Intrapsychic foundations, interpersonal relations, instrumental role, total score.
a. Physical functioning: Commonplace activities.
b. Economic functioning: Occupational role, work functioning, work level, possession of commonplace objects.
c. Social functioning: Interpersonal relations (household, friends, acquaintances, social activity, social network, social initiative, social withdrawal, sociosexual functioning).
d. Psychological functioning: Sense of purpose, motivation, curiosity, anhedonia, aimless inactivity, empathy, emotional interaction, work satisfaction.

Psychometric properties: Interrater reliabilities on conjointly conducted interviews range from .84 to .97 on summary scales. Individual item intraclass correlations range from 0.5 to 0.9. Confirmatory factor analysis conducted. Validity not assessed.

Comparative data: None.

Data analysis: Reports mean scores for individual items.

Quality of Life Interview

Key references: Lehman et al., 1982; Lehman et al., 1986; Lehman, 1988 (9–11).

Purpose: To assess quality of life of severely mentally ill living in board and care homes, hospitals, and other supervised settings.

Patients studied:
a. Severely mentally ill in Los Angeles board and care homes, $N = 278$.
b. Inpatients of a state mental hospital, $N = 99$.
c. Severely mentally ill in supervised community residences, $N = 92$.
(All groups predominantly schizophrenic.)

Type of instrument: Structured interview by trained lay interviewers.

Number of items: 143.

Length of administration: 45 minutes.

Summary of content:
a. Physical functioning: Number of leisure activities.
b. Economic functioning: Current employment status, total monthly financial support, monthly spending money.
c. Social functioning: Frequency of family contacts, frequency of social contacts, frequency of religious activities, legal problems and victimization.
d. Psychological functioning: General perceived health status, general life satisfaction, satisfaction with living situation, family relations, social relations, leisure, work, religious activities, finances, safety, and health.
e. Other: Medical and psychiatric care during the past year.

Psychometric properties: Internal consistency reliabilities range: life satisfaction scales, 0.79 to 0.88 (median reliability = .85); objective quality of life scales, 0.44 to 0.82 (median reliability = .68); reliabilities replicated on two severely mentally ill populations. Test re-test reliabilities (1 week): life satisfaction scales, 0.41 to 0.95 (median reliability = = .72); objective quality of life scales, 0.29 to 0.98 (median reliability = .65). Construct and predictive validity assessed as good by confirmatory factor analysis and multivariate model prediction.

Data analysis: Between group comparisons (inpatient versus outpatient; severely mentally ill versus general population and disadvantaged subgroups in the general population); multivariate predictive model of general well-being.

Comparative data: General population norms on life satisfaction (5); norms for inpatient versus outpatient severely mentally ill.

Quality of Life Checklist

Key reference: Malm et al., 1981 (12).

Purpose: To provide information about which aspects of quality of life are particularly important to patients and natural raters in order to assist in therapeutic planning.

Patients studied: Chronic schizophrenic outpatients, $N = 40$.

Type of instrument: Rating scale completed by a trained interviewer based on a 1 hour, semistructured interview.

Number of items: 93.

Length of administration: 5 to 10 minutes to complete ratings after a 1 hour, semistructured interview.

Summary of content: Scoring: For all areas, ratings are "satisfactory" or "unsatisfactory."
a. Physical functioning: Leisure activities.
b. Economic functioning: Work, vocational rehabilitation, economic dependency.
c. Social functioning: Relationships.
d. Psychological functioning: Knowledge and education, psychological dependency, inner experience.
e. Other: Housing standard, medical care (psychiatric and general), religion.

Psychometric properties: None reported.

Data analysis: Reports of simple frequencies of "satisfactory" versus "unsatisfactory" by items.

Comparative data: None.

Community Adjustment Form

Key reference: Stein and Test, 1980 (13).

Purpose: To assess life satisfaction and other quality of life outcomes in a randomized study of an experimental system of community-based care for the severely mentally ill versus standard care.

Patients studied: Patients seeking admission to a state hospital (50% schizophrenia), $N = 130$.

Type of instrument: Semistructured self-report interview; type of interviewer not specified (probably nonclinical).

Number of items: 140 (approximate).

Length of administration: Not indicated (estimate 45 minutes).

Summary of content:
a. Physical functioning: Leisure Activity Scale (same as Lehman Quality of life Interview).
b. Economic functioning: Quality of living situation; employment history and status; income sources and amounts; free lodging and/or meals.
c. Social functioning: Contact with friends, family; legal problems.
d. Psychological: 21-item life satisfaction scale, self-esteem scale.
e. Other: Medical care, agency utilization.

Psychometric properties: None reported.

Data analysis: Repeated measures comparing two treatment groups. Most scales appear sensitive to differentiate the two treatment groups over time.

Comparative data: Results replicated in Australian study (14) (except for no between-group differences found in life satisfaction in the Australian study).

CHOOSING A MEASURE

Given that none of these quality of life measures has been widely used or accepted as a standard, the choice of a measure must be determined by the investigator's particular purpose and needs. The most comprehensive and psychometrically best-characterized scales are the Oregon Quality of Life Questionnaire and the Lehman Quality of Life Interview. Both cover similar domains of quality of life functioning, are based on comprehensive quality of life models, and have acceptable psychometric properties. They have been used with typical samples of severely mentally ill patients in the United States, which included high percentages of psychotic patients. Both instruments require approximately 45 minutes to administer. Our experience has been that most investigators either do not want to devote this length of time to quality of life assessment or want to include other items not contained in these instruments. Therefore many probably administer subsections of these longer instruments, supplemented by additional items from other sources. If this approach is taken we strongly recommend that at least the original subscales be kept intact. The major argument for using the complete instruments is that each was developed with a comprehensive quality of life model in mind.

The only quality of life measure that has been used in experimental research to date has been the Community Adjustment Form (13,14). This instrument is similar in content to the two just discussed. Unfortunately, no psychometric properties have been reported on the Community Adjustment Form, although it sensitively detected differences between two treatment conditions.

The remaining four instruments have had much more limited usage and are less comprehensive. The Satisfaction with Life Domains Scale is a reasonably well-characterized and brief measure of life satisfaction that has been used with severely mentally ill populations. Since it only measures life satisfaction, measures of other quality of life functioning (physical, social, and economic) would have to be added to provide a comprehensive quality of life assessment. The Quality of Life Checklist was developed specifically for use in a clinic setting and seems particularly adapted to helping clinicians assess the various areas of quality of life functioning. However, it has no known psychometric properties and to our knowledge has only been used in one small study. The Standardized Social Schedule has only been used with chronic neurotic patients in Britain. It has adequate reliability properties, but its factor structure is not stable. Finally, the Quality of Life Scale is a relatively comprehensive and well-characterized instrument, thus similar to the first two discussed. However, it was developed for the more focal purpose of assessing the deficit functional symptoms of schizophrenia and requires administration by a trained clinician. As such it does not fit readily into the mainstream of quality of life assessment and must be viewed as more disease-specific than the others.

Beyond these instrument-specific comments, some general comments and caveats are warranted for the investigator seeking a quality of life measure for the severely mentally ill. First, a major problem with using normative quality of life measures in this population is that floor effects are frequently encountered in social and economic functioning. For these two areas of quality of life functioning, special attention must be paid to instrument sensitivity. Such floor effects are not a typical problem with the severely mentally ill in the quality of life areas of physical functioning and psychological functioning (life satisfaction). Second, significant numbers of these patients have problems with task perseverance and comprehension, therefore pencil-and-paper questionnaires are not recommended. Note that all of the instruments discussed here are interviews. Finally, psychopathology affects patients' ratings of their quality of life. In the only study of this phenomenon, anxiety and depression had significant effects on the patients' perceived life satisfaction (15). Therefore quality of life assessments of these patients should be accompanied by a concomitant assessment of psychopathologic symptoms to reduce the confounding effects of psychiatric syndromes.

USING A MEASURE

There are three situations in which investigators use a quality of life measure in studies of the severely mentally ill: (a) to assess patients' current quality of life to establish a baseline or to compare samples cross-sectionally; (b) to monitor the mediating effects of changes in quality of life on core clinical outcomes, for example, symptom levels and relapse; and (c) to assess quality of life as a primary longitudinal outcome of research interventions. To our knowledge there have been no studies of the utility of quality of life assessments for prescribing interventions.

STATISTICAL CONSIDERATIONS

The types of statistical analyses used for each of the seven measures included in this chapter have been briefly summarized in the sections above. For the most part the data have been analyzed to detect between-group differences using standard univariate or multivariate techniques. Typically data are reported as scale scores or item means or frequencies. Only Lehman has analyzed the data according to a predictive model of quality of life (16). Although such model testing is necessary to advance the field theoretically, most applications will probably rely on more standard between-group comparisons.

DATA INTERPRETATION AND EXTRAPOLATION

Because this field in psychiatric research is new, it is not possible to make specific recommendations about the interpretation of quality of life data. Conceptually quality of life is generally seen as related to, but distinct from, clinical syndromes such as depression and anxiety. Perhaps the most important point about interpretation that can be made at present is the need to distinguish psychological quality of life (for example, life satisfaction or morale) from clinical symptomatology, particularly depression. We know that measures of psychological quality of life functioning are clearly affected by clinical symptomatology (15). However, at least conceptually, life satisfaction and its quality of life equivalents are generally viewed as distinct from clinical syndromes. This distinction has particular relevance with regard to implications for interventions. That is, one might attempt to effect various changes in a patient's environment to improve housing, financial, or work dissatisfaction, whereas one might prescribe a clinical intervention, such as an antidepressant, to alleviate symptoms of depression. Certainly we can foresee the development of an interactive model between quality of life and clinical symptomatology, but at the very least we can say that to adequately interpret quality of life data from psychiatrically impaired populations, one needs to assess both quality of life and clinical syndromes.

For some of the measures described above, there are published norms for different samples of patients, thus allowing some comparison of new patient samples with these samples. For the life satisfaction measures in the Lehman Quality of Life Interview and Satisfaction with Life Domains Scale, there are also national normative data because these measures were based heavily on prior work assessing general quality of life in the United States (5).

AREAS FOR FUTURE IMPROVEMENT

In order to advance quality of life assessment for severely mentally ill persons to the point that more scientifically and clinically meaningful applications can be achieved, several areas need work. First, we need a clearer definition of what quality of life is and what it is not. The existing literature is characterized both by conceptually clear but disparate models of quality of life and by overly broad and vague definitions of the phrase "quality of life." Definitions include life satisfaction, illness-related "deficit states," very comprehensive multidimensional models of well-being, and ill-defined notions that are appealing but vague. Second, with the adoption of a common definition, there needs to be some agreement about how to measure quality of life. This will allow us to begin to accumulate comparable data across studies and populations. Third, we need to compare quality of life data from psychiatrically impaired populations with those from other nonpsychiatric groups, particularly the physically disabled and the general population, in order to establish some normative perspective. Fourth, we need a better understanding of how quality of life varies naturally over time in psychiatric populations, the predictive validity of quality of life measures for subsequent illness course and outcome, and the sensitivity of quality of life measures for detecting treatment effects among these patients, who may at best experience very modest improvements. Finally, there is a need for basic conceptual work to develop better models for integrating quality of life data into a general model of outcome for persons with severe mental illnesses.

The eventual role that quality of life assessment will play in the development and evaluation of policies and programs for the severely mentally ill remains to be seen. The quality of life concept, in both planning and evaluation, fits trends in contemporary thought about the needs of these patients. Instruments, including those presented here, now exist to evaluate their quality of life, although we may expect continued evolution of these measures as more mental health evaluators attempt to assess quality of life. At this juncture, some form of quality of life assessments are being employed in several longitudinal studies of treatment services for the severely mentally ill. As these studies conclude, we will have a better idea of the value of quality of life assessments in planning for our severely mentally ill citizens.

ACKNOWLEDGMENT

Preparation of this chapter was supported by NIMH Grant No. MH43703.

REFERENCES

1. Spring B, Zubin J. Vulnerability to schizophrenic episodes and their prevention in adults. In: Albee GW, Joffe JM, eds. *Primary prevention in psychopathology: The issues*, vol 1. Hanover, NH: University Press of New England, 1977;254–284.
2. Baker F, Intagliata J. Quality of life in the evaluation of community support systems. *Evaluation and Program Planning* 1982;5:69–79.
3. Bradburn NM. *The structure of psychological well-being*. Chicago: Aldine, 1969.
4. Endicott J, Spitzer R, Fleiss J, Cohen J. The global assessment scale: A procedure for measuring overall severity of psychiatric disturbance. *Arch Gen Psychiatry* 1976;33:766–771.
5. Andrews FM, Withey SB. *Social indicators of well-being*. New York: Plenum Press, 1976.
6. Bigelow DA, Brodsky G, Steward L, Olson M. The concept and measurement of quality of life as a dependent variable in evaluation of mental health services. In: Stahler GJ, Tash WR, eds. *Innovative approaches to mental health evaluation*. New York: Academic Press, 1982;345–366.
7. Clare AW, Cairns VE. Design, development and use of a standardized interview to assess social maladjustment and dysfunction in community samples. *Psychol Med* 1978;8:589–604.
8. Heinrichs DW, Hanlon TE, Carpenter WT. The quality of life scale: An instrument for rating the schizophrenic deficit syndrome. *Schizophr Bull* 1984;10:388–398.
9. Lehman AF, Ward NC, Linn LS. Chronic mental patients: The quality of life issue. *Am J Psychiatry* 1982;10:1271–1276.
10. Lehman AF, Possidente S, Hawker F. The quality of life of chronic mental patients in a state hospital and community residences. *Hosp Community Psychiatry* 1986;37:901–907.
11. Lehman AF. A quality of life interview for the chronically mentally ill. *Evaluation and Program Planning* 1988;11:51–62.
12. Malm U, May PRA, Dencker SJ. Evaluation of the quality of life of the schizophrenic outpatient: A checklist. *Schizophr Bull* 1981;7:477–487.
13. Stein LI, Test MA. Alternative to mental hospital treatment: I. Conceptual model, treatment program and clinical evaluation. *Arch Gen Psychiatry* 1980;37:392–397.
14. Hoult J, Reynolds J. Schizophrenia: A comparative trial of community oriented and hospital oriented psychiatric care. *Acta Psychiatr Scand* 1984;69:359–372.
15. Lehman AF. The effects of psychiatric symptoms on quality of life assessments among the chronic mentally ill. *Evaluation and Program Planning* 1983;6:143–151.
16. Lehman AF. The well-being of chronic mental patients: Assessing their quality of life. *Arch Gen Psychiatry* 1983;40:369–373.

Quality of Life Assessments in Clinical Trials, edited by B. Spilker. Raven Press, Ltd. New York © 1990.

28

Inflammatory Bowel Disease

*John W. Garrett, *Douglas A. Drossman, and †Donald L. Patrick

Division of Digestive Diseases and Nutrition, Department of Medicine, University of North Carolina, School of Medicine, Chapel Hill, North Carolina 27599; †Department of Health Services, School of Public Health, University of Washington, Seattle, Washington 98195

The term "inflammatory bowel disease" describes two common medical disorders afflicting up to 500,000 people in this country. Ulcerative colitis, a disease of the colon, presents with rectal bleeding, diarrhea, and pain. Crohn's disease can affect most of the gastrointestinal tract and presents with abdominal pain, diarrhea, vomiting, fever, infection, and weight loss from nutritional disturbances. The health care costs for inflammatory bowel disease patients are considerable: more is spent for the inpatient care of a patient with inflammatory bowel disease than for gallbladder surgery, appendectomy, or peptic ulcer disease (1).

There is growing recognition in the scientific literature that biological processes alone are insufficient to explain a patient's health status, and that we must obtain additional information regarding quality of life and psychosocial issues in order to better understand and manage patients with chronic disease. Since patients with inflammatory bowel disease have a chronic illness with varying degrees of physical and psychosocial impairment, further information is needed regarding their quality of life. Also, because it is unlikely that there will be a cure in the near future, research must be directed toward helping patients to adapt both medically and psychosocially to their illness. The evaluation and treatment of inflammatory bowel disease patients is currently based on the degree of disease activity or its complications. These are relatively crude measures of health status since most patients, even with mild disease activity, experience impairment in their quality of life (2). Existing measures of disease activity are not sensitive enough to fully assess the impact of the disorder, and standardized psychosocial assessments, including subjective experiences, are needed to improve our ability to gather this data. This chapter discusses some of the methodological issues related to the study of health-related quality of life in inflammatory bowel disease and reviews the existing data for this population.

PROBLEMS WITH HEALTH-RELATED QUALITY OF LIFE ASSESSMENT

There is a paucity of information regarding quality of life issues in inflammatory bowel disease. Why is this so? First, health-related quality of life has not been considered relevant to the diagnosis and care of inflammatory bowel disease patients;

TABLE 1. *Some problems with previous behavioral research*

A. Lack of agreement as to terminology, conceptualization, and research design among the behavioral disciplines.
B. Difficulties in obtaining psychosocial data:
  1. Behavioral factors are subjective and cannot easily be defined or measured or validated (e.g., pain, stress, social support, illness behavior).
  2. Information from questionnaires or interviews may not be reliable or valid (e.g., do not account for denial, social compliance).
  3. Information from standardized questionnaires may not be appropriate for the population under study or the questions being asked.
  4. Information from physician case reports is not easily verified by experimental technique (retrospective, uncontrolled, may be biased).
C. Human illness and its effects are multidetermined. It is difficult to limit or control for the contributing psychosocial variables.
D. There is a lack of prospective studies. Data from retrospective or case comparison studies cannot provide information about causation.

disease activity has been considered the standard measure of illness. However, in the last few years, the literature has provided scientific evidence for the inclusion of quality of life as an outcome measure of chronic illnesses (rheumatoid arthritis, heart disease, and chronic lung disease). Second, for inflammatory bowel disease and gastrointestinal diseases in general, quality of life assessment is difficult. The complexity of the cultural and psychosocial influences on human behavior and gut function and the difficulties in designing methodologically sound studies in behavioral research have restricted our ability to understand the interaction between psychosocial and biologic variables in disease and health. It has also been difficult to develop specific criteria for quality of life assessment in inflammatory bowel disease because there is so little information regarding patients' functional status and concerns. Table 1 describes some methodologic problems related to behavioral research, stressing the difficulty obtaining relevant psychosocial information and a lack of standardization in terminology and research design. With regard to inflammatory bowel disease, there are additional factors to consider.

Heterogeneity

Traditionally, ulcerative colitis and Crohn's disease have been studied together, yet these are different medical diseases. Perhaps these two diseases should be evaluated separately with regard to quality of life issues as well. There is considerable clinical variation within each disease. For example, Crohn's disease consists of three anatomic subgroups: ileitis involving the small intestine, colitis involving the large intestine, and ileocolitis. Patients within each group behave differently in terms of their clinical presentation, symptom characteristics, complications, morbidity, and possibly their psychological profiles (1). Further studies with sufficient numbers of patients are needed to determine whether quality of life and other behavioral factors differ for ulcerative colitis, Crohn's disease, and their clinical subgroups.

Limitations of Disease Activity Assessment as a Measure of Quality of Life

Although subjective health measures have been constructed for medical illnesses (cancer [14], chronic obstructive lung disease [15], and arthritis [16]) which more than satisfy accepted reliability criteria (12,13), they have not been used in inflammatory bowel disease. The measures of disease activity in inflammatory bowel disease do not completely correlate with health-related quality of life; these measures were designed to indirectly determine the degree of biologic activity or inflammation. Some subjective measures were incorporated into disease activity indices, but they related more to symptoms than to function, or than to more global dimensions. Investigators assessed patients' symptoms, physical signs, and endoscopic and laboratory studies to globally rate patients as having mild, moderate, or severe disease (3–5).

The most commonly used index of disease activity is the Crohn's Disease Activity Index (CDAI) developed by Best et al. in 1976 (6). This index was used in the National Cooperative Crohn's Disease Study to provide both a uniform set of clinical parameters for evaluation and a quantitative measure of treatment effect in response to prednisone or sulfasalazine. Regression analysis of 18 variables from 1,897 visits of 112 patients yielded eight weighted variables (abdominal pain, bowel habits, general well-being, use of lomotil or opiates, complications, wasting, abdominal mass, and hemoglobin) which correlated with the physician's subjective impression of disease activity based on a 4-point Likert scale (very well, fair to good, poor, very poor). The index correlated with the physician's opinion ($R = 0.7$), but a relation between the patient's global sense of well-being and the index was not assessed.

Other authors have modified the Crohn's Disease Activity Index or used different variables to assess disease activity. The Harvey Bradshaw Index (7) was devised to simplify the Crohn's Disease Activity Index for clinical use. Utilizing five clinical features (abdominal pain, bowel habits, well-being, complications, and abdominal mass), the authors prospectively compared their index with the Crohn's Disease Activity Index in 112 patients and found that the Harvey Bradshaw Index correlated highly ($R = 0.93$) with the Crohn's Disease Activity Index.

In 1984, Myren et al. (8), as part of the International Organization for the Study of Inflammatory Bowel Disease, formulated a 10-item binary scoring system. To provide more flexibility in scoring, Wright et al. (9) developed a similar index, but one in which the items were scored 0 to 3 for absent to severe rather than present or not present as in the Myren study. With the belief that subjective complaints, as used in previous studies, were unreliable, Van Hees et al. (10) used the physical examination and laboratory studies to create a more objective index of activity. The index correlated well ($R = 0.95$) with the physician's assessment, but not unexpectedly, poorly with the Crohn's Disease Activity Index ($R = 0.67$) (8,10) which also included the patient's subjective symptoms.

More recently, Sandler (11) derived from the Crohn's Disease Activity Index an index for use in survey research which does not require direct physician assessment. Three variables taken from the Crohn's Disease Activity Index (stool frequency, abdominal pain, and sense of well-being) correlated well ($R = 0.87$) with the total Crohn's Disease Activity Index.

As noted, all these indices were derived directly or indirectly from the physician's subjective impression of disease activity rather than from the patient's perception of health status or from independent outcome measures such as health care utilization, number of hospitalizations, or functional status. Also, subjective data generally were not included in disease activity assessments since they were felt to be less reliable than objective findings. However, clinicians rely heavily on patients' subjective reports in addition to laboratory data in the assessment of their health status and in making treatment decisions. Only recently have investigators begun to use the functional status and concerns (2) of inflammatory bowel disease patients as health status measures, and to gauge improvement based on specific outcome measures.

An additional problem with current indices of disease activity is that they are based on the amount of tissue damage or inflammation, and do not assess the quality of life of inflammatory bowel disease patients who have minimal inflammation, but suffer from the effects or complications of the disease (e.g., painful rectal strictures). This is in sharp contrast to other disorders (cardiac, lung disease) where pathologic or physiologic measures exist that closely correlate with quality of life. In addition, unlike patients having diseases (e.g., renal failure, cardiac disease, and chronic obstructive lung disease) that may lead to an inexorable decline, inflammatory bowel disease patients show a great deal of variation in disease activity over time. Thus, quality of life assessments can change markedly, and disease activity is not sufficient to explain those eventualities.

Methodological Concerns

Research in inflammatory bowel disease is also difficult because of issues related to patient selection and study design (1). First, there is a cohort effect that restricts the generalizability of research data from population to population. Severely ill patients are overrepresented in referral centers and those with mild disease may be followed primarily by their local physician, or not at all. It is also possible that the clinical status of inflammatory bowel disease patients may vary based on their regional distribution. Thus, it is unlikely that a representative inflammatory bowel disease population exists (17). Second, the available quality of life assessments have been made without healthy or medical comparison groups as controls, making it difficult to judge the specificity of the findings. Finally, the lack of appropriate quality of life measures has slowed the systematic evaluation of quality of life in inflammatory bowel disease. The value of reported quality of life measures in inflammatory bowel disease may be limited since they have generally involved retrospective analyses, assumed that the ability to work is a sufficient measure of quality of life, and traditionally have used nonstandardized measures of uncertain reliability (e.g., unskilled interviewers, poorly validated questionnaires [1]). Given these limitations, what follows is a summary of health-related quality of life and related data pertaining to inflammatory bowel disease patients.

ASSESSMENT OF QUALITY OF LIFE IN INFLAMMATORY BOWEL DISEASE

Historical Overview

The earliest quality of life assessments in inflammatory bowel disease were designed to be a small part of studies describing prognosis in medical patients or some measure of surgical outcome. For the most part, they were global assessments made without standardized scales (Table 2). For example, Bergman and Krause (18) examined the clinical course of 186 Crohn's disease patients treated between 1956 and 1968 and rated patients' general health or quality of life as I, II, or III, for those patients with good general health, reduced ability to work, or those unable to work. After 10 years' observation, 83% of patients (no comparison group) were rated as

TABLE 2. *Quality of life assessment in inflammatory bowel disease:*
Retrospective data

Study/disease	No. of patients entered	Quality of life measure	Results and comments
Bergman and Krause, CD (18)	186	Quality of life 10.5 years after surgery I. Good health II. Reduced ability to work III. Unable to work	 I. 87% II. 9.1% III. 3.6%
Gazzard et al., CD (19)	85	Morbid Anxiety Index (MAI) Eysenck Personality Questionnaire (EPQ) Questionnaire including knowledge of disease, work record, married and sexual life, financial problems Disease activity (clinical and biochemical features)	1. Males tended to be more introverted/neurotic. 2. 74 pts felt well or perfectly well, 11 pts felt poor; only 5 pts gave up work because of disease. 3. Little change in married/family life: 9 thought marriage worse, 19 felt marriage improved, half noted less frequent intercourse. 4. The pt's premorbid personality is the most accurate determinant of outcome.
Hendriksen and Binder, UC (20)	122	Questionnaire of professional, emotional, and family conditions Age and sex matched acute illness patient controls	1. No significant differences in severe family problems (16% pts, 12% controls), frequency of sexual problems (12% vs. 11%), previous treatment for mental disorders (13% vs. 17%), social/physical activities, or absence from work. 2. More inflammatory bowel disease pts with higher socioeconomic status and education (university degrees) (12% pts vs. 2% controls, $p < 0.05$), and fewer unskilled workers (23% vs. 35%).
Sorensen, Olsen, and Binder, CD (21)	106	Personal interview concerning professional conditions, family relations, sex life, living conditions, use of EtOH/tobacco/drugs, and diet. Score kept for social activity (frequent participation, cultural, sports, courses, frequent contact with friends, travel), physical activity. Age and sex matched controls.	1. Family/social: equal numbers married (67% vs. 71%), and had regular sexual activity (72% vs. 73%). 2. Previous psychiatric assistance in 10% pts, 8% controls. 3. No differences in social or physical activity scores. 4. No differences in percent employed, amount of sick leave. 5. Life insurance: 25% CD pts vs. 36% controls. 6. CD pts reported reduced capacity for work (23%) and reduced leisure activities (21%).
Meyers et al., CD (22)	53	Psychosocial survey recording overall satisfaction, physical symptoms, relationships, school, and employment, recreation, sexuality, body image, influence of ileostomy, recurrences.	1. 92% believed first surgery helpful. 2. Patients less symptomatic (18% vs. 48% preop). 3. Improved relations with friends and family (improvement 19% vs. 62% preop). 4. Fewer school/employment difficulties (14% vs. 71%). 5. Improved body image (10% vs. 37%).

CD, Crohn's disease; UC, ulcerative colitis; pts, patients.

quality of life I, 8% quality of life II, and 9% quality of life III. The authors concluded that Crohn's patients had a good quality of life outcome. Gazzard (19) interviewed 85 outpatients with Crohn's disease, and administered the Eysenck Personality Inventory (EPI) and a questionnaire concerning knowledge of disease, work record, marriage and sexual life, financial problems, and worries. They found that most patients live useful, optimistic lives, and that the patient's premorbid personality is the most important determinant of his health prospects. Hendriksen (20) interviewed 122 patients with ulcerative colitis to obtain data on their family as well as their social, emotional, and professional lives and concluded that ulcerative colitis patients adapted well to their condition and suffered few social or professional disabilities as measured by marital status, the frequency of family or sexual problems, leisure activities, physical and earning capacity, the incidence of mental disorders, and the intake of alcohol and other drugs. Sorensen et al. (21) interviewed 106 patients with Crohn's disease regarding family, social, and professional conditions, and found that patients reported little effect on family/social problems or physical activity, but that exacerbations of inflammatory bowel disease strained personal/professional relations. An equal percentage of patients and controls were married and had children, and there were no differences in social and physical activity. Crohn's disease patients had a slightly higher socioeconomic level, and 65% were employed (versus 64% of controls). Only 3% of the Crohn's disease patients were on disability, and both patients and controls had less than 11 sick days annually. Finally, Meyers et al. (22) used a psychosocial survey to assess interpersonal relations, school/job performance, recreational activity, sexuality, and body image in 51 patients 5 to 10 years after their first elective surgery for Crohn's disease. Following surgery, patients noted long-term improvement in the five psychosocial areas as well as physical symptoms, and perceived the operation as having provided long-term improvement in their quality of life.

General Versus Specific Instruments for Quality of Life Assessment

In general, these prior data were limited due to their use of interviews and questionnaires that lacked standardization. Recently, investigators have begun to address quality of life issues in inflammatory bowel disease patients through the development of more standardized specific indices. There has been some controversy as to whether general or disease-specific measures of quality of life should be used. Both measures are important, and each has a specific role in quality of life assessment.

General Measures

General measures such as the Sickness Impact Profile (23), the McMaster Health Index (16), and the Nottingham Health Profile (24) are examples of health profiles developed to cover specific components of health-related quality of life in a systematic and unified manner. These measures are likely to have clinical value as they may uncover symptoms or restrictions in activities that physicians do not elicit from patients, and will permit a more sensitive quantitative assessment of treatment effects than existing disease activity indices. The advantages of general measures are that they permit coverage of several realms of dysfunction, allow comparison between different groups, and several have been extensively validated (25). Disadvantages

TABLE 3a. *Mean Sickness Impact Profile scores: UC and CD outpatients*

Scale	CD	UC	HMO comparison group
Overall	8.64	5.21	3.8
Physical	4.89	3.19	2.0
Psychosocial	10.25	5.60	4.0
Emotional behavior	15.7	7.72	3.6
Sleep and rest	17.46	9.12	7.0
Social interaction	11.76	6.84	5.3

UC, ulcerative colitis; CD, Crohn's disease; HMO, health maintenance organization.
Adapted from Drossman et al., ref. 2.

are that they may be insensitive to changes related to a specific disease (bowel function, abdominal pain), and some (e.g., the Sickness Impact Profile) are designed for medical patients and no normative data are available.

One example of a standardized instrument that has been used in inflammatory bowel disease is the Sickness Impact Profile, a measure of functional status (23). The Sickness Impact Profile, a 136-item self-administered questionnaire, is a behaviorally based measure of sickness-related dysfunction that assesses patient perceptions of performance in 12 areas of activity related to activities of daily living. Patients indicate their level of functioning on the day of the test taking. The categories may be grouped into an overall score, a physical dimensional score (A = ambulation, M = mobility, BCM = body care and movement), a psychosocial dimensional score (SI = social interaction, AB = alertness behavior, EB = emotional behavior, C = communication), and several independent scores (SR = sleep and rest, E = eating, W = work, HM = home management, RP = recreation and pastimes). The test has good convergent and discriminant validity, and has been validated by clinician assessments of patient health status, by scores from other functional assessment instruments, and by independent comparison with objective measures of dysfunction among patients with other medical disorders. It has a test re-test reliability of .92 and an internal consistency of .94. The scale has been shown effective for a variety of clinical and research applications as a health survey instrument, and as a sensitive outcome measure for evaluating treatment regimens and patient progress. Drossman et al. (2) has recently used the Sickness Impact Profile to characterize the functional status in 150 inflammatory bowel disease patients (63 ulcerative colitis, 87 Crohn's disease). Results (Table 3a) indicate: (a) inflammatory bowel disease patients exhibit moderate functional impairment (ulcerative colitis 5.2 ± 6.7, Crohn's disease 8.6 ± 9.8, health maintenance organization comparison group 3.8 ± 5.6, rheumatoid arthritis patients 15.6 ± 9.0) more in the social/psychological realm than in the physical dimensions; (b) Crohn's patients report more dysfunction than those with ulcerative colitis, Crohn's patients scored more dysfunction on the overall functional score ($p < .03$), psychosocial dimensions ($p < .02$), and all individual scales, with significant differences occurring with emotional behavior ($p < .02$), sleep and rest ($p < .02$), and social interaction subscales ($p < .04$), no sex-related differences were noted; (c) Functional status more than disease activity is closely correlated with other ratings of health status. The Sickness Impact Profile showed moderate to good correlation (Table 3b) with other health status measures: patient's and physician's

TABLE 3b. *Sickness Impact Profile: Correlational data*

	Ulcerative colitis		Crohn's disease	
	R=	p<	R=	p<
Overall SIP with:				
Patient's health rating	.35	.009	.51	.0001
Physician's health rating	.33	.01	.37	.0007
Physician visits	[.36	.13]	.41	.001
Hospitalizations	.32	.02	.40	.0002
Surgeries	[−.01	.94]	.28	.07
Disease activity with:				
Overall SIP score	.29	.03	[.10	.42]
Patient's health rating	[.20	.16]	.24	.04
Physician's health rating	.37	,005	.39	.0003
Physician visits	[.05	.71]	.37	.002
Hospitalization	[.12	.39]	[.11	.33]
Surgeries	[.12	.48]	[.05	.76]

SIP, Sickness Impact Profile.
[ ] = Not statistically significant.
Adapted from Drossman et al., ref. 2.

global assessment of health, and health care utilization. In comparison, the physician's rating of disease activity correlated poorly with both measures and with functional status. We believe that the Sickness Impact Profile is a sensitive measure of inflammatory bowel disease patient functional status which may be used in research and clinical care.

Specific Measures

In contrast to the general measures described above, disease-specific measures are useful because they can assess disease-specific issues and are generally less cumbersome to use. Disadvantages include that they may assess only one aspect of health status, and do not permit comparison between groups of patients with different chronic diseases. The Inflammatory Bowel Disease Questionnaire is a new measure of health status devised for clinical trials in inflammatory bowel disease (26,27). The authors developed a health status measure for clinical trials which examined disease-related dysfunction in inflammatory bowel disease patients. The instrument examines four aspects of patient's lives: symptoms directly related to the primary bowel disturbance, systemic symptoms, and emotional and social function. The Inflammatory Bowel Disease Questionnaire was designed to reflect areas of function that are important to patients with the disease, to be responsive to clinically important changes in health status, and to be relatively short and simple to complete. Items were selected from literature review, other quality of life questionnaires, and from the results of an open-ended questionnaire to clinicians caring for inflammatory bowel disease patients. Ninety-seven subjects with inflammatory bowel disease were given the 30-item questionnaire, and results (Table 4) indicate that primary bowel symptoms, systemic symptoms, and altered emotional function were common. Functional and social impairment were less frequent. Apart from primary bowel complaints, patients seldom volunteered other facets of quality of life impairment; this was particularly true for impairment of emotional function. Moreover, although

TABLE 4. *Inflammatory bowel disease symptom questionnaire, spontaneous versus elicited response[a,b]*

Dimension and item	Number of spontaneous responses (%)	Mean[c] importance	Number of elicited responses (%)	Mean importance
Bowel symptoms				
Frequent bowel movements	78 (86.7)	4.3	12 (13.3)	3.6
Loose bowel movements	53 (74.6)	4.0	18 (25.4)	4.4
Abdominal cramps	43 (53.8)	4.0	37 (46.2)	3.5
Pain in the abdomen	45 (69.2)	4.3	20 (30.8)	3.3
Systemic symptoms				
Fatigue	43 (48.9)	4.3	45 (51.1)	3.7
Overall feeling unwell	6 (7.2)	4.0	77 (92.8)	3.7
Feeling worn out	12 (14.6)	3.6	70 (85.4)	3.8
Emotional function				
Frustrated	34 (44.7)	4.0	42 (55.3)	3.6
Depressed	37 (50)	3.8	37 (50)	3.1
Worried about surgery	2 (3.4)	4.5	56 (96.6)	3.7
Social impairment				
Avoiding events where washrooms not close at hand	7 (12.5)	4.0	49 (87.5)	3.1
Cancelling social engagements	7 (14)	3.9	43 (86)	3.5
Functional impairment				
Inability to attend work/school regularly	15 (41.7)	4.0	21 (58.3)	3.9

[a] 97 subjects were asked to list all physical, emotional, and social problems experienced as a result of inflammatory bowel disease. When the subjects had no more "spontaneous" items to volunteer, they were asked to identify any additional items from the problem pool that represented problems for them ("elicited" responses).

[b] Adapted from Mitchell et al., ref. 26.

[c] Subjects rated the mean importance of each item on a 5-point Likert scale from "not very important" to "extremely important."

many patients noted troublesome symptoms, the majority of inflammatory bowel disease patients did not report major disruption in their work or personal lives.

It appears that the Inflammatory Bowel Disease Questionnaire may be useful in future treatment trials, but there were several limitations in the original study. First, the patient population used to develop the instrument was selected for convenience, and results may reflect this selection bias. Not unexpectedly this primarily outpatient population reported a lack of interference of the disease with work or school. Second, ileostomy and proctitis patients were excluded from analysis. Yet these are important groups to study because ileostomy patients may have significant impairment in social or psychologic function due to body image concerns, and proctitis patients often restrict social activities because of symptoms of urgency and tenesmus. These patients can have even greater impairment in function and be more refractory to treatment. Third, lack of a comparison group does not permit us to know the degree of impairment reflected by the scores. This information may be obtained in the future by comparing the scores with those of patients with functional bowel disorders or other chronic conditions. Finally, many items appear to be highly intercorrelated. For example, in the systemic system category, fatigue, feeling unwell, and feeling worn out seem to be similar symptoms, and cluster analysis or other statistical techniques should be considered in the future. The systemic symptom category could also reflect the emotional state. These items could be reported by a depressed population.

TABLE 5. *Patient concerns in inflammatory bowel disease: Numerical ranking and comparison of UC and CD outpatients*

	All (N = 150)	UC (N = 60)	CD (N = 77)	
	Mean (S.D.)	Mean (rank)	Mean (rank)	p<
Sumscore	39.0 (21.1)	37.5	38.0	
1. Having ostomy bag	63.3 (35.2)	61.2 (1)	62.1 (1)	
2. Your energy level	59.1 (31.5)	57.6 (3)	61.2 (2)	
3. Having surgery	55.8 (33.1)	55.7 (5)	55.7 (3)	
4. Feelings about body	55.1 (33.4)	55.5 (6)	50.8 (4)	
5. Loss bowel control	49.9 (36.1)	58.5 (2)	44.9 (6)	.04
6. Developing cancer	46.4 (33.6)	55.9 (4)	39.1 (9)	.005
7. Burden on others	45.4 (36.1)	45.0 (7)	42.5 (7)	
8. Pain	43.2 (29.2)	36.3 (12)	46.6 (5)	.05
9. Producing odors	42.5 (34.6)	43.5 (8)	39.1 (10)	
10. Intimacy	40.0 (33.9)	40.3 (10)	34.3 (11)	
11. Financial difficulties	39.0 (34.9)	31.2 (15)	41.2 (8)	
12. Feeling out of control	36.2 (31.5)	41.7 (9)	31.6 (13)	
13. Attractiveness	35.3 (32.0)	34.5 (14)	31.6 (14)	
14. Perform sexually	34.7 (35.0)	35.6 (13)	29.0 (17)	
15. Dying early	34.5 (32.7)	37.7 (11)	29.9 (16)	
16. Loss of sex drive	33.2 (35.1)	29.2 (17)	33.5 (12)	
17. Feeling alone	28.1 (30.0)	21.5 (19)	30.4 (15)	
18. Feeling dirty/smelly	27.8 (31.8)	30.4 (17)	23.0 (20)	
19. Pass inflammatory bowel disease to others	26.6 (35.0)	21.4 (20)	28.0 (18)	
20. Treated as having a defect	25.1 (28.9)	22.6 (18)	24.6 (19)	
21. Ability to have child	23.5 (32.1)	14.0 (21)	27.4 (21)	.03

UC, ulcerative colitis; CD, Crohn's disease.
Adapted from Drossman et al., ref. 2.

Another example of a disease-specific measure for inflammatory bowel disease is the self-administered 21-item Rating Form of Inflammatory Bowel Disease Patient Concerns Questionnaire (RFIPC) designed by Drossman et al. (2). Recognizing specific worries and concerns is important in order to provide education, to foster the patient's adjustment to the illness, and to insure patient satisfaction and compliance with treatment. Patient concerns may also affect the choice of treatment. For example, in planning for a total colectomy, an adolescent who feels socially stigmatized by an external ostomy is likely to prefer and do better with an ileoanal procedure. A long distance truck driver, on the other hand, may prefer not to make frequent rest room stops, and is likely to adapt better to a Kock pouch. The authors studied inflammatory bowel disease patients by videotape interview to identify specific worries and concerns that might affect treatment planning, patient satisfaction, and adjustment to illness. They then developed a questionnaire that identified and prioritized patients' worries and concerns, and applied it to a sample of 150 inflammatory bowel disease patients (63 ulcerative colitis, 87 Crohn's disease). All patients were asked, "Because of your condition, how concerned are you with . . . ?" The items were rated by patients from 0 to 100 (0 = not at all, 100 = a great deal) on a visual analog scale, and an averaged score of all concerns (sumscore) was also obtained. Major content areas (Table 5) for inflammatory bowel disease patients relate to having surgery (55.8), one's energy level (59.1), and body image issues such as having an ostomy bag (63.3). Ulcerative colitis and Crohn's patients had similar concerns

TABLE 6. *Correlation of concerns sumscore with health status and health care utilization*

	Ulcerative colitis		Crohn's disease	
	$R=$	$p<$	$R=$	$p<$
With health status:				
Sickness Impact Profile	46	.0002	.48	.0001
Patient's health rating	.38	.005	.47	.0001
Physician's health rating	.46	.0003	.23	.05
Physician's disease rating	.44	.0007		NS
With health care utilization:				
Physician visits		NS		NS
Hospitalization	.25	.07	.28	.02
Surgeries		NS		NS

Adapted from Drossman et al., ref. 2.

except that ulcerative colitis patients were more concerned with loss of bowel control and developing cancer, and Crohn's disease patients were more concerned with pain and the ability to have children. Also, patients who took oral steroids, regardless of disease, were more concerned with physical attractiveness (43.5 versus 30.0; $p < .02$), dying early (44.3 versus 27.8; $p < .004$), and being treated as having a defect (30.7 versus 20.5; $p < .04$). The consistency of these findings with clinical expectations provides a degree of validity, and attests to the potential use of this questionnaire as a sensitive measure of patient worries and concerns.

The Rating Form of Inflammatory Bowel Disease Patient Concerns provides an analysis of worries and concerns that can be rank ordered and used in clinical practice to plan patient education or treatment. For research purposes, the items can be averaged to produce a total score (sumscore) or four clinically relevant category scores: disease-related, body-related, inter/intrapersonal, and sex-related. It may also be a valuable measure of health status based on its correlation (Table 6) with other measures of health such as physician and patient global health ratings, functional impairment, disease activity for ulcerative colitis patients, and number of hospitalizations.

There are limitations to the Rating Form of Inflammatory Bowel Disease Patient Concerns in its present form. First, the content areas of the questionnaire are quite diverse, and the category scores are empirically derived. This group is presently analyzing the results of a national mail survey using this instrument and factor analysis will be done to determine whether specific clusterings of dysfunction can be identified. Second, further reliability and validity data are needed. Third, the specificity of the scale and its ability to measure concerns unique to inflammatory bowel disease patients are not established. This could be obtained from patients with other chronic gastrointestinal disorders, such as irritable bowel syndrome.

FUTURE RESEARCH

More information is needed to better characterize quality of life in the inflammatory bowel disease population. We need to determine whether disease-related differences (ulcerative colitis versus Crohn's disease) exist. In addition, we must assess the relationship between disease activity and quality of life, and examine how complications unrelated to disease activity (incontinence, strictures, obstruction, pain, and physical deformity) affect quality of life in inflammatory bowel disease patients. Finally, there are no data regarding health outcomes such as quality of life relative to disease and psychologic variables. Investigations to answer these and other questions will permit us to develop more sensitive measures of illness, particularly for outpatients with mild disease in whom the disease activity indices are insensitive. This work will not only further our understanding of health outcomes in inflammatory bowel disease, but also aid in the determination of health care utilization, medical versus surgical options, resource allocation, and the efficacy of therapeutic trials in the future.

REFERENCES

1. Drossman DA. Psychosocial aspects of ulcerative colitis and Crohn's disease. In: Kirsner J, Shorter L, eds. *Inflammatory bowel disease*. Philadelphia: Lea and Febiger, 1988;209–226.
2. Drossman DA, Patrick DL, Mitchell CM, Zagami EA, Appelbaum MI. Health related quality of life in inflammatory bowel disease: Functional status and patient worries and concerns. *Digestive Diseases and Sciences* 1989;34(9):1379–1386.
3. DeDombal FT, Burton IL, Clamp SE, Goligher JC. Short-term course and prognosis of Crohn's disease. *Gut* 1974;15:435–443.
4. Willoughby JMT, Kumar PJ, Beckett J, Dawson AM. Controlled trial of azathioprine in Crohn's disease. *Lancet* 1971;2:944–947.
5. Talstad I, Gjone E. The disease activity of ulcerative colitis and Crohn's disease. *Scand J Gastroenter* 1976;11:403–408.
6. Best WR, Becktel JM, Singleton JW, Kern F. Development of a Crohn's disease activity index, National Cooporative Crohn's Disease Study. *Gastroenterology* 1976;70(3):439–444.
7. Harvey RF, Bradshaw JM. A simple index of Crohn's disease activity. *Lancet* 1980;1:514.
8. Myren J, Bouchier IAD, Watkinson G, Softley A, Clamp SE, DeDombal FT. The O.M.G.E. multinational inflammatory bowel diseaase survey 1976–1982, a further report on 2,657 cases. *Scand J Gastroenterol* 1984;19(95):1–27.
9. Wright JP, Marks IN, Parfitt A. A simple clinical index of Crohn's disease activity—The Cape Town Index. *S Afr Med J* 1985;68:502–503.
10. Van Hees PAM, Van Elteren PH, Van Lier HJJ, Van Tongemen JHM. An index of inflammatory activity in patients with Crohn's disease. *Gut* 1980;21:279–286.
11. Sandler RS, Jordan M, Kupper L. Development of a Crohn's disease index for survey research. *J Clin Epidemiol* 1988;41:451–458.
12. Ware JE. Methodological considerations in the selection of health status assessment procedures. In: Wenger NK, Matteson ME, Furburg CD, Elinson J, eds. *Assessment of quality of life in clinical trials of cardiovascular therapies*. New York: LeJacq, 1984;87–111.
13. Ware JE, Broom RH, Davis AR, Loht KN. Choosing measures of health status for individuals in general populations. *Am J Pub Health* 1981;71(6):620–625.
14. Spitzer WO, Dobson AJ, Hall J, et al. Measuring QOL of cancer patients. *J Chron Dis* 1981;34:585–597.
15. Kaplan RM, Atkins CJ, Timms R. Validity of a quality of well being scale as an outcome measure in chronic obstructive pulmonary disease. *J Chron Dis* 1984;37(2):85–95.
16. Chambers LW, McDonald LA, Tugwell P, Buchanan WW, Kraag G. The McMaster Health Index Questionnaire as a measure of quality of life for patients with rheumatoid disease. *J Rheumatol* 1982;9(5):780–784.
17. Mendeloff AI, Caulkins BM. The epidemiology of idiopathic inflammatory bowel disease. In: Kirsner J, Shorter L, eds. *Inflammatory bowel disease*. Philadelphia: Lea and Febiger, 1988;1–35.
18. Bergman L, Krause U. Crohn's disease: A long-term study of the clinical course in 186 patients. *Scand J Gastroenterol* 1977;12:937–944.
19. Gazzard BG, Price HL, Libby GW, Dawson AM. The social toll of Crohn's disease. *Br Med J* 1978;2:1117–1119.
20. Hendriksen C, Binder V. Social prognosis in patients with ulcerative colitis. *Br Med J* 1980;281(6240):581–583.
21. Sorensen VZ, Olsen BG, Binder V. Life prospects and quality of life in patients with Crohn's disease. *Gut* 1987;28:382–385.
22. Meyers S, Walfish JS, Sachar DM, Greenstein AJ, Hill AG, Janowitz HD. Quality of life after surgery for Crohn's disease: A psychological survey. *Gastroenterology* 1980;78:1–6.

23. Bergner M, Bobbit R, Carter W, Gibson B. The Sickness Impact Profile: Development and final revision of a health status measure. *Med Care* 1981;XIX(8):787–805.

24. Hunt SM, McKenna SP, McEwen J. A quantitative approach to perceived health. *J Epidemiol Commun Health* 1980;3:281–285.

25. Patrick DL, Erickson P. What constitutes quality of life? Concepts and dimensions. *Clin Nutrition* 1988;7(2):53–63.

26. Mitchell A, Guyatt G, Singer J, Irvine EJ, Goodacre R, Tompkins C, Williams N, Wagner F. Quality of life in patients with inflammatory bowel disease. *J Clin Gastroenterol* 1988;10(3):306–310.

27. Guyatt G, Mitchell A, Irvine EJ, Singer J, Williams N, Goodacre R, Tompkins C. A new measure of health status for clinical trials in inflammatory bowel disease. *Gastroenterology* 1989;96(3):804–810.

Quality of Life Assessments in Clinical Trials, edited by B. Spilker. Raven Press, Ltd. New York © 1990.

29

Renal Replacement Therapies

Atara Kaplan De-Nour

Department of Psychiatry, Hadassah University Hospital, Jerusalem 91120, Israel

End-stage renal disease is the terminal and final phase of several very different conditions. Some of the diseases that lead to end-stage renal disease are hereditary and can be localized only to the kidney, e.g., polycystic kidney disease, or can effect many systems including the kidney, e.g., familial Mediterranean fever. Other diseases that cause end-stage renal disease are not hereditary. Some of them effect only the kidney, e.g., glomerulonephritis and pyelonephritis, whereas in other cases the damage of the kidney is part of a systemic disease, e.g., diabetes. Thus the disease process preceding end-stage renal disease is varied, and the patients go through different stages of disease and differ in comorbidity. Common to all, however, is the nonfunctioning of kidneys which, up to 25 years ago, meant uremia and death. Renal replacement therapy is the solution to nonfunctioning kidneys, but naturally not to the basic disease process that has led to the end-stage renal disease.

Renal replacement therapy now includes several modes of treatment. Hemodialysis was actually the first renal replacement therapy and in most countries it is still the most common. This treatment is usually administered three times a week for a total of about 12 hours a week. It is mostly done in hospitals or centers and is supervised by professional staff. In most countries only a minority of hemodialysis patients in limited care units or, more commonly, at home are supervised by family members. The second mode of renal replacement therapy is peritoneal dialysis. Intermittent peritoneal dialysis is carried out in the hospital and is comparatively rare, but continuous ambulatory peritoneal dialysis is gaining popularity in most countries. The third mode of renal replacement therapy is transplantation, usually from a cadaver donor and less commonly from a living related donor.

End-stage renal disease is a fairly common condition and each year about 50 to 60 new patients per million population will require renal replacement therapy. The availability of renal replacement therapy, however, differs greatly in various countries, from under 50 to over 250 per million population. These huge differences are caused mostly by financial considerations. The differences between countries, however, are not only in the number of patients on renal replacement therapy, but also in the relative proportions of the different modes of treatment. The modes differ not only in cost but also in what each of them requires and entails. Hemodialysis means being hooked up to a machine 12 hours a week and following a strict diet (low sodium, low proteins, and greatly restricted fluid intake). The patients on hemodialysis most often have severe sexual problems and sooner or later will have severe bone problems. Home hemodialysis gives them more freedom and allows them to compensate more easily for food binges, but it imposes a burden on their helper. Continuous ambulatory peritoneal dialysis relieves the patient from being hooked to a machine and from most of the dietary restrictions, but it imposes a grave danger of infection and peritonitis. Transplantation restores the patient's freedom and relieves the dietary restrictions, but imposes the side effects of steroids and the fear of rejection.

Thus renal replacement therapy does offer patients life—and the 5-year survival rate is now more than 50%—but what about the quality of this life?

To a certain extent end-stage renal disease is a unique situation in medicine. We are dealing with a fairly large patient population, more than 100,000 in the countries that are members of the European Dialysis and Transplant Association, who would have been dead but for renal replacement therapy and who may yet survive for many years. All factors that determine or modify patients' quality of life can be studied in end-stage renal disease and its different therapies. Indeed, machine-dependent life and replaced organ-dependent life caught the interest of the behavioral scientists from their beginnings in the early 1960s. By now there are hundreds of articles as well as a number of books on various aspects of quality of life of patients with end-stage renal disease. One would think that we know all there is to know about the quality of life of patients in the different modes of renal replacement therapy. The fact is, however, that we know little about the quality of life of end-stage renal disease patients.

The World Health Organization stated, "Health is a state of complete physical, mental and social well-being and not merely the absence of diseases and infirmity" (1). Therefore, when we speak of quality of life we should actually assess to what extent complete physical, mental, and social well-being has been achieved. However, most studies of end-stage renal disease patients and renal replacement therapy have not addressed *all* three facets of quality of life. Furthermore, different researchers used different definitions of quality of life, therefore very different measures can be found. To make the issue even more complicated, the symptoms of uremia are very similar to the symptoms of depression and medication (e.g., steroids, antihypertensive drugs) and can have massive psychological effects.

Many studies have shown that physical, mental, and social well-being are strongly interrelated and that it is often difficult to discover the directionality; i.e., does the physical condition influence the emotional condition or is it the other way round? But for the sake of clarity, let us first handle each aspect separately.

PHYSICAL CONDITION AND PHYSICAL FUNCTION

Great variability can be found in the physical condition and physical function of end-stage renal disease patients. Some are in very good condition and many are very sick. Yet, amazingly, there are practically no measures for the physical condition of patients receiving renal replacement therapy. In studies of quality of life the subject is often ignored, or at most some biochemical data are given with no commitment as to the relative importance of each factor to the physical condition of the patient. A serious effort to overcome this discrepancy was made by Strauch et al. (2), who developed a standardized list of somatic criteria for comparative assessment of regular dialysis therapy patients. However, the list is long and many units do not have all the data (e.g., nerve conduction or upper gastrointestinal X-rays). We could find no studies that used this standardized list to assess physical condition in patients with end-stage renal disease.

Some studies used the Karnofsky Index Categories to assess the overall physical functional ability (3). Results are contradictory: in Gutman's study only 60% of nondiabetic patients were capable of physical activity beyond self care (4). In Evan's study (5), which also included diabetic patients, the percentage was different: about 70% of in-center hemodialysis patients, just over 70% of continuous ambulatory peritoneal dialysis patients, 85% of home hemodialysis, and just under 90% of transplanted patients. These discrepancies suggest that either the earlier studied group was indeed very much sicker or that the Karnofsky Index is not easily applicable to end-stage renal disease patients.

There should be no doubt, however, that physical function is an important aspect of quality of life. Strong evidence was presented by the group at Washington University School of Medicine in St. Louis (6–8) that improvement of physical function is followed by improvement of psychological condition. It was shown that exercise training improved the physical as well as the psychological condition of dialysis patients, whereas supportive group psychotherapy did not prevent deterioration in patients' psychological condition.

VOCATIONAL REHABILITATION

Vocational rehabilitation of patients with end-stage renal disease received a lot of attention. At face value vocational rehabilitation should be a very simple and reliable outcome measure of quality of life. One should simply count the number of hours the patient works. It seems, however, that it is not such a simple objective measure. One should assess separately at least two aspects: (a) how much the patient can work, and (b) how much he actually does work. Earlier reports of the European Dialysis and Transplant Association clearly showed the big discrepancy between the physician's global (and vague?) assessment of how much the patient can work and how much he actually works. In these reports one of the definitions used was, "Able to work but not working; earning capacity less than social security benefits." In some countries less than 10% of dialysis patients were included in that classification, and in other countries nearly 40% of the patients were in this state. This seems to suggest that how much the patient works is not necessarily a good index for quality of life. The question, perhaps, should be only how much the patient can work. It should be remembered that the physicians are not necessarily very objective raters of their patients' vocational rehabilitation. We had the opportunity to study physicians' assessment of dialysis patients' adjustment and found that in some units the interraters' agreement was very low (9).

One can ask the patients in global terms, as Evans did (5), "Are you now able to work for pay full time, part time or not at all?" The authors regarded this measure as more objective than self-perceived emotional status. This study, however, highlights the complexity of the issue: the correlation between the answer to that question and the functional impairment (Karnofsky) was only 0.42. Furthermore, a very great discrepancy was found between physicians' assessment of no functional impairment and patients' assessment of their ability to work half time or more. As can be seen from Table 1, the patient's feeling of being able to work is not closely linked to his physical condition as assessed by his physician.

TABLE 1. *Patient's feeling and physician's assessment of ability to work*

	Percent of patients with almost normal physical activity (physician's assess.)	Percent of patients able to work half-time or more (patient's assess.)
In-center hemodialysis	44.7	37.2
Home hemodialysis	59.1	59.3
CAPD	47.5	24.7
Transplantation	79.1	74.1

CAPD, continuous ambulatory peritoneal dialysis.

Another way to obtain information about vocational rehabilitation is to use more detailed self-reports, for example the vocational environment section of the Psychosocial Adjustment to Physical Illness Scale (PAIS) (10). In a study carried out a few years ago we obtained seemingly meaningful results: a fairly high variability was found as well as a fairly good agreement between the patient's report and the physician's assessment of their vocational rehabilitation (11). This self-report, however, does not apply well to students, house wives, or to people who for one reason or another do not wish to work.

It seems, therefore, that the patient's actual vocational rehabilitation is not a good measure/index of quality of life. It is influenced not only by the patient's physical and psychological condition but also by external social factors. Often it is not worthwhile for the patient to work. On the other hand, ability to work is to some extent a measure of quality of life. It is, however, very dependent on the patient's physical and emotional condition, and is very difficult to assess. Keeping in mind all these problems, one may suggest that vocational rehabilitation should not be included in studies on quality of life.

SOCIAL FUNCTIONING

Social functioning of patients with end-stage renal disease has received scant attention. Basically two methods are used. More commonly the authors compose a list of social activities that seem to them important and ask the patients about them, or use the list as a self-report. Less common is the use of a questionnaire that has undergone some previous validation test, e.g., the social environment domain of the Psychosocial Adjustment to Physical Illness Scale that inquired into the patient's wish to participate in social activities as well as their actual participation.

Family relations can be regarded as one facet of social relations, possibly the most important one. Chowanec and Binik recently reviewed the literature on end-stage renal disease and the marital dyad (12) and found more than two dozen studies, mostly descriptive and performed on a small number of patients. Only four studies were found where "an interpersonal frame of investigation with standardized procedures had been used." We recently studied couples on hospital, home hemodialysis, and continuous ambulatory peritoneal dialysis (13). On the two adjustment measures (Psychosocial Adjustment to Physical Illness Scale and Brief Symptom Inventory), very strong correlations between patients and spouses were found, suggesting that chronic disease, in this case, end-stage renal disease, is a family affair. It seems that within the marital dyad there is an "infection" of adjustment/maladjustment without knowing, at present, which of the partners is the source and which is the reactor. That, however, does not say much about the patient's ability to interact.

One has to wonder why social functioning received so little attention while vocational rehabilitation so much. Does it reflect our bias that to work is more important than to have fun?

PSYCHOLOGICAL CONDITION

The psychological condition of patients with end-stage renal disease is, on the other hand, certainly the most studied, or rather the most reported, aspect. Binik recently summarized the literature on depression (which is the most common psychiatric problem of end-stage renal disease patients) (14). In this review more than 20 studies were included. The range of depression was from 50% of the patients to barely a few percents. Hardly any study controlled for confounding demographic or medical variables. Different methods were used, from unstandardized clinical evaluations to semistructured clinical interview to standardized psychiatric interview. Practically every imaginable test and self-report was used; e.g., Rorschach and Thematic Apperception Tests were used by few, whereas others preferred the Minnesota Multiphasic Personality Inventory. Other personality or trait measures included Locus of Control, Health Locus of Control, Rotter Sentence Completion Test, and the California Personality Inventory. To measure depression and anxiety very different instruments were used, including the Beck Depression Inventory, the General Health Questionnaire, the Multiple Affective Adjective Checklist, Zung Self Rating Depression Scale and Anxiety Scale, and many others. It is not surprising, therefore, that the information about the patient's psychological condition is often so contradictory.

The problem was highlighted in a recent study by Smith et al. (15) who studied 60 randomized end-stage renal disease patients. Twenty-eight of them (47%) were found to be depressed on the Beck Depression Inventory. Of these only six were also found to be depressed on the Multiple Affect Adjective Checklist. Out of the six that were found depressed on both tests, only three were found to be depressed by a structured psychiatric interview based on the Diagnostic and Statistical Manual (DSM) III.

MEASUREMENT OF QUALITY OF LIFE

One can certainly agree with Binik's statement in his paper on coping with chronic, life-threatening illness that, "Unfortunately, much of the available literature is characterized by multiple methodological flaws. These include over-reliance on non-objective and idiosyncratic measures, inadequate quantification and selection procedures, lack of specification of patient population or comparison groups, and failure to control for psychosocial influences attributable to relevant demographic, medical or response style variables" (16).

What can be done to change this state of affairs?

One should mention that "quality of life" is a fairly recent term. Only in 1977, "it was agreed that it would be desirable to identify the nature of the main determinants of the overall quality of life of Americans and use this as the frame of reference for selecting search targets for the future'' (17). As medicine made great progress in prolonging life—which is very striking in end-stage renal disease—the interest in quality of life of these patients increased. One could suspect also that the heavy cost of these treatments made the questions about quality of life even more central.

In Flanagan's recent paper on measurement of quality of life (18), suggestions for developing quality of life measures for persons with disability were made. Such a study, however, seems to be far away. Until we have such specific measures we have to compromise.

Churchill's global ''time trade-off'' is nearly a despair measure implying that we cannot measure, but it provides very meaningful information (19). The patient is presented with two hypothetical options: the first is to continue in the present health (including its emotional, physical, and social connotations for a lifetime, which are determined from actual data). The second choice is a shorter time (x) in a state of full health. The value x/t is the utility of the health state for the individual ranging from 0 for death to 1.00 for perfect health. Churchills' paper was published recently, but we could not find anyone who used it in end-stage renal disease patients.

Researchers studying quality of life differ in their interests. Some wish to study in depth one facet or another; others are interested in studying the factors that influence the quality of life or in assessing the efficacy of therapeutic interventions. The first issue, therefore, should be declaring what we want to measure, and the second issue should be determining how we measure it. This author suggests that the basic aspects we measure should follow the World Health Organization definition of health (i.e., assess the physical, mental, and social well-being).

Let us take each of these facets and see *how* we do measure. As to physical condition, it seems that we are still far from having a comprehensive measure that will take into account everything, including comorbidity. It might be better, therefore, to opt at present for a global measure like the Karnofsky Activity Scale. To safeguard, at least to some extent, against severe bias, two raters should be used. If the interrater's reliability is high, we have in this measure at least some representation of the patient's physical condition stated in terms which are very meaningful to the patient's quality of life. One can only hope that sooner and not later the nephrologists will develop adequate measures for the physical condition of end-stage renal disease patients.

As to the patient's mental, i.e., emotional condition, there is no doubt that depression and anxiety are the most common problems. We are looking, therefore, for methods to assess depression and anxiety. Semistructured or structured interviews have the drawback of requiring highly skilled manpower, so it is sometimes better to opt for a self-report. Because patients on renal replacement therapy are often extremely sick people, none of the self-reports that include many of the somatic items of depression and anxiety should be used. Three tests which are not too long and exhausting seem to fulfill this requirement. One is the Brief Symptom Inventory (20), which is the shorter version of the Symptom Check List-90 (SCL-90). This test has many advantages: most people like doing it; they feel that they are being asked about important issues. It provides a global measure of psychological distress but also measures by nine separate subscales, some of which are extremely important and often ignored (e.g., hostility). It has been well validated and there are American norms by sex as well as to some extent by age. We could find no validation studies in other languages nor norms from other cultures. We have been using it in end-stage renal disease patients (21,22) but have found no other studies of these patients using the Brief Symptom Inventory. Another possible measure is the Hospital Anxiety and Depression Scale (23). This test is even shorter, has been fairly well validated, and has been translated into many languages.

An even shorter test is the brief Profile of Mood States. It assesses depressive elements and was well validated (24). One could suggest, however, that it "invites" suppression and denial. The Brief Symptom Inventory is certainly much longer than the other two tests mentioned and therefore also more expensive in scoring. Yet the wealth and depth of information provided by the Brief Symptom Inventory should make it the preferred test. The only drawback is that it is and should be a self-report, therefore we would not recommend using it with patients who cannot read.

Testing social well-being is the greatest problem. In this area also lies the great temptation to develop one's own test. The temptation is caused mostly by the fact that every researcher understands social well-being somewhat differently, and is nurtured further by the lack of good, easy to administer tests for social well-being. However, the temptation should be resisted because it is better to use a well-validated test which is not optimal, than to use a private self-made test that taps exactly what one wishes to study but which has not been strictly validated. With this in mind, a compromise is the Psychosocial Adjustment to Physical Illness Scale (10). Among the strong points of this test are that it was devised specifically for patients with physical illness, it is divided into seven domains of life (e.g., domestic environment, social environment), and it inquires into how much the illness interferes in these domains. The test has been very well validated. It has its drawbacks, length being a major one, but all in all it is a satisfactory test for social well-being.

A suggested battery would take 5 minutes of the physician's time for the Karnofsky Activity Scale and up to 30 minutes of the patient's time for the Brief Symptom Inventory and Psychosocial Adjustment to Physical Illness Scale. It would provide the basic information about the patient's quality of life and should be regarded as a core battery. To that one could add other measures according to the specific question. We would like to suggest another measure to be included in all quality of life studies: a measure of social desirability. We found no study of this parameter in end-stage renal disease, nor have we ourselves ever used such a measure. Still one can suggest that it should be part of the routine, that we should have some idea about how much information is suppressed.

A core battery of one kind or another is desperately needed. Furthermore, it should be part of the routine assessment of patients in or about to start renal replacement therapy. Measurement of depression should become a routine-like measurement of blood urea nitrogen (BUN).

A few words should be added about problems in test administration. We have often found end-stage renal disease patients to be angry, hostile, and less than fully cooperative. This problem can be even bigger if patients have already been over-tested, and if they have the feeling that the routine renal replacement therapy they receive ignores their quality of life. It is often much easier to conduct a study if an inside person—a nurse or a social worker—helps with the administration of the tests. This also helps overcome units' resistance; some units regard a study of patients' adjustment as a threat and implied criticism to the unit.

CONCLUSION

One cannot stress enough the urgent need for a core battery to assess quality of life of end-stage renal disease patients. Among the hundreds of published papers one can hardly find a half dozen that studied by the same methods a certain quality of life aspect. This lack of agreement about methods of measuring is at least a partial explanation for the contradictory information. There is not any agreement about the quality of life of patients in renal replacement therapy. Some results are very hard to accept: e.g., in a very large-scale study, American home hemodialysis and transplanted patients were found to be happier than the general American public (5). One can only ask what is wrong with the test or alternatively, what is wrong with the American public? In another study it was found, on the Mental Health Index, that end-stage renal disease patients scored only slightly higher than dermatological patients or patients with arthritis.

The lack of consensus about patients' quality of life is not only an academic problem but also a highly practical one. If we do not know patients' adjustment, how can we study and elucidate the factors that influence adjustment, how can we improve adjustment, or how can we suggest to a patient which of the available renal replacement therapies is better for him? In the last 20 years tremendous progress has been made in the medical and surgical treatment of end-stage renal disease. The impression, however, is that patients' quality of life has not improved. Perhaps our ignorance has contributed to this.

REFERENCES

1. Cassileth BR, Lusk EJ, et al. Psychosocial status in chronic illness. *New Engl J Med* 1984;311:506–511.
2. Strauch MR, Lipke R, Schaffheulle R, Nachbauer B, Strauch R, Lauser G. A standardized list of somatic criteria for comparative assessment of regular dialysis therapy patients. *Int J Art Int Organs* 1978;2(Suppl.).
3. Karnofsky DA, Burchenal JH. The clinical evaluation of chemotherapeutic agents in cancer. In: Maclead CM, ed. *Evaluation of chemotherapeutic agents*. New York: Columbia University Press, 1949;191–205.
4. Gutman RA, Stead WW, Robinson RR. Physical activity and the employment status of patients on maintenance dialysis. *New Engl J Med* 1981;304:309–313.
5. Evans RW, Manninen DL, Garrison LP, et al. The quality of life of patients with end stage renal disease. *New Engl J Med* 1985;312:553–559.
6. Carney RM, McKeith PM, Goldberg AP, Hagberg J, Delznez JA, Huster HR. Psychological effects of exercise training in hemodialysis patients. *Nephron* 1983;33:179–181.
7. Carney RM, Templeton B, Hong BA, et al. Exercise training reduces depression and increases performance of pleasant activities in hemodialysis patients. *Nephron* 1987;47:194–198.
8. Goldberg AP, Geltman EM, Hagberg JM, et al. Therapeutic benefits of exercise training for hemodialysis patients. *Kidney Int* 1984;24:303–309.
9. Kaplan De-Nour A, Czaczkes JW. Bias assessment of patients on chronic dialysis. *J Psychosom Res* 1974;18:217–221.
10. Derogatis LR, Lopez MC. PAIS and PAIS-SR-administration, scoring and procedures manual. *Clin Psychometric Research*, Baltimore, MD, 1983.
11. Kaplan De-Nour A. Psychosocial adjustment to illness scale (PAIS): A study of chronic hemodialysis patients. *J Psychosom Res* 1982;26:11–22.
12. Chowanec GD, Binik YM. End stage renal disease and the marital dyad. *Soc Sci Med* 1981;16:1551–1558.
13. Soskolne V, Kaplan De-Nour A. Psychological adjustment of home hemodialysis, CAPD and hospital patients and their spouses. *Nephron* 1987;47:266–273.
14. Binik YM. Coping with chronic life threatening illness: Psychosocial perspectives on end stage renal disease. *Can J Behav Sci* 1983;15:374–391.

15. Smith MD, Hong BA, Robson AM. Diagnosis of depression in patients with end stage renal disease. *Am J Med* 1985;79:160–166.
16. Binik YM, Devins GM, Orme CM. Psychological stress and coping in end stage renal disease. In: Neufeld RWJ, ed. *Advances in investigation of psychological stress*. New York: Wiley (*in press*).
17. Flanagan JC. The American Institute for Research. The first thirty years. Palo Alto, CA: American Institute for Research, 1976.
18. Flanagan JC. Measurement of quality of life. Current state of the art. *Arch Physiol Med Rehabil* 1987;63:56–59.
19. Churchill DN, Morgan J, Torrance GW. Quality of life in end stage renal disease. *Periton Dial Bull* 1984;20–23.
20. Derogatis LR, Melisaratos N. The brief symptom inventory: An introductory report. *Psychol Med* 1983;13:595–605.
21. Sayag R. Psychosocial adjustment of transplanted and dialysis patients. M.A. Thesis, Tel Aviv University, 1988.
22. Soskolne V, Kaplan De-Nour A. Psychological adjustment of home hemodialysis, continuous ambulatory peritoneal dialysis and hospital dialysis patients and their spouses. *Nephron* 1987;47:266–273.
23. Zigmond AS, Smaith RP. The hospital anxiety and depression. *Acta Psychiatr Scand* 1980;67:361–370.
24. Cella DF, Jacobsen PB, Orav EJ, Holland JC, Silberfarb PM, Rafla S. A brief POMS measure of distress for cancer patients. *J Chron Dis* 1987;40:939–942.

Quality of Life Assessments in Clinical Trials, edited by B. Spilker. Raven Press, Ltd. New York © 1990.

30

Chronic Obstructive Pulmonary Disease

*A. John McSweeny and †Karen T. Labuhn

*Medical College of Ohio, Toledo, Ohio 43699;
†Kaiser-Permanente Center for Health Research,
Portland, Oregon 97215

A BRIEF REVIEW

Chronic obstructive pulmonary disease (COPD) is a debilitating disease of adult life. Although there is some disagreement among pulmonologists as to the precise definition of chronic obstructive pulmonary disease, the term has enjoyed common use in the medical literature for approximately 25 years and almost all pulmonologists would agree that the cardinal feature of the disease is expiratory airflow obstruction (1). The primary clinical signs of chronic obstructive pulmonary disease include chronic cough, chronic expectoration, shortness of breath during physical exertion, and reduction in expiratory airflow as measured by spirometry. In addition, inflammatory damage to lung airways and alveoli are observed during autopsy (2). The major subtypes of chronic obstructive pulmonary disease, chronic bronchitis and emphysema, although representing somewhat distinct syndromes, often exist concomitantly, and both conditions result in subnormal amounts of gas exchange in the lungs and decreased arterial oxygen tension, a condition termed "hypoxemia." Chronic bronchitis is usually associated with airway narrowing and increased resistance to airflow, whereas emphysema is associated with loss of elastic recoil of lung tissue and subsequent loss of air pressure during exhalation.

Chronic obstructive pulmonary disease is relatively common; the prevalence rate for the United States in 1980 was 4.75%. The disease accounts for approximately 2.5% of all deaths in the U.S. and is the fifth leading cause of death (3). The etiology of chronic obstructive pulmonary disease is closely linked to smoking. Indeed, Petty (4) has suggested that the disease would be a fairly minor health problem if people did not smoke. Infection and occupational or environmental air pollution may also be contributing factors in some cases. In addition, males are at higher risk for developing the disease than females (although women are beginning to catch up with men), older persons are at more risk than younger ones, and one or more genetic factors appear to modify susceptibility (3).

The physical effects of chronic obstructive pulmonary disease and hypoxemia are well known and include decreased cardiac efficiency, decreased ability to engage in sustained physical activity, adverse changes in blood chemistry, and chronic shortness of breath (5). More recent studies indicate that chronic obstructive pulmonary disease is associated with cerebral dysfunction as well (6,7). The disease is not reversible and cannot be "cured." However, it can be managed using a combination of approaches. Bronchodilator medications are used to help keep airways open and antibiotics are used to treat or prevent infection. Pulmonary rehabilitation programs, which include patient and family education, breathing training, and systematic exercise help the patient learn how to cope with the effects of the disease as well as how to maximize function (8,9). Finally, supplemental oxygen use can be helpful in returning arterial oxygen levels and blood chemistry closer to normal (9,10).

The preceding is only a cursory overview of the pathophysiology, etiology, epidemiology, and treatment of chronic obstructive pulmonary disease. Interested readers are strongly encouraged to consult other sources. A good introduction may be found in work by Cugell (1), and a more comprehensive treatment is available from Petty (11).

ISSUES IN QUALITY OF LIFE RESEARCH

Definitions

The term "quality of life" has enjoyed colloquial use in the fields of medicine and health for a long time, although its use as a scientific concept is relatively recent. A major conceptual impetus to the scientific application of psychosocial concepts in medicine was provided by the publication of George Engel's (12) paper on the biopsychosocial model of medicine. Using a systems theory framework, Engel argued that the inclusion of psychosocial information in the formulation of medical concepts, research, and patient care serves to make medicine a more "scientific" enterprise when compared with more narrow biomedical models or with nonscientific "holistic" models. Engel's viewpoint has been widely embraced by medical schools, and a new generation of physicians and medical investigators is being trained within the biopsychosocial model.

One result of the intensified interest in psychosocial issues in medicine is the development of the quality of life concept. As might be expected with any relatively new concept, several definitions have been offered. A review of alternative definitions of life quality reveals some commonalities but some variations as well, particularly in terms of comprehensiveness, specificity, and theoretical relevance. Levine and Croog (13), for example, note that many medical researchers have utilized a single variable of human functioning, such as employment, general happiness, or sexual functioning, as an ad hoc indicator of life quality. In contrast, Wenger et al. (14) have provided a detailed definition of life quality that incorporates three basic dimensions (functional capacity, perceptions, and symptoms) and nine subdimensions (daily routine, social functioning, intellectual functioning, emotional functioning, economic status, health status, well-being, life satisfaction, and symptoms related to the disease under study, as well as other diseases). Wenger et al. also provide a fairly detailed set of rationales for the inclusion of each quality of life criterion.

Most definitions fall somewhere between the extremes as just described, and demonstrate some commonality of content. The definition provided by McSweeny et al. (15) is fairly typical. McSweeny et al. composed their definition after a review of the limited literature on the psychosocial aspects of chronic obstructive pulmonary disease, but without the detailed consideration of the definition issues as exemplified by Wenger et al. Four dimensions of life quality are included in McSweeny et al.'s definition: (a) emotional functioning, including mood changes and other psychiatric symptoms; (b) social role functioning, including employment, home management, and social/family relationships; (c) activities of daily living, such as self-care skills and mobility; and (d) the ability to engage in enjoyable activities, such as hobbies and recreation.

Another issue in quality of life research is the perspective from which it is defined. Pearlman and Jonsen (16) note that life quality can be viewed from the vantage point of the patient, of an "onlooker of another's life situation" (i.e., a relative or physician), or of society in general. Many times the perspective issue is reduced to a debate concerning the relative value of "subjective" versus "objective" viewpoints on quality of life, with the usual conclusion that both viewpoints should be considered, although the latter viewpoint is more amenable to scientific study.

McCullough (17) concludes that the perspective issue is quite complex and reflects a more general value issue. He notes that the use of objective measures by clinicians and researchers stems from a "beneficence model" of health care, which assumes that health professionals know "what promotes or protects the best interests of patients." This is a "remarkable claim" according to McCullough. The beneficence model is contrasted with the "autonomy model," which depends on the patients to provide knowledge about what is in their best interests. McCullough concludes that the beneficence and autonomy models have the same final goal: "seeking the greater balance of good over harm for the patient." However, the two models differ in terms of who should decide how to define good or harm, how the goal should be reached (i.e., what treatments should be used), and how the outcome should be measured.

McCullough's work on alternative models of health care and quality of life should sensitize those of us who work with patients to the concept that the patient's viewpoint of what constitutes a good quality of life is at least as valid as what a researcher or clinician might suggest. Pearlman and Jonsen's (16) discussion points out that the patient's "significant others," and even society in general, may hold additional viewpoints on an appropriate definition of quality of life. From a practical standpoint, researchers and clinicians should try to incorporate these different perspectives into their definitions of life quality. This is particularly important when the quality of life definition has potential impact on the treatment of patients.

The preceding discussion points to some of the complexities in the definition of quality of life. The reader is advised to consult Levine and Croog (13) or Wenger et al. (14,18) for more detailed discussions of these issues.

Measurement of Quality of Life

McSweeny et al. (15) reported that the validity and range of measurement devices represented serious methodological problems in the research conducted before 1980 on quality of life and chronic obstructive pulmonary disease. The authors noted a common failure to specify the assessment procedures other than in vague terms such as "psychiatric interview" or "nursing interview." One must suspect that here the interview procedures were as vague as the descriptions. Although an unstructured clinical interview might provide rich clinical information about a single patient, it does not have the requisite psychometric characteristics, e.g., validity and reliability, to permit sound research.

Those studies that did use formal psychometric procedures often used only one or two instruments to assess emotional status, one of which usually was the Minnesota Multiphasic Personality Inventory (19). This inventory has a long history of use in medical research and is the instrument that many medical researchers turn to first when investigating the psychosocial aspects of a medical problem. Unfortunately, this "old favorite" of medical psychologists is inadequate as a single instrument of quality of life. The Minnesota Multiphasic Personality Inventory is concerned primarily with symptoms of personality and emotional disturbance, which makes it useful for psychiatric diagnosis but less useful as a measure of general life quality. Other aspects of quality of life, including social adjustment, activities of daily living, and recreation activities, are not addressed by the inventory or by the studies that used it as a single psychosocial measure. In addition, the original clinical scales of the Minnesota Multiphasic Personality Inventory are heterogeneous in their content, and several, particularly depression (scale 2), include a variety of physical symptoms. Thus, the meaning of a high score on any scale is not always clear without additional analysis (20). This is especially relevant when one considers the frequent finding of depression in chronic obstructive pulmonary disease from the inventory-based studies.

The history of life quality measurement follows the history of the development of the concept of quality of life quite closely. Much of the important work in this area has been accomplished in the last 10 years. Most authors now recommend that several aspects of life quality should be assessed in any study of the concept given its multidimensional nature. In addition, assessment from the multiple perspectives, i.e., those of the patient, the care givers, and the relatives, are suggested. Single perspective, unidimensional, single-instrument evaluations of quality of life are now recognized as inadequate and are becoming rarer.

Psychometricians interested in medical research recently have developed several instruments designed specifically to measure quality of life or similar concepts. This has made it easier for life quality researchers to conduct investigations in the area. These instruments vary in their content, comprehensiveness, and established psychometric characteristics, but several, such as the Sickness Impact Profile (21) and the McMaster Health Index Questionnaire (22), show considerable promise. Six of these instruments are reviewed in Wenger et al. (14), and the basic characteristics of those instruments are illustrated in Table 1. Other reviews are available in Bergner and Rothman (23), Kaplan (24), and Walker and Rosser (25).

The study of quality of life in chronic obstructive pulmonary disease by McSweeny et al. (15) illustrates a typical life quality assessment battery as used in current research. As noted before, these investigators assessed four dimensions of quality of life: (a) emotional functioning, (b) social role functioning, (c) activities of daily living, and (4) recreation. These four dimensions were assessed with data from self-reports and reports from the patient's spouse or a close relative of the patient. The three self-report measures included the Minnesota Multiphasic Personality Inventory, the Profile of Mood States (26), and the Sickness Impact Profile. The Minnesota Multiphasic Personality Inventory served as a measure of psychiatric disturbance, whereas the Profile of Mood States indicated general mood. The Sickness Impact Profile, which contains 12 sections, served as a "broad-band" measure of quality of life. The Katz Adjustment Scale–Form R Relative's version (KAS-R; 27) was used to assess functioning from the perspective of someone who interacted with the patient on a regular basis. These instruments and their use in chronic obstructive pulmonary disease studies are described in more detail elsewhere (15,28).

TABLE 1. *Examples of current assessment methodology*

Instrument	Dimensions examined	Length	Administration
Sickness Impact Profile (SIP)	Physical: ambulation, mobility, body care Psychosocial: social interaction, communication, alertness, emotional behavior Other: sleep/rest, eating, work, home management, recreational pastimes	136 items	Self or interviewer (30 min)
McMaster Health Index Questionnaire (MHIQ)	Physical: mobility, self-care, communication, and global physical functioning Social: general well-being, work/social role performance, social support and participation, and global social function Emotional: self-esteem, findings about personal relationships and the future, critical life events, and global emotional functioning	59 items	Self-administered (20 min)
Nottingham Health Profile (NHP)	Six domains of experience: pain, physical mobility, sleep, emotional reactions, energy, social isolation Seven domains of daily life: employment, household work, relationships, personal life, sex, hobbies, vacations	45 items	Self-administered (10 min)
Psychological General Well-Being Index (PGWB)	Six dimensions: freedom from bodily distress, life satisfaction, sense of vitality, cheerful vs. distressed, relaxed vs. anxious, self control	22 items	Self or interviewer (12 min)
General Health Rating Index (GHR)	Six dimensions: past, present, and future perceptions of health; health-related worry and concern; resistance vs. susceptibility to illness; tendency to view illness as part of life	50 items[a]	Trained interviewer (12 min)
Quality of Well-Being Scale (QWB)	Measures actual performance and preference: self-care, mobility, institutionalization, social activities, reports of symptoms and problems (including mental)	50 items[a]	Trained interviewer (12 min)

[a] Although there are 50 major questions in the QWB, the incorporation of multiple items for multiple days results in total coverage extending to several hundred possible responses.
From Wenger et al., ref. 14, with permission.

Guyatt et al. (29,30) have designed a self-report questionnaire to assess specific aspects of life quality among chronic obstructive pulmonary disease patients. The four dimensions measured include dyspnea, fatigue, emotional functioning, and feeling of control over the disease (mastery). The content of this questionnaire is based on interviews with 100 chronic obstructive pulmonary disease patients about how their lives are adversely affected by their disease, and their spouses' reports. The investigators report adequate stability reliability for the instrument (coefficient of variation less than 12% on test re-test) and good sensitivity to changes produced by drug treatment and respiratory rehabilitation. Since this instrument includes physical symptoms related to the chronic obstructive pulmonary disease process, it may be particularly useful for periodic clinical evaluations of patients' adjustment. Used alone, it would not be comprehensive enough for assessments of quality of life in most research investigations.

The availability of "ready-made" measures of life quality does not relieve investigators of the necessity of considering what instruments are most appropriate for their research purposes. Often it will be advantageous to supplement one of the ready-made quality of life tools with other measures. Investigators and clinicians who wish to assess life quality may wish to consult McSweeny (28) or Ware (31) for specific criteria to guide their choice of instruments.

Methodological Issues in Quality of Life Research

McSweeny et al. (15) noted several methodological problems with previous quality of life research, in addition to problems with measurement. First, many of the studies were restricted by sample size and representativeness. All of the studies that we reviewed had sample sizes of less than 50; most other studies investigated even smaller samples. This fact limits the statistical conclusion validity and external validity (32) of the studies. In less technical terms, conclusions drawn from these studies may not be considered reliable and cannot be generalized to other patients and settings.

A second methodological issue that was noted by McSweeny et al. in all but one of the reports they reviewed was the lack of a comparison group matched in terms of age, sex, social position, and other factors which must be assessed separately from the effects of the disease to insure internal validity (32). Related to this is the fact that patients with various chronic diseases have very similar psychosocial profiles. Casselith et al. (33), for example, studied 758 patients from six different diagnostic groups (arthritis, diabetes, cancer, renal disease, dermatological disorders, and depression) using the Mental Health Index, a multiscale instrument concerned with different aspects of psychological distress and well-being (34). Casselith et al. found no significant differences among the five groups of patients with a diagnosis of a chronic physical disease, but some significant differences did appear with the depressed group. Their findings raised the question of uniqueness in the psychosocial consequences of chronic obstructive pulmonary disease, at least when compared with other chronic diseases. Although more recent studies of quality of life and chronic obstructive pulmonary disease (15,35–37) have employed control groups matched for the sociodemographic variables mentioned previously, they have not included a control group of patients with other chronic diseases. Thus, the uniqueness of the psychosocial aspects of chronic obstructive pulmonary disease remains an open question.

A final problem noted by McSweeny et al. (15) concerned data analysis. Most of the studies in their review contained no formal data analysis or only simple statistics, once again limiting the statistical conclusion validity of the studies. Fortunately, more recent studies have included appropriate methods of statistical data analysis.

REVIEW OF CURRENT FINDINGS

Emotional Disturbances Associated with Chronic Obstructive Pulmonary Disease

Depression

By far the most commonly reported emotional consequence associated with chronic obstructive pulmonary disease is depression. Depressive symptoms, including pessimism, self-dislike, and feelings of sadness have been reported in virtually every study of the psychological aspects of chronic obstructive pulmonary disease as well as in reviews of the literature (38–41). To some extent, this consistency across studies may reflect the fact that many used the Minnesota Multiphasic Personality Inventory as the measure of depression and, as noted earlier, the inventory depression scale contains several items concerned with somatic symptoms. However, depression has been noted as the predominant emotional difficulty in studies that have used instruments other than the Minnesota Multiphasic Personality Inventory, including those that have utilized the perspective of a relative (15,35). Agle and Baum (42) reported "significant" depression in 74% of their patients, whereas McSweeny et al. reported that 42% of their patients were primarily depressed and an additional 7% had symptoms of depression combined with other psychiatric symptoms. The differences between the two studies might reflect differences in patient samples and measurement methods, but the basic finding that chronic obstructive pulmonary disease patients are at high risk for depression is consistent.

Opinions vary as to the causes of depression in chronic obstructive pulmonary disease. Most writers have focused on the psychosocial consequences of the disease such as the loss of pleasurable activities, economic hardship, and difficulties in coping (38,43,44). Others have suggested that physiological factors, including hypoxemia of the limbic system and related brain mechanisms, might also be relevant factors (15). Labuhn (45) tested the relative importance of a variety of psychosocial, medical, and physiological factors in the development of depression in a group of 303 chronic obstructive pulmonary disease patients, using multivariate casual-modeling methods known as path analysis. The results of this study suggest that although physiological factors did play an important role in the development of depression, the depression that chronic obstructive pulmonary disease patients experience is largely a reaction to their situation. This study is described in more detail later.

Other Emotional Disturbances

A variety of other emotional disturbances have been reported in addition to depression. These include anxiety, irritability, hysterical disorders, somatic preoccupation, dependency, and aggressive behavior (15,35,38,39,41,42,46,47). The findings of anxiety and somatic preoccupation appear to be fairly reliable across studies. To some extent, this is because many studies have used the Minnesota Multiphasic Personality Inventory. However, it is not difficult to imagine that anxiety and concern about one's bodily condition would be a common occurrence in chronic obstructive pulmonary disease. Angle and Baum (42), for example, reported disabling anxiety in

96% of their patients, and McSweeny et al. (15) reported somatic preoccupation in 8.7% of their patients, in contrast to 0% in the demographically matched control group.

The findings of hysterical disorders, suspiciousness, and aggressive behavior have been less reliable. Although some of the earlier studies reported hysterical tendencies (46), later studies have not consistently confirmed these results. McSweeny et al. (15) found that 2.7% of their chronic obstructive pulmonary disease patients exhibited primarily hysterical symptoms compared with 1.5% of the older healthy individuals. In addition, the Minnesota Multiphasic Personality Inventory hysteria scale, which is often used as the criterion of hysterical complaints, contains a high number of somatic symptoms. McSweeny et al. also failed to find unusual degrees of suspiciousness or anger, although relatives of the patients did report a moderately high degree of oppositional behavior. The lack of overt hostility is consistent with the clinical picture of the "emotional straightjacket" described by Dudley et al. (48). On the basis of Dudley's (49) classic studies of the psychophysiology of breathing, Dudley et al. (48) suggested that the chronic obstructive pulmonary disease patient learns to avoid the expression of strong emotions, including anger, to prevent the excessive oxygen uptake that occurs in conjunction with physiological arousal. This relationship between dyspnea and emotional status was also observed in a study by Burns and Howell (46), who found that "disproportionately breathless" chronic obstructive pulmonary disease patients had higher rates of emotional distress than the remaining chronic obstructive pulmonary disease patients. In addition, the dyspnea improved with the resolution of emotional disturbance.

Social Role Functioning and Activities of Daily Living

General Discussion

The performance of basic social roles and activities of daily living is often used as a standard for the impact of a disease entity. However, this area is less well represented in the chronic obstructive pulmonary disease literature than is emotional functioning, primarily because of the lack, until recently, of appropriate methods of assessment.

Barstow (43) reported that "major changes" were evident in the "style of living" manifested by the chronic obstructive pulmonary disease patients in her study. These included alterations in bathing, grooming, dressing, eating, sleeping, and mobility. She noticed, for example, that "the mode of dress was altered in favor of less restrictive clothing that was easily slipped on and off." Food intake was decreased by many of the patients because an overdistended stomach interferes with diaphragmatic breathing. Sleep/rest difficulties received particular attention in Barstow's report. Disruptions of sleep because of cough, dyspnea, or restlessness were common. In addition, Barstow reported some sleep changes that were apparently related to endogenous depression.

McSweeny et al. (15) also reported a broad range of disturbances in sleep and rest and activities of daily living. The Sickness Impact Profile was used to present the patient's self-evaluation. In all categories of the Sickness Impact Profile except one, chronic obstructive pulmonary disease patients reported a much higher percentage of impairment than did control subjects. The only category not affected differentially

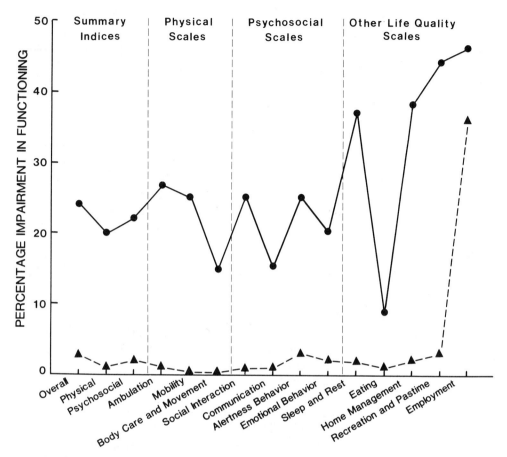

FIG. 1. Mean Sickness Impact Profiles for patients with chronic obstructive pulmonary disease and control subjects. Patients are significantly ($p < 0.001$) more impaired on all scales except employment using paired t-tests ($N = 66$). NOTT, nocturnal oxygen therapy trial. From McSweeny, ref. 15, with permission.

was employment, presumably because the chronic obstructive pulmonary disease and control groups both contained many elderly retired persons. The areas of functioning found most severely affected were home management and sleep/rest. Eating and communication, on the other hand, seemed to be only moderately affected by the disease (Fig. 1). The results from the Katz Adjustment Scale–Form R which represented the relative's viewpoint, indicated that relatives regarded the patient's social role functioning as deficient; they expected less of the patients but still felt dissatisfied with the patients' performance of socially expected activities.

Prigatano et al. (35) also utilized the Sickness Impact Profile and Katz Adjustment Scale–Form R with chronic obstructive pulmonary disease patients who had mild hypoxemia. Their findings were similar to those obtained by McSweeny et al. with severely hypoxemic patients, although, as might be expected, the degree of impairment was proportionately less. One interesting exception was that Prigatano et al. did find significant differences in employment status between chronic obstructive pulmonary disease patients and controls. This appears to be because the control subjects in Prigatano et al.'s study were much more likely to be employed than those in that of McSweeny et al. (15). This, in turn, is the result of a greater proportion of persons younger than 65 among the patients and controls in the Prigatano et al. study. In summary, employment status is more likely to be a significant issue for younger patients than for older patients and may be affected even in those who have small reductions in PaO_2.

Another noteworthy study is Hanson's (50) questionnaire survey of approximately 130 chronic obstructive pulmonary disease patients. Her survey included 40 questions about 11 areas, including several aspects of social role functioning and activities of daily living such as employment, self-care, home/personal business, marriage, care of grandchildren, and dependency on others. Hanson's results were consistent with those of McSweeny et al. (15) and Prigatano et al. (35) in that she found a general negative effect of chronic obstructive pulmonary disease across the different categories in her survey. One interesting aspect of her study is that her questionnaire was bipolar, i.e., it allowed respondents to indicate a positive impact of chronic obstructive pulmonary disease on different life areas as well as a negative impact. In fact, a few individuals did indicate a positive effect, ranging from 28% for care of grandchildren to 40% for marriage. One might be tempted to conclude that there is some benefit to adversity, but the meaning of her results are unclear given the lack of a comparison sample.

Sexton and Munro (37) recently reported findings from a study of quality of life among female chronic obstructive pulmonary disease patients. In this study, 72 women with diagnosed chronic obstructive pulmonary disease and 40 demographically similar women who had no chronic illness were compared on their perceived health status, problems of daily living, amount of subjective stress, and life satisfaction. The questionnaire used for this study included demographic and illness-related questions as well as adapted versions of the Subjective Stress Scale (51) and the Life Satisfaction Index (52) which Sexton and Munro (36) had tested in an earlier study of chronic obstructive pulmonary disease spouses' quality of life. In comparison with their healthy controls, the female patients were found to have lower perceived health status, more subjective stress, and less life satisfaction. They also reported more problems in daily living. Major problems included shortness of breath and fatigue, loneliness and depression, and restricted household and social activities.

Sexual Functioning

One topic not assessed in detail in the McSweeny et al. (15) and Prigatano et al. (35) studies was sexual functioning. Other investigators, however, have paid more attention to this important aspect of quality of life. In one of the earlier studies on the topic, Kass et al. (53) reported that 19% of their male chronic obstructive pulmonary disease patients were impotent. More recent studies have suggested even higher rates of sexual dysfunction among men. Fletcher and Martin (54), for example, reported that 30% of their chronic obstructive pulmonary disease patients were impotent and that an additional 5% had ceased intercourse because of dyspnea. Frequency of intercourse for the remaining 65% of their patients fell to 16% of predisease levels.

Sexton and Munro's (36) study of the impact of chronic obstructive pulmonary disease on the spouse's life also provides evidence of sexual dysfunction associated with the disease. These investigators compared the subjective experiences of 45 wives of male patients with those of 30 age-matched women whose husbands had no chronic illness. The patients' wives reported significantly fewer marital relations than did the comparison wives. Fifty-four percent of the chronic obstructive pulmonary disease wives no longer engaged in sexual relations. Forth-eight percent of these wives, versus 15% of the controls, stated that they had no desire for sexual relations. The wives of the patients also gave significantly lower ratings on their own health status, and this may account for their lack of sexual interest. Health differences between these two groups of age-matched wives could also be due to stressors related to living with a chronic obstructive pulmonary disease patient, however. The patients' wives reported many difficulties with sleeping due to their husbands' breathing problems. They also had taken on many extra responsibilities and had given up many of their own social activities because of their husbands' illnesses.

Only limited data exist concerning sexual functioning in female chronic obstructive pulmonary disease patients, although it is probably safe to assume that the factors that affect sexual functioning in men affect sexual functioning in women as well. One self-report study concerning sexual fuctioning in a mixed sex (62% men, 38% women) sample was conducted by Hanson (50). She found that among the 11 life areas assessed in her study, sexual functioning was the area most consistently rated as being negatively affected by chronic obstructive pulmonary disease. Thus, Hanson's results are consistent with the more objective findings from Fletcher and Martin (54) and Kass et al. (53), and also suggest that chronic obstructive pulmonary disease presents problems for sexual functioning for women as well as for men. Unfortunately, Hanson did not report results separately for men and women, and we are still left in some doubt. Clearly, the sexuality of female chronic obstructive pulmonary disease patients is a neglected area and in need of further research.

One controversy in the area of sexuality and chronic obstructive pulmonary disease concerns whether the problems that are observed are largely secondary to a past history of marital and sexual difficulties or to the relatively immediate physical effects of the disease. Kass et al. (53) reported on a sample of 90 men and 10 women and concluded that the sexual problems associated with chronic obstructive pulmonary disease patients were *not* primarily due to the effects of the disease. Rather, such problems were the results of life-long behavior patterns. The presence of a wife who was angered by the level of support required by her husband was also mentioned as a common problem in the maintenance of good sexual functioning. The authors provided five case histories (all were of men) to illustrate their conclusions.

In contrast to Kass et al.'s report are the more recent findings of Fletcher and Martin (54). Fletcher and Martin carefully assessed erectile dysfunction in relation to cardiopulmonary, hormonal, and neurovascular dysfunction. They concluded:

> Data from this study suggest that sexual dysfunction and erectile impotence can accompany COPD in the absence of other known causes of sexual problems. Furthermore, sexual dysfunction tended to be worse in those subjects with more severe pulmonary function impairment as assessed by pulmonary function tests, blood gases, and exercise tests (p. 420).

Fletcher and Martin did note that several of their subjects who were impotent by nocturnal penile tumescence had high T-scores on some Minnesota Multiphasic Personality Inventory scales, but only one of their 20 subjects clearly had psychogenic impotence. In the remainder, chronic obstructive pulmonary disease was responsible for both sexual dysfunction and emotional disturbance independently, or at least some of the psychological distress was secondary to sexual failure brought on by the chronic obstructive pulmonary disease.

In summary, chronic obstructive pulmonary disease has a documented negative effect on sexual functioning in men and probably in women as well. Although psychosocial factors play an important role in sexual functioning, the sexual dysfunctioning associated with chronic obstructive pulmonary disease is closely linked with cardiopulmonary dysfunction and hypoxemia.

Hobbies and Recreational Activities

As was true for social role functioning and activities of daily living, only limited data exist concerning hobbies and recreational activities. McSweeny et al. (15) noted that their patients with chronic obstructive pulmonary disease reported severe restrictions in recreation and other leisure time activities. The Sickness Impact Profile results suggested a reduction of 40% to 50% in pleasurable activities, which is certainly an important aspect of life quality. Indeed, the recreation and pastimes category showed the greatest level of impairment relative to the other categories on the Sickness Impact Profile when compared with the control group. The results from the Katz Adjustment Scale–Form R indicated that relatives also recognized decrements in the free-time activities of the patients.

The study by Prigatano et al. (35) produced results similar to those of McSweeny et al., with the exception that the effects were less severe. A reduction of 30% to 40% in pleasurable activities was seen in the mildly hypoxemic patients on the Sickness Impact Profile. This was, again, the most impaired category on this test. In addition, the Katz Adjustment Scale–Form R results indicated that the relatives were aware of the problem.

That there is a significant loss of pleasurable activities in chronic obstructive pulmonary disease is relevant to theories of depression which suggest that the loss of reinforcers is a major contributing factor in the development of depression (55). Therefore, it is possible that helping chronic obstructive pulmonary disease patients to maintain old hobbies and develop new ones might ameliorate the negative impact of the disease on emotional status.

QUALITY OF LIFE AND ITS RELATIONSHIP TO OTHER FACTORS

Introduction

McSweeny et al. (15) noted that there was considerable variability in the life quality of patients with chronic obstructive pulmonary disease. This raises the question of what factors might improve or worsen emotional functioning and other aspects of life quality in these patients. Suggested psychosocial, behavioral, neuropsychologic, and physiologic factors, as well as the practical implications of this area of research, will be discussed.

Psychosocial and Behavioral Factors

Various psychosocial factors, both in the chronic obstructive pulmonary disease patient's immediate family and in the community and health care system, influence the patient's quality of life, as do behavioral factors such as smoking and self-care practices. Some of these factors that have been highlighted in the chronic obstructive pulmonary disease literature are discussed below.

Psychosocial Assets and Social Support Resources

A number of investigators have studied chronic obstructive pulmonary disease patients' psychosocial assets and social support resources in relating to quality of life. Sandhu (41) defines psychosocial assets as "those individual characteristics and social supports that allow coping with or modifying one's environment." After reviewing the chronic illness literature, he concluded that psychosocial assets seem to "play a major, perhaps central, role in the patient's ability to cope adaptively." Sandhu noted that high assets correlate with positive outcome in medical treatment, whereas low assets typically are associated with a variety of poor outcomes, including increased morbidity and mortality.

Investigations among asthma and chronic obstructive pulmonary disease patients indicate that patients who have stronger psychosocial assets require less medication and adapt to life changes more readily (56), respond more positively to group therapy (57), and have less dyspnea, better regimen compliance, and longer survival time (38). It is important to recognize that the concept of psychosocial assets includes psychological characteristics of the patient, such as emotional stability and coping style, as well as the amount of support the person receives from external sources. Thus, although chronic obstructive pulmonary disease patients' psychosocial assets do predict outcomes that are relevant to quality of life, it is unclear how much of the impact is related to the patients' internal psychological resources and how much is related to external social supports.

Recently, investigators have used more precise measures of external support. They also have attempted to study social support in relation to other factors which influence quality of life. Jensen (58) studied the impact of social support and various risk factors in chronic obstructive pulmonary disease patients' symptom management. He found that social support and life stress predicted the number of hospitalizations better than did the patient's demographic characteristics, the severity of the illness, or previous hospitalizations. Labuhn (45) found that married chronic obstructive pulmonary disease patients had better exercise tolerance than did single, widowed, or divorced patients, even controlling for age, disease severity, and neuropsychological functioning. Marriage did not have a significant influence on patients' depressed mood states, but it indirectly contributed to patients' physical and psychosocial functioning through its impact on their exercise capacity.

Two additional studies provide evidence concerning personal social supports and chronic obstructive pulmonary disease patients' quality of life. Barstow (43) conducted home interviews with patients to assess their problems and coping strategies. The patients in this study identified the presence of a supportive spouse as the most important factor for successful coping. Sexton and Munro (37) had similar findings in their study of female chronic obstructive pulmonary disease patients. Ninety-five percent of the married patients identified their husbands as important sources of support. The husbands provided instrumental support by helping out with various household activities, treatments, and other things needed. About half of the chronic obstructive pulmonary disease women talked their problems over with their husbands. They also turned to friends, relatives, and children for emotional support.

In addition to personal supports, structural supports such as economic security and community resources contribute to the life quality of chronic obstructive pulmonary disease patients and their families. Economic security had been found to be related to life satisfaction in several studies. In a study of 163 chronic obstructive pulmonary disease patients and their spouses, Young (59) found that patients' monetary savings and health insurance, as well as their personal resources (positive illness perceptions, knowledge of the illness, regimen compliance, and religion) predicted better adaptation. The female chronic obstructive pulmonary disease patients in Sexton and Munro's (37) study identified financial concerns as one of their major problems. Similarly, the wives in Sexton and Munro's (37) earlier study had greater life satisfaction if they were satisfied with the amount of money that was available.

The availability of community resources was not directly related to Young's (59) patients' self-adaptation, but it did have a significant impact on the adaptation of the patients' spouses. Only 20% of Young's chronic obstructive pulmonary disease patients reported that they received assistance from persons other than their spouses, children, and parents, and this may account for the greater importance of community support for the spouses. About two-thirds of the spouses in Sexton and Munro's (36) study said that they relied on their sons and daughters for help. Forty-six percent of these wives identified the physician as an important source of support. Thirty-seven percent also relied on friends and 34% relied on neighbors.

Findings from the above studies have suggested that most chronic obstructive pulmonary disease patients rely heavily on their immediate families for support, whereas family members may rely on each other as well as professional and community resources. It is important to consider the implications of these findings for patients who live alone as well as the quality of life of patients' families. Additional investigations are needed to examine chronic obstructive pulmonary disease family's social support needs in more detail, and to evaluate the effectiveness of interventions directed toward mobilizing supports.

Family Functioning

Chronic obstructive pulmonary disease, like most chronic illnesses, has a negative impact on the family's functioning and quality of life as well as the identified patients' quality of life. In the above section, we discussed some of the problems that spouses of patients experience. The manner in which family members interact with each other in attempting to deal with the illness influences the patient's adjustment of life quality. The family's response also can influence the course of the illness as well as the happiness of the family unit itself (60).

Bruhn (61) points out that chronic illness is more likely to be disintegrative than integrative for families. As duties and responsibilities are taken away from the ill person and are assumed by another, the ill person experiences a sense of loss, while the other family member is overburdened. Sexton and Munro's studies (36,37) indicate that this is the case in many chronic obstructive pulmonary disease families. About one-third of these investigators' female patients said they felt lonely and depressed, despite the support given by their husbands and families. The major problems of patients' wives were being worried over their husbands' physical condition and his negative attitudes and irritability, and coping with the loss of their own freedom. Less than one-third of the wives said they shared problems with their husbands. Most were afraid that this would result in their husbands' having an attack of breathlessness.

Chronic obstructive pulmonary disease patients and their family members often have different perceptions about the patients' capabilities and the problems posed by the illness. Guyatt et al. (29,30) had 36 pairs of patients and their significant others complete identical questionnaires about problems posed by the illness. The questionnaire included 108 items related to dyspnea, mastery, fatigue, sleep disturbance, emotional problems, social problems, and cognitive function. The patients identified more of the items as problematic than did their significant others ($p < .02$), but the significant others attached greater importance to the problems they identified. Only 17 items were identified as problematic by equal numbers of patients and significant others, and correlations between the patients' and relatives' total scores were moderate in strength.

In Guyatt et al.'s studies, the severity of patients' airflow limitation was not significantly related to their identified problems. These investigators emphasize the importance of physicians asking patients and their families about their views of illness-related problems, rather than relying on physical disease indicators. This seems to be good advice, because if chronic obstructive pulmonary disease patients and their family members do not share their perceptions of these problems, it will be difficult for them to find mutually acceptable solutions. Differing views and expectations can contribute to the patients' isolation and depression, as well as to the spouses' subjective stress. A potential scenario is that the chronic obstructive pulmonary disease patient and spouse may achieve a kind of shared lifestyle that limits the quality of life for both (36).

Smoking

Cigarette smoking has serious implications for chronic obstructive pulmonary disease patients' quality of life. Continued smoking contributes to the physical disease process and exacerbates the patients' respiratory symptoms. When persons with chronic obstructive pulmonary disease quit smoking or substantially reduce their smoking rates, the decline in lung function is much less rapid, and in some cases returns to that associated with normal aging (62–64). In comparison with current smokers, ex-smokers have less sputum production, fewer chest infections, easier breathing, and greater tolerance for physical activities (62,64). As a result, they may perceive themselves to be physically healthier and more comfortable than do current smokers (65). Chronic obstructive pulmonary disease ex-smokers also are more capable of performing physical and psychosocial activities associated with everyday living, and may be more emotionally adjusted (35).

Most persons with diagnosed chronic obstructive pulmonary disease are aware that smoking contributes to their lung disease, and they report that they have been advised to quit smoking (66). Most of these persons say that they want to quit smoking, but they have little confidence in their ability to quit. Seventy-five percent of the current smokers in the study by Pederson et al. (66) stated that they wanted to quit smoking, but only 20% were certain they would quit within 6 months. In a review of the literature on physician advice to quit smoking, Pederson (67) found quitting rates of 20% to 56% for chronic obstructive pulmonary disease patients. Other investigators have found that from two-thirds to three-fourths of the patients in respiratory rehabilitation programs eventually quit smoking (68). However, Mausner (69) found that most persons with chronic obstructive pulmonary disease make multiple attempts to quit smoking before achieving success.

Labuhn et al. (70) interviewed 136 chronic obstructive pulmonary disease patients about their experiences with quitting smoking and found results similar to Mausner's (69). Both ex-smokers and current smokers reported multiple relapses. The most frequently used methods to quit smoking were cold turkey and gradual cutting down. Few individuals used self-help materials, received counseling on quitting strategies, or participated in smoking cessation programs. Most of the patients were not aware of the available resources for smoking cessation, and 50% of the current smokers requested that information be sent to them.

The reasons for chronic obstructive pulmonary disease patients' particular difficulties in quitting smoking are complex. The insidious nature of the disease is one factor. Symptoms develop over a period of years, and patients often are not aware of the seriousness of their lung condition until the disease is fairly far advanced. After diagnosis, the physician might not give strong enough messages about the need to quit smoking, or he might give inadequate information about quitting methods (67,71). Most patients are long-term heavy smokers. If they are addicted to nicotine, as is often the case, they have uncomfortable withdrawal symptoms when they try to quit, and this may lead to emotional arousal and increased respiratory distress. Under these circumstances, it is not surprising that most patients are not successful in the initial attempts to quit smoking.

Social factors also play an important role in patients' continued smoking. Cigarette smoking is an integral part of most patients' lifestyle. It is associated with many daily activities, and it is used for various reasons including pleasure, tension reduction, relief of boredom, and just habit. If the chronic obstructive pulmonary disease patient's spouse smokes and is unwilling to stop, quitting is particularly difficult. Not only is the patient continually confronted witih cues to smoke, but if successful in his quitting attempts, he still must deal with the problem of second-hand smoke (37).

Clinically based interventions to assist patients to quit smoking and avoid relapse are badly needed. Interventions need to address the biological aspects of smoking addiction (withdrawal symptoms) as well as psychosocial and lifestyle issues. Physicians will be more successful in their intervention efforts if they provide specific advice on how to quit (67,72) and if they emphasize how smoking cessation can improve the patients' quality of life. Self-efficacy (confidence in one's ability to carry out recommended quitting strategies) is an important factor in quitting (65,73). Patients with low self-efficacy or those who live with other persons who smoke may receive more benefit from specific skills training (such as that provided in smoking cessation programs) than from printed self-help materials. Future studies on patients' smoking cessation attempts need to focus more on the role of emotional arousal during the quitting process (66) as well as self-efficacy (65).

Coping Strategies

The specific coping strategies that chronic obstructive pulmonary disease patients use to deal with the illness also affect their quality of life. Both cognitive and behavioral coping strategies are important. Fagerhaugh (74) discusses "routing" as a basic behavioral strategy that patients can use to conserve energy while carrying out their daily activities. Routing includes planning the number and types of activities that are needed; making judgments about when to delete, postpone, or condense activities; and anticipating obstacles and planning solutions. Halcomb (75) emphasizes the lifestyle changes that are necessary in order for patients to improve their physical and mental well-being. Patients need guidance in learning how to mobilize support resources and deal with family and marital problems, as well as how to prevent and manage disease symptoms. Effective intervention should give the patient a sense of control over the environment. Stollenwerk (76) also suggests that patients' spiritual resources be assessed for their potential as a coping resource. In a study of self-care practices among chronic obstructive pulmonary disease patients, she found that patients' values and spiritual beliefs affected their decisions regarding self-care, as well as their attitudes and emotional stability. Stollenwerk encourages professionals to become better aware of patients' values in order to assist individual patients to achieve their own goals.

Neuropsychologic, Physiologic, and Demographic Factors

We previously discussed research findings concerning the impact of chronic obstructive pulmonary disease on patients' quality of life. Physiological factors related to the disease process account for some of the limitations in life quality. There is ample evidence that respiratory functioning itself has a significant impact on patients' functioning. When bronchodilators are prescribed for symptomatic relief of breathing problems, temporary improvements in patients' functional capacity and emotional states often are seen (30). Oxygen treatment also may result in improved functioning for some, though not all patients (35,77–79).

McSweeny et al. (15) and Prigatano et al. (35) examined life quality in regard to various sociodemographic and disease-related variables, using simple correlation and multiple regression techniques. McSweeny et al. found strong correlations between their quality of life measures and chronic obstructive pulmonary disease patients' age, socioeconomic status, neuropsychological status, and exercise capability. Less robust, but significant relationships also were noted between life quality and specific indicators of chronic obstructive pulmonary disease such as oxygen transport. McSweeny et al. offered the heuristic model pictured in Fig. 2 to help explain the interrelationships between quality of life measures and the predictor variables they studied.

Prigatano et al.'s (35) investigation supports the results of McSweeny et al. and produced some other interesting findings. Chronic obstructive pulmonary disease patients' quality of life was found to be negatively related to smoking history, but not to recent life changes. In addition, Prigatano et al. discovered that neuropsychological functioning, exercise capability, and pulmonary function variables were more strongly related to physical aspects of life quality than they were to psychosocial aspects of life quality, as measured by the Sickness Impact Profile scales. In contrast, mood and emotional functioning, measured by the Minnesota Multiphasic Personality Inventory and the Profile of Mood States, were more strongly related to psychosocial aspects of quality of life. These findings demonstrate some of the complex interrelationships that exist between various aspects of quality of life, as well as

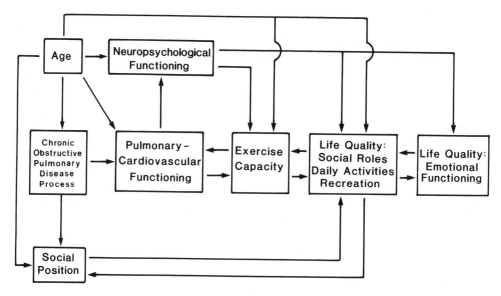

FIG. 2. Heuristic model for interrelation of chronic obstructive pulmonary disease and other variables affecting life quality. From McSweeny, ref. 15, with permission.

between life quality and other spheres of functioning in chronic obstructive pulmonary disease patients.

Guyatt et al. (30) investigated the severity of airflow limitation and age compared to reported emotional disturbances in chronic obstructive pulmonary disease. Severity of airflow limitation was found to have a modest relationship to emotional functioning, which is consistent with the findings of McSweeny et al. (15). In addition, Guyatt et al. found that older patients reported fewer emotional problems than younger patients. This is not consistent with other studies of chronic obstructive pulmonary disease (15,45), but does agree with the results of a study involving patients with several other chronic diseases (33). The reasons for the discrepant findings concerning the relationship of age to reported psychological distress remain unclear.

In a dissertation study, Labuhn (45) further investigated the relationships between life quality and other aspects of functioning in chronic obstructive pulmonary disease. Specifically, her study focused on testing a multivariate model for explaining patients' depressed mood states. The model (shown in Fig. 3) included five sociodemographic variables and five disease-related variables. The two quality of life indicators were perceived illness dysfunction, measured by the Sickness Impact Profile, and depressed mood, measured by the Profile of Mood States. To test the model, data from the McSweeny et al. and Prigatano et al. studies were combined into one data set, and path analysis (80) techniques were applied. Figure 3 and Table 2 show the standardized regression coefficients for linkages in the hypothesized model. Table 2 also includes a summary of the direct, indirect, and total effects of each predictor variable on depressed mood.

Findings from this study indicate that perceived illness dysfunction, which reflects patients' difficulties in carrying out their daily physical and psychosocial activities, makes the largest contribution to depressed mood. Neuropsychological impairment directly contributes to depressed mood, and it also has a negative impact on exercise

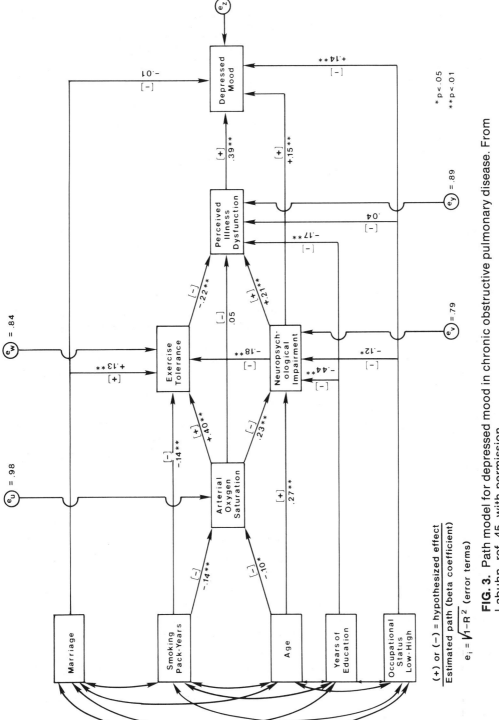

FIG. 3. Path model for depressed mood in chronic obstructive pulmonary disease. From Labuhn, ref. 45, with permission.

(+) or (−) = hypothesized effect
—————————————————————
Estimated path (beta coefficient)

$e_i = \sqrt{1-R^2}$ (error terms)

* p < .05
** p < .01

TABLE 2. *Direct, indirect, and total effects of predictors on the NOTT and IPPB patients' depressed mood scores*

Predictor variable	Direct effect	Indirect effect	Total effect
Perceived illness dysfunction	+0.39	0.0000	+0.3900
Neuropsychological impairment	+0.15	+0.0973	+0.2473
Exercise tolerance	0.00	−0.0858	−0.0858
Arterial oxygen saturation	0.00	−0.1007	−0.1007
Occupational status (low-high)	+0.14	−0.0453	+0.0947
Education (low-high)	0.00	−0.0751	−0.0751
Age	0.00	+0.0834	+0.0834
Smoking pack-years	0.00	+0.0274	+0.0274
Marriage	−0.01	−0.0112	−0.0212

Adapted from Labuhn, 1984.

tolerance, physical functioning, and psychosocial functioning. Neuropsychological impairment also serves as an important intervening variable between depressed mood and disease severity (as measured by oxygen saturation), education, and age. Exercise tolerance has only a small effect on depressed mood, but it also contributes to life quality by influencing patients' physical and psychosocial functioning. Oxygen saturation has no direct affect on the quality of life measures, but it indirectly affects life quality by its influence on patients' exercise tolerance and neuropsychological functioning.

Additional analysis from Labuhn's study suggests that the relative contribution of predictor variables to chronic obstructive pulmonary disease patients' quality of life may change as the disease progresses. For instance, psychosocial factors appear to be more important in explaining depressed mood when patients have mild to moderately severe disease, but physiological and neuropsychological factors are more predictive of depressed mood for patients with advanced disease. Overall, quality of life is never a simple function of disease severity. A wide range of adjustment is seen at all stages of the disease.

Practical Applications

The fact that there is an interrelationship between psychosocial and physiological factors in chronic obstructive pulmonary disease has been exploited infrequently in the clinical situation, if we are to judge from the number of published reports. Those reports that we were able to locate all came from the United Kingdom.

The earliest report is by Clark and Cochrane (81), who employed the personality theory, and assessment procedures of Eysenck (82,83) to help predict which chronic obstructive pulmonary disease patients would show higher-than-expected CO_2 tension (P_{CO_2}) from that predicted from forced expired volume in 1 second (FEV_1). The authors noted that according to Eysenck, extraversion is related to the degree of excitation in the central nervous system. Thus, they reasoned that extraversion should be related to the excitability of the neural network controlling respiration. This hypothesis remains untested, however.

Rutter (84) examined the usefulness of several psychological and physiological variables to predict outcome in an evaluation of a management program for chronic obstructive pulmonary disease patients that included medical treatment, physical therapy, and breathing training. She found that the psychological variables had significant but limited value for predicting outcome as assessed by medical measures of disease severity. Psychological variables, in contrast, were highly useful in predicting the vocational adjustment and work record after management, whereas physiological variables had very limited prognostic value.

Four relatively recent articles (85–88) have focused on exercise capability as an outcome of treatment and rehabilitation. These studies have produced remarkably consistent results. Psychological factors, including mood, attitudes, and beliefs, are important predictors of outcome as assessed by exercise-capability tests. Indeed, the reports indicate that psychological variables are at least as important, and perhaps even more so, than initial ventilatory status. Patients who feel better about themselves, their situation, and the future will participate more actively in therapies and will subsequently benefit more.

IMPLICATIONS OF QUALITY OF LIFE RESEARCH

Implications of Research in Chronic Obstructive Pulmonary Disease

The investigations reviewed in the preceding sections underline the importance of psychological factors in the experience of chronic obstructive pulmonary disease and the patient's ability to cope with life and to benefit from rehabilitation and treatment. Thus, it would seem axiomatic that psychological variables should be included as outcome variables in most patients and as predictor or moderator variables in some patients, when medical and rehabilitative interventions for chronic obstructive pulmonary disease are evaluated. In addition, as the research by Dudley (49) and Clark and Cochrane (80,81) demonstrates, psychological factors may also be useful in explaining some aspects of respiration in chronic obstructive pulmonary disease that cannot be otherwise explained. Future research should include formal evaluations of psychological interventions for patients that are aimed at ameliorating the psychological consequences of chronic obstructive pulmonary disease as well as at improving the process and outcome of treatment and rehabilitation programs.

Clinical Implications

General Comments

Clinicians who care regularly for patients with chronic obstructive pulmonary disease will not be surprised that researchers have found that many of their patients are unhappy, anxious, obstreperous, and unable to manage social transactions appropriate to their age and socioeconomic situation. Perhaps the more important finding, however, is that quality of life is not simply a function of the patient's cardiopulmonary pathophysiology. Rather, the ability of the patient to cope is influenced by age, social position, and neuropsychological status as well. Thus, the older and more disadvantaged patient is likely to have more social impairment and subjective distress. At the same time, changes in mental abilities may make the patient less able to understand treatment and be less cooperative and flexible in seeking alternative sources of satisfaction.

Current research leads to the prediction that the patient with the poorest life quality is the least likely to respond to traditional intervention because of the disease-associated features of advanced age, low social position, depressed cognitive set, and neuropsychological deficit. This prediction is borne out by one study by Pattison et al. (57) that attempted to use insight-oriented group psychotherapy with patients. Several of the persons in this program became openly hostile to the implication that they might have a "psychological problem," and others showed little or no benefit. Grant, a frequent writer in the area of chronic obstructive pulmonary disease and quality of life, has commented that a cognitive behavioral-oriented therapy should be more efficacious with chronic obstructive pulmonary disease patients than insight-oriented therapy (Grant, *personal communication*). In addition, Rosser et al. (89) obtained encouraging results with individual psychotherapy. In general, however, the utility of psychotherapy with chronic obstructive pulmonary disease patients requires additional investigation.

A more fruitful approach might be to integrate psychosocial supports into a multimodal pulmonary rehabilitation program, a suggestion made also by Dudley et al. (90). Psychological interventions that are part of standard patient education and rehabilitation programs are less obtrusive, more acceptable to patients, and have greater potential for success than does traditional psychotherapy. A program devised by the American Lung Association of West Virginia (91), for example, includes both didactic lectures concerning the psychosocial effects of chronic obstructive pulmonary disease and how to cope with them, and structured group exercises for patients with the disease and their families. This program puts a particular emphasis on "depersonalizing" the emotional effects of chronic obstructive pulmonary disease by attributing them to the disease process and teaching patients how to maximize access to activities that would yield psychological reinforcement. This program has been adopted for use with patient support groups (Better Breathers Clubs) in the Toledo area and has been enthusiastically received.

Some Suggestions for Pulmonary Clinicians

A goal of this chapter has been to point out the importance of psychosocial factors in the lives of chronic obstructive pulmonary disease patients. At the beginning of the chapter, we noted that this was consistent with Engel's (12) biopsychosocial model for the science and profession of medicine. As Sandhu (41) has noted, this model may also be used fruitfully as a guide to the management of the patient with chronic obstructive pulmonary disease. To begin with, the physician will want to assume an empathetic, understanding, and encouraging (when appropriate) attitude toward patients and their families. Patients and family members should feel confident that their doctor will listen to their concerns, respond to questions about the psychosocial issues, and give them advice (or provide for the other health care professionals to do so) on how to best cope with the "slings and arrows of [their] outrageous fortune" (92) as well as to maximize the rewards and pleasures that are available to them. This requires regular appointments, even when the patient appears to be functioning well. The physician will need to recognize and deal with psychological defenses; possess good interpersonal skills; and demonstrate time, willingness, and ability to listen.

Pulmonary clinicians may find it useful to include an evaluation of psychosocial functioning in their comprehensive assessment of patients with chronic obstructive pulmonary disease. This should always include an interview of the patient and, if possible, relatives concerning emotional functioning, social role functioning, activities of daily living, sexuality, and recreational pastimes. Current smoking behavior should also be periodically assessed and addressed. For some patients it may be useful to consult a clinical psychologist or psychiatrist for suggestions concerning a formal assessment that includes psychometric measures. The areas assessed and specific instruments to be used could include several of those mentioned in earlier sections of this chapter. The Minnesota Multiphasic Personality Inventory could be used to provide a good overview of psychological adjustment and psychopathology, whereas the Sickness Impact Profile may be used to obtain a broad view of the patient's psychosocial and physical behavioral functioning. The Profile of Mood States may be used to assess mood, and the Berle Index may be employed to assess psychosocial status. The Million Behavioral Health Inventory (94) is a relatively new instrument that has not been used systematically in research with chronic obstructive pulmonary disease patients but has demonstrated utility with adult medical patients in general. It is a relatively brief (150 items versus 566 for the Minnesota Multiphasic Personality Inventory) test of personality and emotional functioning developed specifically for use with physically ill patients. Twenty scales are grouped into four basic categories: basic coping styles, psychogenic attitudes, psychosomatic correlates, and prognostic indices.

Computer scoring and interpretation programs exist for several psychological tests including the Minnesota Multiphasic Personality Inventory and Million Behavior Health Inventory, and many can be used on a personal computer. Most of these programs have the patina of validity but, in fact, their quality varies greatly. As experienced computer users and psychometricians, we strongly recommend against using a computerized interpretation of a psychological test unless the reader is already well familiar with the test instrument and its interpretation. If this is not the case, a psychologist or psychiatrist who is familiar with the test should be consulted.

Once the assessment is completed, an intervention plan should be developed. Many times, patients and relatives may be already functioning relatively well and may require only simple advice and reassurance from their physician concerning the conduct of their lives. Many patients and relatives will also find peer support groups to be very helpful. In the United States these include the Better Breathers Clubs, which are supported by the local chapters of the American Lung Association. These groups usually include discussions of psychosocial issues as well as educational programs concerning medical aspects of chronic obstructive pulmonary disease. Practical information, such as the location of restaurants with no-smoking policies, is often available through these groups.

As noted previously, psychosocial issues may also be handled efficaciously in a rehabilitation or patient education program. These are usually based in the respiratory therapy department of a local hospital. Many, but not all, of these programs do address psychosocial issues. Therefore, the physician or nurse may wish to visit the program and review it before referring patients to it.

A few patients (and relatives) will require referral to a mental health professional. Because the problems of the chronic obstructive pulmonary disease patient are unique and somewhat different from the typical psychiatric patient, it will be important to choose a mental health professional who is familiar with medical illness and the problems it presents. If psychotropic medication is indicated, familiarity with the interaction between psychotropic drugs and the drugs used in the management of chronic obstructive pulmonary disease is essential, as is knowledge of the effects of the psychotropic drugs on respiration. The reader should consult Dudley and Sitzman (94) for further details on the use of psychotropic medications.

CONCLUSIONS

The goal of this chapter has been to underline the importance of psychosocial factors in chronic obstructive pulmonary disease. It is our hope that physicians will wish to incorporate a biopsychosocial model in their clinical and research efforts. Similarly, we hope that the chapter may encourage interested behavioral scientists and clinicians to bring their talents to bear on understanding and ameliorating the many problems faced by patients with chronic disease.

The psychosocial management of the chronic obstructive pulmonary disease patient has received brief treatment in this chapter. For further suggestions, the reader is advised to consult Dudley et al. (90,95), Grant and Timms (96), McSweeny and Grant (97), and Sandhu (41).

REFERENCES

1. Cugell DW. COPD: A brief introduction for behavioral scientists. In McSweeny AJ, Grant I, eds. *Chronic obstructive pulmonary disease: A behavioral perspective*. New York: Marcel Dekker, 1988;1–18.
2. Petty TL. Definitions, clinical assessment, and risk factors. In: Petty TL, ed. *Chronic obstructive pulmonary disease*, 2nd ed. New York: Marcel Dekker, 1985;1–30.
3. Tockman MS, Khoury MJ, Cohen BH. The epidemiology of COPD. In: Petty TL, ed. *Chronic obstructive pulmonary disease*, 2nd ed. New York: Marcel Dekker, 1985;43–92.
4. Petty TL. Early diagnosis and therapeutic interventions. In: Petty TL, ed. *Chronic obstructive pulmonary disease*, 2nd ed. New York: Marcel Dekker, 1985;429–440.
5. Hodgkin J. *Chronic obstructive pulmonary disease*. Park Ridge, Illinois: American College of Chest Physicians, 1979.
6. Grant I, Prigatano GP, Heaton RK, et al. Progressive neuropsychological impairment in relation to hypoxemia in chronic obstructive pulmonary disease. *Arch Gen Psychiatry* 1987;44:999–1006.
7. Prigatano GP, Grant I. Neuropsychological correlates of COPD. In: McSweeny AJ, Grant I, eds. *Chronic obstructive pulmonary disease: A behavioral perspective*. New York: Marcel Dekker, 1988;39–57.
8. Petty TL. Pulmonary rehabilitation. In: Petty TL, ed. *Chronic obstructive pulmonary disease*, 2nd ed. New York: Marcel Dekker, 1985;340–354.
9. Petty TL. Medical management of COPD. In: McSweeny AJ, Grant I, eds. *Chronic obstructive pulmonary disease: A behavioral perspective*. New York: Marcel Dekker, 1988;87–103.
10. Petty TL. Long-term outpatient oxygen therapy. In: Petty TL, ed. *Chronic obstructive pulmonary disease*, 2nd ed. New York: Marcel Dekker, 1985;375–388.
11. Petty TL. Chronic obstructive pulmonary disease, 2nd ed. New York: Marcel Dekker, 1985.
12. Engel GE. The clinical application of the biopsychosocial model. *Am J Psychiatry* 1980;13:535–543.
13. Levine S, Croog SH. What constitutes quality of life: A conceptualization of the dimensions of life quality in healthy populations and patients with cardiovascular disease. In: Wenger NK, Mattson ME, Furberg CD, et al., eds. *Assessment of quality of life in clinical trials of cardiovascular therapies*. New York: LeJacq, 1984;46–58.
14. Wenger NK, Mattson ME, Furberg CD, et al. Preface and overview: Assessment of quality of life in clinical trials of cardiovascular therapies. In: Wenger NK, Mattson ME, Furberg CD, et al., eds. *Assessment of quality of life in clinical trials of cardiovascular therapies*. New York: LeJacq, 1984;1–22.
15. McSweeny AJ, Grant I, Heaton RK, et al. Life quality of patients with chronic obstructive pulmonary disease. *Arch Intern Med* 1982;142:473–478.
16. Pearlman RA, Jonsen A. The use of quality-of-life considerations in medical decision making. *J Am Geriatr Soc* 1985;33:344–352.
17. McCullough LB. The concept of quality of life: A philosophical analysis. In: Wenger NK, Mattson

ME, Furberg CD, et al., eds. *Assessment of quality of life in clinical trials of cardiovascular therapies.* New York: LeJacq, 1984;25–36.

18. Wenger NK, Mattson ME, Furberg CD, et al. Assessment of quality of life in clinical trials of cardiovascular therapies. *Am J Cardiol* 1984;54:908–913.

19. Dahlstrom WG, Welsh GS, Dahlstrom LE. *An MMPI Handbook*, rev. ed., Minneapolis: University of Minnesota, 1972.

20. McSweeny AJ. Assessing the quality of life in patients with chronic obstructive pulmonary disease. In: Wenger NK, Mattson ME, Furberg CD, et al., eds. *Assessment of quality of life in clinical trials of cardiovascular therapies.* New York: LeJacq, 1984;250–265.

21. Bergner M, Bobbitt RA, Carter W, et al. The Sickness Impact Profile: Development and final revision of a health status measure. *Med Care* 1981;12:787–805.

22. Chambers LW, MacDonald LA, Tugwell P. The McMaster Health Index Questionnaire as a measure of the quality of life for patients with rheumatoid disease. *J Rheumatol* 1982;9:780–784.

23. Bergner M, Rothman ML. Health status measures: An overview and guide for selection. *Annu Rev Public Health* 1987;8:191–210.

24. Kaplan RM. Quality of life measurement. In: Karoly P, ed. *Measurement strategies in health psychology.* New York: Wiley-Interscience, 1985.

25. Walker SR, Rosser RM. *Quality of life: Assessment and applications.* London: Ciba Foundation, 1988.

26. McNair DM, Lorr M, Droppleman LF. *Manual for the Profile of Mood States.* San Diego, Educational and Industrial Testing Service, 1971.

27. Katz MM, Lyerly SB. Methods of measuring adjustment and behavior in the community: I. Rationale, description, discriminative validity, and scale development. *Psychol Rep* 1963;13:503–535.

28. McSweeny AJ. Quality of life assessment in neuropsychology. In: Tupper DE, Cicerone K, eds. *The neuropsychology of everyday life.* Amsterdam: Kluwer, 1989.

29. Guyatt GH, Berman LB, Townsend M, et al. A measure of quality of life for clinical trials in chronic lung disease. *Thorax* 1987;42:773–778.

30. Guyatt GH, Townsend M, Berman LB, et al. Quality of life in patients with chronic airflow limitation. *Br J Dis Chest* 1987;81:45–54.

31. Ware JE. Methodological considerations in the selection of health status assessment procedures. In: Wenger NK, Mattson ME, Furberg CD, eds. *Assessment of quality of life in clinical trials of cardiovascular therapies.* New York: LeJacq, 1984.

32. Cook TD, Campbell DT. *Quasi-experimentation: Design and analysis issues for the field settings.* Chicago: Rand-McNally, 1979.

33. Casselith BR, Luck EJ, Strouse TB, Miller DS, Brown LL, Cross PA, Tenaglia BS. Psychosocial status in chronic illness: A comparative analysis of six diagnostic groups. *N Engl J Med* 1984;311:506–511.

34. Veit CT, Ware JE. The structure of psychological distress and well-being in general populations. *J Consult Clin Psychol* 1983;51:730–742.

35. Prigatano GP, Wright EC, Levin D. Quality of life and its predictors in patients with mild hypoxemia and chronic obstructive pulmonary disease. *Arch Intern Med* 1984;144:1613–1619.

36. Sexton DL, Monro BH. Impact of a husband's chronic illness (COPD) on the spouse's life. *Res Nurs Health* 1985;8:83–90.

37. Sexton DL, Monro BH. Living with a chronic illness: The experience of women with chronic obstructive pulmonary disease (COPD). *West J Nurs Res* 1988;10:26–44.

38. Dudley DL, Glaser EM, Jorgenson BN, et al. Psychosocial concomitants to rehabilitation in chronic obstructive pulmonary disease, part I: Psychosocial and psychological considerations. *Chest* 1980;77:413–420.

39. Greenberg GD, Ryan JJ, Bourlier PE. Psychological and neuropsychological aspects of COPD. *Psychosomatics* 1985;26:29–33.

40. McSweeny AJ. Quality of life in relation to COPD. In: McSweeny AJ, Grant I, eds. *Chronic obstructive pulmonary disease: A behavioral perspective.* New York: Marcel Dekker, 1988;59–85.

41. Sandhu HS. Psychosocial issues in chronic obstructive pulmonary disease. *Clin Chest Med* 1986;7:629–642.

42. Agle DP, Baum GL. Psychosocial aspects of chronic obstructive pulmonary disease. *Med Clin North Am* 1977;61:749–758.

43. Barstow RE. Coping with emphysema. *Nurs Clin North Am* 1974;9:137–145.

44. Post L, Collins C. The poorly coping COPD patient: A psychotherapeutic perspective. *J Psychiatry Med* 1981–82;11:173–182.

45. Labuhn KT. An analysis of self-reported depressed mood in chronic obstructive pulmonary disease. (Doctoral Dissertation, University of Michigan, 1984.) *Diss Abst Int* 1984;45:524B.

46. Burns BH, Howell JBL. Disproportionately severe breathlessness in chronic bronchitis. *Q J Med* 1969;38:277–294.

47. Kinsman RA, Yaroush RA, Fernandez E, et al. Symptoms and experiences in chronic bronchitis and emphysema. *Chest* 1983;83:755–761.

48. Dudley DL, Wermuth C, Hague W. Psychosocial aspects of care in the chronic obstructive pulmonary disease patient. *Heart Lung* 1973;2:289–303.
49. Dudley DL. Psychophysiology of Respiration in Health and Disease. New York: Appleton-Century-Crofts, 1969.
50. Hanson EI. Effects of chronic lung disease on life in general and sexuality: Perceptions of adult patients. *Heart Lung* 1982;11:435–441.
51. Chapman JM, Reeder LG, Massey FJ. The relationship of stress, tranquilizers and serum cholesterol levels in a sample population under study for coronary heart disease. *Am J Epidemiol* 1966;83:537–547.
52. Neugarten B, Havinghurst R, Tobin S. The measurement of life satisfaction. *Gerontol* 1961;16:134–143.
53. Kass I, Updegraff K, Muffly RB. Sex in chronic obstructive pulmonary disease. *Med Aspects Hum Sex* 1972;6:33–42.
54. Fletcher EC, Martin RJ. Sexual dysfunction and erectile impotence in chronic obstructive pulmonary disease. *Chest* 1982;81:413–421.
55. Costello CG. Depression: Loss of reinforcers or loss of reinforcer effectiveness? *Behav Ther* 1972;2:240–247.
56. De Araujo G, Van Arsdel PP, Holmes TH, et al. Life change, coping ability and chronic intrinsic asthma. *J Psychosom Res* 1973;17:359–363.
57. Pattison EM, Rhodes RJ, Dudley DL. Response to group treatment in patients with severe chronic lung disease. *Int J Group Psychother* 1971;21:214–255.
58. Jensen PS. Risk protective factors, and supportive interventions in chronic airway obstruction. *Arch Gen Psychiatry* 1983;40:1203–1207.
59. Young RF. Marital adaptation and response in chronic illness: The case of COPD. (Doctoral dissertation, Wayne State University, 1981.) *Diss Abstr Int* 1982;42:4947A.
60. Litman TJ. The family as a basic unit in health and medical care: A social behavioral overview. *Soc Sci Med* 1974;8:495–519.
61. Bruhn J. Effects of chronic illness on the family. *J Fam Pract* 1977;4:1057–1060.
62. Fletcher C, Peto R, Tinker C, et al. The natural history of chronic bronchitis and emphysema. Oxford: Oxford University Press, 1976.
63. Hughes JA, Hutchinson D, Bellang DE, et al. The influence of cigarette smoking and its withdrawal on the annual change in lung function in pulmonary emphysema. *Q J Med* 1982;51:115–124.
64. Petty TL. Pulmonary medicine. *JAMA* 1985;254:2271–2273.
65. Devins GM, Edwards PJ. Self-efficacy and smoking reduction in chronic obstructive pulmonary disease. *Behav Res Ther* 1988;26:127–135.
66. Pederson LL, Wanklin JM, Baskerville JC. The role of health beliefs in compliance with physician advice to quit smoking. *Soc Sci Med* 1984;19:573–580.
67. Pederson LL. Compliance with physician advice to quit smoking: A review of the literature. *Prev Med* 1982;11:71–84.
68. Dudley DL, Aickin M, Martin CV. Cigarette smoking in a chest clinic population—Psychophysiologic variables. *J Psychosom Res* 1977;21:367–375.
69. Mausner JS. Cigarette smoking among patients with respiratory disease. *Am Rev Resp Dis* 1970;102:704–713.
70. Labuhn KT, Koon KA, Lewis CK. *An exploratory survey of COPD patients' smoking cessation attempts: Preliminary findings.* Paper presented at the University of Virginia Nursing Research Colloquium, Charlottesville, 1988.
71. Rose G, Hamilton PJS. A randomized controlled trial of the effect on middle-aged men of advice to stop smoking. *J Epidemiol Comm Health* 1978;32:275–281.
72. Flaxman J. Behavioral prevention of COPD: Smoking control. In: McSweeny AJ, Grant I, eds. *Chronic obstructive pulmonary disease: A behavioral perspective.* New York: Marcel Dekker, 1988;163–181.
73. Candiotte MM, Lichtenstein E. Self-efficacy and relapse in smoking cessation programs. *J Consult Clin Psychol* 1981;49:648–658.
74. Fagerhaugh S. Getting around with emphysema. In: Strauss AL, ed. *Chronic illness and quality of life.* St. Louis: Mosby, 1975.
75. Halcomb R. Promoting self-help in pulmonary patient education. *Respir Ther* 1984;14:49–54.
76. Stollenwerk R. An emphysema client: Self care. *Home Healthcare Nurse* 1985;3:36–40.
77. Heaton RK. Psychological effects of oxygen therapy for COPD. In: McSweeny AJ, Grant I, eds. *Chronic obstructive pulmonary disease: A behavioral perspective.* New York: Marcel Dekker, 1988;105–121.
78. Heaton RK, Grant I, McSweeny AJ, et al. Psychologic effects of continuous and nocturnal oxygen therapy. *Arch Int Med* 1983;143:1941–1947.
79. Petty TL. Home oxygen in advanced chronic obstructive pulmonary disease. *Med Clin North Am* 1981;65:615–627.
80. Asher HB. *Casual modeling.* Beverly Hills, CA: Sage, 1976.

81. Clark RJH, Cochrane GM. Effect of personality on alveolar ventilation in patients with chronic airways obstruction. *Br Med J* 1970;1:273–275.
82. Eysenck HJ. *The structure of human personality*, 2nd ed. London: Methuen, 1960.
83. Eysenck HJ, Eysenck SBG. *Manual of the Eysenck Personality Inventory*. London: University of London Press, 1964.
84. Rutter BM. *The prognostic significance of psychological factors in the management of chronic bronchitis. Psychol Med* 1979;9:63–70.
85. Geddes DM. Chronic airflow obstruction. *Postgrad Med J* 1984;60:194–200.
86. Morgan AD, Peck DF, Buchanan DR, et al. Effects of attitudes and beliefs on exercise tolerance in chronic bronchitis. *Br Med J* 1983;286:171–173.
87. Morgan AD, Peck DF, Buchanan DR, et al. Psychological factors contributing to disproportionate disability in chronic bronchitis. *J Psychosom Res* 1983;27:259–261.
88. Webber BA. Living to the limit: Exercise for the chronic breathless patient. *Physiotherapy* 1981;67:128–130.
89. Rosser R, Danford J, Heslop A, et al. Breathlessness and psychiatric morbidity in chronic bronchitis and emphysema: A study of psychotherapeutic management. *Psychol Med* 1983;13:93–110.
90. Dudley DL, Glasser EM, Jorgenson BN, et al. Psychosocial concomitants to rehabilitation in chronic obstructive pulmonary disease, part II: Psychosocial treatment. *Chest* 1980;77:544–551.
91. Carlson J, Hoy R, McSweeny AJ, et al. *Your guide to better breathing: Instructor's manual*. Charleston, WV: American Lung Association of West Virginia, 1981.
92. Shakespeare W. The tragedy of Hamlet, Prince of Denmark. In: Harrison GB, ed. *Shakespeare: The complete works*. New York: Harcourt, Brace and World, 1603/1952;880–934.
93. Millon T, Green CJ, Meagher RB. *Millon Behavioral Health Inventory Manual*, 3rd ed. Minneapolis: National Computer Systems, 1982.
94. Dudley DL, Sitzman J. Psychobiological evaluation and treatment of COPD. In: McSweeny AJ, Grant I, eds. *Chronic obstructive pulmonary disease: A behavioral perspective*. New York: Marcel Dekker, 1988;183–235.
95. Dudley DL, Glaser EM, Jorgenson BN, et al. Psychosocial concomitants to rehabilitation in chronic obstructive pulmonary disease, part III: Dealing with psychiatric disease. *Chest* 1980;77:667–684.
96. Grant I, Timms RM. Psychiatric disturbances in chronic obstructive pulmonary disease. In: Bondow RA, Moses KM, eds. *Manual of clinical problems in chronic obstructive pulmonary disease*. Boston: Little, Brown, 1985.
97. McSweeny AJ, Grant I. *Chronic obstructive pulmonary disease: A behavioral perspective*. New York: Marcel Dekker, 1988.

Quality of Life Assessments in Clinical Trials, edited by B. Spilker. Raven Press, Ltd. New York © 1990.

31

Cancer

*Ivan Barofsky and †Paul H. Sugarbaker

*Institute of Social Oncology, Silver Spring, Maryland 20904;
†Cancer Institute, Washington Hospital Center, Washington, DC 20010

Cancer consists of 100 or more separate diseases. Thus, it is not surprising that asking how to measure quality of life among cancer patients reflects much of the ongoing debate in measuring quality of life in general. Progress toward this goal requires an understanding of how quality of life has been assessed in the past and how quality of life is changed.

Quality of life assessment originated with political efforts to evaluate social programs meant to enhance the quality of an individual's existence (1). In a medical context, quality of life assessment would be expected to evaluate the qualitative outcome of medical care. These assessments would help clarify the views and values of clinicians and patients so that a consensus evolves concerning the risks and benefits inherent in the modern treatment of the cancer patient.

Major changes in a person's quality of life occur by technical innovation, without any formal assessment of quality of life. The same would occur following the introduction of innovative cancer treatment (e.g., substituting a radical mastectomy for a lumpectomy in early breast cancer, or introducing a new chemotherapy regimen). This suggests that a formal quality of life assessment is secondary to the evolution of medical treatment, and functions best when it modulates this process. Quality of life assessments, therefore, are an absolute necessity for the ethical conduct of cancer medicine. However, the formal assessment of quality of life needs to be established.

Patients are being asked to make a judgment when they participate in a quality of life assessment. They are asked how satisfied they are with their lives or how much their lives have changed as a result of cancer treatment. All judgments can be perceived as consisting of two elements: a descriptive statement (information), and some value or weight associated with that statement. Theories differ in terms of how these elements are combined and what factors are included in the judgment process. A wide variety of theories of the judgment process exist (2), each of which fits this two-component model.

The two-component model can be used to understand the design of the major population-based, health-related quality of life assessments. Each measure differs primarily in how the weightings are generated. Weightings of descriptors in the Quality of Well-Being Scale (3) are generated from representatives of the general public. Clinicians are the source of the weights of the descriptors in the Sickness Impact Profile (4). Statistical procedures indirectly weighted descriptors in RAND's General Health Rating Index (5). Descriptors themselves often come from available instruments (e.g., the Health Interview Survey of the National Center for Health Statistics [6]), although they may be generated in other ways as well (e.g., a panel of patients, or physicians and nurses).

This chapter reviews the development of quality of life issues in cancer treatment. It also illustrates how a formal quality of life assessment leads to changes in the qualitative consequences of cancer treatment. The wide range of cancer-specific quality of life assessments that are currently available are described to assist the reader in selecting among available instruments.

DEVELOPMENT OF QUALITY OF LIFE EVALUATIONS OF CANCER TREATMENT

Major advances in the surgical treatment of cancer patients occurred 100 to 150 years ago following the development of general anesthesia and methods for controlling sepsis (7). Such changes in surgical procedures lead to an improvement in patients' quality of life (e.g., reduced operative pain and anticipatory anxiety), which then contributed to the acceptance of the new modality. Improvements in quality of life for other major cancer treatment modalities (e.g., radiation, drugs) also contributed to their acceptance. For example, the discovery that X-rays could be used to treat cancer occurred within months of its initial discovery (8). Patients with cancerous skin lesions improved without the adverse physical trauma and cosmetic consequences of surgery.

Progress in the acceptance of new cancer therapies is critically dependent on their quality of life consequences. These consequences can either facilitate or impede the acceptance process. It might be asked whether it is necessary to formally assess quality of life, since if survival is extended, the patient's quality of life is presumably enhanced.

The assumption that people universally perceive healthy survival as the best quality of life state and death the worst is not correct. Torrance (9) found that subjects rate an extremely limited life as worse than death itself. Sutherland et al. (10) introduced the concept of "maximum endurable time," which is a time interval within which an individual will endure a particular state, but beyond which they use different criteria to determine their preferences. *These points suggest that death and complete health are not extremes of a linear continuum for quality of life states.*

Cancer treatments produce adverse effects and diminish the quality of life, even as the patient's survival is extended. This can be illustrated by the relationship between tumor control, treatment complications, and treatment dose (11; Fig. 1). Increases in treatment dose raise the probability of tumor control, while increasing the probability of complications (Fig. 1). As tumor control reaches maximum so does the probability of a complication. The smaller the area between these two functions, the more toxic the treatment.

Thus, formal assessment of quality of life is important because mere extension of survival is not directly correlated with an improved or optimum quality of life, and because maximum tumor control is associated with maximum tolerated drug dose, and therefore with maximum toxicity. Escalation of a drug's dose or intensity of radiation is limited by complications or adverse effects on quality of life.

Quality of life assessment establishes the limits within which cancer care occurs, although treatment decisions are often independent of quality of life considerations.

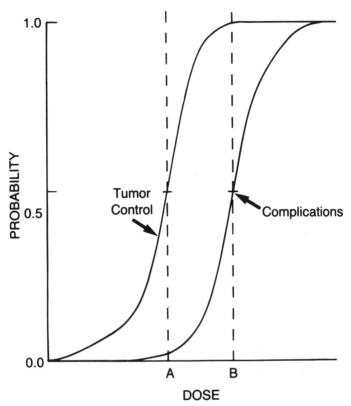

FIG. 1. The probability of tumor control and complications as a function of treatment dose. The intersection between the dotted lines and the functions represent the point where 50% of the subjects respond. The distance between the two doses (A and B) are a measure of the therapeutic index. Adapted from Hellman (1985).

This can be illustrated by patients with cancer of the middle or lower third of the rectum (12), where surgical excision involves sacrifice of the anal sphincter. Patients have a post-surgery colostomy, and a majority of the males are impotent. Alternative operative procedures have made sphincter sparing a feasible alternative for a limited number of patients. These patients would not require a colostomy. Still, no clinician would ordinarily attempt surgery that would improve the patient's quality of life (i.e., bowel hygiene and care) if it was at the cost of shortened survival.

Williams and Johnston (12) demonstrated the advantage of a formal quality of life assessment in this situation when they found only 30% of the patients who received a sphincter-sparing procedure were incontinent, whereas 100% of the colostomy patients were. In addition, 83% of the sphincter-spared patients returned to a previous job, whereas only 40% of the colostomy patients returned to work. Finally, 30% of the spincter-spared patients reported impaired sexual functioning, compared to 67% of the colostomy patients.

Formal quality of life assessments in cancer treatment help determine the balance between an optimal therapeutic effect on patient survival, and an acceptable quality of life outcome. Fig. 2 shows that there is an optimal treatment that may initially produce a decrease in quality of life (e.g., the patient who feels well but requires a surgery) or an increase in it (e.g., patients with pain whose quality of life improves

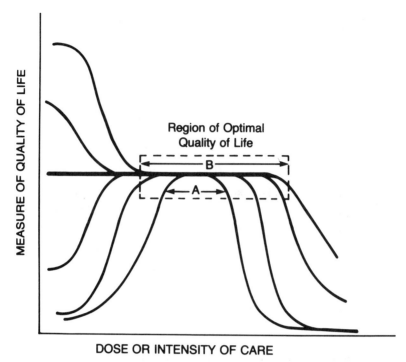

FIG. 2. A measure of quality of life as a function of treatment dose. The figure illustrates that low treatment doses can have no impact, decrease, or even improve quality of life, but that with continued increases in dose or intensity of care, a region of optimal quality of life emerges only to be followed by a reduction of quality of life at higher treatment doses or intensity of care. The length of the region of optimal quality of life is an indirect measure of the therapeutic index of the treatment. In this figure Treatment B has a higher therapeutic index than Treatment A.

following treatment). Continued increments in the level of treatment would eventually decrease quality of life.

FORMAL ASSESSMENT OF QUALITY OF LIFE IN THE DEVELOPMENT OF CANCER TREATMENT

Quality of life assessment is applicable to a wide range of clinical situations in oncology (e.g., determining the impact of a treatment, characterizing the nature of terminal illness). The development of limb-sparing procedures for soft tissue sarcomas helps explain how quality of life assessments affected the development of a new cancer treatment.

Soft tissue sarcomas arise in the soft tissues of the body. Although soft tissues comprise 50% of the body weight, sarcomas are relatively rare, comprising only 0.7% of all reported cancers (13). Soft tissue sarcomas are characterized by a tendency to aggressively invade surrounding local tissue and a tendency to form micrometastases in the lung early in their clinical course. Increasing the amount of tissue removed decreases local recurrence, but also increases the likelihood that the patient will experience impaired function. This creates a dilemma for clinicians.

TABLE 1. *Selected history of the development of treatment for extremity soft-tissue sarcoma: The NCI experience[a]*

1. Initiation of the Extremity Soft-Tissue Sarcoma Protocol: May, 1975.
2. Quality of Life Study: January 1977–August 1978, Sugarbaker et al., 1982 (ref. 16).
3. Initial Summary of Data: Rosenberg, Costa, Kent, et al., 1978 (ref. 15).
4. Initial Functional Assessment: Lampert et al., 1984 (ref. 18).
5. Endocrine Studies: Shamberger et al., 1981 (ref. 17).
6. Completion of Extremity Soft-Tissue Sarcoma Protocol: April, 1981.
7. Modification of Radiotherapy Procedures: Tepper et al., 1982 (ref 20).
8. Modification of Surgical Procedures: Sugarbaker and Nicholson, 1984 (ref. 19).
9. Final Functional Assessment: Hicks et al., 1985 (ref. 21).
10. NIH Consensus Conference: 1985.

[a] Many of the events listed sequentially here occurred concurrently. Also publication date does not necessarily correspond to date of completion of the study. This history refers only to the protocol that compared amputation and limb-sparing procedures.

Rosenberg et al. (14,15) stated, "local surgical excision followed by adjuvant therapy can produce levels of local control equivalent to that of major radical surgical excisions without the morbidity of the latter procedures." The assumption in this study was that the limb-sparing procedure would produce less morbidity (i.e., a better quality of life) than an amputation.

In an attempt to address this issue, Sugarbaker, Barofsky, et al. (16) designed a study that included a battery of standard assessments (e.g., the Sickness Impact Profile), study-specific assessments (e.g., the Treatment Trauma Scale), and clinical assessments (e.g., mobility). What was found unexpectedly was that limb sparing did not necessarily produce a better quality of life outcome than amputation. Radiotherapy was found to disrupt sexual functioning and mobility. Disruption in sexual functioning was confirmed by endocrinological studies (17), and impairment in mobility was confirmed by functional assessments (18). Rosenberg et al. modified the limb-sparing surgery (14), radiotherapy (20), and physical therapy that patients received. Hicks et al. (21) then showed that patients who received the modified limb-sparing procedures had significantly improved function as compared to patients who were assessed in the study by Sugarbaker et al. (16). Finally, a National Institutes of Health Consensus Conference (22) was held to confirm and extend these conclusions (Table 1).

Few quality of life studies of the cancer patient link the outcome of an assessment with modification of a treatment regimen as clearly as the sarcoma studies (Table 1). The strong desire of the principal investigator to demonstrate qualitative advantages (i.e., less morbidity) of the limb-sparing procedure insured that the procedural changes required among the several disciplines would occur.

Quality of life assessment can lead to change in cancer care in two ways. The history of sarcoma studies reviewed in Table 1 represents a single step procedure where the quality of life assessment was an integral part of the treatment development process. Most quality of life studies, however, contribute to change in cancer care through a multistep process. First, the assessment of quality of life occurs and then the development of a consensus for change occurs. This is followed by a diffusion of this innovation through the cancer care system. Limited usage of cytotoxic agents, following Priestman's (23) studies of the quality of life of breast cancer patients receiving chemotherapy in Great Britain (see this section), illustrates this second model. Irrespective of the method, practitioners respond to the challenge of inno-

TABLE 2. *Types of quality of life assessments used in cancer studies*

1. Population-based assessments:
   —Indexes (Quality of Well-Being Index)
   —Profiles (Sickness Impact Profile)
2. Psychosocial assessments:
   —Coping (Psychosocial Adjustment to Illness Scale)
   —Depression (Beck Depression Scale)
3. Global assessments:
   —Karnofsky Scale
   —Spitzer's Quality of Life Index
4. Cancer-specific assessments:
   —Functional Living Index–Cancer
   —Quality of Life Index–Padilla
   —Linear Analogue Self-Assessment
   —EORTC-Lung Quality of Life Questionnaire
   —Anamestic Comparative Self-Assessment
   —Stage II Breast Cancer Questionnaire
   —Time Without Symptoms of Disease and Subjective Toxic Effects (TWIST)

vation by modifying the innovation and shaping it into a form that they can incorporate into their practice (24). The same process is expected to occur following a quality of life assessment.

CANCER-SPECIFIC QUALITY OF LIFE ASSESSMENTS

Quality of life assessments have become an integral part of medical research. A review of the Medline literature since 1966 revealed quality of life as a descriptor or text term in over 4,000 references (25). Much of this increase in interest has occurred since the mid-1970s. In the area of cancer, there is an ever increasing number of papers, reviews (26–30), and published symposia (31–34) on quality of life.

Table 2 summarizes the types of self-administered assessments that have been used in various cancer quality of life studies. Cancer-specific interview protocols are not included and are not discussed in this review. Population-based instruments that address health policy issues have been used in a wide range of cancer studies (35). Psychosocial instruments provide estimates of normative coping and adjustment (16). Some of these instruments (e.g., the Psychosocial Adjustment of Illness Scale) provide norms for cancer patients (36), whereas others have been modified to be suitable for cancer patients (e.g., the Profile of Moods Scale; [37]). Another group of instruments, global quality of life assessments, have been developed using cancer patients to establish the instrument's reliability and validity, although they can be used for a wide variety of patient groups (38,39). A final group of instruments or methods has been developed and used only in studies of the cancer patient. These instruments are described further (Table 3).

The construction of a quality of life assessment reflects the developer's view of how best to combine the two major components of a judgment into an assessment instrument. In the Quality of Well-Being Index, respondents indicate the presence or absence (yes or no) of a symptom or functional state within the preceding 3 to 8 days. The respondent is carefully asked not to make any judgment of the importance of these events but only to report whether they occurred. The Sickness Impact Profile, as a behavioral checklist, also asks only if the described behavior occurred.

TABLE 3. *The content of cancer-specific quality of life assessments*[a]

				Assessments			
		FLIC	QOLI-P	LASA-P	LASA-S	QOLQ	BCQ
	N =						
Dimensions		22	23	25	31	42	30
Global well-being		9.1%	21.8%	—	3.2%	9.5%	10.0%
Treatment, disease, or health issues		9.1%	17.4%	—	—	—	13.3%
Physical functions, signs, and symptoms		18.2%	34.8%	40.0%	61.3%	57.1%	50.0%
Psychological variables		27.3%	—	20.0%	19.4%	11.9%	13.3%
Social variables		36.4%	26.1%	40.0%	16.1%	21.4%	13.3%

[a] The classification system was empirically derived. Representative items included in each dimension are provided below:

1. Global well-being: Happiness, self-satisfaction, fear of future, feeling well, positive about future, feeling good, life satisfaction, etc.
2. Treatment, disease, health: Hardship of cancer, adjustment to colostomy, confidence in treatment, health care, hospital services, information, etc.
3. Physical functions (signs and symptoms): Nausea, vomiting, pain, strength, sleep, energy, appetite, constipation, swallowing, activities of daily living, etc.
4. Psychological variables: Coping, depression, thinking, appearance, self-care, worry, irritability, nervousness, loneliness, frustrated, stress, etc.
5. Social variables: Recreation, leisure, housework, friends, fun, privacy, sexual relationships, relationships with others, vacations, work, etc.

FLIC, Functional Living Index–Cancer, QOLI-P, Quality of Life Index–Fadilla; LASA-P, Linear Analogue Self Assessment–Priestman; LASA-S, Linear Analogue Self Assessment–Selby; QOLQ, EORTC–Lung Group Quality of Life Questionnaire; BCQ, Stage II Breast Cancer Questionnaire.

The valuation of these descriptors is then left to a different process. Both of these instruments, therefore, disaggregate the normal judgment process and reconstruct quality of life judgments, but now in terms of indexes or profiles.

Most cancer-specific quality of life assessments do not disaggregate the judgment process, as described above. Instead, a patient is asked to scale the content or topic at issue. Campbell et al. (40) conceptualized quality of life judgment as having an affective and cognitive component. This has stimulated a philosophical debate about whether quality of life is an emotional or rational phenomenon (41). It also resulted in the content or domains of quality of life being scaled along bad–good or satisfied–dissatisfied dimensions. In contrast, the contents of most cancer-specific quality of life assessments are scaled in terms of the frequency of events (e.g., how often do you feel depressed?; never–continually), or in terms of the qualitative consequences of events (e.g., How well do you feel today?; extremely poor–extremely well).

Table 3 shows that six representative cancer-specific quality of life assessments are diverse in content, even when the items are clustered in broad subcategories. The more the assessment is designed for a specific type of cancer or cancer treatment, the more likely that the assessment contains items that measure physical signs or symptoms of toxicity (e.g., nausea, vomiting, pain, strength, fatigue, activities of daily living, swallowing, dyspnea). Diversity in scaling used in cancer-specific quality of life assessments also exists. Thus, in the Functional Living Index–Cancer (42) there are 13 different scales for 22 items, whereas only four scales are used in EORTC-Lung (43) measure.

Scaling of content or descriptors, however, is not to be confused with the valuation process. When cancer patients indicate the intensity of the pain they feel, this is not same as indicating the importance that the particular intensity of pain has for them. Valuations reflect broader assessments that may include multiple scaled items. None of the instruments included in Table 3 include valuations, although some consider value-related issues indirectly (see below).

FUNCTIONAL LIVING INDEX–CANCER

The Functional Living Index–Cancer, probably more than any other cancer-specific quality of life assessment, has made quality of life assessment an accepted activity among cancer researchers. The index's known psychometric properties and promotion by a practicing oncologist have led to its rapid inclusion in a wide variety of clinical trials and cancer care studies (42). However, it also has been found to be difficult to administer and often has failed to detect expected differences in clinical trials (44).

The Functional Living Index–Cancer was developed by a iterative process; 250 items generated by a panel of patients and clinicians were administered to 175 patients, followed by a questionnaire scaled down to 42 items administered to 312 patients, and finally a 20-item questionnaire administered to 175 patients. A fourth run of the index, as part of a validation study, resulted in two new items being added to produce the final 22-item version. After the second run, a factor analysis was performed and items with the highest factor loadings were included in the next version of the questionnaire.

The resultant questionnaire was distinguished by its relatively small number ($N = 4$) of items dealing with physical signs or symptoms; two items dealt with pain and two dealt with nausea. Since some cancer treatments produce neither pain nor nausea, using the Functional Living Index–Cancer in a clinical trial evaluating such treatments would inevitably mean that approximately 9% to 18% of the items on the questionnaire would contribute in a random way to detecting differences between treatments. This is one of the trade-offs an investigator makes when using a standardized instrument. He or she trades-off using an assessment tool with known psychometric characteristics against having an instrument with sufficient specificity and sensitivity to detect differences in the treatment arms of a clinical trial. On the other hand, the method used to generate the items in the instrument reflects the major concerns of cancer patients, although certain relevant topics are not included as a result of this process (e.g., no items deal with sexual activity). Still, the Functional Living Index–Cancer tracks the natural history of cancer and its treatment, and is an appropriate component of any testing battery.

As mentioned above, the Functional Living Index–Cancer uses 13 different scales for the 22 items. It is not clear whether this adds richness, complexity, or both to the judgment task of the respondent. Additional research needs to be done with the index. What would happen, for example, if the descriptors or content areas of the index are kept constant and the items rephrased so that fewer scales could be used? Would this increase or reduce the sensitivity or specificity of the instrument?

An additional research issue has to do with scoring the Functional Living Index–Cancer. Investigators are asked to add up the scaled scores for each of the 22 items and use this composite measure as a quality of life indicator. The assumption in this method is that each item on the questionnaire has equal weight, an assumption that Perloff and Persons (45) have shown can produce a significant bias in any resultant index. Yet, establishing the relative importance of each item on the questionnaire is done in a valuation exercise. Thus, it is important to generate a valuation system with the Functional Living Index–Cancer that reflects the preferences of cancer patients in general, and patients with specific types of cancer.

QUALITY OF LIFE INDEX–PADILLA

The Quality of Life Index–Padilla is a modification of a 10-item quality of life assessment originally developed by Presant et al. (46). The initial version of the index was a 14-item instrument (47), which has been modified and expanded into a 23-item questionnaire for colostomy patients only (48).

Padilla et al. (48) were interested in using quality of life as an outcome measure of nursing practice. Items were selected to reflect this intent and did not include all quality of life domains (Table 3). Padilla claims that one cluster of items, identified by factor analysis, can be labeled as "psychological well-being." Three of the items (happiness, satisfaction, and general quality of life), however, have traditionally been used as global measures of quality of life (40). It is not clear if these items of well-being are any more or less psychological in nature than items labeled as physical well-being are physical in nature (strength, fatigue, ability to work, health, and perceived usefulness).

The authors organized the 14 items into three subgroups: general physical condition, important human activities, and general quality of life. These constructs are used to generate a model of the relationship between nursing practice and quality of life. The usefulness of this model depends on the precision with which it can be translated into hypotheses to test, or used to interpret data. The artificial nature whereby the items were originally selected for inclusion on the Quality of Life Index–Padilla assessment decreases the chances that operationalizable constructs will result. On the other hand, this effort recognizes that quality of life assessments can be used for quality assurance purposes. This indicates the potential for facilitating change that a quality of life assessment offers by making it an outcome measure of clinical practice.

LINEAR ANALOGUE SELF-ASSESSMENT–PRIESTMAN

Priestman and Baum (49) reported one of the earliest efforts at developing a breast cancer-specific quality of life assessment. The efforts of several groups (50,51) has resulted in a significant lower usage of adjuvant chemotherapy for breast cancer in Great Britain than in other countries. The original impetus for developing the Linear Analogue Self-Assessment–Priestman was a desire by the investigators to supplement standard measures of physical status (e.g., the Karnofsky Scale; 38) with measures of the patient's feelings and subjective response to treatment. Their work represents the original application of the visual analogue self-assessment technique to cancer patients.

The Linear Analogue Self-Assessment technique consists of drawing a 10 cm line for a given variable, with the ends of the line labeled with words that describe the extremes of the variable. The patient draws a line at that point on the 10 cm line that reflects his or her feelings. These scores are then summed to give an overall index.

In a cross-sectional pilot study using the technique for 10 variables, Priestman and Baum (49) found that the sum of Linear Analogue Self-Assessment–Priestman scores for women with advanced breast cancer varied with treatment and whether or not they were responding to treatment. This was followed by a prospective study of 100 recurrent or metastatic breast cancer patients who were randomized to receive either endocrine or cytotoxic chemotherapy, in which a 25-item Linear Analogue Self-Assessment questionnaire, the Linear Analogue Self-Assessment–Priestman (Table 3), was used. The results of this study (52) revealed that patients who received cytotoxic agents experienced more adverse reactions, but also had an improved well-being due to greater tumor shrinkage when compared to the hormonally treated patients. An additional analysis of responders and nonresponders receiving chemotherapy demonstrated that adverse reactions experienced by both groups became intolerable to patients who did not experience an objective response. As a result of this study, Priestman et al. (53) stated that patients may be expected to tolerate the adverse reactions of cytotoxic agents as long as some objective response occurs. In the absence of tumor regression, clinicians should consider either terminating or altering the treatment regimen to avoid undue distress.

Priestman and Baum (49) quantified the qualitative outcome of different treatments with a simple instrument and described the limits of these treatments. Simple assessment instruments or test batteries can lead to useful data if the clinical phenomena being studied are sufficiently robust. Priestman and Baum (49) compared metastatic cancer patients who responded or did not respond to therapy, while Sugarbaker et al. (16) compared patients treated by amputation or limb sparing. Clearly, the more sharply drawn the experimental question, the more explicit is the value or preference issue. In these situations a detailed identification of values or preferences may not be necessary, and assessments based on descriptors alone may suffice.

LINEAR ANALOGUE SELF-ASSESSMENT–SELBY

Selby, Boyd, et al. (54) have also utilized the Linear Analogue Self-Assessment method to develop a cancer-specific quality of life assessment. Their assessment instrument differed from the one developed by Priestman and Baum (49) in that formal methods were used to select items, to determine the relevance of these items to the patients who were being assessed, and to establish the instrument's reliability and validity. Eighteen of the items reflect content areas found on the Sickness Impact Profile (55). This seems to be an attempt by the authors to insure that their instrument is comprehensive. Like the Linear Analogue Self-Assessment–Priestman, the Linear Analogue Self-Assessment–Selby is designed for breast cancer patients. Originally Selby et al. (54) reported a 31-item instrument, but this has been reduced to a 29-item instrument in their most recent report (56).

Items on the Linear Analogue Self-Assessment–Selby are scaled according to events which happened within the last 24 hours. In contrast, identical items on the Functional Living Index–Cancer use a 2-week period as the time base (e.g., items on nausea). By limiting the time base to 24 hours, respondents have the opportunity to base their responses on recalled events; in contrast, recall over a 2-week period becomes increasingly impressionistic and constructed. The differences in these two tasks underscore the variations in data generated by these two seemingly identical quality of life assessments.

Boyd et al. (56) reported that the physical functioning items on the Linear Analogue Self-Assessment–Selby were able to discriminate among patients who did or did not have metastatic disease, whereas items reflecting treatment-related toxicities were able to discriminate patients who received chemotherapy or not. Finally, scores on psychological and social health items were similar for patients receiving chemotherapy, independent of their disease status.

Clearly, the Linear Analogue Self-Assessment–Selby has the psychometric capacity to detect differences between respondent characteristics. Since the Selby instrument is limited to describing the status of the patient, inferences about the significance of the observed changes remain conjectural. There is no reason, however, why an investigator could not determine the preferences of the respondents for any observed outcomes with an ancillary study.

EORTC–LUNG GROUP QUALITY OF LIFE QUESTIONNAIRE

The EORTC–Lung Group Quality of Life Questionnaire is an excellent example of a carefully constructed assessment instrument. It represents an application of methodology developed by Ware et al. in the Health Insurance Study (57). This 42-item questionnaire includes three open-ended questions all summarized on both sides of one legal-size page. As shown in Table 3, it predominantly measures physical signs and symptoms or functional states, and does not address treatment regimen or disease-specific issues.

The methodological importance of the EORTC–Lung Group Quality of Life Questionnaire is its approach to generating scales and indexes. The authors (58) have selected items that can be combined into 15 nonoverlapping scales, indexes, or single items. This procedure reduces the number of scores that are required to define a variable yet increases the range of values for any one variable. It also increases the reliability of the summary scores, since they are now based on a larger data base. It also provides a convenient method of dealing with missing data, since a variable may still be defined based on items to which the patient responded. Also, by using positive and negatively worded items for the same variable, the investigator can further increase the precision of his assessment. These procedures increase the chances of the assessments being valid. The methods used to generate composite scores were Likert's method of summated ratings (59) or Guttman's Scalogram Analysis (60).

Major scales or indexes of EORTC–Lung Group Quality of Life Questionnaire are functional status, symptoms of lung cancer, side effects of treatment, fatigue and malaise, psychological distress, sense of well-being/satisfaction, and social interaction. Measures of internal consistency (i.e., Chronbach's alpha) ranged from 0.69 for social interaction to 0.95 for symptoms of lung cancer. The validity of the overall tool was established in three ways. First, a series of factor analyses were performed with representative items from each of the variables. If these items loaded in different factors, then this suggested the presence of construct validity. Next, a multitrait scaling technique was used to test for item-discriminant validity, and the results supported the distinctiveness of the scales studied. Finally, intercorrelations between each of the scales were also performed revealing correlations ranging in strength from 0.21 to 0.58, suggesting modest but distinct relationships between the variables.

The psychometric characterization of this instrument reflects a distinct theoretical orientation toward how to incorporate valuations into a quality of life assessment. Bush (61) stated the alternatives as *relative preferences or relative frequencies* approaches. The EORTC–Lung Group Quality of Life Questionnaire was designed to be consistent with a relative frequencies approach to the valuation task.

ANAMESTIC COMPARATIVE SELF-ASSESSMENT

The Anamestic Comparative Self-Assessment is not so much an assessment instrument as it is an assessment method. In contrast to the Quality of Well-Being Index, which disaggregates and then "constructs" a measure of well-being, the Anamestic Comparative Self-Assessment directly assesses well-being (62). Respondents are asked to select the best and worst periods of their lives. Numbers are then assigned to these extremes (usually $+5$ to -5), making a scale that is a totally self-defined measure of well-being. No single patient's scale is like that of any other patient. The impact of treatment and disease on well-being is measured by asking patients to indicate where on their scale they were just prior to the onset of their illness, what their well-being was when they experienced symptoms, and what it was when they were diagnosed. Difference scores are calculated to compare individuals.

Anamestic Comparative Self-Assessment measures covary with changes in performance status, estimated life expectancy, and changes in a patient's attitude toward their disease (63). This suggests that the instrument can track important clinical phenomena. Its major weakness is that the assessment is sensitive to immediate events or circumstances that may be unrelated to the patient's disease or treatment. In addition, the scores may be biased by the clinical investigator during the process of facilitating the patient's scaling activities. A third limitation is that having obtained a measure, there is no way to determine what produced it.

The Anamestic Comparative Self-Assessment provides a very simple and direct method of measuring the value structure of a respondent. Its simplicity, as documented above, is also its limitation. Whether procedural changes can enhance its usefulness remains to be determined.

The Anamestic Comparative Self-Assessment is not the only attempt to incorporate patient values into the design of a quality of life assessment. Ferrans and Powers (63) reported the development of a 32-item quality of life index for dialysis patients which scaled a wide range of quality of life domains in terms of satisfaction/dissatisfaction and importance. The assessment of importance immediately distinguishes their instrument from many others because it assesses patient's values.

STAGE II BREAST CANCER QUESTIONNAIRE

The Anamestic Comparative Self-Assessment, the Ferrans and Power's importance scaling, and the Stage II Breast Cancer Questionnaire each incorporate valuation issues in the administration or development of their respective instruments. The Stage II Breast Cancer Questionnaire was developed by Levine et al. (64). In this questionnaire, patients were asked to rate the importance of 99 statements which described being a breast cancer patient. These items fell into seven categories, and the highest rated items in each of these categories were selected to generate a final questionnaire consisting of 30 items. The item that received the highest endorsement was feeling positive about the future (4.44 of a 5.0 range). Thus, the process whereby items were selected represents a valuation process. Table 3 indicates the category of items included.

Comparison of the Stage II Breast Cancer Questionnaire with a number of standard quality of life assessment instruments revealed that it and the Karnofsky were most likely to detect changes over time when patients received one of two chemotherapy treatments. This suggests that the Stage II Breast Cancer Questionnaire can track important clinical phenomena, better than the RAND emotional and physical measure and Spitzer's Quality of Life Index (74). Like these other measures, the Stage II Breast Cancer Questionnaire weights each item equally and sums scores for each item to give a total score.

TIME WITHOUT SYMPTOMS OF DISEASE AND SUBJECTIVE TOXIC EFFECTS OF TREATMENT (TWIST)

Gelber and Goldhirsch (65) have developed a general methodological approach to quality of life assessment rather than a specific instrument. The TWIST measures the total time that patients are without symptoms while receiving cancer treatment. Since the toxic symptoms patients experience vary as a function of the disease severity and type of treatment, each study has its own set of criteria to determine when the patient is symptom-free.

Gelber and Goldhirsch (65) illustrate how to use their method with a representative patient who refused treatment during the 12th month of participation in a clinical trial. This patient was nauseous and vomited from the second cycle to the fourth cycle, and lost her hair from the third to the 11th cycle, after which she did not need a wig. She had a second mastectomy performed at 18 months, and is alive and well in the 64 month after-study entry. The TWIST score is calculated by subtracting from the 64 months survival period the 3 months the patient was without hair, the 10 months she had chemotherapy-induced symptoms, and the 3 months associated with having and recovering from a mastectomy. The final TWIST score is 48. Calculating the cumulative TWIST score at successive time intervals makes it possible to generate TWIST Kaplan-Meir functions comparable to functions generated for overall survival or disease-free interval data.

The TWIST measures the time that patients are free of subjective symptoms. The assumption made is that the quality of symptom-free time at the onset of treatment, post-initial treatment, and post-treatment following recurrence is the same, independent of what has transpired prior to its measurement. Thus, in the example given the patient had no symptoms after dropping out of treatment following double mastectomies and failing on chemotherapy.

Figure 3 illustrates the variety of patterns that emerge when the entire time course for a variety of patients receiving the same basic treatment are considered (66). The figure illustrates the diversity of events that occur over time and also at any one time. Although adding time has a superficial appearance of objectivity, it actually masks the interactions that occur between time intervals as a function of the patient's disease and its treatment.

Another concern with the TWIST methodology is the arbitrary nature of defining a subjective toxic effect. This can be illustrated by comparing what Gelber and Goldhirsch (65) list as toxic to what Levine et al. (64) found to be the most important

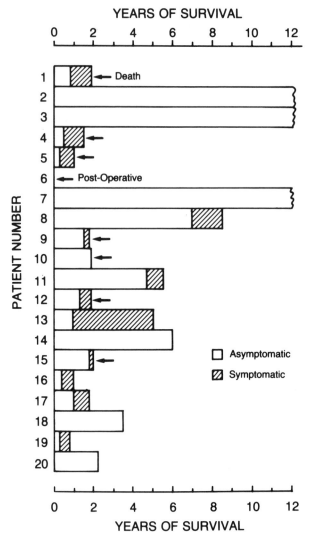

FIG. 3. The natural history of colorectal cancer following major hepatic resections. The figure illustrates the great diversity of outcomes for patients with a common disease, and emphasizes again the importance of valuing the time in particular states.

concerns of breast cancer patients. Clinicians and patients do not necessarily agree on what is an adverse effect (67). The issue is who should define an adverse effect.

Goldhirsch et al. (68) are sensitive to the above concerns, stating in a more recent paper, "This 'all-or-none' analysis was somewhat unrealistic, as it assigned no value to both the period of life with toxicity and to the period following systemic relapse" (77; pp. 36). Using their version of the two-component model of a quality of life assessment, they then generated a quality-adjusted TWIST measure (Q-TWIST). The Q-TWIST consists of weighted estimates of the time with toxicities, plus the period of time associated with relapse. Knowing the time with toxicities, without toxicities, and in relapse for the three arms of the study being evaluated, the authors were able to display each component separately in survival plots. Using arbitrary values for weightings (i.e., utility coefficients ranging from 0 to 1.0) they were also able to perform threshold analyses so that it is possible to display in one graph what treatment a patient would select depending on the weightings applied to the time with toxicities and the time in relapse.

Goldhirsch et al. (68) respond to the criticism concerning the arbitrary nature of adding components of the TWIST (see above) by suggesting that different time periods can be weighted differently (i.e., the time periods can be discounted). This approach, although applicable for groups of patients, would become unmanageable if many time periods were involved and if used for individual patient decisions.

The Q-TWIST methodology creates a framework within which values (or utilities) of individual patients can be used to assess preferences among several treatments. The Q-TWIST methodology makes no statement on how to assess the values of cancer patients. Some methods for estimating values are based on reference groups (55,61,69), and others involve direct patient assessments (70). Llewellyn-Thomas et al. (71) have demonstrated that values are less dependent on the assessment method used than on the components of the judgment task itself (such as the type of material involved, or order of presentation of tasks [71]). Thus, more will have to be learned about how preferences are made before the usefulness of the Q-TWIST in determining individual patient treatment preferences will be established.

The TWIST and Q-TWIST methodologies represent a major attempt to incorporate quality of life issues in the decision-making processes in clinical trials. The authors are particularly intent on separating the statistical analysis of a clinical trial from the clinically relevant treatment decisions that would use the Q-TWIST methodologies. The success of this method is critically dependent on the assumption that different time intervals during a clinical trial can be added. Also of concern is the fact that the database used to illustrate the Q-TWIST methods includes a no-treatment observation group. It is important to demonstrate that the Q-TWIST methodology is useful for clinical trials comparing standard and experimental treatments.

METHODS OF INCORPORATING VALUES INTO QUALITY OF LIFE ASSESSMENTS

Psychometric evaluations of cancer-specific quality of life studies show them to have acceptable reliability and validity (27). This provides important support for further development of disease-specific instruments (72). The two-component model of the judgment process is helpful in organizing and understanding the significance of different strategies for developing quality of life assessments. At least four methods exist for incorporating values into a quality of life study assessment.

The first method involves structuring the clinical research so that an obvious value preference is incorporated into the study. Asking who is better off—an amputee or someone whose limb is spared, or someone who has a colostomy or someone whose anal sphincter is spared—sometimes has obvious answers. The assessment need only confirm the existence of the valued outcome; no assessment of preference may be needed. Yet as the limb and anal sphincter-sparing studies quoted above indicate, the answers to these questions usually reflect relative advantages of one procedure over the other. Under these circumstances direct assessment may be necessary, especially if the clinician wishes to select between two or more treatment options. On the other hand, if the purpose of the assessment is to monitor and improve the

TABLE 4. *Components of a quality of life judgment*

Affective dimensions	Cognitive dimensions	
	Satisfied	Dissatisfied
Good:	Achievers	Aspirers
Bad:	Resigners	Frustrated

quality of care provided, then the relativistic outcome may be needed to stimulate modification of the treatment regimen.

The second method of incorporating a patient's values into quality of life studies involves manipulating the testing methods so that preferences are incorporated into the design of the assessment instrument. For example, in the Anamestic Comparative Self-Assessment we learn of the patient's most and least preferred states. These states are then used to create a preference scale to judge current events (e.g., being diagnosed, receiving treatment). In the Ferrans and Powers (63) study, respondents scale single items in terms of satisfaction and importance. This is an approximation of what is usually a multicomponent preference evaluation. Finally, the item selection procedure in the Levine et al. (64) study insures that patient preferences have been considered when structuring a quality of life assessment.

The third method, the relative frequency approach, takes advantage of statistical procedures to order quality of life outcomes; the fourth approach, direct valuation or relative preference approach, was discussed above.

THE PSYCHOLOGY OF QUALITY OF LIFE ASSESSMENT

Szalai (73) was the first to point out that when someone is asked, "How are you?" they are, in effect being asked to make a personal quality of life assessment. The phrase represents a quality of life assessment because it requires that the person reflect about current and past events, and value these events in some global manner. This everyday event involves the same two-component process found in all quality of life assessments, and would be expected to be influenced by the same factors that ordinarily influence judgments.

It has been observed that cancer patients report better qualities of life than would be expected from an independent assessment of the impact of their disease and its treatments (27). There are several explanations of this observation. De Haes and von Knippenberg (27) suggest that a patient's response may reflect perceptual restructuring, i.e., expecting less, the patient feels that he or she is doing well. Helson and Bevan's adaptation theory would account for this phenomenon (74).

An alternative explanation, reflecting a more psychopathological perspective, suggests that patients tend to respond in a socially desirable way (75) and provide responses they think the physician (or the interviewer) wants to hear. Hurny et al. (75) found that increasing age (up to age 60) and having a chronic illness increased the chance of a socially desirable response.

Another explanation of cancer patients' more positive perception of their quality of life than anticipated reflects a cognitive perspective. Campbell et al. (40) suggest that a quality of life judgment contains a cognitive and affective component, each of which can change independently of the other. Table 4 illustrates the four aspirational outcomes. Studies which demonstrate that cancer patients remain satisfied may simply be masking the negative affective changes which will occur concurrently and which require independent assessment. As de Haes and von Knippenberg (27) point out, the same explanation could account for the observation by Irwin et al. (76), who found that patients who received radiation rated their quality of life as being as satisfying as "normal" persons, but who did not assess the affective dimension of these judgments.

Whether the quality of life of a major proportion of cancer patients is indeed comparable to noncancer patients or healthy persons remains controversial. What is obvious is that the cancer patient is not passively responding to his or her state, but is actively processing events and circumstances of their existence.

Cognition is usually described as a two-stage process. In the first stage, information is interpreted and in the second stage the judgment is produced (77). How the interpretation or framing of information affects judgments of cancer patients can be illustrated by the Sanger and Reznikoff (78) study. These authors studied breast cancer patients who received either a modified radical or segmental mastectomy. They asked each patient to retrospectively rate their satisfaction with their body appearance prior to their surgery, and the importance each of several body parts had to them. They also asked each of the patients if they were aware of the existence of alternative surgical procedures, and found that all 20 of the women who had the modified radical mastectomy were not aware, prior to their surgeries, that an alternative surgery existed. What they found was that the women who had the modified radical mastectomy rated their preoperative breast as more satisfying to them than the women who had the segmental mastectomy. Analysis of covariance was used to separate preoperative from postoperative satisfaction scores. Subsequent analyses revealed that segmental mastectomy patients experienced significantly less change in satisfaction in their postoperative breast then the modified radical mastectomy patients.

Clearly, questions about alternative surgical procedures or retrospective ratings of satisfaction with body parts provides a context within which judgments concerning current satisfaction with body parts may be made. Why else would two groups of women, with presumably similar features, rate their past appearance so differently? How the inferences drawn from the study would change if a different context existed for the patients remains a worthwhile research task.

Llewellyn-Thomas et al. (71) have been studying the effect of various methodological factors on the values assigned to various health states by cancer patients. They found that order of presentation of tasks, type, and amount of material involved in the valuation task, and the valuation method (standard gamble, or category ratings) each influenced the values generated. They suggest that patients adopt various heuristics as aids in making judgments. Heuristics are cognitive techniques that people use to simplify the task of making judgments, but which can also result in the person using less of the available information in the judgment. What rules or tricks cancer patients use when generating values have yet to be determined, as well as whether their heuristics are different from what noncancer patients use or persons without illness use. Whatever the outcome, it seems likely that cancer patients use such cognitive devices when making judgments, and that understanding their role will be an important part of understanding quality of life judgments by cancer patients.

Although it has been argued that cancer treatment leaves cancer patients intellectually normal (79), it is becoming increasingly obvious that this assumption may require direct empirical evaluation for particular types of cancer patients. Thus, a heavily pretreated patient being asked to participate in a phase 1 study, the elderly, the metastatic patient treated with a multidrug regimen, all may have impaired neurological functions that will alter their cognition. The neuropsychology of quality of life assessment remains a relatively unexplored research area, although there are sufficient reports in the literature to warrant its serious study (80,81).

CONCLUSIONS

The major focus of this chapter provides a conceptual foundation to organize and understand the assessments used to measure the cancer patient's quality of life. This chapter also illustrates how a quality of life assessment can become part of the social and political events that lead to treatment innovation and development. Also documented was what is known about the psychology of a quality of life assessment for cancer patients.

REFERENCES

1. Barofsky I. Quality of life assessment: Evolution of the concept. In: Ventaffrida V, Yancik R, van Dam FSAM, Tamburini M, eds. *Quality of life assessment and cancer treatment*. Amsterdam: Elsevier, 1986;11–18.
2. Hammond KR, McClelland GH, Mumpower J. *Human judgment and decision making*. New York: Praeger, 1980.
3. Kaplan RM, Anderson JP. A general health policy model: Update and applications. *Health Serv Res* 1988;23:203–235.
4. Bergner M, Bobbitt RA, Kressel S, Pollard WE, Gilson BS, Morris JR. The Sickness Impact Profile: Conceptual foundations and methodology for the development of a health status measure. *Int J Health Serv* 1976;6:393–415.
5. Ware JE. Methodological considerations in the selection of health status assessment procedures. In: Wenger NK, Mattson ME, Furberg CD, Elinson J, eds. *Assessment of quality of life in clinical trials of cardiovascular therapies*. New York: Le Jacq, 1984;87–111.
6. *Health Interview Survey Procedure: 1957–1974*. Series 1, no. 11, National Center for Health Statistics, United States Department of Health, Education and Welfare. DHEW (HRA) 75-311.
7. Rosenberg SA. Principles of surgical oncology. In: DeVita VT, Jr., Hellman S, Rosenberg SA, eds. *Cancer: Principles and practice of oncology*. Philadelphia: Lippincott, 1985;215–225.
8. Jackson SM. *Radiation oncology: A handbook for residents and the allied health professions*. St. Louis: Green, 1985.
9. Torrance GW. Health states worse than death. In: van Eimeren W, Engelbrecht R, Flagle CD, eds. Third International Conference on System Science in Health Care. Berlin: Springer, 1984;1085–1089.
10. Sutherland HJ, Llewellyn-Thomas HA, Boyd NF, Till JE. Attitudes towards quality of survival: The concept of "maximal endurable time." *Med Decis Making* 1982;2:229–309.
11. Hellman S. Principles of radiation therapy. In: DeVita VT, Jr., Hellman S, Rosenberg SA, eds. *Cancer: Principles and practice of oncology*. Philadelphia: Lippincott, 1985;227–255.
12. Williams NS, Johnston D. The quality of life after rectal excision for low rectal cancer. *Br J Surg* 1983;70:219–225.
13. *Cancer Patient Survival Report #5*, United States Department of Health Education and Welfare, Publ. No. (NIH) 77-992, 1976.
14. Rosenberg SA. Soft tissue sarcoma of the extremities. In: Sugarbaker PH, Nicholson TH, eds. *Atlas of extremity sarcoma surgery*. Philadelphia: Lippincott, 1984;1–17.
15. Rosenberg SA, Kent H, Costa J, Webber BL, Young R, Chabner B, Baker AR, Chretien PB, Cohen MH, de Moss EV, Sears HF, Seipp C, Simon R. Prospective randomized evaluation of the role of limb-sparing surgery, radiation therapy and adjuvant chemotherapy in the treatment of adult soft-tissue sarcomas. *Surgery* 1978;84:62–69.
16. Sugarbaker PH, Barofsky I, Rosenberg SA, Gianola FJ. Quality of life assessment of patients in extremity sarcoma clinical trials. *Surgery* 1982;91:17–23.
17. Shamberger RC, Sherins RJ, Rosenberg SA. The effect of postoperative and adjuvant chemotherapy and radiotherapy on testicular function in men undergoing treatment for soft tissue sarcoma. *Cancer* 1981;47:2368–2374.

18. Lampert MH, Gerber LH, Glatstein E, Rosenberg SA, Danoff JV. Soft tissue sarcoma: Functional outcome after wide local excision and radiation therapy. *Arch Phys Med Rahabil* 1984;65:477–480.
19. Sugarbaker PH, Nicholson TH. *Atlas of extremity sarcoma surgery.* Philadelphia: Lippincott, 1984.
20. Tepper J, Rosenberg SA, Glatstein E. Radiation therapy technique in soft tissue sarcomas of the extremity—Policies of treatment at the National Cancer Institute. *Int J Radiat Oncol Biol Phys* 1982;8:263–273.
21. Hicks JE, Lampert MH, Gerber LH, Glatstein E, Danoff J. Functional outcome update in patients with soft tissue sarcoma undergoing wide local excision and radiation. *Arch Phys Med Rehabil* 1985;66:542–543.
22. National Institutes of Health Consensus Conference. Limb-sparing treatment of adult soft-tissue sarcomas and osteosarcomas. *JAMA* 1985;254:1791–1794.
23. Priestman T. Evaluation of quality of life in women with breast cancer. In: Aaronson NK, Beckmann JH, eds. *The quality of life of the cancer patient.* New York: Raven Press, 1987;193–200.
24. Fennell ML, Warnecke RB. *The diffusion of medical innovations: An applied network analysis.* New York: Plenum, 1988.
25. Roberts G. A study of the literature on clinical aspects of quality of life. *Centre for Medicines Research* 1988;6:(2)6.
26. Clark A, Fallowfield LJ. Quality of life measurement in patients with malignant disease: A review. *Ann R Soc Med* 1986;79:165–169.
27. de Haes JCJM, van Knippenberg FCE. Quality of life of cancer patients: Review of the literature. In: Aaronson NK, Beckmann JH, eds. *The quality of life of the cancer patient.* New York: Raven Press, 1987;167–182.
28. Fayers PM, Jones DR. Measuring and analyzing quality of life in cancer clinical trials: A review. *Stat Med* 1983;2:429–446.
29. Selby P. Measurement of quality of life in cancer. In: Walker SR, ed. *Quality of life: Assessment and application.* Lancaster: MTP Press, 1987;203–247.
30. van Dam FSAM, Linssen ACG, Couzijn AL. Evaluating quality of life: Behavioral measures in clinical cancer trials. In: Staquet M, Sylvester R, Buyse M, eds. *The practice of clinical trials.* New York: Oxford University Press, 1983.
31. Aaronson NK, Beckmann JH. *The quality of life of the cancer patient.* New York: Raven Press, 1987.
32. Katz S. The Portugal Conference: Measuring quality of life and functional status in clinical and epidemiological research. *J Chron Dis* 1987;40:459–650.
33. Takeda F. *Quality of life in cancer patients.* Saitama, Japan: Diamond, 1985.
34. Ventaffrida V, Yancik R, van Dam FSAM, Tamburini M. *Quality of life assessment and cancer treatment.* Amsterdam: Elsevier, 1986.
35. Schmale AH, Morrow GR, Schmitt MH, Adler LM, Enelow A, Murawski BJ, Gates C. Well-being of cancer survivors. *Psychosom Med* 1983;45:163–169.
36. Derogatis LR. The Psychosocial Adjustment to Illness Scale (PAIS). *J Psychosom Res* 1986;30:77–91.
37. Cella DF, Jacobsen PB, Orav EJ, Holland JC, Silberfarb PM, Rafla S (for Cancer and Leukemia Group B, Brookline, Massachusetts). A brief POMS measure of distress for cancer patients. *J Chron Dis* 1987;40:939–942.
38. Karnofsky DA, Buchenal JH. The clinical evaluation of chemotherapeutic agents in cancer. In: Macleod CM, ed. *Evaluation of chemotherapeutic agents.* New York: Columbia, 1949;191–205.
39. Spitzer WO, Dobson AJ, Hall J, Chesterman E, Levi J, Shepherd R, Battista RN, Catchlove BR. Measuring the quality of life of cancer patients. *J Chron Dis* 1981;34:585–597.
40. Campbell A, Converse PE, Rodgers WL. *The quality of American life.* New York: Sage, 1976.
41. Veenhoven R. *Conditions of happiness.* Dordrecht: Reidel, 1984.
42. Schipper H, Clinch J, McMurray A, Levitt M. Measuring the quality of life of cancer patients: The Functional Living Index–Cancer: Development and validation. *J Clin Oncol* 1984;2:472–483.
43. EORTC Lung Cancer Cooperative Group (1982): *Protocol 08825: Induction versus induction plus maintenance chemotherapy in small cell lung cancer.* Brussels: EORTC Data Center, 1982.
44. Ganz PA, Haskell CM, Figlin RA, La Sota N, Siau J. Estimating the quality of life in a clinical trial of patients with metastatic lung cancer using the Karnofsky Performance Status and Functional Living Index–Cancer. *Cancer* 1988;61:849–856.
45. Perloff JM, Persons JB. Biases resulting from the use of indexes: An application to attributional style and depression. *Psychol Bull* 1988;103:95–104.
46. Presant CA, Klahr C, Hogan L. Evaluating quality of life in oncology patients: Pilot observations. *Oncol Nurs For* 1981;8:26–30.
47. Padilla GV, Presant C, Grant MM, Metter G, Lipsett J, Heide F. Quality of life index for patients with cancer. *Res Nurs Health* 1983;6:117–126.
48. Padilla GV, Grant MM. Quality of life as a cancer nursing outcome variable. *Am Nursing Sci* 1985;8:45–60.

49. Priestman T, Baum M. Evaluation of quality of life in patients receiving treatment for advanced breast cancer. *Lancet* 1976;1:899–901.
50. Maguire GP. Monitoring the quality of life in cancer patients and their relatives. In: Symington T, Williams AE, McVie JG, eds. *Cancer-assessment and monitoring.* Edinburgh: Churchill Livingstone, 1980;40–52.
51. Morris T, Greer HS, White P. Psychological and social adjustment to mastectomy: A two-year follow-up. *Cancer* 1977;40:2381–2387.
52. Baum M, Priestman TJ, West RR, Jones EM. A comparison in subjective responses in a trial comparing endocrine and cytotoxic treatment in advanced carcinoma of the breast. In: Mouridsen HT, Palshof T, eds. *Breast cancer—Experimental and clinical aspects.* Oxford: Pergamon, 1980;223–226.
53. Priestman T, Baum M, Priestman S. The quality of life in breast cancer patients. In: *Proceedings of the First EORTC Workshop on Quality of Life,* Amsterdam, 1981.
54. Selby PJ, Chapman JAW, Etazadi-Amoli J, Dalley D, Boyd NF. The development of a method for assessing the quality of life of cancer patients. *Br J Cancer* 1984;50:13–22.
55. Bergner M, Bobbitt RA, Carter WB, Gilson BS. The Sickness Impact Profile: Development and final revision of a health status measure. *Med Care* 1981;19:787–806.
56. Boyd NF, Selby PJ, Sutherland HJ, Hogg S. Measurement of the clinical status of patients with breast cancer: Evidence for the validity of self assessment with linear analogue scales. *J Clin Epidemiol* 1988;41:243–250.
57. Stewart AL, Ware JE, Brook RH. Advances in the measurement of functional status: Construction of aggregate indexes. *Med Care* 1981;19:473–488.
58. Aaronson NK, Bakker W, Stewart A, van Dam FSAM, van Zandwijk N, Yarnold JR, Kirpatrick A. Multidimensional approach to the measurement of quality of life in lung cancer clinical trials. In: Aaronson NK, Beckmann JH, eds. *The quality of life of the cancer patient.* New York: Raven Press, 1987;63–82.
59. Likert R. A technique for the measurement of attitudes. *Arch Psychol* 1932;140:1–55.
60. Guttman LA. A basis for scaling qualitative data. *Am Soc Rev* 1944;9:139–150.
61. Bush JW. Relative preferences versus relative frequencies in health-related quality of life evaluation. In: Wenger NK, Mattson ME, Furberg CD, Elinson J, eds. *Assessment of quality of life in clinical trials of cardiovascular therapies.* New York: Le Jacq, 1984;118–139.
62. Bernheim JC, Buyse M. Amnestic comparative self-assessment, a method to measure the subjective quality of life of cancer patients. *J Psychosoc Oncol* 1983;4:25–38.
63. Ferrans CE, Powers MJ. Quality of life index: Development and psychometric properties. *Am Nurs Sci* 1985;8:15–24.
64. Levine MN, Guyatt GH, Gent M, De Pauw S, Goodyear MD, Hryniuk WM, Arnold A, Findlay B, Skillings JR, Bramwell VH, Levin L, Bush H, Abu-Zahra H, Kotalik J. Quality of life in stage II breast cancer: An instrument for clinical trials. *J Clin Oncol* 1988;6:1798–1810.
65. Gelber RD, Goldhirsch A. A new endpoint for the assessment of adjuvant therapy in postmenopausal women with operable breast cancer. *J Clin Oncol* 1986;4:1772–1779.
66. Adson MA, van Heerden JA. Major hepatic resections for metastatic colorectal cancer. *Ann Surg* 1980;191:576–583.
67. Slevin ML, Plant H, Lynch D, Frinkwater J, Gregory WM. Who should measure quality of life, the doctor or the patient? *Br J Cancer* 1988;57:109–112.
68. Goldhirsch A, Gelber RD, Simes RJ, Glasziou P, Coates AS. for the Ludwig Breast Cancer Study Group. Costs and benefits of adjuvant therapy in breast cancer: A quality-adjusted survival analysis. *J Clin Oncol* 1989;7:36–44.
69. Torrance GW. Health status index models: A unified mathematical view. *Manag Sci* 1976;22:990–1001.
70. McNeil BJ, Varady PD, Burrows BA, Adelstein SJ. Measures of clinical efficacy: Cost-effectiveness calculations in the diagnosis and treatment of hypertensive renovascular disease. *N Engl J Med* 1975;293:216–221.
71. Llewellyn-Thomas HA, Sutherland HJ, Tibshirani R, Ciampi A, Till JE, Boyd NF. Describing health states: Methological issues in obtaining values for health states. *Med Care* 1984;22:543–552.
72. Barofsky I, Sugarbaker PH. Health status indexes: Disease specific and general population measures. *Proceedings of the Public Health Conference on Records and Statistics,* June, 1978, Washington, D.C. DHEW (PHS) 79-1214, 1979;263–269.
73. Szalai A. The meaning of comparative research on the quality of life. In: Szakau A, Andrews FM, eds. The quality of life: Comparative studies. Beverly Hills, California: Sage, 1980;7–21.
74. Helson H, Bevan W. *Contemporary Approaches to Psychology.* Princeton, NJ: Van Nostrand, 1967.
75. Hurny C, Piasetsky E, Bagin R, Holland J. High social desirability in patients being treated for advanced colorectal or bladder cancer: Eventual impact on the assessment of quality of life. *J Psychosoc Oncol* 1987;5:19–29.
76. Irwin PH, Gottlieb A, Kramer S, Danoff B. Quality of life after radiation therapy: A study of 309 cancer survivors. *Soc Indicators Res* 1982;10:187–210.

77. Tversky A, Kahneman D. The framing of decisions and the psychology of choice. *Science* 1981;211:453–458.
78. Sanger CK, Reznikoff M. A comparison of the psychological effects of breast-saving procedures with the modified radical mastectomy. *Cancer* 1981;48:2341–2346.
79. Barofsky I. Issues and methods in the psychosocial assessment of the cancer patient. In: Bradley LA, Prokop CK, eds. *Medical psychology: A new perspective.* New York: Academic, 1981;55–65.
80. Adams F, Larson D, Goepfert H. Does depression in head and neck cancer mask organic brain disease? *Otolaryngol Head and Neck Surg* 1984;92:618–624.
81. Carr I. The Ophelia syndrome: Memory loss in Hodgkin's disease. *Lancet* 1982;1:844–845.

Quality of Life Assessments in Clinical
Trials, edited by B. Spilker. Raven
Press, Ltd. New York © 1990.

32

Chronic Rheumatic Disease

Matthew H. Liang, Jeffrey N. Katz, and Katherine S. Ginsburg

*Departments of Rheumatology/Immunology and Medicine, Robert B.
Brigham Multipurpose Arthritis Center, Brigham and Women's Hospital,
Harvard Medical School, Boston, Massachusetts 02115*

The more than 100 diverse rheumatic disorders (Table 1) are bound together by musculoskeletal complaints and disability. With few exceptions, their cause is unknown, primary prevention is not possible, and cure is not possible. Most forms of arthritis do not shorten life span. For practical purposes, it is useful to think of four common patterns of rheumatic disability: rheumatoid, osteoarthritis, spondylitis, and systemic rheumatic disease disabilities.

Rheumatoid disability (rheumatoid arthritis, seronegative polyarthritis, juvenile arthritis, psoriatic arthritis, Reiter's syndrome) arises in conditions with polyarticular synovitis such as rheumatoid arthritis and juvenile rheumatoid arthritis. Rheumatoid arthritis is the most common chronic inflammatory disease leading to disability, and rheumatoid disability is characterized by multiple joint involvement, chronicity, variable symptoms of disability, and occasional systemic symptoms such as fatigue, fever, and weight loss.

Features of rheumatoid disability reflect the person's age and social role. In children, polyarthritis affects biological, psychological, and social growth and development. It may interfere with the attainment of educational and career goals, and the acquisition of skills required for a job and family life. In adolescence it may interfere with emancipation from parents, interacting with peers, self-esteem, and body image.

Polyarthritis in young adults affects the critical issues of that stage which are separation from parents and home, training, career choice, achieving economic independence, peer relationships, and finding a mate. In middle age, polyarthritis may affect career development, raising a family, family relationships, or return to work when children are grown. Polyarthritis occurring in older persons accentuates the aging process and accelerates physical dependency. The deformities associated with chronic arthritis contribute to psychosocial disability and physical limitation.

Osteoarthritis disability, with its involvement of the small joints of the hand or of the weight-bearing joints of the lower extremity and back, is characterized by onset in middle or old age, lack of systemic symptoms, and mono- or pauci-articular involvement.

Osteoarthritis disability unfolds slowly, paralleling the aging process, thus its psychosocial impact is not as apparent as rheumatoid disability. Indeed, many individuals (and physicians) assume that musculoskeletal symptoms from osteoarthritis are

TABLE 1. *Classification of the Rheumatic Diseases*

I. Diffuse connective tissue diseases
    A. Rheumatoid arthritis
    B. Juvenile rheumatoid arthritis
        1. Systemic onset (Still's disease)
        2. Polyarticular onset
        3. Pauci-articular onset
    C. Systemic lupus erythematosus
    D. Systemic sclerosis
    E. Polymyositis/dermatomyositis
    F. Necrotizing vasculitis and other vasculopathies
        1. Polyarteritis nodosa group (includes hepatitis B associated arteritis and Churg-Strauss allergic granulomatosis)
        2. Hypersensitivity vasculitis (includes Schönlein-Henoch purpura, hypocomplementemic cutaneous vasculitis, and others)
        3. Wegener's granulomatosis
        4. Giant cell arteritis
            a. Temporal arteritis
            b. Takayasu's arteritis
        5. Mucocutaneous lymph node syndrome (Kawasaki disease)
        6. Behçet's disease
        7. Cryoglobulinemia
        8. Juvenile dermatomyositis
    G. Sjögren's syndrome
    H. Overlap syndromes (includes undifferentiated and mixed connective tissue disease)
    I. Others (includes polymyalgia rheumatica, panniculitis (Weber-Christian disease), erythema nodosum, relapsing polychondritis, diffuse fasciitis with eosinophilia, adult onset Still's disease)

II. Arthritis associated with spondylitis
    A. Ankylosing spondylitis
    B. Reiter's syndrome
    C. Psoriatic arthritis
    D. Arthritis associated with chronic inflammatory bowel disease

III. Degenerative joint disease (osteoarthritis, osteoarthrosis)
    A. Primary (includes erosive osteoarthritis)
    B. Secondary

IV. Arthritis, tenosynovitis, and bursitis associated with infectious agents
    A. Direct
        1. Bacterial
            a. Gram-positive cocci (staphylococcus and others)
            b. Gram-negative cocci (gonococcus and others)
            c. Gram-negative rods
            d. Mycobacteria
            e. Spirochetes including Lyme disease
            f. Others including leprosy and mycoplasma
        2. Viral including hepatitis
        3. Fungal
        4. Parasitic
        5. Unknown, suspected (Whipple's disease)
    B. Indirect (reactive)
        1. Bacterial (includes acute rheumatic fever, intestinal bypass, postdysenteric-shigella, Yersinia, and others)
        2. Viral (hepatitis B)

V. Metabolic and endocrine diseases associated with rheumatic states
    A. Crystal-induced conditions
        1. Monodosium urate (gout)
        2. Calcium pyrophosphate dihydrate (pseudogout, chondrocalcinosis)
        3. Apatite and other basic calcium phosphates
        4. Oxalate

  B. Biochemical abnormalities
    1. Amyloidosis
    2. Vitamin C deficiency (scurvy)
    3. Specific enzyme-deficiency states (includes Fabry's, Farber's, and others)
    4. Hyperlipoproteinemias (types II, IIa, IV, and others)
    5. Mucopolysaccharidoses
    6. Hemoglobinopathies (Sickle cell disease and others)
    7. True connective tissue disorders (Ehlers-Danlos syndrome, Marfan's sign, osteogenesis inperfecta, pseudoxanthoma elasticum, and others)
    8. Hemochromatosis
    9. Wilson's disease (hepatolenticular degeneration)
    10. Ochronosis (alkaptonuria)
    11. Gaucher's disease
    12. Others
  C. Endocrine diseases
    1. Diabetes mellitus
    2. Acromegaly
    3. Hyperparathyroidism
    4. Thyroid disease
    5. Others
  D. Immunodeficiency diseases, primary immunodeficiency, acquired immunodeficiency syndrome (AIDS)
  E. Other hereditary disorders
    A. Arthogryposis multiplex congenita
    2. Hypermobility syndromes
    3. Myositis ossificans progressiva

VI. Neoplasms
  A. Primary (e.g., synovioma, synoviosarcoma)
  B. Metastatic
  C. Multiple myeloma
  D. Leukemia and lymphoma
  E. Villonodular synovitis
  F. Osteochondromatosis
  G. Other

VII. Neuropathic disorders
  A. Charcot joints
  B. Compression neuropathies
    1. Peripheral entrapment (carpal tunnel syndrome and others)
    2. Radiculopathy
    3. Spinal stenosis
  C. Reflex sympathetic dystrophy
  D. Others

VIII. Bone, periosteal, and cartilage disorders associated with articular manifestations
  A. Osteoporosis
    1. Generalized
    2. Localized (regional and transient)
  B. Osteomalacia
  C. Hypertrophic osteoarthropathy
  D. Diffuse idiopathic skeletal hyperostosis (includes ankylosing vertebral hyperostosis—Forestier disease)
  E. Osteitis
    1. Generalized (osteitis deformans—Paget's disease of bone)
    2. Localized (osteitis condensans illii; osteitis pubis)
  F. Osteonecrosis
  G. Osteochondritis (osteochondritis dissecans)
  H. Bone and joint dysplasias
  I. Slipped capital femoral epiphysis
  J. Costochondritis (includes Teitze's syndrome)
  K. Osteolysis and chondrolysis
  L. Osteomyelitis

TABLE 1. *Continued*

IX. Nonarticular rheumatism
    A. Myofascial pain syndromes
        1. Generalized (fibrositis, fibromyalgia)
        2. Regional
    B. Low back pain and intervertebral disc disorders
    C. Tendinitis (tenosynovitis and/or bursitis)
        1. Subacromial/subdeltoid bursitis
        2. Bicipital tendinitis, tenosynovitis
        3. Olecranon bursitis
        4. Epicondylitis, medial or lateral humeral
        5. DeQuervain's tenosynovitis
        6. Adhesive capsulitis of the shoulder (frozen shoulder)
        7. Trigger finger
        8. Other
    D. Ganglion cysts
    E. Fasciitis
    F. Chronic ligament and muscle pain
    G. Vasomotor disorders
        1. Erythromelagia
        2. Raynaud's disease or phenomenon
    H. Miscellaneous pain syndromes (includes weather sensitivity, psychogenic rheumatism)

X. Miscellaneous disorders
    A. Disorders frequently associated with arthritis
        1. Trauma (the result of direct trauma)
        2. Internal derangement of joints
        3. Pancreatic disease
        4. Sarcoidosis
        5. Palindromic rheumatism
        6. Intermittent hydrarthrosis
        7. Erythema nodosum
        8. Hemophilia
    B. Other conditions
        1. Multicentric reticulohistiocytosis (nodular panniculitis)
        2. Familial Mediterranean fever
        3. Goodpasture's syndrome
        4. Chronic active hepatitis
        5. Drug-induced rheumatic syndromes
        6. Dialysis-associated syndromes
        7. Foreign body synovitis
        8. Acne and hydradenitis suppurativa
        9. Pustulosis palmaris et plantaris
      10. Sweet's syndrome
      11. Other

an inevitable part of aging. In old age, it is the most common form of chronic arthritis and a major reason for dependence and being homebound.

Spondylitis disability (ankylosing spondylitis, spondylitis associated with psoriasis, inflammatory bowel disease, juvenile arthritis, Reiter's syndrome, etc.) is characterized by stiffness or restrictive movement of the spine, with occasional involvement of the peripheral joints, most commonly the shoulder, hip, or knee. The disability is characterized by male predominance, onset in young and middle-age adults, and by the episodic nature of the peripheral arthritis. Spondylitis disability is compatible with good function except when it involves peripheral joints, in which case it can affect mobility. Usually physical mobility and independence are maintained. Spondylitis in young adult males may affect self-esteem, body image, leisure activities, and peer relationships, particularly in the exercise and physique-conscious milieu of the 1980s.

Systemic rheumatic disease disability is illustrated by the functional problems which occur in systemic rheumatic diseases such as systemic lupus erythematosus, scleroderma, Sjögren's syndrome or disease, polymyositis, vasculitis, and some patients with rheumatoid arthritis. Except for the latter, arthralgias are more common than arthritis and much of the disability is due to other organ involvement such as lung or heart, or from constitutional symptoms such as fatigue and decreased endurance. These disabilities affect work capacity and socialization. Self-esteem and body image may be impaired by medications such as steroids or the disease process itself (tight skin and contractures of the joint). Additional problems include the sense of stigmatization and victimization from having a rare disease, and the fear of relapse or death.

As the preceding discussion suggests, rheumatic diseases vary in their clinical expression, yet each has a major effect on function. Thus, the medical management is directed toward preserving and restoring function with medications, rehabilitation measures, surgery, or psychosocial interventions. In 1949, the importance of function was recognized with the development of the American Rheumatism Association Functional Classes (2). Since then, hundreds of ad hoc, nonstandardized, loosely defined assessments of activities of daily living have been used by clinicians. In 1977, attempts to assess health status or quality of life by questionnaires expanded tremendously. A wealth of descriptive literature exists on the psychometrics of these instruments, and their application to clinical trials is increasing. It is our goal to review the work done in measuring function and health status in the rheumatic and musculoskeletal diseases, some conceptual limitations to their use, and future research directions.

DEFINITIONS

The terms used in describing the impact of arthritis on the individual can be defined as follows: *Impairment* is demonstrable anatomic loss or damage, a physiologic state. Examples include a limited range of motion or a number of inflamed joints. An impairment may not cause functional limitations, for instance, a patient with a loss of 10° of elbow extension without other joint impairment usually will not have problems dressing or feeding himself. *Disability* is the functional limitation caused by an impairment which interferes with what a patient needs or wants to do. Physical *function* is the complex integrated physical ability dependent on physical integrity of the joints and an intact neuromotor system to perform tasks needed for activities of daily living, that is to care for oneself, to play, to work, etc. When the activities of daily living concept is extended beyond essential activities in the home and community, the term instrumental activities of daily living is used. These include using a telephone, shopping for groceries, etc. The lack of ability to do instrumental activities of daily living suggests a need for special services. *Health status* or *quality of life,* an ephemeral concept, embodies the dimensions of physical, social, and emotional function.

Functional diagnosis is the systematic evaluation of a patient who has a functional limitation, in order to understand the determinants of that limitation. Difficulty doing

TABLE 2. *Quality of life and health status measures in rheumatic disease*

Rheumatoid disability

Sickness Impact Profile (SIP) (4)
Index of Well-Being (IWB) (5)
Functional Status Index (FSI) (7)
Health Assessment Questionnaire (HAQ) (10)
Modified Health Assessment Questionnaire (MHAQ) (11)
Arthritis Impact Measurement Scales (AIMS) (9)
Convery Polyarticular Disability Index (8)
Lee Functional Status Instrument (12)
Toronto Functional Capacity Questionnaire (13)
McMaster Health Index Questionnaire (MHIQ) (14)
MACTAR Questionnaire (15)
RAND Health Insurance Study (6)

Spondylitis

Dougados Functional Index (16)
Daltroy Functional Status for the Spondyloarthropathies (17)

Childhood rheumatic disease

Hoskins and Squires Test (26)
Basic Gross Motor Assessment (27)
Denver Developmental Screening Test (28)
Newington Children's Hospital JRA Evaluation (32)
Adapted Health Assessment Questionnaire (33)

sit-to-stand transfers, for example, may be caused by weak quadriceps, ligamentious laxity, and pain from patellofemoral osteoarthritis.

Function is a complex phenomenon. Disability arises when there is a discrepancy between ability and need, when one's capabilities are not sufficient for independence. This is dependent on whether there is an actual or perceived need for a specific function, a patient's expectations, his/her motivation, and the support system. Function changes over the course of people's development in terms of what they are capable of doing and what they wish or need to do. In children and adolescents, rapid change and maturation of cognitive, behavioral, emotional, and psychological function are the rule whereas in adult life, those capacities are stable but life circumstances are changing.

HEALTH STATUS AND QUALITY OF LIFE MEASUREMENT

The instruments for measuring health status or quality of life (Table 2) cover a variety of dimensions of health, including physical, social, and emotional functioning. Some instruments are general health status measures which have been applied to rheumatic disorders (4–6). Others are measures developed for rheumatic diseases, particularly rheumatoid arthritis, the numerically most important chronic polyarthritis (7–15). Measures of function emphasizing those affected by arthritis of the spine are available (16,17). Only one instrument assesses patient priorities (15). Only one assesses patient satisfaction with their functional level (11). Even with these gaps, a diverse literature demonstrates the potential of health status measurement both in clinical work and as a research tool.

These newer instruments are as reliable as traditional measures of improvement in clinical status, such as traditional measures used in rheumatic diseases (based on anthropometric approaches or laboratory tests such as 25-yard walk time or erythrocyte sedimentation rate). Health status instruments are interchangeable in their ability to measure major clinically significant improvement, but have varying ability to demonstrate changes in subdimensions such as social and global function (18–20). Other studies indicate that measures of function or health status predict mortality and correlate with utilization of health services (21,22). A simple functional questionnaire is an economic and efficient technique for case finding and has been applied in developing countries for diagnosis of community burden (23).

A description of health status or quality of life and physical function measures follows: The Arthritis Impact Measurement Scales, a health status or quality of life instrument developed for rheumatoid arthritis, has 48 multiple-choice questions with nine subscales measuring physical, social, and mental health status (9). The possible range of scores on each subscale is 0 to 10; subscale results are averaged to obtain a total score. The scale is self-administered and takes 15 to 20 minutes to complete, and has been used in a number of studies on rheumatic disease.

The Functional Status Index measures dependence, pain, and difficulty experienced in the performance of 18 activities of daily living (7). Each activity is rated between 0 and 4 on each dimension. Studies on patients with rheumatoid arthritis show validity and a high degree of interobserver reliability. In self-assessed format, it takes 10 to 20 minutes to complete.

The Index of Well-Being (5) evaluates mobility, physical activity, and social activity. An interviewer determines what the patient did and did not do because of illness during the last 6 days. Scoring for particular levels of function is based on preference weights derived from normals and have been validated in rheumatoid arthritis patients (24). The interview requires a trained assessor, and takes 20 minutes to complete. The instrument has been validated, but may not be as sensitive as other measures to changes seen in patient status during a clinical trial in rheumatoid arthritis (19). Major limitations are the complexity of the instrument and the requirement for a specially trained interviewer.

The McMaster Health Index Questionnaire measures the quality of life in patients with rheumatoid disease (14). It measures physical function in physical activities, self-care activities, mobility, communication, and global physical activity. A social index combines general well-being, work performance, material welfare, support and participation with friends and family, and global social function. The emotional index measures feelings about personal relationships, self-esteem, thoughts concerning the future, critical life events, and global emotional function. It contains 59 items, is self-administered, and takes about 15 to 20 minutes to complete.

The McMaster Toronto Arthritis Patient Preference Disability Questionnaire (MACTAR) was developed for use in clinical trials in rheumatoid arthritis (15). Using a semi-structured interview, patients are asked to designate key functional activities based on their own preferences, and the five activities that rank highest are evaluated. At the end of a study period patients are asked if their ability to perform the ranked activities has improved, worsened, or stayed the same. This technique may be more sensitive to small changes when compared with conventional standardized questionnaires. The problems in evaluating each patient in a different way are formidable, and this approach requires further investigation.

The RAND Health Insurance Study Batteries assess four dimensions: social, psychological, and physical functioning, as well as general health perceptions (6). Specific scales in each area of function include social interaction and social participation in community and family; anxiety, depression, and self-control; activities of daily living, role activities, household tasks, leisure, and physical activity. The instrument is administered by an interviewer and requires at least 60 minutes to complete. The complete RAND batteries have not been used in the rheumatic diseases but the General Health Perceptions portion has been used in a clinical trial of auranofin versus placebo and did not show change, whereas the Current Health Assessment showed some change. The Arthritis Impact Measurement Scale anxiety and depression versions are shortened versions of the anxiety and depression sections of the full RAND instrument.

The Sickness Impact Profile contains 136 items on patient status (4). Questions are answered true or false. Scores for items use predetermined weights based on rater panel estimates of relative severity of the dysfunction. Three of the categories (ambulation, body care, and mobility) may be aggregated into a physical dimension; and four categories (emotional behavior, social interaction, alertness behavior, and communication) may be aggregated into a psychosocial dimension. Five categories are independent (work, sleep and rest, eating, home management, and recreation and pastimes). The Sickness Impact Profile is available in a self-administered form or can be administered in an interview. It requires up to 30 minutes to complete as an interview. It has been validated in a number of disorders, including arthritis. A total score is computed by summing categories and then standardizing to a percentage of the maximum. The instrument may accurately reflect change for groups of arthritis patients, but appears to be relatively insensitive to changes in individual patients (25).

The Health Assessment Questionnaire (10), a self-administered instrument, exists in two formats, a short form that requires 3 minutes to complete, and a longer version requiring 20 minutes. The short form is composed of 24 questions on activities of daily living and mobility. The answers to the short form yield a summated index between 0 and 3 on a continuous scale. The questionnaire is a validated instrument that has been used in a clinical trial of rheumatoid arthritis (19), and was incorporated into the 2nd National Health and Nutrition Examination Study. It is a predictor of health services utilization (21). The longer version adds additional questions relating to pain, global severity, income, job change, cost of medical care, and side effects of therapy.

The Modified Health Assessment Questionnaire (11) evaluates physical function through eight questions instead of 24, and adds new scales for change in function, satisfaction, and pain in the performance of each of these activities. It can be completed in less than 5 minutes. Reliability and validity of the Modified Health Assessment Questionnaire and the Health Assessment Questionnaire are comparable. The instrument has been used in clinical trials and observational studies of rheumatoid arthritis and osteoarthritis.

The Toronto Functional Capacity Questionnaire assesses function in personal care, upper extremity activities, mobility, work, and leisure activities (13). The instrument is administered by an interviewer, and requires approximately 18 minutes to complete. Weighting of responses is based on preferences derived from panels of occupational and physical therapists and rheumatologists. Reliability and validity have been demonstrated. The instrument has been shown to be sensitive to change in clinical trials (15).

Evaluation of Children and Adolescents with Rheumatic Disorders

The evaluation of physical function and health status in young patients is far less developed than the measures available to assess health status of adults with rheumatic diseases. These measures are modified adult measures and are not designed to evaluate children developmentally. Conceptually, the achievement of developmental milestones is a central theme in assessment of children, and health is conceptualized as achieving normal development and participating fully in developmentally appropriate physical, psychological, and social activities.

The Hoskins and Squires Test for Gross Motor and Reflex Development gives a Motor Quotient computed by having a clinician rate on a scale of 1 to 4, an infant's ability to perform 60 voluntary physical tasks (26). The motor age is established by finding the highest level where the child can perform at least 50% of the required voluntary skills. The assessment covers children from birth to 5 years. Norms for the assessment were derived from a literature search. The instrument has been tested for interrater reliability and item validity.

The Basic Gross Motor Assessment (27) is based on normative data from 1,260 children aged 5 to 12 and takes children through seven standardized tasks such as standing on one leg with eyes open and then closed, tandem walking, and throwing bean bags at a target. The clinician is asked to rate performance from 0 (unable) to 3 (good with no deviations). The instrument has been tested for reliability, content, construct, and concurrent validity.

Denver Developmental Screening Test instruments consist of a prescreening parental questionnaire and an observational screening test for children from 1 month to 6 years, 3 months and is scaled for age (28–30). The areas covered are personal-social, fine motor-adaptive, language, and gross motor. The questionnaire and test are simple and brief. They are designed to assess whether the child has achieved age-norm milestones developmentally. A cross-cultural study of the test emphasizes the impact of cultural differences on patterns of development (31).

The Newington Children's Hospital Juvenile Rheumatoid Arthritis Evaluation (32) is a two-dimensional index under development that measures quality of motor performance on a scale of 0 to 4 (0 = unable to perform; 1 = performs with significant influence of abnormal joint function; 2 = performs with moderate stiffness or joint deviation; 3 = performs with mild stiffness or joint deviation; 4 = performs with normal motor patterns) against chronological age at which the task is normally mastered. The index assumes that central nervous system development is normal and that tasks are sequentially learned. Fifty-eight motor tasks are included and are weighted equally. The instrument is designed to evaluate children 1 to 6 years old.

Instruments have been developed which comprehensively measure physical, social, and psychological functioning or health status in young subjects.

The Adapted Health Assessment Questionnaire for Children is an instrument based on the adult questionnaire (33). It has been studied in juvenile rheumatoid arthritis patients and parents and healthy controls to determine if children and/or parents can reliably self-report pain, disability, and psychosocial impact and whether the reports correlate with functional performance noted by a physical or an occupational therapist (34). Age and grade level matched controls were used to establish normal standards for the measured activity of daily living tasks. The school grade level range was 2 to 11. Reliability and validity testing is in progress.

The RAND Health Insurance Study instrument is directed at a general population and not specifically for use in rheumatic diseases (6). Questions for children up to age 13 focus on physical function in self-care activities, mobility, and role activities, such as going to school or play. Social relations and parental concerns are covered for 5 to 13 year olds. It has not been used in childhood rheumatic disease and is untested for its ability to distinguish degrees of disability.

LIMITATION OF QUALITY OF LIFE MEASURES

Selecting the measures for use in a clinical trial is like making a bet; it is an attempt to anticipate and measure the multiple dimensions of health and the consequences of therapies prescribed. To some degree the instruments listed are interchangeable but as discussed above, the dimensions covered by each instrument vary and have differential sensitivity to change. Nearly all of the instruments have been developed and tested in adults with rheumatoid arthritis and as such, the experience with the performance of these measures in other arthritic conditions such as osteoarthritis and the spondyloarthropathies is limited, as is their reliability and validity in the very young or very old. The Arthritis Impact Measurement Scale, for instance, must be used with care in children (35). The Pain and revised Physical Disability subscales of the Arthritis Impact Measurement Scale are the most reliable and valid components. The Mobility and Activities of Daily Living subscale probably need modification. The Household Activity subscale may not be appropriate for male patients, and the Activities of Daily Living subscale may be insensitive to mild disability (36). Instruments developed in one setting need modification when used in another culture (37).

Not all costs and benefits of interventions are measurable or predictable. We spend a great deal of energy deciding what items should be included in a questionnaire, but cannot anticipate the complete consequences of an intervention in the short or long run. There are many examples in the rheumatic diseases to illustrate that outcomes require continued assessment. Corticosteroids for rheumatoid arthritis improved patients' sense of well-being and reduced synovitis dramatically, but it was not until a decade after the introduction of steroids that patients suffered considerable morbidity and mortality from excess steroid therapy. Quality of life in patients treated with steroids shows major improvement in the first few months of therapy. However, the instruments we have would not capture the disfiguring effects of steroids which distress so many patients, nor the disability from steroid-induced fractures, nor the mortality resulting from increased susceptibility to infection.

Function is relative. Psychometrically sound instruments assume that function can be measured with the same standard instrument. However, patients' function is relative to their age, sex, motivation, social supports, priorities, and goals, and to their needs for daily living, work, and recreation. Because function is relative, a small change in an individual's function may make a lot of difference. The small change may be totally adequate for the person's needs, yet not meet statistical norms.

Covering a range of functional activities in a comprehensive questionnaire provides breadth at the sacrifice of depth. The measurement of specific functions in questionnaires is too crude for monitoring patients. For example, function of the carpal metacarpal joint may be assessed by a question on difficulty with fastening buttons or doing zippers. The hand surgeon needs to measure and detect more subtle change which might be more appropriately derived from measurement of grip and pinch strength and standardized dexterity measures.

Questionnaires cannot make a specific etiologic diagnosis or replace a clinical evaluation of the subtle, interrelated components of function such as motivation, neuromuscular competency, cognitive ability, joint integrity, availability of environmental modifications and social supports, and the like. Also, self-reported function can be unreliable and can overestimate or underreport observed performance (23,34). Even with reliable responses, the information is too general to be useful in the individual patient. For example, in a patient with difficulty walking, the problem may be due to motivation, pain (structural or inflammatory or both), muscle strength, impairment of the nervous system, stability of the joint, and more.

Another limitation of health status questionnaires is the unresolvable issue of whether each item should be equally weighted. From a clinical perspective, not all activities of daily living are equal for a patient, and the technology of deriving weights leaves the clinician dissatisfied.

Willingness-to-pay as a method for eliciting preferences in rheumatic disease, in our experience, has had response rates of less than 50% (38,39). We explain this on the basis that patients cannot understand the task, are hostile to the type of question, or have little idea of how much is spent on specific health care items.

The preferences of a group may not be those of the individual. Inasmuch as function is relative, so are values placed on it. The preferences expressed by healthy, reasonable individuals are not those of the sick and the anxious. Preferences of the sick and anxious do not remain constant during the vicissitudes of rheumatic illnesses which are characterized by chronicity and an unpredictable waxing and waning course. Values change with time, and experiences of illness or personal circumstances change because people learn, adjust, or accommodate over the course of illness. No system for patient preference measurement takes into account this dynamic state.

The analysis of patient preference in decision making fails to address the "confusion" and sense of crisis which is part of the illness experience. Whereas some patients see their illness experience as an area in which they can and should exert control of their fate, many do not wish to take responsibility for determining their "fate" by expressing preference.

SELECTION OF APPROPRIATE MEASURES FOR CLINICAL STUDIES

The goal of medical care is to do no harm, to relieve pain and suffering, and to improve and maintain one's physical, social, and emotional function. Thus, any evaluation of an intervention, whether it is medication, surgery, or a program with elements of these, should examine if these goals are achieved and to what extent. Some interventions relieve symptoms and improve function promptly, whereas others may take time or require that a patient be rehabilitated from some stable level of function. In the same light, known and unknown negative effects can occur immediately or as a delayed or cumulative consequence. For a medical intervention designed to treat a root cause or primary mechanism of joint destruction, such as synovitis, one should see evidence of improved inflammation. To the degree that psychosocial dysfunction results from the rheumatic condition, one would expect improvement of these parameters. However, prolonged psychological symptoms or innate traits are not likely to be helped by attention to synovitis alone. In fact, a discrepancy between one's perceived function and objective signs of disease is often a clue that there is something else going on which needs attention.

General health status measures are preferred to arthritis-specific ones for questions of health policy in which decision makers must allocate resources to different conditions. The use of such scales in a clinical trial can help the investigator relate the findings to other diseases and the policy maker to understand the trade-offs in resource allocation. The use of a general health status measure may not capture the specific outcomes seen in a disorder but usually there is little empirical data to know *a priori*. The best approach is to examine each item to determine if there is sufficient coverage of all relevant dimensions for a specific disorder, if these items are sufficiently scaled to spread out individuals on a continuum, and if the items are possibly symptoms seen as part of the disease complex. On this latter point, depression and inability to get going in the morning are frequently seen in inflammatory arthritis such as rheumatoid arthritis; this cannot be considered a specifically psychoaffective symptom. There is temptation to take a scale from a general measure to be used in a specific study. Authors of instruments recoil at the thought and would argue from a psychometric point of view that disaggregating the scale will not insure reliability or validity. This is particularly true if the index results in one score; omitting a subscale will not allow one to compute the score. We support this and would also add that in the actual conduct of trials, leaving out one or two subscales does not really save much time or measurably reduce the burden to the patient.

Arthritis-specific scales usually provide better coverage of dimensions of health thought to be important in a particular condition. The advantage of using an arthritis-specific scale is that clinicians may have a better sense of what changes on the scale mean, and they may have been used in other studies for comparison. All health status measures measure a broad number of variables but not in any great depth. A glance at the nine-volume *Mental Measurements Yearbook* shows countless scales for any psychoaffective symptom or cognitive skill, all of which have been tested for reliability and validity. Unfortunately, sophisticated scales to measure any specific psychological trait or symptom may be too long for application in a clinical trial where a host of independent variables are being measured.

Our approach in selecting measures for clinical trials in rheumatic conditions, specifically inflammatory arthritis, is to have a detailed clinical understanding of the range of benefits and adverse reactions that might be expected, and to get the best measure for each of the positive and negative attributes of the intervention. Traditional anthropometric measures should be supplemented by measures of physical function and health status. The battery should include a general health status measure if the results are to be used in health policy. If available, a disease-specific health status measure such as the Arthritis Impact Measurement Scale, the Modified Health Assessment Questionnaire, and the Health Assessment Questionnaire should also be used. The evaluation should include some measure of whether patients are satisfied with their state and global evaluations of whether they felt better and whether the treatment was worth it considering all the positive effects on disease and negative effects, and the effort required for monitoring the drug or following the recommendations of the prescription.

Indirect and direct costs should be evaluated after efficacy has been determined. The most expensive portion of health care is hospitalization or institution-based care followed by diagnostic tests, X-rays, drugs, etc. Health care costs paid for by insurance or out-of-pocket are poorly remembered and there should be validation against objective data. Hospital costs, being the most important part of the cost, should include information on length of stay and cost based on some relative value scale rather than charges that are idiosyncratic and variable from region to region. Hospitalization rates and length of stay are biased by recent changes in health financing and may not reflect clinical necessity.

We have used and compared the Sickness Impact Profile, Index of Well-Being, Functional Status Index, Arthritis Impact Measurement Scale, and Modified Health Assessment Questionnaire in a variety of descriptive and evaluative studies. In addition, using joint replacement surgery as a model, we have studied the performance and relative measurement sensitivity of these instruments. All the instruments correlated highly with one another and demonstrated change. We found that of the five instruments, the Functional Status Index had the most missing data. The Arthritis Impact Measurement Scale, Functional Status Index, and Sickness Impact Profile were equally efficient in detecting improvement in mobility, but the Health Assessment Questionnaire and Index of Well-Being were about a half as efficient as the other three instruments. For pain evaluation, the Arthritis Impact Measurement Scale was more sensitive than the Health Assessment Questionnaire. The Index of Well-Being and Sickness Impact Profile do not have a pain subscale. With regard to social function the Sickness Impact Profile, Index of Well-Being, and Health Assessment Questionnaire were more sensitive than the Arthritis Impact Measurement Scale. For global function the Sickness Impact Profile, Arthritis Impact Measurement Scale, and Index of Well-Being were more efficient than the Functional Status Index or Health Assessment Questionnaire.

From a practical point of view the Index of Well-Being is an arduous questionnaire to administer, somewhat counterintuitive and artificial for patients, and requires resources to train interviewers. However, it has the advantage of being a ratio scale with a true zero point (which is not terribly relevant in rheumatic diseases, in general), thus making it the best instrument for calculating quality-adjusted life-years, a prerequisite for cost-benefit studies. In a controlled drug trial in rheumatoid arthritis, it displayed the smallest change of the techniques used to measure change (19). The omission of pain as a dimension makes it less desirable as a single instrument in rheumatic disorders since pain is a central concern for patients (42,43).

The Sickness Impact Profile is much easier to understand by patients, is self-administered, and has been used in numerous rheumatic disorders. It results in one score. Its only disadvantage is that it contains questions related to continence and communication which are not relevant to rheumatic disorders. Nevertheless, we use the complete instrument.

The Functional Status Index enables a patient to disaggregate their function along three dimensions of dependence, pain, and difficulty experienced. This is not always understood or possible for patients. In elderly patients, there was poor compliance and response rates with this question (44). We found the same in a study of patients undergoing total joint arthroplasty (20).

The Arthritis Impact Measurement Scale is convenient to use and of the arthritis scales is probably the most widely used next to the Modified Health Assessment Questionnaire or Health Assessment Questionnaire in published studies. The Modified Health Assessment Questionnaire is convenient and assesses patient satisfaction with their level of functioning.

Because there are no perfect measures of function or health status, careful consideration of likely outcomes and which instruments provide the best coverage is necessary. Multiple measures and serial assessment of outcome using different approaches, such as combining questionnaires with open-ended interviews about the same outcome, may be necessary when the sensitivity of an instrument is unknown. No instrument will help a weak study design. Thus, blinded evaluation, randomization, and definition of "meaningful" effect are essential.

FUTURE RESEARCH DIRECTIONS

Questionnaires quantitatively measure physical function and health status in rheumatic disease patients. Their limitations are inherent to their form and attempt to circumscribe a boundless and sometimes amorphous dimension of impact on the average patient. Development of such instrumentation has gone as far as it can except perhaps for developing specific items for different types of rheumatic disease disability. Evaluating patient priorities and their satisfaction with their state provides additional areas for future research, but we are nearly there. Ultimately, if patient care and outcome are to be improved, attention to function must be incorporated in the daily practice, and tools for its screening, follow-up, and diagnosis need to be developed. It is likely that these will come from improved understanding of epidemiology of function in the rheumatic diseases, the natural course of functional decline, and if, in fact, there are critical points in which intervention might make a difference.

To know a functional problem exists is only the start, and physicians at all levels need to have improved understanding of where and what can be done to improve function. Recent attempts to more equitably reimburse physicians for cognitive work will certainly create some incentive for this.

Increasingly, policy makers are looking to health status measurement as a way to assess the quality of care delivered by individual physicians or institutions. Mortality rates are too insensitive and likely reflect case-mix rather than physician or institution performance. Health status measures are reliable, valid, and may be more sensitive to differences. Validity, however, is a property specific to a particular characteristic an instrument is designed to measure. Health status measures demonstrate patient improvement in studies of the clinical efficacy of total joint replacement surgery and of certain medications. None of the measures, however, have been shown to be valid indicators of physician or institution performance.

The applicability of health status measures in evaluating physician performance is an area worthy of investigation. Even if changes in health status correlate with an independent assessment of the quality of care, careful interpretation is required. Much of the dysfunction identified in health status measures (e.g., social function) involves a complex interaction of disease process and the environment. How broad is the physicians' mandate to intervene in these spheres and how accountable are physicians or institutions for reversing these impairments?

We feel that the most valuable aspect of health status measures is their ability to capture the human condition. It is acknowledged that social and emotional function, and the interplay between impairment and needs, are critical to patients. At issue, among other things, is whether physicians can be held accountable for problems that stem from diverse causes, for problems resulting from innate personality characteristics, or for reckless health behavior such as excess alcohol or smoking.

Many aspects of health status, functional measure, and preference measure will not surrender to multivariate techniques. Improved patient evaluation must become more quantitative, but functional and health status questionnaires, like the left brain, provide the vocabulary without the richness, the nuance. Statistics are normative and the emphasis is on similarities; patient care is humanistic and the emphasis is on differences. Psychometric approaches alone are not miscible with individual patient care, but the interaction between the two domains is a necessary and desirable goal for all we seek to accomplish with clinical investigation.

SOURCES OF INFORMATION

Potential users are encouraged to contact the source person for updated information on content and scoring.

Adapted Child Health Assessment Questionnaire (ACHAQ)
ES Shear, MSW
Children's Hospital Medical Center
Special Treatment Center–Juvenile Arthritis
Elland and Bethesda Avenues
Cincinnati, OH 45229
513/559–4676

Arthritis Impact Measurement Scales (AIMS)
Robert F. Meenan, MD
Boston University School of Medicine
80 E. Concord Street
Boston, MA 02118
617/638–5180

Denver Developmental Screening Test (DDSDT)
W. K. Frankenburg
(*The Denver Developmental Screening Test Manual,* 1970.)
Denver: University of Colorado Press

Functional Status Instrument (FSI)
Alan M. Jette, PT, PhD
Massachusetts General Hospital
Institute of Health Professions
15 River Street
Boston, MA 02108–3402
617/726–8009

Health Assessment Questionnaire (HAQ)
James F. Fries, MD
Department of Medicine
Stanford University
HRP 109C
Stanford, CA 94305–5091
415/723–6003

Index of Well-Being (IWB)
Robert Kaplan, PhD

University of California, San Diego
La Jolla, California 92023

McMaster Health Index Questionnaire
Larry Chambers, PhD
Educational Center Aging & Health
Health Sciences Center, Room 1N1
McMaster University
1200 Main Street W
Hamilton, ON L8N 3Z5 Canada
416/525–9140, ext. 2136

McMaster Toronto Arthritis Patient Preference Disability Questionnaire
   (MACTAR)
Peter Tugwell, MD
Department of CE & B, Room 2C16, HSC
McMaster University
1200 Main Street W
Hamilton ON L8N 3Z5 Canada
416/525–9140

Modified Health Assessment Questionnaire (MHAQ)
Theodore Pincus, MD
Division Rheumatology-Immunology
Vanderbilt University
B-3219 Medical Center N
Nashville, TN 37232

RAND Health Insurance Study Batteries
Robert H. Brook MD
RAND Corporation
P.O. Box 2138
Santa Monica, CA 90406
213/393–0411, ext. 7368

Sickness Impact Profile (SIP)
Marilyn Bergner, PhD
Department of Health Policy and Management
The Johns Hopkins University
Room 606624 N. Broadway
Baltimore, MD 21205
301/955–6546

Toronto Functional Capacity Questionnaire (TFCQ)
Hugh A. Smythe, MD, FRCPC
Department of Medicine
University of Toronto
St. 647, Wellesley Hospital
Toronto, ON M4Y 1J3 Canada

ACKNOWLEDGMENT

We gratefully acknowledge the expert assistance of Jacqueline Pepe, Mary Scamman, Lisa Bail, and Wendy Gross in the preparation of this manuscript.

This work was supported by the National Institutes of Health, Grants nos. AM36308 and RR05669.

REFERENCES

1. Classification of the rheumatic diseases. In: Schumacher HR, ed. *Primer on the rheumatic diseases.* Atlanta, GA: Arthritis Foundation, 1988;81–83.
2. Steinbrocker O, Traeger CH, Battman RC. Therapeutic criteria in rheumatoid arthritis. *JAMA* 1949;140:659–662.
3. Liang MH, Jette AM. Measuring functional ability in chronic arthritis: A critical review. *Arthritis Rheum* 1981;24:80–86.
4. Bergner M, Bobbitt RA, Pollard WE, Martin DP, Gilson BS. The Sickness Impact Profile: Validation of a health status measure. *Med Care* 1976;14:57–67.
5. Kaplan RM, Bush JW, Berry CC. Health status: Types of validity for an index of well-being. *Health Serv Res* 1976;11:478–507.
6. Brook RH, Ware JE, Davied-Avery R, et al. Overview of adult health status measures fielded in RAND's health insurance study. *Med Care* (Suppl.). 1979;17:1–131.
7. Jette AM. Functional Status Index: Reliability of a chronic disease evaluation instrument. *Arch Phys Med Rehabil* 1980;61:395–401.
8. Convery FR, Minteer MA, Amiel D, Connett KL. Polyarticular disability: A functional assessment. *Arch Phys Med Rehabil* 1977;58:494–499.
9. Meenan RF, Gertman PM, Mason JH. Measuring health status in arthritis: The Arthritis Impact Measurement Scales. *Arthritis Rheum* 1980;23:146–152.
10. Fries JF, Spitz P, Kraines RG, Holman HR. Measurement of patient outcome in arthritis. *Arthritis Rheum* 1980;23:137–145.
11. Pincus T, Summey JA, Soraci SA, Jr., Wallston KA, Hummon NP. Assessment of patient satisfaction in activities of daily living using a modified Stanford Health Assessment Questionnaire. *Arthritis Rheum* 1983;26:1346–1353.
12. Lee P, Jasani MK, Dick WC, Buchanan WW. Evaluation of a functional index in rheumatoid arthritis. *Scand J Rheumatol* 1973;2:71–77.
13. Helewa A, Goldsmith CH, Smyth HA. Independent measurement of functional capacity in rheumatoid arthritis. *J Rheumatol* 1982;9:794–797.
14. Chambers LW, MacDonald LA, Tugwell P, et al. The McMaster Health Index Questionnaire as a measure of quality of life for patients with rheumatoid disease. *J Rheumatol* 1982;9:780–784.
15. Tugwell P, Bombardier C, Buchanon WW, Goldsmith CH, Grace E. The MACTAR Questionnaire— An individualized functional priority approach for assessing improvement in physical disability in clinical trials in rheumatoid arthritis. *J Rheumatol* 1987;14:446–451.
16. Dougados M, Gueguen A, Nakache J-P, Nguyen M, Mery C, Amor B. Evaluation of a functional index and an articular index in ankylosing spondylitis. *J Rheumatol* 1988;15:302–307.
17. Daltroy L, Larson MG, Roberts WN, Liang MH. A measure of functional status for the spondylo-arthropathies (*submitted*).
18. Meenan RF, Anderson JJ, Kazis LE, Egger MJ, Altz-Smith M, Samuelson CO, Jr., Willkens RF, Solsky MA, Haynes SP, Blocka KL, Weinstein A, Guttadauria M, Kaplan SB, Klippel J. Outcome assessment in clinical trials: Evidence for the sensitivity of a health status measure. *Arthritis Rheum* 1984;27:1344–1352.
19. Bombardier C, Ware J, Russell IJ, Larson M, Chalmers A, Read JL, the Auranofin Cooperating Group. Auranofin therapy and quality of life in patients with rheumatoid arthritis: Results of a multicenter trial. *Am J Med* 1986;81:565–578.
20. Liang MH, Larson MG, Cullen KE, Schwartz JA. Comparative measurement efficiency and sensitivity of five health status instruments for arthritis research. *Arthritis Rheum* 1985;28:542–547.
21. McNevitt MC, Yelin EH, Henke CJ, Epstein WV. Risk factors for hospitalization and surgery for rheumatoid arthritis: Implications for capitated medical payments. *Ann Intern Med* 1986;105:421–428.
22. Mitchell DM, Spitz PW, Young DY, et al. Survival, prognosis, and causes of death in rheumatoid arthritis. *Arthritis Rheum* 1986;29:706–714.
23. Liang MH, Phillips E, Scamman M, Lurye CS, Keith A, Cohen L, Taylor G. Evaluation of a pilot program for rheumatic disability in an urban community. *Arthritis Rheum* 1981;24:937–943.
24. Balaban DJ, Sagi PC, Goldfarb NI, Nettler S. Weights for scoring the quality of well-being (QWB) instrument among rheumatoid arthritis: A comparison to general population weights. *Med Care* 1986;24:973–980.
25. Deyo RA, Inui TS. Towards clinical applications of health status measures: Sensitivity of scales to clinically important changes. *Health Serv Res* 1984;19:275–289.

26. Hoskins TA, Squires JE. Developmental assessment: A test for gross motor and reflex development. *Phys Ther* 1973;53:117–125.
27. Hughes JE, Riley A. Basic gross motor assessment: Tool for use with children having minor motor dysfunction. *Phys Ther* 1981;61:503–511.
28. Frankenburg WK, Dodds J, Fandal A. The Denver Developmental Screening Test manual. Denver: University of Colorado Press, 1970.
29. Frankenburg WK, Camp BW, VanNatta PA. Validity of the DDST. *Child Dev* 1971;42:475–485.
30. Frankenburg WK, Camp BW, VanNatta PA, Demersseman JA: Reliability and stability of the DDST. *Child Dev* 1971;42:1315–1325.
31. Williams PD, Williams AR. Denver Developmental Screening Test norms: A cross-cultural comparison. *J Ped Psych* 1987;12:39–55.
32. Rhodes V, Pumphrey K. *Juvenile rheumatoid arthritis evaluation*. Newington, CT: Newington Children's Hospital, 1988.
33. Shear E, Howe S, Levinson J, Lovell D. Pilot project to develop and validate a childhood disability scale. *Arthritis Rheum* 1988;31:5152.
34. Spiegel JS, Hirshfield MS, Spiegel TM. Evaluating self-care activities: Comparison of a self-reported questionnaire with an occupational therapist interview. *Br J Rheum* 1985;24:357–361.
35. Coulton CJ, Zborowsky E, Lipton J, et al. Assessment of the reliability and validity of the Arthritis Impact Measurement Scales for children with juvenile arthritis. *Arthritis Rheum* 1987;30:819–824.
36. Potts MK, Brandt KD. Evidence of the validity of the Arthritis Impact Measurement Scales. *Arthritis Rheum* 1987;30:93–96.
37. Kirwan JR, Reeback JS. Stanford Health Assessment Questionnaire modified to assess disability in British patients with rheumatoid arthritis. *Br J Rheum.* 1986;25:206–209.
38. Thompson MS, Read JL, Liang MH. Willingness-to-pay concepts for societal diseases in health. In: Kane RL, Kane RA, eds. *Values and long term care*. Lexington MA: DC Health, 1982;103–105.
39. Thompson MS, Read JL, Liang MH. Feasibility of willingness-to-pay measurement in chronic arthritis. *Med Decis Making* 1981;4:195–215.
42. Kazis LE, Meenan RF, Anderson JJ. Pain in the rheumatic diseases: Investigation of a key health status component. *Arthritis Rheum* 1983;26:1017–1022.
43. Liang MH, Rogers M, Larson M, et al. The psychosocial impact of systemic lupus erythematosus and rheumatoid arthritis. *Arthritis Rheum* 1984;27:13–19.
44. Liang MH, Partridge AJ, Larson MG, Gall V, Taylor JE, Master R, Feltin M, Taylor J. Evaluation of comprehensive rehabilitation services for elderly homebound patients with arthritis and orthopedic disability. *Arthritis Rheum* 1984;27:258–266.

Subject Index